Neale's Common Foot Disorders:
Diagnosis and Management

For Churchill Livingstone

Publisher: Mary Law
Project Editor: Dinah Thom
Copy Editor: Andrew Gardiner
Production Controller: Mark Sanderson
Sales Promotion Executive: Hilary Brown

Neale's Common Foot Disorders:
Diagnosis and Management

A GENERAL CLINICAL GUIDE

Edited by

Donald L. Lorimer BEd (Hons) MChS

Head of School, Durham School of Podiatric Medicine, New
College, Durham; Chairman of Council, Society of Chiropodists,
UK

FOURTH EDITION

CHURCHILL LIVINGSTONE
EDINBURGH LONDON MADRID MELBOURNE NEW YORK AND TOKYO 1993

CHURCHILL LIVINGSTONE
Medical Division of Longman Group UK Limited

Distributed in the United States of America by Churchill
Livingstone Inc., 650 Avenue of the Americas, New York,
N.Y. 10011, and by associated companies, branches and
representatives throughout the world.

First published 1993
  Reprinted 1994

ISBN 0-443-04470-8

British Library Cataloguing in Publication Data
A catalogue record for this book is available from the British
Library.

Library of Congress Cataloging in Publication Data
Neale's common foot disorders: diagnosis and management: a
  general clinical guide.—4th ed./edited by Donald
  L. Lorimer.
      p.   cm.
    Rev. ed. of: Common foot disorders. 3rd ed. 1989.
    Includes bibliographical references and index.
    ISBN 0-443-04470-8
    1. Podiatry. 2. Foot—Diseases. I. Lorimer,
Donald L.   II. Neale, Donald.   III. Common foot
disorders.   IV. Title: Common foot disorders.
    [DNLM: 1. Foot Diseases—diagnosis. 2. Foot
Diseases—therapy. WE 890 N348]
  RD563.C65   1993
  617.5'85—dc20
  DNLM/DLC   92-48834
  for Library of Congress   CIP

Produced by Longman Singapore Publishers (Pte) Ltd.
Printed in Singapore

The
publisher's
policy is to use
**paper manufactured
from sustainable forests**

Contents

Contributors

Eric G. Anderson MB ChB MSc FRCS (Edin) FRCS (Glas)
Consultant Orthopaedic Surgeon, Western Infirmary, Glasgow, UK

Alan S. Banks DPM
Podiatrist, Peachtree Podiatry Group, Atlanta, Georgia, USA

Alison M. Barlow MSc MChS
Senior Lecturer in Podiatry, University College, Salford, UK

James A. Black MChS
Podiatrist, Orthopaedic Foot Clinic, Western Infirmary, Glasgow, UK

Richard J. Bogdan MS DPM FACFO
Sports Podiatrist, Concord, California, USA

Patricia M. Boyd DPodM BApplSc(Pod)
Lecturer, Queen Margaret College, Edinburgh; Podiatrist, Fitness Assessment and Sports Injury Centre, University of Edinburgh, Edinburgh, UK

Susan J. Braid MSc FChS
Senior Lecturer in Podiatry, University College, Salford, UK

Michael I. D. Cawley MD FRCP
Consultant Rheumatologist, Southampton General Hospital, Southampton, UK

Alistair J. Clark MChS
Senior Lecturer, Durham School of Podiatric Medicine, New College, Durham, UK

Michael Davies MB FRCP
Senior Lecturer in Medicine and Consultant Physician, Royal Infirmary, Manchester, UK

Manesty S. K. Forster BSc (Hons) MChS
Senior Lecturer, Durham School of Podiatric Medicine, New College, Durham, UK

Gwen French DPodM MChS
Principal Lecturer, Division of Podiatric Medicine, University of Westminster, London; Formerly Head of Chiropody Department, Greenwich District Hospital, London, UK

Margaret Johnson DPodM PhD
Senior Lecturer, Durham School of Podiatric Medicine, New College, Durham, UK

Donald L. Lorimer BEd (Hons) MChS
Head of School, Durham School of Podiatric Medicine, New College, Durham; Chairman of Council, Society of Chiropodists, UK

John C. McDermott BSc PhD
Senior Lecturer in Microbiology, Department of Science and Dietetics, Queen Margaret College, Edinburgh, UK

E. Dalton McGlamry DPM
Podiatrist, Peachtree Podiatry Group, Atlanta, Georgia, USA

Iain M. M. Macmillan MB ChB MRCGP
Ladywell Medical Centre, Edinburgh; Lecturer, Edinburgh School of Chiropody

Rae M. Morgan BSc (Pharm) PhD MRPharmS
Senior Lecturer in Pharmacology, School of Health Sciences, University of Sunderland, Sunderland, Tyne and Wear, UK

Donald Neale OBE FChS
Formerly Principal, Edinburgh Foot Clinic and School of Chiropody, Edinburgh, UK

J. A. Raeburn MB ChB PhD FRCP (Edin)
Professor of Clinical Genetics, University of
Nottingham; Clinical Director, Genetics
Directorate, Nottingham Genetic Services,
Nottingham, UK

George C. Rendall BSc (Hons) DPodM
Lecturer, Department of Podiatry and
Radiography, Queen Margaret College,
Edinburgh, UK

Peter Sandercock MB MRCP
Consultant Neurologist, Department of Clinical
Neurosciences, Western General Hospital,
Edinburgh, UK

A. G. J. Saunders MCSP
Formerly Lecturer, Department of Physical

Therapy, Queen Margaret College, Edinburgh,
UK

Louis A. Smidt FChS
Formerly Principal, London Foot Hospital and
School of Chiropody; Unit General Manager
(Community), Bloomsbury Health District,
London, UK

Barbara Wall BSc FChS DPodM
Senior Lecturer in Podiatric Medicine, University
of Westminster, London, UK

Michael Whiting MA DPodM FChS
Dean of Faculty of Health, University of
Brighton, Falmer, Brighton, UK

Preface to the Fourth Edition

In preparing this fourth edition there have been two considerations of central concern. They were, first, to maintain the original concept of the book as a clinically orientated guide to the diagnosis and management of foot disorders and, second, to incorporate recent developments which have emerged in the practice of podiatry. These aims have placed limitations on what it has been possible to include within the scale of the book but, with the introduction of new contributors for several of the chapters, the opportunity has been taken to revise the content in the light of the changing body of knowledge available. The introduction of new contributors has also provided the opportunity for a critical appraisal of existing theories.

The most notable result of this has been the changes made to Chapters 2 and 5 which have been revised to bring them into line with recent developments in biomechanics and pathomechanics based on the research of the past few years. Similarly, Chapters 6 and 7 (on Skin and Subcutaneous Tissues and The Human Nail and its Disorders) have undergone major revision and now present the latest state of knowledge on these subjects which are of critical importance to podiatrists. Chapters 8 and 9 have also been revised completely and demonstrate the major contribution which podiatrists now make to the provision of health care for the diabetic and the elderly.

A major change which is reflected throughout the text is the change of title from 'chiropodist' to 'podiatrist'. This change has become accepted throughout the world and is now recognized in the all-graduate status of the pre-state registration courses in the United Kingdom. This recent move to graduate status in the profession of podiatry is now strongly demonstrated in the scientific approach to the presentation of information in this new edition.

There have been other changes of nomenclature. The term 'corn' has been replaced by 'heloma'; but in some instances where two terms are in current use the argument for a choice between one term and the other has been less clear and in those cases both terms have been retained. An example of this is the use of 'hindfoot' and 'rearfoot' where both forms seem to have equal currency.

For most patients and practitioners, conservative management allied to ambulatory foot surgery remains the major emphasis of treatment. Revisions to the text in these areas have taken account of advances in therapeutic methodology and, where methods previously included have now been shown to have fallen short of expectations, they have been omitted. The rate of change in recent years has been very rapid and the revisions to the text demonstrate this.

Increasingly podiatrists have become part of the medical team, recognized for their special expertise in providing effective therapies, coupled with an ability to recognize the responsibilities of independent practice. The chapters providing the essential medical knowledge necessary to the podiatric practitioner have been fully revised by their authors to ensure that the reader has access to the latest information available.

It is also recognized that the increasing complexity of systemic drug therapy makes it essential for podiatrists to be aware of possible drug interactions and to monitor the effects of systemically administered drugs in their patients so that, when necessary, treatment may be modified. Indeed, many instances already exist where the podiatrist has been the first to detect the early symptoms of fixed drug reactions. With this in mind the chapter on Clinical Pharmacology has been totally restructured to help the reader to continue to develop this important aspect of the podiatrist's role.

Lastly, some minor reordering has been undertaken to bring related topics together within the same chapter. An example of this is in Chapter 18 where nail surgery has now been included with digital bone surgery. Colour photographs have also been introduced to this chapter, greatly improving the value of the illustrations.

Donald Neale set high standards when he planned, compiled and edited the first edition of *Common Foot Disorders*. With the assistance of his co-editor, Isobel Adams, he ensured that those same standards were met in the second and third editions. It is believed that the changes which have been made for this fourth edition will further enhance the value of this textbook to students and practitioners alike, while maintaining the high standards set by Donald Neale. In recognition of the contribution his book has made to the education and practice of podiatry the title has now been changed to *Neale's Common Foot Disorders*.

Durham, 1993   D. L. L.

Preface to First Edition

Most books about the feet have naturally enough been written by medical authors for medical readers and they have dealt mainly with the major deformities and acute traumatic injuries and with their surgical management. Most everyday foot troubles, however, develop from biomechanical anomalies which only gradually become symptomatic, though they may ultimately be quite disabling in their cumulative effects. They only seldom reach the physician or surgeon and are generally treated by chiropodists, for whom there has recently been a relative dearth of literature. This book has been compiled to help to fill that need and it has been written with a clinical orientation.

There is abundant evidence that the common foot disorders cause a great deal of pain and disability. Numerous surveys have shown how prevalent they are among all groups of the population from school children to the elderly. They require specialised knowledge and skills for their effective management. The evolution and development of a chiropodial profession specialising in this field is sufficient testimony to the need.

In Great Britain, the training of a state registered chiropodist is broadly based on the medical sciences. It equips him to provide a comprehensive service of diagnosis and treatment virtually from the cradle to the grave and to identify those cases which require medical or surgical investigation and treatment. The scope of practice of the chiropodist has steadily enlarged within recent years and his therapeutic methods have become more efficient and durable. Developments in the field of mechanical therapy and the capacity to undertake minor surgical procedures under local anaesthesia have particularly increased his range and effectiveness.

It is in the public interest that this expansion should continue since it is a wasteful use of other costly skills and facilities if physicians and surgeons are unnecessarily burdened with cases within the competence of chiropodists. Heavy demands on hospital beds and operating theatres place a premium on effective methods of foot care which obviate or postpone the need for admission to hospital or which enhance post-operating care.

The diagnosis and management of the common foot disorders require the application of a variety of manual skills which cannot be taught or learnt solely from books. Such practical techniques as clinical examination, operating, and applying dressings can be mastered only through repeated practice under the guidance of clinical teachers. While they are all necessarily based on scientific principles, their application to individual cases is more art than science. There is no way of acquiring such skills other than by instruction from expert clinicians and practice in the techniques involved. It is impracticable to attempt to include much detailed instruction of that kind in a general text and it is properly left to the clinical teacher who has the dominant role in establishing the required levels of practical expertise.

This book attempts no more than to encapsulate current concepts on the origins, diagnosis and conservative management of the common foot disorders, while relating this particular field to the general medical and surgical conditions which bear directly upon it. The willing cooperation of so many different disciplines in its preparation is indicative of such collaboration in the clinical field.

Edinburgh, 1981   D. N.

Acknowledgements

In preparing the fourth edition the Editor has been faced with the twin challenges of continuing the emphasis started, so successfully, by Donald Neale and of continuing the necessary process of revision of knowledge about foot disorders and their management. In both of these areas the help and advice given freely by Donald Neale has been invaluable. The contributors to previous editions have also carried out revision of continuing chapters.

Much new material appears in this edition and the Editor gratefully acknowledges the expert help of the following authors:

Miss Pat Boyd and Mr George Rendall for rewriting Chapter 2 and for the major revisions to Chapter 5.

Mr Eric Anderson in co-operation with Mr Jim Black for revisions to Chapter 3 and also Mr Jim Black for the revision made to Chapter 13.

Mr Michael Whiting for the major revisions made to Chapter 6.

Dr Margaret Johnson for the reorganization and updating of Chapter 7.

Mrs Barbara Wall for the major revision to the chapter on the management of diabetic patients.

Miss Gwen French, together with Mrs Sue Braid and Mrs Alison Barlow, for their work in revising the chapter on the ageing foot.

Dr Rae Morgan for the revisions to Chapter 12 on Clinical Pharmacology.

Dr Alan Banks for his help in producing the colour photographs for Chapter 18.

In addition, I would like to acknowledge the invaluable help given by Mrs Manesty Forster in preparing new line drawings and revising others. The help of my wife, Mrs Eileen Lorimer, in assisting with proof-reading is also gratefully acknowledged.

Special mention should also be made of the generous advice given by Mr Keith Rome and Mr Peter Ball in the preparation of this fourth edition. Together with the comments received from Schools of Podiatry in the United Kingdom, this help was invaluable in shaping developments in the new volume.

The Editor would wish to place on record his grateful thanks for all the assistance and advice given by members of staff of Churchill Livingstone.

1. The common foot disorders: their nature and origins

Donald L. Lorimer   Donald Neale

The foot, although not numbered among the organs vital for survival of the human being, has a major role in a series of complicated activities centred around mobility. The ability of the human being to function effectively over a wide variety of activities is often restricted when the foot does not provide a sound interface with the ground. As a result there have been many studies, all attempting to put into precise scientific terms the normal range of activity of the foot. These studies have added greatly to understanding, and later chapters in this text have been modified substantially to accommodate the changes but, as yet, such studies have not produced a model from which all abnormal function can be measured.

The common foot disorders which are the concern of the podiatrist can be classified into three broad categories according to their nature and origins:

1. those arising from biomechanical factors
2. those caused by infection
3. those representing manifestations in the foot of general or systemic disease.

The effects of ageing may exacerbate any conditions already present or give rise to new ones.

Most foot disorders are complex in their aetiology and pathology and involve the skeletal components of the foot as well as its soft tissues, therefore the groups listed above are by no means mutually exclusive. Infections and general disease are not always involved as causes of disorders, but biomechanical factors are always present since the foot and lower limb are constantly involved in the mechanical functions of providing support and locomotion. In all assessments and diagnoses and in the formulation of management plans of patients with foot disorders, these biomechanical factors should be considered fully, even when they do not appear to be contributory. Failure to do so may prolong or exacerbate conditions caused initially by other factors. For example, a diabetic ulcer or a septic toe may respond more readily to treatment if the relevant biomechanical factors are properly evaluated.

THE BIOMECHANICAL BASIS OF FOOT DISORDERS

The biomechanical causes of foot disorders can be subdivided as follows:

1. primary intrinsic defects—occurring within the foot—which affect the structure and function of the foot
2. primary extrinsic defects—occurring outwith the foot—which affect the structure and function of the lower limb
3. stress factors—including occupation, weight and footwear
4. direct trauma.

Each of these subdivisions requires close attention. The principal functions of the foot are to serve as a base supporting the body in stance and as a lever in locomotion. The foot also serves as an auxiliary hand, as in swimming and kicking a football, but in such activities it is not serving its true function in weight-bearing. The range of function demanded from the foot varies from the fine balance of the ballet dancer to the propulsion required in the athlete. The mechanical stresses placed on the foot by these extremes of activity, as with the everyday activities of standing and walking, depends ultimately, although by no means only, on the mechanical efficiency of the human foot.

In considering this mechanical efficiency it must be remembered that the foot is no more than the final component of the entire neuromuscular and skeletal system which supports and moves the body. The *kinetic chain*, as it is called, consists of the whole lower limb including the foot and its joints, the ankle, knee and hip joints. Structural and functional abnormalities in the various links of this chain are reflected in the behaviour of the foot on weight-bearing and function and, similarly, malfunction in the foot may also be reflected in symptoms in the knee, hip and lower back.

Primary intrinsic defects

Some primary intrinsic defects which affect the normal structure adversely are:

— malalignments between the hindfoot (rearfoot) and the forefoot which cause abnormal pronation or supination or otherwise interfere with midtarsal and subtalar motion in locomotion
— metatarsus adductus and metatarsus primus adductus, which dispose to hallux abducto valgus and claw toes
— tarsal synostoses which inhibit normal ranges of movements at the subtalar and midtarsal joints
— inadequate development of the sustentaculum tali which deprives the talus of sufficient bony support from the calcaneum.

The effects of such defects are discussed in Chapters 4 & 5. In Chapter 2, the normal function of these structures is discussed.

Primary extrinsic defects

Some primary extrinsic defects which affect the normal alignment and posture of the lower limbs adversely are:

— genu varum and genu valgum

— abnormal internal or external rotation of the femora or the tibiae
— coxa vara or coxa valga
— limb length discrepancy.

Such conditions need to be recognised as the underlying causes of their associated foot disorders and their significance is discussed in Chapter 4. Their management as primary conditions is the responsibility of the paediatrician and orthopaedic surgeon, but frequently the podiatrist is involved. Quite often the podiatrist is the first practitioner to diagnose these conditions.

Other stress factors

The function of the foot in the gait cycle depends upon a series of stages occurring within a range of normal motion. Abnormal stress interferes with this sequence of events and this may initiate or exacerbate foot disabilities. Such stresses may derive from occupational demands, excessive weight-bearing and footwear faults.

Certain occupations, such as postal delivery, impose abnormal stresses due to the carrying of loads, coupled with excessive hours and the need for occupational footwear. Persons working in hot atmospheres or on hot surfaces (e.g. bakers) may also suffer detrimental effects. Steps that can be taken to ameliorate such factors should be considered as part of the management.

Excessive weight-bearing

This may be due not only to occupational hazards but also to obesity. Excessive body weight imposes added stress on both musculoskeletal and cardiovascular systems. Reduction of weight or of excessive load carrying is essential in the management of such cases.

Footwear faults

Ill fitting and unsuitable footwear which is used persistently, affects the functioning of the foot in the gait cycle. The following are the most common and significant ways.

Impaction. Impaction of the toes is caused by

pressure applied distally which occurs if the shoes are too short or the foot elongates excessively on weight-bearing. It can also occur if the foot is allowed to slip forward because of inadequate retaining mechanisms or forced forward because of high heels or sloping heel seats. Impaction is a contributory factor in the causation of nail disorders (Ch. 7), mallet and hammer toes, claw toes and hallux rigidus. By restricting free movement of the toes and the metatarsal joints, the joint area becomes overloaded, resulting in superficial plantar lesions as well as a range of painful deeper conditions (Ch. 5).

Constriction. Constriction of the forefoot results from wearing shoes which are too narrow or pointed. The resultant transverse pressure deflects the toes and contributes to hallux abducto valgus and deformities of the lesser toes. The pressure may also restrict the circulation to the forefoot, particularly where this may be already impaired by vascular disease. Impaction and contriction frequently occur simultaneously as a result of wearing high heeled and pointed shoes.

Excessive heel height. This disrupts the normal gait cycle by transferring weight rapidly from the heel to the forefoot, missing out midstance. Similarly, it transfers the weight-bearing capability from the lateral aspect of the foot to the medial border of the forefoot. In such a shoe, the foot is usually allowed to slip forward thus adding impaction and constriction to the stresses on the forefoot.

Shallow toe spaces. In certain designs of shoe, insufficient depth is allowed in the forepart so that even if they are long enough, the shoes exert dorsal pressure on the toes and in particular the nails.

Abnormal wear. This is an indication of some structural or functional disorder. It is said the 'the shoe is the mirror of the foot' and that it should be studied to identify abnormal wear patterns. This is discussed in Chapter 3.

Direct trauma

In recent years podiatrists have become more involved in the management of sports injuries and as a result have had to deal with minor acute trauma. Many of the conditions dealt with in Chapter 10 cause acute pain to the athlete and the rapid and effective treatment given by podiatrists has resulted in the development of this area of practice.

Major acute trauma lies outwith the scope of this text but many acute conditions, such as fractures of bones in the foot, sprains of the ankle, bruises, contusions and lacerations, are treated effectively by podiatrists. Acute trauma to nails is a common cause of onychogryphosis.

The most common direct trauma results from biomechanical malfunction. The pain and discomfort arises mainly from the secondary lesions of the skin and soft tissues. Such lesions should never be treated without seeking the underlying causes.

Nail disorders

These constitute a special category in themselves since they present, in small compass, examples of injury, infection and disease. Situated as they are in areas of great sensitivity, some nail conditions give rise to acute pain and require early and expert attention. Modern techniques of treatment can provide comprehensive care and cure for such conditions, which are described fully in Chapter 7.

INFECTIONS

Manifestations of bacterial, viral and mycotic infections may all be seen in the foot. The various forms are discussed in Chapter 6 and appropriate treatments are described in Chapter 11.

Bacterial infection

This may arise as a primary condition but it occurs most commonly as a complication of helomata, bursitis and onychocryptosis. In most cases, the invading organisms are staphylococci, which result in a well circumscribed area of inflammation, possibly accompanied by pus formation; this responds well to local antiseptic treatment. Other organisms, such as streptococci, produce spreading infections with cellulitis which may require systemic antibiotic therapy.

Viral infection

This is commonly seen in children as verruca pedis on the surface contact areas. However, it may occur anywhere on the foot in any age group. Verrucae may be acutely painful, but respond well to local treatment. They are discussed in detail in Chapters 6 & 11.

Mycotic infection

The mycotic infections which affect the feet manifest themselves as tinea pedis and onychomycosis. Though not a major cause of concern, tinea pedis requires prompt recognition and treatment in order to minimise cross infection, particularly within communities such as schools, sports clubs and swimming clubs where there are communal facilities for changing.

Control of infection

The eradication of infection where it presents clinically, and the prevention of cross infection to other patients and to themselves, are fundamental objectives of all practitioners. Public awareness of the risks of infection by blood borne viruses, coupled to an extending range of invasive techniques practised by podiatrists, has created a need to apply measures of infection control (Ch. 15).

GENERAL AND SYSTEMIC DISEASE

Dependent as it is on the rest of the body for its nutrition and innervation, the foot is necessarily affected by disease of the major systems, making it essential that the podiatrist can recognise and assess such problems. This is necessary for two reasons: first, so that the effects of such systemic conditions can be assessed relative to the patient's foot condition and account therefore taken of limits which may be necessary on local therapeutic regimes; second, the podiatrist, by virtue of the time spent with the patient, may well be the first to see prodromal symptoms of systemic disease, and so can pass the patient on for early treatment and, hopefully, cure. Several chapters in the text describe the lower limb manifestations of systemic disease processes, covering circulatory, neurological, metabolic and rheumatic disorders (Chs 20–23). Chapter 19 outlines hereditary influences which may predispose to deformity.

In many instances of existing disease processes, it is necessary to deduce the cause from the medicines a patient is receiving. For this purpose Chapter 10 has been revised extensively. Podiatrists should be alert, also, to drug reactions and the chapter points this out.

The management of patients at special risk because their foot problems derive from an underlying systemic disease is well exemplified in Chapter 8.

THE EFFECTS OF AGEING

The ageing process, although a natural effect, produces degeneration of the body tissues and functions. Much of the work of the podiatrist is with the elderly, who easily acquire foot problems which give rise to much pain and loss of mobility. The effective management of foot conditions in the elderly makes a valuable contribution to their quality of life but requires a special understanding of the ageing processes which are taking place. These specific problems are discussed in Chapter 9, which has been revised extensively.

APPROACHES TO MANAGEMENT

Effective management strategies depend on a comprehensive examination of the patient in order to establish a sound diagnosis on which to base the treatment. In Chapter 3, the methodology for examination is discussed and additional routines are introduced in association with specific purposes, such as the administration of local anaesthetics. A good diagnostic routine has two principal elements, the first of which is careful interrogation of the patient by listening to their answers and subsequently checking statements made by them through further questions and by use of standard reference material, e.g. the Monthly Index of Medical Specialities (MIMS), which lists indications and contraindications for the use of drugs. The second element is the accurate recording of answers, avoiding ambiguous abbreviations and ensuring that all subsequent changes are recorded.

Establishing a diagnosis entails much more than merely attaching a label to a condition. It includes the taking of a case history, the assessment of the presenting problem, its likely response to treatment and the possible prognosis. It must also lead to a conclusion as to the overall effect of the disorder on the patient, which may range from being merely inconvenient to absolutely crippling and potentially dangerous to life and limb. The practitioner should always remember that it is not simply lesions on feet that are being treated, but the whole patient.

The podiatrist may be the first professional to be consulted and because of this must accept the responsibility to *recognise* the presence and possible significance of any manifestations in the lower limb of general or systemic disease, to *relate* such findings to any treatment given and to *refer* the patient for any further investigations as may be appropriate. Foot disorders vary in complexity, intensity and duration; their onset may be insidious or acute. The range of clinical problems with which the podiatrist may be confronted necessitates a flexible approach by the practitioner. Although constantly faced with established and chronic deformities, it is also essential to be able to cope with any acute condition, such as a spreading cellulitis.

Podiatrists have at their disposal a wide range of therapeutic techniques together with supporting services from other disciplines. Clinical skill lies in the ability to match diagnostic analysis with a synthesis of therapeutic measures for the benefit of the patient.

The incidence of adult chronic conditions, such as pes planus, hallux abducto-valgus and digital deformities, is particularly high, however such deformities alone are often not painful—adaptation having taken place in the bones and joints. The significance of these conditions usually lies in the attendant chronic symptoms, such as helomata, callosities, bursitis, local infections, ulcerations and nail conditions. These superficial lesions, in contrast, *are* often acutely painful and disabling, needing effective long term treatment to control them. Nevertheless they are only symptoms of an underlying dysfunction and cannot be cured except by controlling the primary condition.

Recent advances in methods of treatment have brought to the podiatrist the means to control more effectively many of the common foot disorders. These advances have rendered obsolete much of the reliance on temporary and repetitive palliative measures which were formerly the core of practice.

2. Structure and function

Patricia M. Boyd   George Rendall

EVOLUTIONARY DEVELOPMENT

'Structure is the ultimate expression of function.'
(John Hunter)

The human foot presents a remarkable example of the truth of this saying. Only a brief summary of the evolutionary changes which have produced the contemporary human foot need be given here.

The primitive pentadactyl limb, common to all vertebrates, consists of three segments. The proximal segment has one bone (humerus, femur) and the intermediate segment two bones (radius and ulna, tibia and fibula). The distal segment (hand, foot) originally contained nine bones in its more proximal part (carpus, tarsus), and five more intermediately (metacarpus, metatarsus) with five digits (fingers, toes) each having three phalanges. The bones of the hand and foot were all arranged symmetrically about the midline, the five digits projecting distally in a symmetrical fan-shaped form. The central 'ray' was the longest, as it still is in the human hand. All four limbs were used for support and locomotion, the hands and feet projecting laterally as primitive fins and paws.

The gradual change over comparatively recent evolutionary time from quadrupedal to bipedal stance and gait necessitated and induced major structural adaptations to this primitive form. The adoption of an upright posture necessitated both the lumbar curve in the spine and the development of the heel to provide posterior support and stability upon which the upright body could be balanced. The development of the heel gave rise to the uniquely arched formation of the human foot.

Another major adaptations was the increase in size of most of the tarsal bones in response to the posterior shift of the weight-bearing stresses, and the fusion of two lateral tarsal bones to form the cuboid. A third important change was the closer approximation of the formerly atavistic first metatarsal segment to the second, with which it became more firmly tied. The first segment became longer and stronger as the feet came to point more directly forward and required greater capacity for leverage. The hallux thus lost its prehensile role and the foot as a whole lost much of its mobility as it became necessarily more rigid in adapting to its role as a lever in locomotion.

THE BIOMECHANICS OF STANCE AND GAIT

The function of the foot is to act as an interface between the body and supporting surface in stance and gait. It is the platform upon which the body rests in standing, walking and running and is ideally designed to adapt to the range of stresses imposed on it by human locomotion. Foot function must vary both to accommodate these stresses and to enhance locomotor efficiency during gait. The foot is, at appropriate times, a shock absorber, a mobile adapter and a rigid lever.

The stability and behaviour of the weight-bearing foot are influenced by the manner in which the body weight is transmitted to it by the tibia through the trochlear surface of the talus. The body weight is transmitted to the foot through this saddle articulation, then inferiorly to the calcaneus and lateral column and anteriorly to the navicular and medial column. Any movements occurring in the tibia are also transmitted into the foot.

Although the plantar surface of the foot is in

firm contact with the ground, movement within the foot, principally *pronation* and *supination*, can occur allowing the body and lower limb to move above it. Pronation is a triplanar movement involving *abduction* (transverse plane), *eversion* (frontal plane) and *dorsiflexion* (sagittal plane). Supination also occurs in three planes, its components being *adduction, inversion* and *plantarflexion*. These movements take place at the *subtalar* and *midtarsal* joints in response to ground reaction forces from below, transverse and frontal plane motions of the tibia and femur from above and eccentric and concentric contraction of muscles. Sagittal plane movements of the lower limb are accommodated by dorsiflexion and plantarflexion of the ankle joint and the metatarsophalangeal joints.

Ground reaction occurs in three planes and is entirely dependent on the force applied by the foot above. This will vary with the mass of the patient, the speed of walking, the stability/mobility of the contact limb and the interaction of the foot with the supporting surface (e.g. concrete will tend to give higher forces than sponge rubber). Ideally, reaction forces are minimised at heel strike and maximised in propulsion in order to reduce impact trauma and maximise propulsive efficency. As a general rule, subtalar pronation is associated with structural mobility and force reduction, whilst supination is associated with structural stability and force transmission.

The subtalar joint is often described as a *torque translator* because of its ability to alter the direction of forces between the leg and foot. For example, internal rotation of the tibia effects adduction of the talus due to its firm articulation with the tibia and fibula at the ankle joint. Adduction is resisted by ground reaction but permitted by the subtalar joint, which pronates to allow the talus and calcaneus to rotate in opposite directions in response to the action and reaction forces from above and below. The perceived movements are talar adduction with plantarflexion and calcaneal eversion — a one directional three plane rotation described as closed chain subtalar pronation. These movements in the rearfoot do not occur in isolation from the rest of the foot. Calcaneal eversion and talar plantarflexion produce frontal plane

ground reaction forces under the 1st ray, which supinate the forefoot around the longitudinal axis of the midtarsal joint to keep the foot plantargrade. Transverse and sagittal plane reaction forces pronate the oblique axis of the midtarsal joint, increasing forefoot adaptability and shock absorption. Internal rotation therefore increases the ability of the foot to adapt and absorb shock from ground reaction forces.

External rotation of the tibia also has a direct but opposite effect on the foot, helping to supinate the subtalar joint. Transverse plane reaction forces adduct the forefoot, supinating the oblique axis of the midtarsal joint. Abduction and dorsiflexion of the talus induce calcaneal inversion thereby prompting lateral ground reaction forces, which pronate the forefoot around the longitudinal axis of the midtarsal joint. External rotation, therefore, helps to lock the forefoot making it a rigid lever for propulsion.

Reaction and internal rotation are a passive result of the effect of gravity. External rotation and muscle contraction are antigravitational. Muscular contraction is generally perceived as a shortening of a muscle belly to initiate movement. In terms of the gait cycle, muscular contractions occur in three ways:

- *isometric contractions*, which maintain stability without movement
- *eccentric contractions*, which act as a brake, slowing down and controlling movements (the muscle belly will actually *lengthen* under tension throughout its contraction)
- *concentric contractions*, which initiate movement acting to change the direction of movement against the influence of gravity or other forces.

Antagonistic muscles may also act to damp down excessive movement caused by contraction of the opposing group of muscles (see also p.13).

These features combine to form a complex mechanism which allows for alterations in body posture whilst maintaining a plantargrade foot as a base upon which to stand, walk and run.

Standing

The function of the foot in standing is to act as a base, supporting the body above it, and to maintain both intrinsic and postural stability with the minimum expenditure of energy. *Intrinsic stability* is achieved by interlocking the joints under the influence of compression from the opposing forces of bodyweight and ground reaction. To achieve *postural stability* it is necessary to maintain the centre of mass or gravity within the base of stance (Fig. 2.1).

Postural stability

Base of stance can be defined as that area of the body in contact with the supporting surface plus all the area contained within its margin. In quadrupedal stance, a large area is contained within the four feet, so producing a wide base of stance. In bipedal stance, the base of stance consists of the feet and the ground in between. The foot as a base of stance is predominantly a rigid structure acted upon by the muscles of the leg.

The *centre of gravity* is that part of a body around which all of its mass acts. During stance in humans, the centre of gravity lies within the pelvic girdle. A plumb line dropped from the centre of gravity in stance would hang between the feet and slightly ahead of the tibia, through which the body mass is transmitted to the feet. The foot extends well beyond this point and loading is principally on the heel and forefoot, with the centre of gravity occurring fairly centrally within the base of stance. The advantages of this are clear in terms of stability and energy conservation. The centre of gravity lies slightly ahead of the ankle joint's axis of motion and also ahead of the knee joint. If the centre of gravity moves forward and threatens stability, the triceps surae undergo contraction to pull the tibia back and restore stability. This large muscle group undergoes frequent minimal contracture to maintain postural tone and stability and, as long as the centre of gravity remains in front of the ankle and knee joint axes, other groups, including the anterior muscles of the leg and thigh, should remain at rest.

Human balance mechanisms are highly refined and thus balance maintenance seems effortless in spite of a relatively narrow base of stance. When balance systems fail, however, it is necessary to apply these principles of static stance in order to

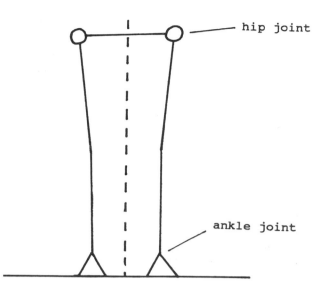

CENTRE OF MASS. STATIC, ANTERIOR VIEW.

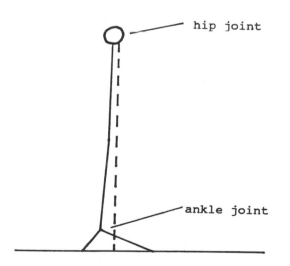

CENTRE OF MASS. STATIC, LATERAL VIEW.

Fig. 2.1 Centre of mass static in anterior view (above) and lateral view (below).

prevent falls. Use of a walking stick or frame increases stability in such cases by substantially increasing the margins of the base of stance.

Intrinsic stability and subtalar neutral position

In stance, the foot is normally a rigid structure

with the subtalar joint in its neutral position and the midtarsal joint locked. The simplest definition of subtalar joint neutral postion is, 'that position of the joint in which the foot is neither supinated nor pronated' (Root, Orien & Weed 1977). Functional rigidity is achieved by locking the midtarsal joint in maximal pronation when the subtalar joint is in neutral or supinated. Normally at this time the planes of the hindfoot and forefoot are parallel. Ideally, a bisection line of the posterior surface of the calcaneus is vertical when the subtalar joint is in neutral. This position is also achieved during locomotion when the weight bearing foot reaches the end of midstance. Variations from vertical, either inverted or everted, show some mechanical anomaly which may lead to symptoms of pain or deformity (see Ch. 5).

Locking of the midtarsal joint is achieved through a combination of controlled loading from above and ground reaction forces in different directions from below. Sagittal plane ground reaction forces create a dorsiflexion moment to lock the oblique axis of the midtarsal joint. Frontal plane ground reaction forces create an evertory moment to lock the longitudinal axis of the midtarsal joint. Normal postural tone in the triceps surae balances these forces through plantarflexion of the ankle (sagittal plane) and inversion of the calcaneus (frontal plane). Stability is achieved when all forces and moments within the foot are in equilibrium (see Fig.2.4 on p.11).

Walking

The lower limb represents what Steindler (1964) designated a *kinetic chain*—a series of links free to move on each other but also capable of combining into a stable column to support the body. The chain is said to be *open* when the distal link is free to move and *closed* when it is fixed in weight-bearing. When open, the distal links move on the proximal; when closed the proximal links move on those more distal. During the stance phase, the loaded lower limb is a closed kinetic chain in which the foot is fixed as a stable base over and upon which the lower limb and the body are swung forward. During the swing phase, the unloaded lower limb is an open kinetic chain with its separate segments swinging freely forward in relation to the body above it.

The foot is required to be a stable base during stance. This may also be said of walking but here foot function must vary throughout the gait cycle in order to reduce the force of impact, adapt to

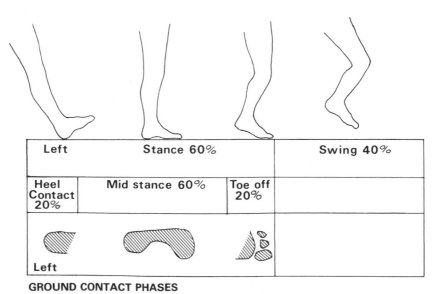

GROUND CONTACT PHASES

Fig. 2.2   The walking cycle showing stance and swing phases and the weight-bearing areas of the plantar surface.

variations in its relationship with the body above and the supporting surface below, and maximise efficient transference of energy.

For purposes of analysis it is convenient to divide the walking gait cycle into four distinct but consecutive phases. These are *contact, midstance* and *propulsion* (which combined are described as the *stance* phase), and the *swing* phase. The foot functions as a shock absorber in contact and a rigid lever in propulsion. Midstance is a period of functional transfer and stabilisation as the centre of gravity passes over the loaded foot. The swing phase permits the foot to recover from propulsion and reposition itself in preparation for contact. The swinging limb also has an important function in pelvic rotation and changing the position of the centre of gravity (Fig. 2.2).

Contact

Heel strike signals the end of the swing phase and the beginning of the contact phase. Force reduction in the contact phase is essential to minimise the potentially harmful effects of impact, so the foot and lower limb act as a shock absorber during this period. Contact force is reduced by a combination of factors. The subtalar joint pronates 4–6°, the tibia rotates internally, the ankle plantarflexes and the knee flexes. The heel pad and elastic plantar components, plantar aponeurosis, deltoid, spring, long and short plantar ligaments all assist in absorbing shock, but the major shock absorbing features within the foot are controlled pronation of the subtalar joint and controlled plantarflexion of the ankle joint. Flexion of the knee joint also contributes significantly to shock absorption during gait.

Pronation occurs as a result of lateral ground reaction force at heel strike (creating an evertory moment around the subtalar joint). Plantarflexion occurs as a result of posterior reaction forces on contact (creating a plantarflexion moment around the ankle joint). Control is given by medial/anterior resistance from contraction of the tibialis anterior (creating an invertory and dorsiflexion moment). These factors reduce force by extending the period of deceleration as the foot strikes the ground (Fig. 2.3).

Fig. 2.3

Force (N) = Mass (Kg) × Acceleration (ms⁻²)

$$\text{Acceleration (ms}^{-2}) = \frac{\text{Change in velocity (ms}^{-1})}{\text{Time (s)}}$$

e.g.

$$\frac{50 \text{ Kg} \times 10 \text{ ms}^{-1}}{1 \text{ s}} = 500 \text{ N}$$

$$\frac{50 \text{ kg} \times 10 \text{ ms}^{-2}}{2 \text{ s}} = 250 \text{ N}$$

The components of force are mass, change in velocity and time. Increasing mass or change in velocity increases force. Increasing time reduces force.

Moments are turning forces which rotate levers (e.g. the bones of the foot) around axes (e.g. joints). Rotation will continue to occur until moments in a certain direction equal moments in the opposite direction, at which time they are said to be in equilibrium. In gait, equilibrium is normally achieved when the foot is flat on the supporting surface, at which time it is said to be plantargrade (Fig. 2.4).

Fig. 2.4 Moments or turning forces are a product of force × distance (the length of the lever arm). Moments can therefore be changed by altering either the force or the length of the lever arm, e.g. 500 Newtons × 0.20 metre = 100 Nm; 500 Newtons × 0.10 metre = 50 Nm; i.e. the moment reduces in direct relation to the length of the lever.

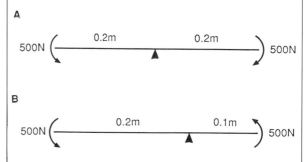

In A, the clockwise and anticlockwise moments are equal, i.e. there is equilibrium.

In B, shortening the clockwise moment arm by half reduces the resultant moment by half, therefore the lever will turn in an anticlockwise direction.

Midstance

The midstance phase begins as the metatarsals make ground contact, become fully weight-bearing and the opposite foot leaves the ground. The foot in early midstance is a *mobile adapter*, capable of achieving stability despite variations in the supporting surface and the postion of the body and lower limb relative to it. This is facilitated to a large degree by pronation of the subtalar joint and the associated talocalcaneal motions. Plantarflexion and adduction of the talus increase the congruency or parallelism of the planes of motion of the two articular facets of the midtarsal joint so that the calcaneocuboid and talonavicular joints can move as one. This unlocks the oblique axis of the midtarsal joint (see Midtarsal joint, Subtalar joint, pp 15–16).

Eversion of the calcaneus twists the medial side of the forefoot against the ground to produce inversion, unlocking the longitudinal axis. Pronation also increases mobility in the medial and lateral columns. Shock absorption continues in early midstance and is provided by muscles lengthening under tension to control yielding motions at the knee, ankle, tarsal and midtarsal joints.

As midstance progressess, foot function changes and the need for stability and, ultimately, rigidity supplants that for adaptability and shock absorption. Towards the end of midstance, when the weight-bearing limb is directly over the foot, the subtalar joint resupinates to achieve subtalar neutral position, prior to heel lift. The body passes over and anterior to the foot as it prepares for propulsion. The ankle joint dorsiflexes by 10° to coincide with 10° of extension of the hip, allowing the centre of gravity to pass ahead of the base of support with the heel in ground contact. Resupination is assisted by the increasing tension on the triceps surae and by external rotation of the femur and tibia. The rotations are transferred to the talus via the ankle joint and, when countered by ground reaction forces, facilitate supination of the subtalar joint and locking of the midtarsal joint. Midstance may therefore be considered a transfer phase which enables the mobile shock absorber to become a rigid lever.

Propulsion

In the propulsive phase, rigidity is essential to maximise efficient transfer of energy and to minimise risk of injury to joints. As the heel leaves the ground, the subtalar joint supinates rapidly due to the action of the triceps surae and tibialis posterior. The planes of rotation around the two articular facets of the midtarsal joint become less parallel and the lateral border of the forefoot is twisted against the ground so that the forefoot becomes locked to the rearfoot (see Midtarsal joint, p.15). The foot is rigid, the arch height increases and loading is concentrated on the metatarsal heads and the distal pads of the toes. This area of contact provides the fulcrum for toe off. Subtalar joint and midtarsal joint axes rotate toward the sagittal plane to minimise their vulnerability to reaction moments (Fig. 2.5). Finally, the first ray is plantarflexed by contraction of the peroneus longus and by the stabilising action of the plantar fascia (Fig. 2.6). This stabilises the medial column to maximise propulsive stability. The foot then leaves the ground and the swing phase begins as the opposite foot enters the stance phase (Fig. 2.7).

Swing

During the swing phase the foot is clear of the ground as the limb swings past its neighbour, preparing to resume weight-bearing at heel strike, and so the gait cycle is repeated. Swing phase provides the foot with an opportunity to recover in preparation for the next stance phase and also assists the forward movement of the centre of gravity. The forward rotation of the pelvis associated with the swinging limb also initiates the external rotation which is so important to the stance limb in late midstance.

Double support phase. At toe off and heel strike, both feet are simultaneously in ground contact for approximately 10% of the walking cycle. This period of double support becomes shorter with increased speed of walking until eventually in running there is no double support phase and both feet are off the ground in float phase.

Fig. 2.5 Lever length can be changed by altering the angle of application of the force. The further the angle of application is from 90°, the smaller will be the perpendicular (turning) component of the force.

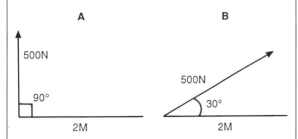

In diagram A, the 500 N clockwise force pulls at 90° 2 m from the fulcrum, giving a moment of 500 N × 2 m = 1000 Nm.

In diagram B, the 500 N clockwise force pulls at only 30° from parallel, reducing its vertical pull and therefore its moment. In this case we find the vertical component by the calculation:

500 N × 2 m × sin 30° = 1000 Nm × 0.5 (i.e. sin 30°) = 500 Nm.

Thus the moment *reduces* as the line of action of a force moves away from the perpendicular to the lever.

This is used to advantage in the gait cycle. Turning the axis of rotation of a joint toward the reaction forces *reduces* perpendicularity to these forces, and therefore reduces resultant moments around joints. The effect is to reduce joint stress and increase stability in propulsion.

Muscle action

During these alternating phases, the muscles of the lower limb act both from their proximal to their distal attachments, and vice versa, according to the needs of the moment. A muscle may act either by shortening and bringing its attachments closer together (isotonic/concentric contraction), or by maintaining its length unchanged and its attachments stable under tensile stress (isometric contraction), or by a controlled elongation which damps down and checks the moving apart of its attachments under a tensile force (eccentric contraction). Collectively, the muscles of the lower limb effect and control movement in the following ways:

1. Prime movers contract isotonically to move apart, e.g. the triceps surae muscle group acts on

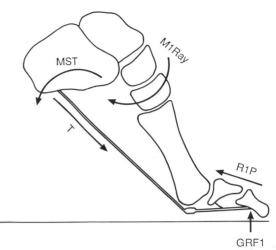

Fig. 2.6 Hick's windlass. JH Hick (1954) described a mechanism by which pivoting around the metatarsal heads raises the medial longitudinal arch. Ground reaction force (GRFI) anterior to the metatarsal heads dorsiflexes the 1st toe, creating tension in the plantar aponeurosis (T). This pulls the toe back, producing a reaction force at the 1st metatarsophalangeal joint (RIP) and a plantarflexion moment around the joints of the 1st ray (MIRay). Tension in the aponeurosis produces a supinatory moment around the subtalar joint (MST).

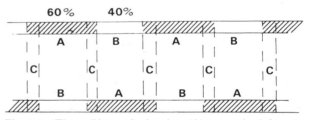

Fig. 2.7 The walking cycle showing: (A) successive left and right stance phases (60%); (B) successive right and left swing phases (40%); (C) successive periods of double support (10%).

the calcaneus from the lower leg to plantarflex the foot.

2. Antagonists resist the pull of the prime movers, thus checking and controlling the movement, e.g. the quadriceps extend the knee for heel contact while the hamstrings check this action.

3. Synergists stabilise the attachments from which prime movers and antagonists are acting e.g. the short digital flexors fix the toes firmly to the ground and so provide a stable base from which the long extensors and flexors can act.

4. Fixators stabilise intervening joints to ensure

that the desired movement occurs at the appropriate articulation, e.g. the triceps surae group stabilises the ankle once the leg has begun to swing forward. This action prevents further dorsiflexion at the ankle and thus ensures that this movement is transferred to the metatarsophalangeal joints so that the heel is raised and the body is tilted forward.

Biomechanically, the act of walking is a repeated series of muscular actions designed to keep the body's centre of gravity off-balance just forward of its base, represented by each foot alternately. The force of gravity is thereby utilised to assist forward movement and this makes for maximum economy in the expenditure of muscular energy. In locomotion, the contractural tone of muscles powerfully reinforces the inert tension of ligaments in binding together the parts of the foot and restraining hypermobility of joints. The tendons of the tibialis posterior and the peroneus longus undersling the tarsus mediolaterally and so provide a dynamic tarsal cradle. The plantar intrinsic muscles similarly provide tensile support longitudinally against the thrust of weight-bearing forces. The transverse head of the adductor hallucis reinforces and guards the transverse intermetatarsal ligaments. The peroneus longus also stabilises the first metatarsal. Muscles thus assist in maintaining structural stability under maximum load while simultaneously initiating and controlling movements.

Joint movements in the lower limb

During the gait cycle, the body's centre of gravity is translated through space in a smooth undulating line of progression; joint motions and muscle action work together to produce an energy-efficient and smooth pattern of gait.

The major displacements of the limbs occur in the sagittal plane as the limbs move backwards and forwards. Most of the muscle activity occurs to control these motions and therefore muscles tend to contract at the beginning and end of the stance and swing phases.

The muscles also control the subtle movements of pelvic tilt and rotation and the transverse and frontal plane motions of the lower limb and foot.

The pelvis. The pelvis pivots in the transverse plane from side to side allowing first one leg and then the other to swing forward. This gives length to the stride. The abductor muscles of the weight-bearing hip support the pelvis, allowing the swinging limb to have ground clearance to follow through. The pelvis also rotates forward with the swinging limb and, as it does so, the weight-bearing hip joint is stabilised in the transverse plane by its external rotators. In this way pelvic movement assists external rotation of the weight-bearing lower limb.

The hip and knee. The hip extends as the limb begins to bear weight and the body passes over the foot in stance phase, then flexes to begin swing phase. Flexion is initiated by the iliopsoas and tensor fascia latae. Simultaneously, the knee flexes to aid clearance of the foot during swing. The swinging limb is controlled by the hamstrings as it prepares for contact. The quadriceps retard flexion of the knee after contact until the centre of gravity moves anteriorly to the knee joint.

The knee joint flexes and extends twice in the gait cycle. Flexion occurs just after heel contact to absorb shock and again during swing to allow for foot clearance. Extension occurs at heel strike and during midstance, as the body passes directly over the weight-bearing limb.

The hip and knee joints also rotate slightly on their vertical axes, medially as they flex and laterally as they extend. Pronation of the subtalar joint includes internal rotation of the tibia and femur along with knee flexion, to produce shock absorption as the limb becomes loaded in early stance. External rotation of the femur and tibia assists supination at the tarsal joints, encouraging rigidity for leverage at toe off.

The ankle. The ankle joint moves through rapid plantar flexion at heel contact. The movement is controlled by the tibialis anterior muscles contracting eccentrically to prevent foot slap and reduce the force of impact. The ankle then dorsiflexes as the body passes over the weight-bearing limb, reaching 10° beyond the vertical. Rapid plantar flexion follows with heel lift initiated by contraction of the triceps surae group. Once again, dorsiflexion of the ankle occurs to give toe clearance during swing. The tibialis anterior muscles again facilitate this movement, this time contracting concentrically.

The subtalar joint. The subtalar joint functions in three planes, with substantial frontal and transerve plane and limited sagittal plane motion. The movements available are pronation and supination. (Motion occurs in all three planes or not at all. The subtalar joint has no ability to isolate movement in one plane and act, for example, as an evertor.) In gait, from a position of slight supination at heel strike, the subtalar joint rapidly pronates in the contact and early midstance phases. Pronation is instigated by lateral ground reaction force. When combined with plantarflexion of the ankle and resisted by eccentric contracture of the tibialis anterior, subtalar joint pronation increases the period of deceleration which occurs in the transition from swing to stance. This has the effect of reducing contact forces (Fig. 2.3).

After 25% of the duration of the stance phase, the subtalar joint resupinates, reaching neutral shortly after the swing and stance limbs pass each other at 50% of the stance phase. The subtalar joint continues to supinate and at 80% of the stance phase, when the gastrocnemus contracts and the heel lifts, the calcaneus becomes markedly inverted, a position it retains for the remainder of the stance phase. (Note that the percentage figures given are approximate. Clinical observation indicates significant variation around these figures in apparently normal subjects.)

The subtalar joint can be considered the key to foot function throughout the stance phase of the gait cycle. Whereas the ankle joint can move largely in isolation from the other joints, subtalar joint motion tends to have a major influence on other joints within the foot, particularly the midtarsal joint and first and fifth rays.

Subtalar joint pronation increases midtarsal and forefoot mobility, enhancing the adaptability needed in early midstance. Subtalar supination reduces midtarsal mobility, thereby encouraging rigidity in propulsion.

The midtarsal joint. The midtarsal joint is a triplanar joint with two axes and two degrees of freedom. The longitudinal axis of the midtarsal joint runs close to the sagittal and transverse planes and therefore permits motion primarily in the frontal plane (i.e. inversion/eversion). The oblique axis runs diagonally across all three planes allowing most of its motion in the transverse and sagittal planes.

As the ankle and subtalar joint are the interface between the foot and the rest of the body, so the midtarsal joint interfaces the rearfoot and forefoot. Midtarsal joint function is important for propulsive stability as the forefoot is the contact zone during the propulsive phase. Midtarsal joint function is also highly dependent on subtalar joint function. Subtalar joint pronation leads to adduction and plantarflexion of the talus and eversion of the calcaneus. This increases forefoot adaptability in the following ways:

1. The talus becomes less congruous with the navicular, reducing the stability of the medial column.

2. The oblique axis of motion of the midtarsal joint is lowered, thereby increasing the sagittal plane component of its range of motion.

3. The planes of motion of the talonavicular and calcaneocuboid joints are normally opposed when the subtalar joint is in neutral. Talo-calcaneal movements associated with subtalar joint pronation increase the congruency, or parallelism, of the axes of motion of these two joints and thereby increase their freedom to move in parallel. This is described as unlocking of the oblique axis of the midtarsal joint.

From early midstance the subtalar joint gradually moves from pronation to supination. At about 60% of the stance phase duration, the calcaneus becomes inverted by the contracting triceps surae. Calcaneal inversion at heel lift twists the lateral side of the forefoot against the ground, effecting an evertory reaction force. These opposing moments (inversion of the calcaneus, eversion of the lateral column) screw the foot tight at the calcaneocuboid joint. This is often described as locking of the longitudinal axis of the midtarsal joint in pronation.

External rotation of the leg in propulsion encourages subtalar joint supination by adducting the talus. This effects a transverse plane ground reaction force (adduction) in the forefoot. Adduction twists the forefoot against the abducting talus, locking the oblique axis of the midtarsal joint in supination.

The forefoot. The ankle joint plantarflexes at ground contact and then dorsiflexes until the triceps surae contract to plantarflex the ankle joint, lifting the heel and beginning the propulsive phase. This normally occurs with the ankle in about 10° of dorsiflexion. Plantarflexion of the ankle in propulsion allows the foot to pivot around a fulcrum at the interface of the metatarsal heads and the supporting surface, resulting in digital dorsiflexion and its reaction in the Hick's windlass (Fig. 2.7) metatarsal plantarflexion. The loaded metatarsal slides back over the sesamoids, assisted by contraction of the peroneus longus muscle which inserts into its base. Eccentric contraction of the flexor digitorum longus helps to stabilise the first ray and the medial column.

Weight distribution in locomotion

Weight distribution through the foot in locomotion is determined by the skeletal structure of the foot and its relationship to the moving body above and the ground below.

The ankle, knee and hip joints provide for extension and flexion of the limb in the sagittal plane. The hip and peritalar joints facilitate rotatory motions, the former for internal and external rotation of the thigh and leg on a vertical axis, the latter for pronatory and supinatory rotation of the foot on a roughly longitudinal axis (see Appendix 1).

At heel strike, the foot is slightly inverted and the posterior lateral rim of the heel of the shoe first makes contact with the ground. It is at this stage in the walking cycle that shock absorption is most required within the foot and this is provided by the greater degree of mobility afforded to the small tarsal joints as the foot pronates. As weight is transferred progressively from the opposite foot, the hindfoot pronates at the subtalar joint to allow all the metatarsal heads to make contact with the ground and become fully weight-bearing. This movement is accompanied by some corresponding internal rotation of the tibia and talus. By the middle of the stance phase, the foot is fully loaded with the entire weight of the body.

As the foot progresses through the midstance phase, its function changes into that of a rigid lever to propel the body forwards. This involves supination of the foot with corresponding external rotation of the tibia; the heel leaves the ground and the final force at toe off is concentrated on the plantar surfaces of the medial metatarsals and the hallux. This is the time of maximum loading of the forefoot and maximum stresses on the plantar soft tissues. It is during this period in the stance phase that mechanical defects, from wherever they originate, have the maximum ill effects on the structure and function of the forefoot.

Variable factors affecting stance and gait

The normal variable factors which are of most clinical significance are shape, contour and mobility. These are inter-related and together determine the foot type, which is also related to the build of the body. All these factors have a bearing on the management of the patient.

Variations of shape

These are of importance in shoe fitting but they are also more indicative of the foot type than any other variable. There are three readily identifiable shapes: the short broad foot, the long narrow foot and the triangular foot.

The short broad foot is subject to constriction from footwear of inadequate width and girth. Two further classifications exist related to the bisection lines of the forefoot and the calcaneus, namely the rectus foot and the adductus foot (Fig. 2.8).

The long narrow foot is more likely to be structurally unstable and is subject to impaction of the forefoot from footwear which is too short or which does not restrain the narrow foot from moving forward inside the shoe.

The triangular foot has a broad forefoot and a narrow heel and is the most vulnerable of the three types.

In a rectus foot shape, the forefoot bisection through the second metatarsal, and the hindfoot bisection through the calcaneus, are parallel to each other and the foot is straight. Because of

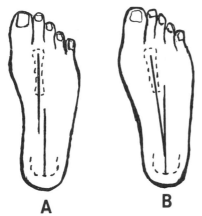

Fig. 2.8   (A) Rectus foot shape; (B) adductus foot shape.

this, if the foot suffers abnormal subtalar joint pronation, any forefoot deformity tends to develop in the sagittal plane, e.g. hallux limitus or hallux rigidus (Fig. 2.8A).

An adductus foot shape is one where the forefoot bisection is adducted relative to the hindfoot bisection and the metatarsals are angled towards the midsagittal plane. This foot shape tends to develop forefoot deformities in the transverse plane, e.g. hallux abductovalgus, if abnormal subtalar joint pronation occurs (Fig. 2.8B).

Variations of intrinsic mobility

Normal feet vary in their range of intrinsic mobility. The totality of movement within all the tarsal joints determines the degree to which the shape and contour of the feet change under the stress of weight-bearing. They may be relatively rigid, showing little or no change on weight-bearing, or relatively mobile, showing some lowering of the longitudinal arch and some consequential elongation whilst still remaining structurally stable. The former type has relatively little

instrinsic capacity for shock absorption, the latter considerably more.

The term *hypermobility* indicates abnormal ranges of movement at joints. In the foot, on weight-bearing, this produces excessive pronation and flattening, thereby significantly increasing its overall length. The breadth across the metatarsal heads may also be increased by splaying of the metatarsals. The term hypermobility is also applied to those metatarsal segments (specifically the first and fifth rays) where the range of movement at the proximal articulations is so marked as to affect the capacity of the metatarsal heads to accept their normal share of the weight-bearing load (see Ch. 5).

Variations in the metarsal formula

It is difficult to gain agreement as to what constitutes the normal parabola of the metatarsal heads in the frontal plane, but there can be no doubt that variations do occur. Clinically the most significant is the short first metatarsal, usually accompanied by a short first toe. Like hypermobility, which may also be present, it may render the segment relatively incompetent for its essential weight-bearing function, causing some compensatory overloading of the adjacent metatarsal heads. The short first toe may be the cause of a mistaken measurement when footwear is being fitted, in which case the adjacent toes may suffer from impaction from a short shoe. Shortness of the fifth or any other metatarsal may similarly overload its neighbour.

Variations in the angle of gait

The angle of gait is the deviation of the long axis of each foot from the sagittal plane (Fig. 2.9). The normal is for the long axes of the feet to be nearly

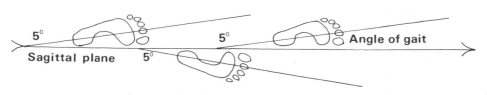

Fig. 2.9   The angle of gait.

parallel or slightly out-toed. Marked in-toeing may arise from internal tibial or femoral torsion, from internal rotation of the hip joint, from bow legs or, in children, from active compensation for knock knees. Marked out-toeing may arise from external tibial or femoral torsion, or knock knees in adults. Whether or not these variations are significant clinically depends on their origins and on other variable factors such as age, weight and occupation.

FURTHER READING

Close J R, Todd F N 1959 The phasic activity of the muscles of the lower extremity and the effect of tendon transfer. Journal of Bone and Joint Surgery 41–A: 189

Du Vries H L 1978 Surgery of the foot, 4th edn. Mosby, St Louis

Hicks J H 1953 The mechanics of the foot II. The joints. Journal of Anatomy 87: 345

Hicks J H 1954 The mechanics of the foot II. The plantar aponeurosis. Journal of Anatomy 88: 25

Hicks J H 1955 The mechanics of the foot IV. The action of the muscles on the foot in standing. Acta Anatomica 27: 180

Jahss M H 1982 Disorders of the foot, Vols I & II. Saunders, Philadelphia

Jones F W 1943 Structure and function as seen in the foot. Baillière Tindall & Cox, London

Lake N C 1943 The foot, 3rd edn. Baillière Tindall & Cox, London

Mann R, Inman V F 1964 Phasic activity of the intrinsic muscles of the foot. Journal of Bone and Joint Surgery 46–A: 469

McMinn R 1982 Colour atlas of the foot and ankle. Wolfe, London

Morton D J 1935 The human foot. Columbia University Press, New York

Root M L, Orien W P, Weed J H 1977 Normal and abnormal function of the foot. Clinical Biomechanics, Vol II. Clinical Biomechanics Corporation, Los Angeles

Schuster R O 1975 Personal communication

Sgarlato T E 1981 Compendium of podiatric biomechanics. California College of Podiatric Medicine, San Franciso

Siebel M O 1989 Foot function—A programmed text. Williams & Wilkins, Baltimore

Steindler A 1964 Kinesiology of the human body. Thomas, Springfield, Illinois

Vincent O T 1968 The mechanics of the foot. The Chiropodist 23: II (Nov) 397–425

Williams M, Lissner H R 1977 Biomechanics of human motion. Saunders, Philadelphia

3. Examination and assessment

Eric G. Anderson   James A. Black

Patient—one who suffers.

Establishing a diagnosis as a basis for treatment depends upon two sets of information, the *subjective symptoms* and the *objective signs*. Symptoms are those abnormal features of which the patient has personal experience. Signs are those detectable by a skilled observer with the help of various types of apparatus. The more information that can be made available from these sources, the more reliable is the diagnosis likely to be. Most of the foot disorders described in this book can be diagnosed by clinical examination, though some require laboratory or radiographic investigation as outlined in later pages.

For examination purposes, foot disorders can be conveniently sub-divided into the superficial lesions of the skin and soft tissues, structural and functional disorders and local manifestations of general or systemic disease. All three aspects need to be considered. Most of the superficial lesions are local symptoms of an underlying disorder and they cannot be treated effectively in isolation. However, it is practical to diagnose them separately since they need specific treatment over and above that required for the underlying fault.

The management of the foot problem cannot be divorced from that of any concurrent general or systemic disorder. Examination of the foot must include recognition of local signs and symptoms of more remote origins in order that fuller investigation may be instituted. This is particularly important when the foot disorder is the first presenting symptom of a more general pathology, as pes cavus may be in spina bifida, or as a swollen interphalangeal joint may be in rheumatoid arthritis. Depending on the findings, the patient may have to be referred for a full orthopaedic, circulatory, neurological or other general examination. In such circumstances, it is clearly impossible for the primary examination to explore all the possibilities of pathology remote from the foot. But the clinician must accept the responsibility to *recognise and record* clinical features of potential significance, to *relate* them to any local treatment that may be necessary, and to *refer* the patient for appropriate specialist examination with a summary of his reasons for doing so.

The foot is an integral part of the kinetic chain. It provides the musculoskeletal system with the mechanical interface between the ground and the lower limb, producing the leverage and propulsion necessary for walking and running whilst at the same time smoothing out the gross movements of locomotion, acting as an effective shock absorber and providing the subtle and delicate balance necessary to adjust to uneven terrain and changes in ground surface. It is important to realise that the leg and foot frequently mirror symptoms from one to the other, and each in turn can be the aetiological factor which results in symptoms experienced elsewhere in the kinetic chain. For example, anterior knee pain should not be diagnosed without a thorough examination of the foot, and conversely alterations in foot posture should not be considered without reference to the structural alignment of the legs, e.g. genu valgum or genu varum.

The lower limb must therefore undergo similar scrutiny so that the structural relationships between the foot and the lower limb can be appreciated. The position of the foot relative to the leg and the body planes must be ascertained, and also the ranges of motion of the hips, knees and the joints of the foot.

During the examination, all clinical observations, measurements and symptoms should be carefully noted in the patient's records. The method of referral to the clinician and all other relevant information, both medical and surgical, including possible drug therapy, must be similarly detailed. The practitioner must be meticulous in writing up case histories. Litigation alleging incompetence and negligence is ever increasing and no effort should be spared irrespective of the contraints of time to ensure that records are complete and up to date. It is also worthy of note that as more records become stored on computer, all such data must be available for inspection under the Data Protection Act. Individual comment relating to the patient should therefore always be of a professional nature.

Before commencing clinical examination, it is essential to put the patient at ease. Patients are not infrequently anxious, if not frightened, and consider the surgery a hostile environment, with the therapist an adversary. Whilst each consultation is just another in the day's work for the therapist, it is a major event for the patient. Reassurance and consideration are paramount. Simple things like the welcoming smile, ensuring the patient is comfortably seated, and not uncomfortably hot because no one has offered to take their coat, will ensure that clinical examination becomes a two-way exchange with information eagerly sought and willingly given. Time spent on this exercise, though sometimes abused, is never wasted, since it helps to quickly establish the relative significance of the complaint.

This exercise is of course even more important when children are the patients, and further reference is made to their particular requirements in Chapter 4.

CLINICAL EXAMINATION PROCEDURES

Before commencing any examination, there are two important features to be considered. These are the positioning and the exposure of the patient. When carrying out the initial examination with the patient seated, it is much more comfortable for the patient to be seated at a higher level than the examiner. This allows the patient to rest with a slightly flexed hip and knee which is more comfortable than sitting with an extended knee.

Ideally the whole limb being examined ought to be exposed, but in practice it is usually sufficient only to expose the leg from above the knee distally. The proximal parts of the limb can be examined in more detail if indicated. It is important to be able to see the knee and the patella, especially when the patient stands, and in order to do so, trouser legs have to be rolled up, not just pushed up. If they can't go up they have to come down. Both legs and feet should always be exposed and examined regardless of the complaint.

It is also helpful to the examiner to follow a set pattern of examination. This is good practice and helps to ensure that nothing is missed out. It is logical to proceed from the superficial (skin and soft tissues) to the deep structures (bones and joints) and thence from the local to the general.

Case history

Patients complain of symptoms; these may be local, e.g. pain, swelling, deformity, difficulty with footwear, or more general, such as abnormality of gait, or symptoms related to other body systems. The purpose in taking a history is to find out as much as possible about these symptoms and to use the information, together with the clinical findings, to determine first the necessary investigations, and then to arrive at a diagnosis. Then, and only then, can a treatment plan be formulated and a prognosis given. The symptoms of which the patient initially complains are the *presenting symptoms*, and it can be disconcerting to the patient if they are not examined first. They should always be given priority without prejudice to the coverage of other and possibly more important symptoms.

The salient features of symptoms are:

1. *Site and radiation of pain*: where is it, and does it go anywhere?
2. *Onset*: when, and the circumstances concerning it; gradual or sudden; relationship

to an event, e.g. injury, sport, change of occupation or footwear.

3. *Nature*: severity and extent; is the pain sharp, dull, fiery, or just bearable discomfort?
4. *Influencing factors*: those that aggravate or relieve, e.g. exercise, rest, elevation. What is the duration of exercise tolerance? It is frequently the case that changes in body position provoke foot pain which then diminishes, or even disappears, with exercise, e.g. patients will often complain of pain when first rising from bed, the pain subsequently easing on mobility.
5. *Duration*: constant or intermittent?
6. *Relationship to general health*: e.g. are the symptoms related to any known health problem, such as diabetes mellitus, generalised arthropathy, circulatory or neurological deficiency, etc.?

To complete the history, it is worth enquiring as to the patient's past history and to social circumstances, particularly if the working environment is involved in their complaints.

Clinical signs

1. Skin

Texture: coarse or fine, dull or shiny
Colour: pallor, cyanosis, erythema, pigmentation, gangrene
Temperature: cool, warm or distinctly hot. (Use the back of the hand and compare with the other limb)
Humidity: dry, sweaty, areas of maceration
Elasticity
Hyperkeratosis (callosities)
Hair: presence or absence, fine or coarse
Integrity: fissures, (heel or interdigital clefts), ulcers
Dermatoses: eczema, psoriasis.

2. Nails

Structure: ridged, cracked, thickened
Extent: overgrown, onychogryphotic, stunted, ingrowing
Subungual abnormality: swelling, pigmentation.

3. Swellings

Tenderness: local, radiating
Consistency: hard, firm, soft, fluctuant
Adherence: to skin, to underlying soft tissue, to bone
Transillumination
Temperature.

4. Vascular status

Despite all the modern sophisticated methods of measuring blood flow, the basic clinical signs have stood the test of time and in the overwhelming majority of cases, still provide both adequate and reliable information on the vascularity of the limb.

Skin colour and temperature. Whilst the relatively avascular foot may be pale and cool, the dysvascular foot, which may also be neuropathic, may be fiery red, especially at the extremities, sometimes tinged with a purplish suffusion.

Blanching of the tip of a toe with finger pressure will in the former instance result in a slow return of colour and, in the latter, in an excessively rapid flush of colour. Blanching also tends to occur on elevation, just as congestion does on prolonged dependency. Dependency may also result in cyanosis, more indicative of venous insufficiency.

The arterial pulses are palpated as shown in Figure 3.1; the dorsalis pedis is just lateral to the extensor hallucis tendon at the base of the first metatarsal; the anterior tibial is at the front of the ankle; and the posterior tibial is just behind and below the medial malleolus, with the foot slightly inverted. Pulses should be palpated with the middle three fingers, avoiding too much pressure, which might obliterate them. The thumb should never be used to feel for a pulse.

Oedema of the ankle and foot, when it is 'pitting', is a sign of more generalised cardio-vascular insufficiency. Brawny oedema does not 'pit' and is usually due to lymphatic insufficiency.

5. Neurological status

The same principles apply to both the neurological and vascular examinations. Both the efferent (motor) and the afferent (sensory) systems must be examined.

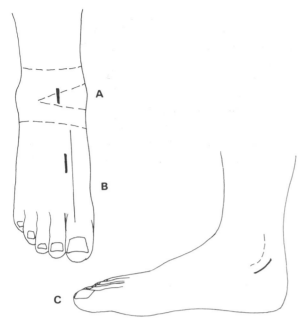

Fig. 3.1   Arterial palpation points for (A) anterior tibial, (B) dorsalis pedis, (C) posterior tibial.

Motor assessment. Muscle power is measured according to the Oxford (MRC) scale, as follows:

0—no muscle activity
1—muscle twitch without moving segment
2—segment moved with gravity eliminated
3—segment moved against gravity
4—segment moved against gravity and resistance
5—full power.

In practice, it is impossible to measure the power of every muscle and so muscles are examined (mostly) in functioning groups. This is particularly true more proximally in the leg. In the lower leg and foot, the following should be tested:

- Toe dorsiflexion (extension)—extensor hallucis longus and extensor digitorum longus
- Toe plantarflexion (flexion)—flexor hallucis longus and flexor digitorum longus
- Invertors—tibialis anterior and tibialis posterior; each of these can be tested separately by holding the foot in dorsiflexion or plantarflexion respectively when applying a resistance

- Evertors—peroneal muscles
- Ankle dorsiflexors—tibialis anterior, peroneus tertius together with the toe extensors
- Ankle plantarflexors—calf muscles via the tendo Achilles. This group consists of two muscles, the soleus, whose origins are entirely within the lower leg, and the gastrocnemius, which has its origins on the distal femur. When spastic contraction is a problem, the origins of the contracture can be determined by testing ankle flexion with and without the knee bent; increased dorsiflexion on knee bending indicates the gastrocnemius as the tighter structure.

Sensory assessment. Sensation has several modalities of which touch, proprioception and pain appreciation are the most relevant to foot care, but temperature and vibration sense provide important information for the specialist. Accurate neurological testing is highly-specialised and time-consuming, but it is important that the examiner can determine areas of gross sensory diminution or loss, and whether there has been any loss of position sense. The reflexes at the knee and ankle should be tested, as should the plantar (Babinski) responses.

6. *Others soft tissues*

Tendons, ligaments, and fibro-fatty pads all require attention. It is necessary to note any local signs of tenderness along the structure, especially at points of attachment to bone, at localised swellings and at areas revealing crepitus on movement. Auscultation over tendons might also indicate a tenosynovitis. The plantar aponeurosis should be palpated for abnormal nodules and tenderness especially at its insertion into the calcaneus. The fibro-fatty subcutaneous tissue which forms the heel pad and the metatarsal pad should be examined to determine its integrity. It diminishes in thickness in the dysvascular and /or ageing foot, allowing bony prominences to be readily palpable subcutaneously. Lacking the shear absorbing capacity of the pads, the bony prominences are a potent source of pain in these people.

Some clinical signs are clearly of more importance than others and demand more urgent attention. Of these, the most important are those of inflammation. Classically they have been described as 'rubor, calor, et dolor' — redness, warmth and pain. Inflammation does not necessarily mean infection — there can be many reasons for its presence — but certain features should be recorded:

— whether acute, subacute, or chronic
— if infective and localised, is it resolving or suppurating?
— if infective and spreading, whether there is lymphangitis or lymphadenitis present; the former appears as longitudinal reddish streaks in the skin, and the latter as tender swellings at the site of the lymph nodes at the back of the knee and in the groin.

Any acute or subacute inflammatory lesion requires at least temporary priority in treatment over any associated deformity. Any spreading infection requires immediate reference for further investigation and treatment.

7. Local signs of systemic disease

The history and clinical signs elicited may point to the presence of systemic disease, and these of course require further referral. Reference should be made to subsequent chapters covering the respective systems, but the following text outlines signs and symptoms that should give rise to suspicion.

Circulatory. (see Ch. 20)
Arterial
  intermittent claudication
  rest pain
  abnormal pulses
  abnormal skin colour, texture or temperature
  abnormal nails
  incipient or established gangrene.
Venous
  pain and swelling associated with thrombophlebitis or thrombosis varicose eczema pigmentation atrophie blanche.
Central
  pitting oedema
  breathlessness.

Neurological. (see Ch. 23)
Almost every neurological symptom requires further investigation, but particularly:
  unexplained weakness
  ataxia
  spasticity
  absent or exaggerated reflexes
  any loss of sensory modality.
Other general conditions may necessitate referral for further investigation and treatment, e.g.
  obesity
  suspected diabetes mellitus
  gout
  rickets
  osteo- or rheumatoid arthritis
  generalised skin disorders
(see Chs 6, 21 and 22).

8. Footwear

Footwear should also be examined during the patient's first visit and points of note recorded. The footwear should be checked for size, shape, style, suitability and indications of abnormal wear. Abnormal wear on the soles and heels often gives the best indication of the weight-bearing pathway during the gait cycle. Distortions of the uppers also give indications of abnormal frontal plane motion during gait. Points to note are:

A. *Heel wear*
  a. Excessive wear at back—calcaneal gait
  b. Excessive wear at front—broken shank, pes plano-valgus
  c. Excessive wear on lateral side—foot inverted: pes cavus, hallux rigidus, painful site
  d. Excessive wear on medial side—foot everted: pes plano-valgus.
B. *Heel and sole wear*
  a. Excessive on lateral side—foot inverted: pes cavus, hallux rigidus, painful site
  b. Excessive on medial side—foot everted: pes plano-valgus
  c. Lateral heel to medial sole—normal, but if excessive, feet are abducted
  d. Lateral heel to lateral sole—feet adducted and inverted

e. Medial heel to medial sole—feet everted and abducted.

C. *Sole wear*
   a. Excessive across tread—pes cavus
   b. Excessive at tip—short shoes
   c. Excessive under hallux—hallux rigidus
   d. Excessive under lateral side—metatarsus varus (adductus).

D. *Bulging of heel counters*
   a. At back—short shoes
   b. At medial side—hindfoot varus, metatarsus varus (adductus)
   c. At lateral side—hindfoot valgus.

E. *Bulging of uppers*
   Splay foot, hallux valgus, hammer toes, claw toes.

F. *Bulging of toe puff*
   Short shoes, uppers too shallow, hypermobile foot.

Biomechanical examination

Joints

Assessment of the joints of the foot, their range and direction of motion is crucial and no accurate diagnosis of the mechanics of the foot can be established without this information. Motion within their normal ranges should be pain-free and unrestricted. Features significant of joint pathology are: pain or movement or limitation of movement, (note any crepitus, subluxations or dislocations); deformity affecting either or both osseous components of the joint; tenderness on palpation indicating inflammation, suggestive of arthritis or sprain.

The *ankle joint* is a hinge joint and, irrespective of the position of the axis of motion, the only free movement permitted is that of plantarflexion and dorsiflexion. The range of motion may vary widely between individuals with 20° to 30° of dorsiflexion available in some cases, and between 30° and 50° of plantarflexion. The range of motion should be assessed with the knee extended and the subtalar joint in its neutral position. It is possible to measure the angles between the long axis of the leg and the lateral border of the foot in both plantarflexion and dorsiflexion to determine the total range of motion. For normal function during walking, there should be at least 10° of dorsiflexion available (Fig. 3.2). Limitation of dorsiflexion may be caused by a tight gastrocnemius, determined by dorsiflexing the foot whilst the knee is fully extended), or by a tight soleus (if limitation persists with the knee flexed). Restriction may also occur as a result of anatomical variations or if there is joint damage.

Because it is easily observed, the ankle joint also provides a ready means of identifying rotational variations in the lower limb. With the patient supine, this may be done by measuring the positions of the malleoli relative to the frontal plane with an orthogauge (Fig. 3.3). The orthogauge is a rectangular sheet of rigid transparent plastic on which is marked the relevant angular and linear components for biomechanical examination.

The *subtalar joint* (talocalcaneal) provides the foot with triplane motion of inversion with adduction and plantarflexion, and eversion with abduction and dorsiflexion. In examining the subtalar joint, interest should concentrate on the total range of motion, its neutral position, and the amount of inversion and eversion from the neutral position. It is considered normal to have twice the range of inversion available as for eversion. Evaluation of the position of subtalar neutral can be assessed by palpation, by observation and by

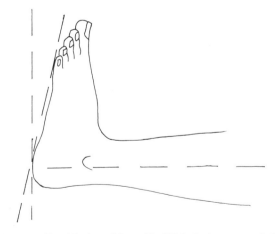

Fig. 3.2 Dorsiflexion of the ankle. With the knee extended and the foot in neutral position, the angle between the long axis of the leg and the lateral border of the foot should be at least 10° less than a right angle. If dorsiflexion is limited, test the range again with the knee flexed.

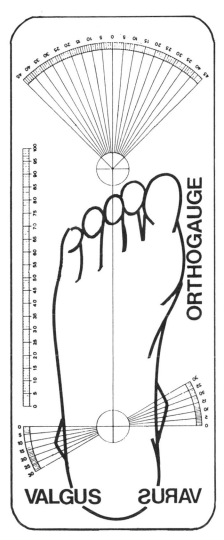

Fig. 3.3 Measurement of rotational torsions by orthogauge. The patient lies supine with the knee axis on the frontal plane and the foot at a right angle to the leg. The angle between a line through the tips of the malleoli and the frontal plane is measured by holding the orthogauge perpendicular to the leg. (Courtesy of Orthogait, Glasgow)

measurement, and all three methods must be used to establish the position accurately.

The significance of the neutral position of the subtalar joint, or any other joint, is that from this position the foot will move maximally in a given direction. When applied to foot mechanics, the neutral position of the subtalar joint allows the practitioner to evaluate the relationship of the forefoot to the rearfoot and the foot to the leg.

Evaluation of the subtalar joint
A. By palpation. With the patient prone and the

knee in full extension, the foot is dorsiflexed to 90° on the leg by applying pressure to the fourth and fifth rays, and the subtalar joint is inverted to its maximum. By palpating the joint about one thumb's breadth anterior to the distal margins of the medial and lateral malleoli, the lateral aspect of the head of the talus will be felt. This method is then repeated with the joint in maximum eversion and the medial aspect of the talar head will be felt. When the head of the talus cannot be palpated on either the medial or lateral sides, the subtalar joint is in its neutral position.
B. By observation. It is possible to evaluate the neutral position by noting the curvatures just above the lateral malleolus and at the lateral aspect of the calcaneus. In neutral, these curves should match each other (Fig. 3.4). In eversion of the calcaneus, the curvature on the calcaneus is more exaggerated than that of the leg; with inversion, the curvature is reduced. The neutral position also approximates with the lowest point on the arc of movement of the plantar aspect of the heel.
C. By measurement (Fig. 3.5).
  a. With the patient prone to secure full muscular relaxation, and the foot extending beyond the leg rest, the leg is rotated to bring the back of the heel horizontal. The back of the heel and the lower third of the leg are marked with separate bisection lines.

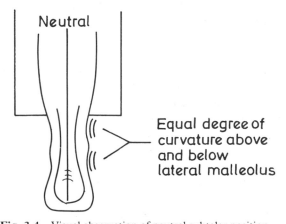

Fig. 3.4 Visual observation of neutral subtalar position. Normally, the curves just above and below the lateral malleolus match each other. In calcaneal eversion, the lower curve is exaggerated; in calcaneal inversion, it is reduced.

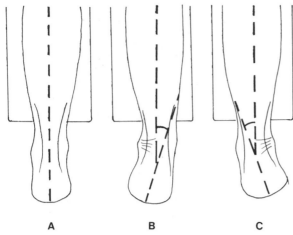

Fig. 3.5 Assessment of neutral subtalar position: (A) bisection of back of leg and back of heel; (B) inversion angle (right foot); (C) eversion angle (right foot).

b. The heel is swung into full inversion and into full eversion, care being taken to keep the foot perpendicular to the leg and to avoid any frontal plane movement in the ankle joint. At each extreme, the angles between the bisection lines are measured and added together to give the total range of movement.

Neutral position is at two-thirds from full inversion and one-third from full eversion, plus or minus two degrees.

c. With the subtalar joint placed in its neutral position, the back of the heel is again bisected. The angle, if any, between this bisection and that of the leg denotes the degree of possible subtalar varus or valgus of the calcaneus. If there is no angulation, the calcaneus is vertical and the foot normal.

This method also indicates the degree of wedging or posting required in an orthotic appliance. Examples:

Inversion angle	Eversion angle	Total range	Neutral position	Indications
21	9	30	20	Normal
27	6	33	22	5 varus
18	15	33	22	4 valgus

d. A convenient alternative method of measuring subtalar varus or valgus is by the use of an orthogauge. When applied with its centre line coinciding with the

bisection line on the back of the leg and its transverse plane reference point on a level with the subtalar joint, degrees of subtalar varus or valgus are indicated by the calcaneal bisection line and can be measured by the protractor component of the orthogauge (Fig. 3.6).

The *midtarsal joint* is made up of the talonavicular and calcaneocuboid articulations which act as

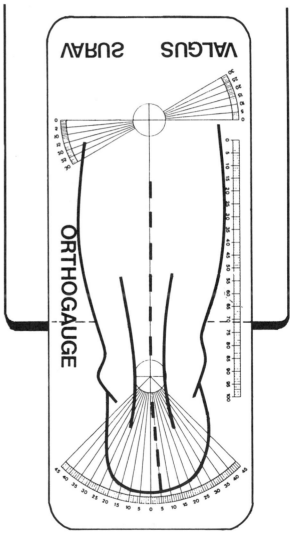

Fig. 3.6 Measurement of subtalar varus or valgus by orthogauge. The centre line is placed over the bisection line marked on the leg. Degrees of subtalar varus or valgus are indicated by the calcaneal bisection line and can be measured by the protractor component. (Courtesy of Orthogait Glasgow.)

a single functional unit. Movements of the midtarsal joint are dependent upon the shape of the articular surfaces and the restraint of the ligamentous structures. Of particular importance to the functioning of the midtarsal joint is the shape of the head of the talus. The talonavicular joint is similar anatomically to a ball and socket joint and the shape of the articular surface of the head of the talus largely dictates the amount of movement available.

Clinical examination should seek to determine the ability of the forefoot to adjust to the position of the hindfoot once the position of 'foot-flat' has been established during the gait cycle. It is therefore important that the range of movement should be assessed with the hindfoot in neutral, and supinated, and pronated. In the normal foot, when the subtalar joint is in its neutral position, the forefoot assumes a position where its plantar aspect is parallel to the transverse plane of the hindfoot. More motion is available during pronation of the hindfoot, and less motion when the subtalar joint is supinated. If, however, there are changes in the position of the axis of motion of the midtarsal joint, then the position of the forefoot relative to the hindfoot can also be changed. The forefoot may assume a position inverted or everted to the hindfoot; these abnormalities profoundly affect the normal mechanics of the foot and need to be evaluated (Fig. 3.7).

Pain on movement of the midtarsal joint with limitation of inversion may be suggestive of osteoarthrosis, rheumatoid arthritis, or a tarsal synostosis.

The structure of the tarsometatarsal joints is such that it is difficult to isolate and evaluate their individual movements. It does however allow for clinical evaluation of the range of plantarflexion and dorsiflexion of the first and fifth rays, and whether such motion is excessive, or whether they are fixed in positions of dorsiflexion or plantarflexion relative to the transverse plane of the forefoot. Transverse motion of these units is practically non-existent, but it is possible to quantify any abduction or adduction of the first and fifth rays respectively.

The relationship of the forefoot to the hindfoot in the transverse plane is also quantifiable, and the practitioner can evaluate relative adduction or

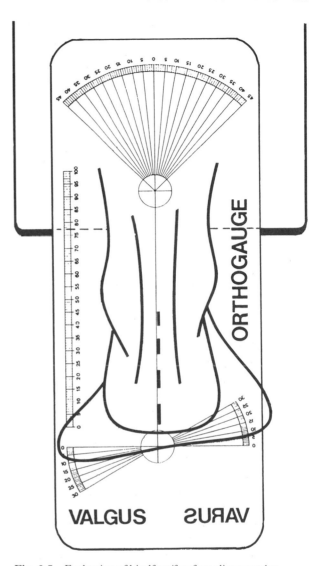

Fig. 3.7 Evaluation of hindfoot/forefoot alignment by orthogauge. With the foot held in its neutral subtalar position, the orthogauge is placed with its centre line on the calcaneal bisection line. Degrees of forefoot varus or, by reversing the orthogauge, of forefoot valgus, are then evaluated by reference to the plantar aspect of the forefoot. (Courtesy of Orthogait, Glasgow.)

abduction by using a goniometer, an orthogauge or a tractograph.

The metatarsophalangeal joints should be assessed individually, then collectively. The range of motion of each should be noted, although only the first and fifth can be quantified. Any change in the integrity of the joints' surfaces, as in Freiberg's infraction, should be recorded. Test each of the joints for pain-free movement, noting any discrepancies in their motion. Note particularly any degree of hallux valgus, hallux limitus or rigidus, or hallux flexus; any possible subluxations or dislocations; and any toe deformities. The state of the metatarsophalangeal joints is critical to the diagnosis and prognosis of all forefoot disorders.

If this evaluation of the position and movements of the joints of the foot is carried out with precision and the details noted, then an accurate assessment of function can be made, especially when it is coupled with other forms of investigation where initial examination has indicated potential pathology.

One must also be aware of the differences between individuals and whether there is generalised joint laxity, hypermobility, or hypomobility from joint stiffness. Both present problems for the clinician as it is virtually impossible to restrict generalised excessive movements within joints, and joints will not move beyond the limits imposed on them by their inherent anatomy. Where there is joint hypermobility, it is a recognised feature on X-ray that the articular surfaces are rounded and larger, and in hypomobility the articular surfaces tend to be smaller and more rectangular in shape, thereby restricting motion. Both conditions frequently result in pathology.

Gait analysis

Analysis of the patient's gait is often necessary in order to develop a complete picture of the events taking place, particularly during the stance phase of gait. Gait analysis can be carried out both by visual observation of the patient walking, and by other mechanical methods described later in this chapter. The two methods differ because the first observes the sequence of events from heel strike to toe-off, while the second examines the distribution of forces acting on the feet. It is helpful to use video equipment, but if this is not available, then careful observation with the naked eye can reveal fundamental gait characteristics. Every person's gait pattern is specific to the individual and it reflects not only leg length but the compensations which may be necessary relative to the anatomical positions of the feet and legs. A treadmill is also very useful since the visual parameters of the practitioner do not alter and cadence can be

controlled at a constant rate. If no treadmill is available, a long well lit corridor will usually suffice. It is important during this form of gait analysis to allow the patient a good five minutes walking before beginning serious observation because patients are usually very self-conscious about being observed.

The normal sequence of events which the clinician wishes to observe is as follows: prior to heel strike, the foot is supinated; it then pronates through to 'foot-flat' when the ground reaction forces reverse the rotation; the foot then supinates to become a rigid lever prior to take-off. Any alteration in these events necessitates further investigation. Abnormalities of a biomechanical nature are often only marginally abnormal so that excessive pronation, early heel lift and other subtle changes take a trained eye to detect. It is frequently a help if more than one practitioner can observe the patient at the same time. After careful observation of the gait, it is then necessary to assess whether any apparent anomalies are of any functional significance and are related to the patient's symptoms. Many anatomical variations necessitate compensatory movements during walking which may not contribute to pathological symptoms.

FURTHER INVESTIGATIONS

Gait analysis

The clinical examination of gait has already been described, and here are mentioned those items of equipment which can add to the basic knowledge already acquired. Many new sophisticated devices are now available but for clinical use in the surgery simple tests can still provide most, if not all, of the information needed to treat patients. Devices are available for both the static and the dynamic evaluation of the foot in gait.

Static evaluation

1. The *plantarscope* shows how the plantar skin blanches under load; the pattern can be adjusted in some cases by the examiner to near normal by manipulating the foot and/or the leg of the patient. This can give a useful indication of the possible cause for the complaint (Fig. 3.8).

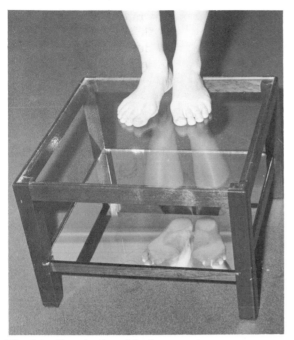

Fig. 3.8   Examination of the feet on a plantarscope demonstrates weight distribution to the plantar surfaces.

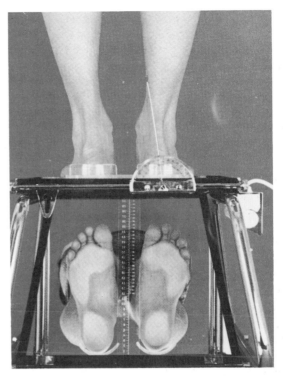

Fig. 3.9   Examination of the feet on the podometer reveals foot size and calcaneal deviation as well as pattern of weight distribution.

2. The *podometer* is a more elaborate form of the above device, combining measurement of the foot size and calcaneal deviation with the reflected image of the foot (Fig. 3.9).

3. The *pedobaroscope*. This device incorporates an internally illuminated sheet of plate glass, upon which is placed a plastic or, preferably, card interface. The patient stands on this interface and a grey scale image of the reflected light that is produced is assessed. The grey image is calibrated electronically and projected on a VDU screen as a colour image which can be photographed, stored on videotape, or printed out as hard copy. It has a very high resolution, recording the pressure under areas of the foot as small as 2 mm × 3 mm.

Dynamic evaluation

1. The simplest of these devices is to dust the patient's foot with chalk and walk him over a black surface. The resulting footprints will give a rough idea of high pressure areas, alignment of the foot, and, if timed over a given distance, the cadence (in steps/minute).

2. The *Harris & Beath mat* is a rubber mat surfaced with tall ridges forming large squares, crossed by smaller ridges forming smaller squares, and even smaller ridges forming even smaller squares. The mat is inked, and covered with a sheet of paper over which the patient walks. Only the highest pressures record all 3 levels of ridge, these areas appearing darker. The print is, of course, a mirror image print which only shows the areas of maximum pressure during the stance phase of gait and is therefore not time-related. It can also be used for static prints, and is undoubtedly the most useful tool for everyday use in the clinic. Much helpful information can be gleaned from good prints (Fig. 3.10).

3. The *dynamic pedobarograph* is mainly a research tool and is a dynamic variant of the pedobaroscope. It works on the same principles, but like many other methods of measuring foot pressures and forces, if it is not understood properly it may produce very attractive pictures which give quite erroneous information. It is, however, reliable in that the results have been shown to be accurate and repeatable, and it has much the best resolution of any such apparatus.

Fig. 3.10 The Harris and Beath mat provides mirror image prints of the pressure areas in standing or on walking.

4. The *Musgrave forceplate system* has been refined to produce a higher resolution, and is a mat of transducers placed on the floor, across which the patient walks. The Musgrave system, like many others, produces computer-generated pictorial results as well as a reading of the pressure between the foot and the ground in kilograms per square centimetre ($kg\,cm^{-2}$). This enables foot pressures to be evaluated before and after treatment regimes (Figs 3.11 & 3.12).

5. The '*E. Med*' is a similar device of German origin, and produces an output not dissimilar to the Musgrave system, but of higher resolution. The apparatus is highly sophisticated and also expensive; an insole version is also being developed.

6. The *electrodynagram* utilises pressure transducers applied directly to the skin and thus can be worn inside footwear. In theory this is the ideal method to measure pressure, but of course it is

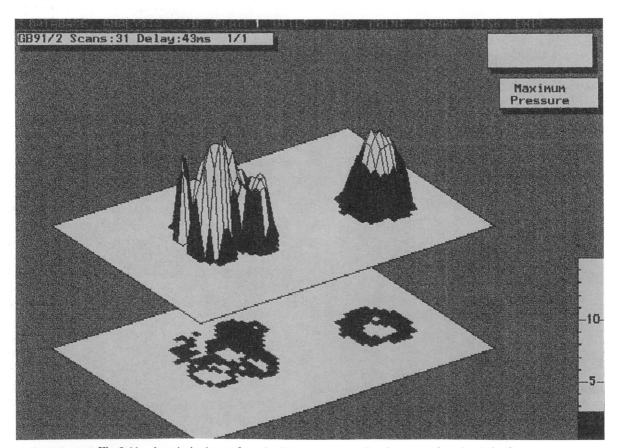

Fig.3.11   A typical printout from the Musgrave system showing areas of maximum load.

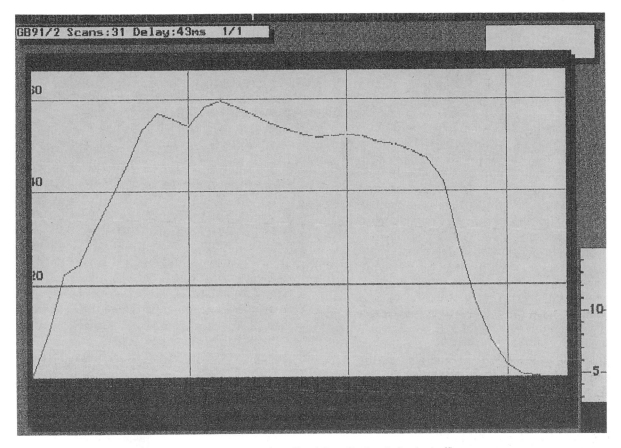

Fig. 3.12 A visual representation of load from 'heel strike' to 'toe off'.

subject to the effect of that specific footwear. The transducers are wired to a miniature recorder and the results are obtained via a computer. The repeatability of results using this method has been called into question by some centres, and the fact that there are transducers and wire leads under the foot may affect the gait pattern.

7. The *force plate* can also provide information about ground reaction forces in 3 directions, but the interpretation of these is complex and very much a matter for the researcher. A more useful clinical system is the *video vector*, utilising both a force plate and video recording of the patient walking. A computer provides a visible vector superimposed on the image of the walking patient on the screen.

8. *Videography* can be very helpful in that pictures can be replayed at leisure, as fast or as slow as one wishes, down to 1 frame at a time.

This is a very instructive way of examining the foot disposition during gait. Like any of these dynamic systems, it does need space, not always readily available, and it is expensive. Video can be combined with use of the treadmill, which allows the patient to run at different speeds on different inclines, as well as walk.

It is important to realise that most of these dynamic systems are sophisticated research tools. For the surgery, a Harris & Beath mat is probably the most useful single item. It can be used statically or dynamically, and takes up little space. It can be obtained as a kit in a box, complete with ink roller to spread the ink, and paper. It is important, too, to realise that static information must not be assumed to be an indication of what is occurring dynamically. The two modes are quite different, and if dynamic information is what is wanted, then data must be obtained in that form.

X-rays

Although many disorders of the foot can be safely diagnosed and treated without radiographic examination, some may need further investigation. This should, however, be supplementary to a thorough clinical examination. The main indications for radiographic examination of the foot are injury, deformity, swelling and pain which cannot be explained by clinical findings. These indications are not absolute: for example, the deformity of hallux valgus can be readily recognised on clinical examination; X-ray examination would only be necessary if surgical treatment was being contemplated.

X-rays and safety

X-rays can be very helpful to the clinician, but they can also be dangerous. Strict precautions should always be enforced when X-rays are being taken, and they are ignored at peril. Although modern X-ray machines produce little scatter of rays, and the intensity of X-rays is inversely proportional to the square of the distance from source, a lead apron should always be worn, or retreat behind a screen undertaken. For small increases in distance away from the source, there are large decreases in X-ray intensity. Those involved with X-rays also require to have their exposure to rays monitored regularly.

X-ray techniques

Plain radiographs are most commonly taken, but other more specialised techniques are available, each with its particular indications.

A. Plain X-rays. Most radiological departments, if asked for X-rays of a foot, will provide non-weight-bearing anteroposterior (dorsoplantar) and oblique views. When suspecting diseased bone, or checking on a previously defined fracture, these may be adequate, but in general, assessment of foot structure ought to be made with standing views. Weight-bearing views are also useful when evaluating the mechanical status of the foot. Lateral weight-bearing radiographs enable the practitioner to determine the extent to which variations exist in the relationship between forefoot and hindfoot.

Standing anteroposterior and lateral views, together with an oblique view, will cover most eventualities, although the weight-bearing metatarsal profile view is helpful in determining the relative positions of the metatarsal heads and status of the sesamoids of the hallux. It is taken with the aid of a perspex stand which supports the feet in normal toe-out, with heels and toes both elevated by 30° (adjustable) wedges. Other plain films can be taken to show specific areas of the foot, such as the axial views for the subtaloid joint or the calcaneus. Most departments can now also provide 'microfocal' or 'macro' views which present a much magnified view while still retaining a high resolution of bone structure. (Fig. 3.13A & B; Fig. 3.14 A & B).

B. Tomograms. These X-rays are taken with the purpose of finding out more about the three dimensional characteristics of a lesion. The head of the X-ray tube swings in an arc as the X-ray plate moves below, allowing one spot to be kept in

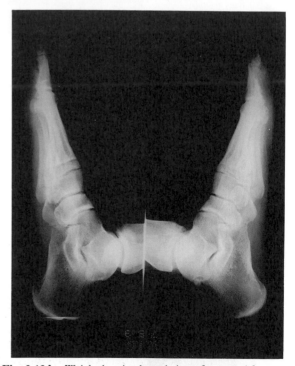

Fig. 3.13A Weight-bearing lateral view of a normal foot. Note the smooth CYMA line and the calcaneal inclination angle of 20°.

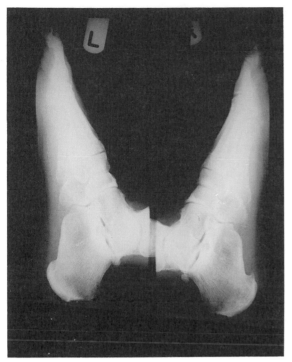

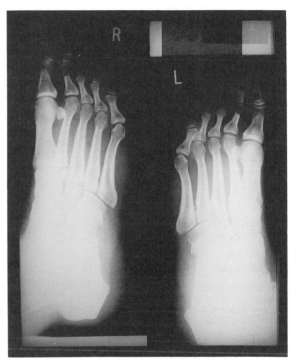

Fig. 3.13B Weight-bearing lateral view of forefoot valgus with a high angle of inclination of the calcaneus and interrupted cyma line.

Fig. 3.14 A Non weight-bearing oblique view.

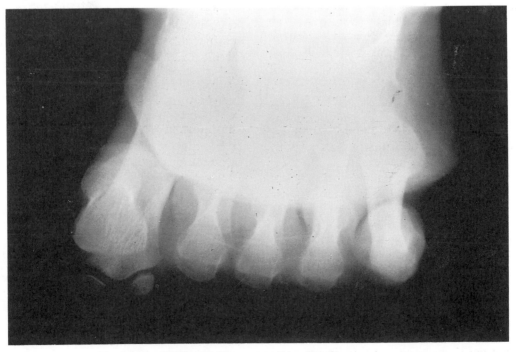

Fig. 3.14B Weight-bearing metatarsal head profile.

focus while the surrounding area remains blurred. By taking sequential exposures at, for example, 1cm intervals through the lesion, a series of pictures can be obtained which will give an idea of the whole.

C. Contrast films. Normal cavities, e.g. joints, or abnormal ones and sinuses can be injected with radio-opaque dye to enable the position and shape of the cavity to be outlined either on plain films, or with tomograms. This is of use in determining the course of a sinus track, or arthrograms can outline soft tissue structures within the joint, e.g. the menisci in the knee.

D. Computerised axial tomography (CT scan). These are simply tomograms which the computer reassembles to give a cross-sectional picture of the part being studied. They are still two dimensional, but with a high resolution of structure. Unfortunately the design of the scanner does not permit true weight-bearing scans of the foot to be carried out. To date it has probably proved of most value in the foot in assessing fractures of the calcaneus and in determining the exact extent of tarsal coalitions.

E. Magnetic Resonance Imaging (MRI). This is a relatively new, non-invasive technique which is not strictly radiological. It involves exciting the structures of the cell nucleus with a magnetic field, and imaging the result. Longitudinal body cuts are then available in a three dimensional format. It is of most use in determining the integrity of soft tissue structures, such as tendons and nerves, and in assessing the extent of soft tissue tumours (Fig. 3.15).

Interpretation

Interpretation does need experience and skill, but there are some basic principles of interpretation common to all forms of radiological imaging which can help the novice. First, always look at the whole X-ray. You can usually tell the sex of the patient, if the name on the label is legible. Films show not only bone, but other soft tissue shadows, especially on CT scans, and they provide much valuable information. It should be remembered, too, that in infants, the bones of the foot are represented by cartilaginous precursors, which may or may not contain centres of

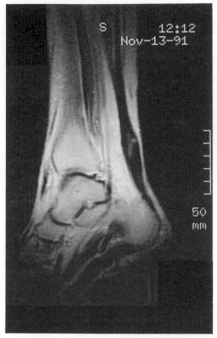

Fig. 3.15 MRI showing degeneration within the tendo achilles.

ossification, and thus the true 'shape' of the bone cannot be seen. In practice clinical examination of the foot will suggest where the abnormality is; nevertheless the whole film must be studied as multiple abnormalities are not uncommon. More specifically, look for:

1. Loss of continuity of bone cortex (e.g. fractures—but know where normal epiphyses and apophyses are to be found)
2. Abnormal bone shape (e.g. developmental disorders or, more commonly, previous operations or old trauma)
3. Alteration of relative position of bones (e.g. dislocations)
4. Extra bones (e.g. accessory ossicles, extra digits or rays)
5. Fusion of bones (e.g. congenital synostoses)
6. Alteration in bone quality (or density), either local or general (e.g. disuse osteoporosis, periarticular porosis in rheumatoid disease)
7. Expansions or outgrowths of bone (e.g. osteophytes, exostoses or tumours)
8. Joint changes (e.g. osteo- or rheumatoid arthritis).

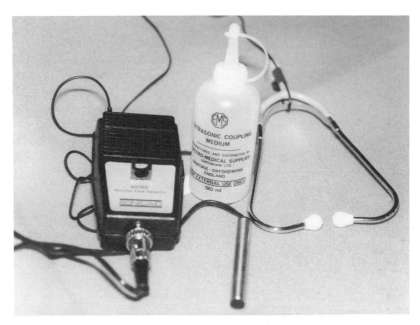

Fig. 3.16   Ultrasonic apparatus for detection of arterial pulsation.

More than one of the above may be present; e.g. a fracture may have occurred through osteoporotic bone in a patient with a hallux valgus, where the hallux has a subungual exostosis.

Arterial pulse wave detection (Fig. 3.16)

The portable Doppler ultrasonic instrument may be used to detect the presence or absence of arterial flow in peripheral vessels in patients who, for example, have oedema preventing manual palpation of arteries. In some cases, the Doppler ultra-sound technique will demonstrate normal flow in instances where pulses are palpable but appear diminished.

CLINICAL LABORATORY TESTS

Simple but useful tests can be carried out on body fluids and discharges, giving useful and sometimes essential information which may assist the clinician to reach a diagnosis or in planning appropriate treatment.

Urine

A midstream urine sample can be examined physically, biochemically and bacteriologically. Physical examination can determine volume, colour and specific gravity. The deposits may be examined microscopically for cells, casts and crystals, etc. (Fig. 3.17) (Casts in urine). Biochemical examination using Multistix (Ames) can determine specific gravity, pH, and the

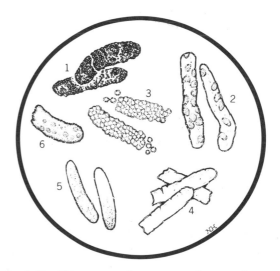

Fig. 3.17   Urinary casts: 1. coarse granular casts; 2. epithelial cell casts; 3. red blood cell casts; 4. waxy casts; 5. hyaline casts; 6. casts with pus cells.

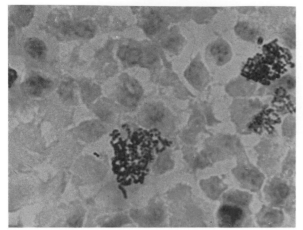

Fig. 3.18 Pus from nail bed infected with *Staphylococcus aureus*. Gram film (× 100 objective).

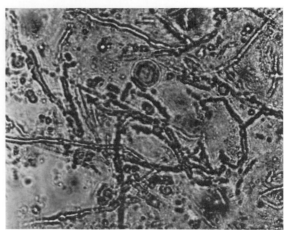

Fig. 3.19 Tinea pedis: nail infected with *Trichophyton rubrum*. KOH preparation (× 40 objective).

presence of the following: proteins, glucose, ketones, bilirubin, blood, nitrites and urobilinogen. The bacteriological examination of urine using microscopes and culture techniques determines the morphology of infecting organisms and their sensitivity to antibiotics.

Blood

Haematological studies show the cell count and the morphology of the cells. The erythrocyte sedimentation rate (ESR) gives a non specific indication of the presence of a disease process, such as infection. Biochemical examination for glucose, electrolytes, urates and many other more esoteric tests are readily available from the laboratory. Simple clinical testing which does not replace conventional laboratory methods includes the dextrostix test for glucose. This is done using a drop of whole blood from a skin prick and should be carried out exactly according to the manufacturers' instructions. Bacteriological examination of blood is sometimes required if there is suspicion of systemic infection.

Discharge

Bacteriological examination of pus and other discharges from wounds is carried out for the purposes stated previously (Fig. 3.18). The importance of obtaining anaerobic cultures should not be overlooked, particularly with wounds of the feet which are not healing.

Skin and nail

Scrapings can be examined for confirmation of fungal infections and should be collected in the following manner:

1. Skin. Clean the area with 70% alcohol. Scrape the active edge of the lesion with a scalpel. Place the scales in a Petri dish. The roof of vesicles should be clipped off with appropriate tissue nippers.

2. Nail. After removing the thickness of the affected nail, scrapings should be taken from the advancing edge of the infection. Cotton wool swabs should not be used as the strands may resemble hyphae (Fig. 3.19).

FURTHER READING

Alexander I J 1990 The foot: examination and diagnosis. Churchill Livingstone, New York
Collee J G, Fraser A G, Duguid J P, Marmion B P (eds) 1989 Mackie & McCartney Practical medical microbiology, 13th edn (Microscopy and technical methods). Churchill Livingstone, Edinburgh

Gamble F O, Yale I 1975 Clinical foot roentgenology, 2nd edn. Krieger, New York
Hicks J H 1953 The mechanics of the foot 1. The joints. Journal of Anatomy 87: 345
Ketwick J E 1982 Clinics in sports medicine. Saunders, Philadelphia

Kapandji I A 1988 The physiology of the joints, 5th edn. Churchill Livingstone, Edinburgh

McRae R 1983 Clinical orthopaedic examination, 2nd edn. Churchill Livingstone, Edinburgh

Mann R A, 1982 Biomechanics of running, Symposium on the foot and leg in running sports, Mosby, St Louis

Office practice of laboratory medicine 1987 Medical Clinics of North America 71 (4)

Roche Scientific Services 1975 Urine under the microscope. Roche, Basle

Root M L, Orien W P, Weed J R 1977 Biomechanical examination of the foot. In: Clinical biomechanics, Vol I. Clinical Biomechanics Corporation, Los Angeles

Sgarlato T E 1978 Compendium of podiatric biomechanics. California College of Podiatric Medicine, San Francisco

Wright D G, Desai S M, Henderson W H 1964 Action of the subtalar and ankle joint complex during the stance phase of walking. Journal of Bone and Joint Surgery 46–A

4. The growing foot

Eric G. Anderson

NORMAL GROWTH AND DEVELOPMENT

In the embryo, the limb buds appear about the fourth week of intrauterine life, becoming segmented into proximal, intermediate, and distal parts by the sixth week and digitated by the seventh. By the ninth week the thigh, leg and foot are recognisable entities. Ossification begins first in the larger bones of the leg and foot, extending gradually to the smaller bones. By the seventh month, the longitudinal arching of the skeleton of the foot is present. At birth, the skeletal framework is predominantly cartilage, but centres of ossification are present in the calcaneus, talus, cuboid, metatarsals and phalanges (see Ossification timetable, Appendix 2). The infant's foot is thus highly malleable. This is important for two reasons. It allows some congenital deformities to be corrected more easily, but it also means that the feet may be deformed by premature or abnormal stresses of weight-bearing.

Abnormalities of intrauterine development of the foot will manifest themselves as congenital deformities. Some anomalies are characterised by failure of formation of parts, or extra parts, and must have their origin within the first few weeks of fetal development. Other deformities may be attributed to the abnormal intrauterine development of a basically normal foot. Little is known of the factors that control shape, form and size other than that they are genetically determined, but are capable of being modified by other influences. For example, the basis form of a bone is determined by the cellular tissue from which it is developed, but is then modified by pressures and stresses from surrounding tissues, such as developing muscles and the external environment. Deform-ities of the foot may be caused by imbalance of the action of muscles inserted into the developing foot. This is seen in extreme form when there is paralysis of muscle groups, as in spina bifida, but some deformities may be due to more subtle imbalance. Moreover, a foot deformity may itself contribute to abnormal development of muscles; thus it is uncertain if the abnormal calf muscula-ture found in children with talipes equinovarus is a cause or effect of the deformity.

At birth, the foot usually appears flat because of a fatty pad which is gradually absorbed as growth proceeds rapidly during the first year. Muscles are developed by the habit of kicking. The legs there-fore should not be restricted by tight clothing, coverings or bedclothes. At about 9 to 10 months of age the infant starts to crawl, then learns to stand, at first with support and then unaided. Between 12 and 15 months the child begins to walk with assistance and gradually acquires proficiency with practice. Some children never crawl; they shuffle along on their bottoms and tend not to walk until they are nearer 2 years old. At first the stance is uncertain with the feet widely spaced and variously abducted or adducted, while the gait is slow and deliberate. The processes of adopting an upright posture and learning to walk unaided depend upon the gradual development of neuromuscular pathways and coordination and should not be unduly or artificially stimulated, particularly in heavy babies, lest the immature foot is overloaded.

The child's foot is not a small-scale model of the adult foot. It is relatively shorter and wider, tapering towards the heel because the hindfoot is less fully developed than the forefoot (Fig. 4.1).

The shape of the foot is not finally determined

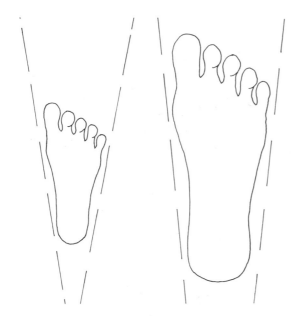

Fig. 4.1   The different proportions of the immature and the mature foot.

until growth ceases about the twentieth year; however adult shoe size is usually reached by age 14. The growth rate of tissues in general is irregular, being very rapid in the first two or three years of life, slowing down at about age four, and spurting briefly at about seven. Thereafter growth is retarded until puberty when the rate accelerates sharply, continuing into late adolescence. During this long growing period, footwear must be constantly adapted to current needs, being discarded when outgrown rather than when outworn. Maximum barefoot activity on suitable surfaces such as carpets, grass and sand should be encouraged as a means of stimulating muscle activity and development.

Most children are born with feet which, with normal growth and development, become both structurally stable and functionally efficient. They are subject thereafter only to the normal hazards of later life, e.g. infection, injury and disease. In some children, however, genetic and ontogenic abnormalities occur pre- and post-natally giving rise to deformity and disability.

Those conditions present at birth are termed congenital disorders, those that manifest later, developmental disorders. If these occur within the foot, they can be considered *intrinsic* defects, and *extrinsic* if the effects on the foot are simply

secondary to deformity elsewhere. The lower limbs, like other parts of the body, may also be affected by developmental defects occurring elsewhere, particularly those involving neuro-muscular disturbances, such as spina bifida. The foot condition is then only part of a larger diagnostic and management problem. Foot disorders arising from systemic diseases are discussed in later chapters.

CONGENITAL ABNORMALITIES

These may arise from two sources, (i) adverse genetic factors, and (ii) adverse environmental factors acting on the developing fetus. Examples of the latter are drugs, e.g. thalidomide, and infections such as German measles. Some authorities believe that intrauterine pressure or abnormal fetal position may play a part in the development of some deformities. Most are probably multifactorial in origin. They vary widely in degree from mild to severe, and therapeutic measures likewise range from conservative mechanical correction to complex reconstructive surgery. They may require prolonged supervision, and with those conditions affecting the whole child, integrated care by several specialists is often required.

Full correction of some cases is not possible, and residual deformity remains as a chronic feature in adult life, requiring continuous supervision and management by means of special footwear, appliances, and appropriate podiatric treatment.

Anatomical anomalies: excesses, deficiencies and fusions

1. Polydactyly (Fig. 4.2)

This term denotes the presence of additional digits on the hand or the foot. On the foot, two or more whole or rudimentary digits may develop from one metatarsal, or there may be complete supernumerary metatarsal segments. Depending on the nature and extent of the abnormality, selective amputation at an early age is indicated to ensure optimum function and to facilitate shoe fitting in childhood and adult life. As in any operation on the foot, it is important that the

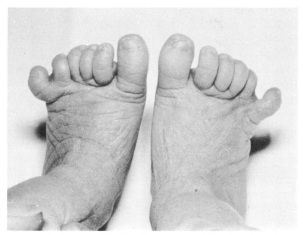

Fig. 4.2 Polydactyly. The hands were similarly affected.

resulting scar is situated away from pressure areas.

2. Syndactyly

This term denotes total or partial fusion of neighbouring digits. There may be a congenital absence of one or more of the corresponding metatarsals. In its mildest forms, it appears as no more than the conjoined webbing of adjacent toes. It is very common in a partial form between the second and third toes. Surgery is rarely indicated as it is difficult to achieve a satisfactory result.

3. Accessory bones (Fig. 4.3)

The importance of recognising these accessory ossicles is to be able to distinguish them from fragments of bone resulting from injury.
The commonest ones are:

* *os trigonum*—a vestigial bone which lies posterior to and sometimes attached to the talus (Fig. 4.4)
* *accessory navicular*—this lies medial to the medial end of the navicular, almost as an extension of it, and should be distinguished too from the sesamoid sometimes present in the tendon of the posterior tibial tendon
* *os vesalii*—is much more rarely found at the base of the fifth metatarsal.

The os trigonum rarely gives rise to symptoms. Pain experienced over an accessory navicular may

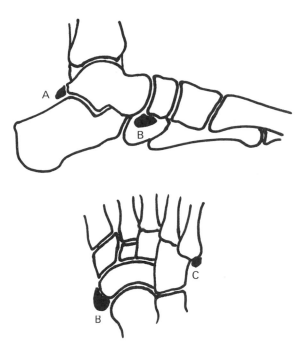

Fig. 4.3 Accessory bones. (A) Os trigonum. (B) Accessory navicular. (C) Os vesalii.

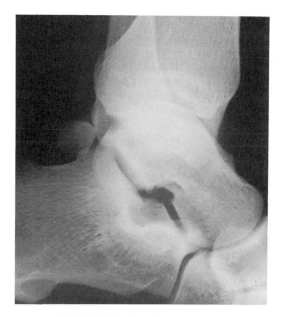

Fig. 4.4 Os trigonum.

not simply be due to its presence, or just direct pressure upon it, but to abnormal stress applied to it by an overactive posterior tibial tendon trying to stop the foot hyperpronating.

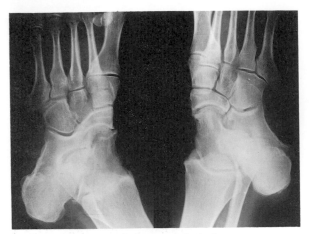

Fig. 4.5 Calcaneo-navicular bar.

4. Tarsal coalitions

In this condition there is an anomaly of ossification in which adjacent tarsal bones are fused together. Fusion may be partial or complete, and may be bony (synostosis) or cartilagenous (synchrondrosis).

The most common coalition occurs between the calcaneus and the navicular with union across the midtarsal joint (Fig. 4.5).

In a talocalcaneal coalition, fusion occurs between the sustentaculum tali and the talus.

Children with tarsal coalitions may never be aware they have them. On rare occasions they are responsible for acutely distressing painful symptoms, and surgery is necessary for adequate relief. Between these two extremes are most children who have little trouble until they enter a growth spurt, when they develop the classical symptoms of the 'spastic flat foot'. This is a painful contraction of the peroneal muscles, and occurs as a protective mechanism. This results in a fixed everted abducted foot which resembles a flat foot, and from which it must be distinguished.

Diagnosis is not always easy. Examination reveals tender, taut and prominent peroneal tendons, and attempts to invert the foot will be painfully resisted. Specialised X-rays or a CT scan may be necessary to demonstrate the fusion.

Initial treatment consists of resting the foot, in a below-knee plaster of Paris cast if necessary, and reserving surgery for those with recurrent or intractable pain.

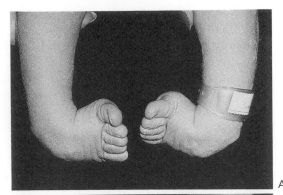

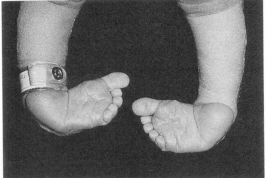

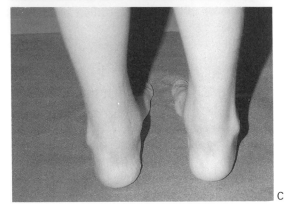

Fig. 4.6 Talipes equino-varus. (A, B) The new born child. (C) Same child aged 6 years 3 months.

Structural deformities

(i) Congenital talipes equino-varus (CTEV) (Fig. 4.6)

This is the commonest form of structural deformity, often known simply as club foot. The foot is plantarflexed and inverted, with the forefoot adducted. The talus has been described as the hub of the deformity, with an abnormal neck directed both plantarwards and varus. Other structural anomalies are secondary to this. Two types are recognised: those which respond to early strapping in a corrected position, and those, the resistant talipes, which do not. This latter group require surgical treatment and this is performed between the ages of 3 and 6 months. The initial operation is one of elongation of the tendo Achilles and a release of the right medial structures of the hindfoot to allow the foot to align as near normally as possible around the talus. Further surgery may be required at a later date if correction has been less than complete. Then, bony operations are required, either taking wedges from the calcaneus or fusing the peritalar joints. The fusing of hindfoot joints is always something to avoid if at all possible, as the consequences, especially in a growing foot, for the function of the forefoot are considerable. A club foot can cause much trouble in adulthood, when pressures are maldistributed over the foot, often excessively along the outer border of the foot, producing painful callosities, and making provision of comfortable insoles and bespoke footwear essential.

(ii) Talipes calcaneo-valgus

The 'opposite' condition to CTEV, this is considered by many to be a postural manifestation, and virtually always corrects with conservative manipulation and strapping. It is important, however, to recognise that this condition is associated in a few with congenital dislocation of the hip, and deformity of the tibia.

(iii) Vertical talus

This is rather a rare deformity, known by several alternative names, such as 'rocker-bottom foot', and is primarily caused by a dislocation of the talonavicular joint. There are secondary structural effects which result in an equinus position of the calcaneus and a valgus dorsiflexed forefoot. Correction is surgical, and is aimed at reducing the dislocation of the talonavicular joint. The older the child the more likely is bony correction or fusion to be necessary.

(iv) Metatarsus adductus

This condition is quite common in infants, and is found with a normal hindfoot. The great majority resolve spontaneously, but it is impossible to pick out the cases which will not. In these cases surgical release of tight medial structures can be carried out.

DEVELOPMENTAL CONDITIONS

Extrinsic structural conditions

(i) Hip

a. Persisting femoral anteversion. This is one of the commonest 'variants' of normal (Fig. 4.7). The angle between the neck of the femur and the frontal plane is greatest at birth, and as the child develops and learns to walk, this angle decreases. The normal 'toe-out' attitude of the foot is the result, but in a not insignificant number of the population, this process is either arrested or never quite occurs, resulting in an in-toeing or 'hentoed' gait. Whilst often quite an embarrassment to its owners, especially at a young age when they tend to trip over their feet, it is rarely the cause of symptoms, and needs no treatment.

b. Coxa vara and coxa valga (Fig. 4.8). The inclination of the neck of the femur to the shaft varies through the growing years, the normal

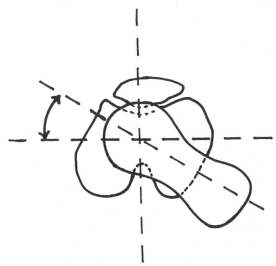

Fig. 4.7 The femoral anteversion angle.

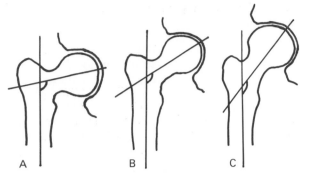

Fig. 4.8 Coxa valga (A) and coxa vara (C) compared with normal inclination angle between femoral neck and shaft—125° in adult (B).

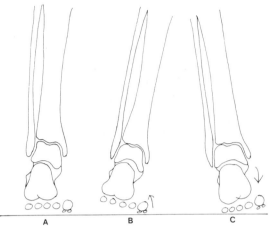

Fig. 4.9 Genu valgum and genu varum . (A) Normal alignment of right leg and foot (from front). (B) In genu valgum the foot is everted as it bears weight and the forefoot supinates to the horizontal. (C) In genu varum the foot is inverted as it bears weight and the hindfoot pronates to bring the forefoot to the horizontal.

angle in the adult being 125°. If less than this, the femoral shaft is abnormally adducted and the limbs are relatively shorter (coxa vara). If the angle is greater, the shaft is abducted, and the limbs relatively longer (coxa valga).

These deformities result in a malalignment of the femora, which must be compensated for at the knees to allow the individual to stand with the feet in a normal attitude. The consequence is a compensatory angular deformity of either genu valgum or genu varum respectively. They inevitably affect both gait and stance, especially if they are unilateral, as this tends to render the limb lengths unequal.

(ii) Knee-genu valgum and genu varum

Normal development of the child sees the varus bow legs of the infant straighten, and often 'over-correct' into distinct valgus, or knock knee, at about age 6. The vast majority of these realign to the normal adult position of around 8° valgus. Persisting deformity in either direction is often associated with rotational deformity and always with altered posture of the feet. For example, genu valgum is associated with an abducted inverted foot on weight-bearing unless actively compensated, which often happens, resulting in the need for the forefoot to supinate. The converse of course applies with genu varum (Fig. 4.9). The treatment in severe cases is surgical realignment by means of osteotomy, but not infrequently the deformity is accepted and then the foot must be encouraged orthotically to adopt as normal a functioning posture as possible.

(iii) Torsions

These may occur as a result of abnormal joint alignment (as described above in relation to the hip) or to a built-in twist in the bones of the lower leg themselves. While internal torsions tend to be self-correcting, external torsions are not. The alignment of the legs is clearly reflected in the posture adopted by the feet, as for example in the inturned leg; the natural adduction is compensated by attempted abduction of the foot and its consequent pronation. With external torsions, however, the feet are still used in abduction, with a consequent hyperpronation and strain on the posterior tibial tendon. The alignment of the legs can be clearly seen by examining first the position of the patellae. A line projected forwards from the mid-point of the patella and at right angles to its transverse plane should normally intersect the foot between the second and third toes. Secondly, the line of the ankle joint axis, as visualised by projecting a line through the malleoli, can be compared with the patellar line. Whilst this latter indicates rotation at and above the knee, the former demonstrates the rotation of the whole leg, or when compared with the patellar line, that rotation due solely to the tibia.

(iv) Leg length discrepancy

It is important to realise two features about leg length. First, that up to 1 cm difference in true length is considered a normal variation. Secondly, that with normal clinical measuring techniques, leg length cannot be measured to an accuracy much greater than 1 cm. This discrepancy can be 'true' due to congenital underdevelopment, underdevelopment as a result of disease such as poliomyelitis, trauma, and even surgical treatment. Apparent discrepancy exists where the limbs are actually the same length, but because of the alignment of one or other, are functionally different.

The effects of limb length discrepancy are either to cause a compensatory pelvic tilt, and secondary spinal scoliosis, or to make the individual walk on his toes in order to effectively lengthen his leg. This latter, of course, will in time result in an adaptive shortening of the tendo Achilles.

The importance of these conditions is that they impose abnormal stresses on the foot, particularly on the talus in stance phase. These in turn may result in compensatory or adaptive changes in the function and structure of the foot with growth, and it is these which are important for the podiatrist.

Extrinsic functional conditions

These conditions affect function by virtue of an imbalance in the muscle control of the respective joints. Most of them are neurological diseases although there are some primary muscular disorders to be considered.

The effects of the imbalance can be likened to a segmented flag pole supported in the upright position by guy ropes attached at different heights and directions. The loss of any one or more guy ropes will have a profound effect on both the stability and the shape of the pole. So it is with the leg and foot. The positions and functions of the foot are infinitely variable depending on exactly which muscle or muscle groups are inactive, partly active, or even spastic or contracted. There is no virtue, therefore, in considering their effects in detail: it is more appropriate to highlight particular points of relevance.

(i) Cerebral palsy (CP)

CP or brain injury results in an upper motor neurone type of paralysis of widely varying extent, from that which is indistinguishable to the untrained eye to the tragic spastic dysarthric who is unable to do anything for himself. CP can be found in different forms, most commonly as a spastic paralysis, but also as athetoid, ataxic or atonic. Surgery has little part to play in their treatment, and must be considered in relation to the child as a whole, and not just to a particular deformity. Inevitably this means that for the podiatrist, foot care may become the primary treatment. Like all of this group of conditions, however, there is great need for a team approach to management and integration of all modalities of therapy, so that the maximum benefit may be gained from each.

(ii) Spina bifida cystica

This is a congenital disorder where there has been a failure of fusion of the posterior spinal elements. It is only the severe cases that make the headlines, but like CP, it can be found in all degrees from fatal to minor bony deformity that exists unbeknown to the patient. The level in the spine at which the lesion occurs relates in some measure to the effects on the patient, but does not equate with their function. In high spinal lesions, total paralysis occurs, and the foot is a malleable flaccid object. The problems arise in the foot in those with sacral lesions, where an imbalance primarily affects the muscles of the foot, resulting in deformity which can be very difficult to manage.

(iii) Charcot-Marie-Tooth disease

(iv) Anterior poliomyelitis

These are described in Chapter 23.

(v) Muscular dystrophies

These are probably primary muscle disorders, the

best known of which is the progressive hereditary Duchenne type. This results in an increasing wasting of the muscles, with a life expectancy rarely exceeding 20 years.

Intrinsic structural conditions

(i) Flat foot

This commonly used term can mean all things to all men. It is therefore necessary to define what is meant by flat foot. The arch of the foot can be made to disappear in two ways: the whole structure can simply collapse in a sagittal plane, or the foot can rotate so that the arch seems to disappear, i.e. the foot pronates (Fig. 4.10).

The collapsed foot is relatively uncommon and seems to be more prevalent in males. It gives rise to no symptoms other than anxiety to relatives who may notice that the foot is flat. Arch supports are of no benefit, and can be quite painful if used.

The hyperpronated foot is another matter altogether. Before considering the pathology to be primarily in the foot, the presence of more proximal causes must first be sought, as described above. Generalised joint hypermobility is sometimes associated with this condition, and renders it important to ensure that adequate treatment is undertaken as soon as the diagnosis is made. Treatment is orthotic: in the pre-school child with a Salop ankle-foot orthosis, and in the older age groups with either a Yates-Helfet heel cup or simple Rose-Schwartz heel meniscus (Fig. 4.11). In each case the object is to maintain the foot in a neutral position while growth takes place.

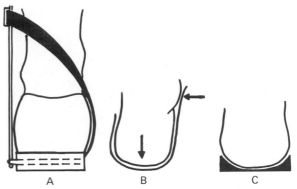

Fig. 4.11 (A) Salop ankle-foot orthosis. (B) Yates-Helfet heel cup. (C) Rose-Schwartz heel meniscus.

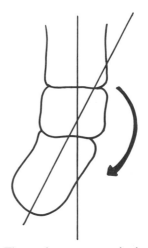

Fig. 4.12 The turning moment on heel strike in the pronating foot.

The tendo Achilles is often noted to be shortened also, but this is probably an adaptive shortening consequent upon the valgus attitude of the calcaneus produced by the hyperpronation. Only rarely does the tendon need lengthening.

If untreated, the hyperpronated foot may cease to be mobile and become fixed. Each step then produces a turning moment at the ankle on heel strike and increasing pain over the medial ligamentous structures as the body weight falls with the area of support of the calcaneus. Surgery may then be required (Fig. 4.12).

(ii) Cavus foot

The high arched foot can also be considered as

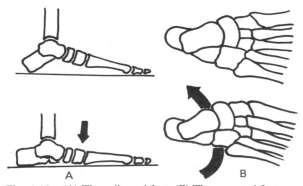

Fig. 4.10 (A) The collapsed foot. (B) The pronated foot.

different entities. The arch may be simply elevated in the sagittal plane as a result of muscle imbalance and is associated with an increased inclination of the calcaneus. The presence of muscle imbalance suggests neurological disorder, and in many patients brisk reflexes in both upper and lower limbs would tend to confirm this and further suggest that the primary pathology may be intra-cerebral. In others it is clearly a consequence of one of the extrinsic functional conditions described above.

Just as the flat foot could be produced by hyperpronation, so the cavus foot can be produced by excessive supination. The most frequently seen cause of this is where the first metatarsal is fixed in a plantarflexed position at the tarsometatarsal joint. This type of cavus foot is more likely to result in a fore to hindfoot malalignment, which if the foot is unable to compensate, may require orthotic treatment.

The third type is simply called idiopathic, aetiology unknown, but there is more than a suggestion of a neurological element in many cases.

It is the neurologic and idiopathic types of cavus foot which produce the greater problems in the long term. As the foot arches, the heel and the metatarsal heads become the primary weight-bearing areas, with a tendency for the first metatarsal head to take more than its fair share. Treatment is directed to straightening out secondarily clawed toes, the lesser toes by flexor to extensor (Girdlestone) tendon transfers, the hallux by a Robert Jones transfer of the long extensor into the metatarsal neck with fusion of the interphalangeal joint. The tight plantar structures can be released by stripping their origins from the calcaneus (Steindler). In older children where the deformity is more fixed, a wedge can be removed from the dorsum of the tarsus to straighten out the foot, or a chevron osteotomy performed to lower the forefoot. The management of the adult cavus foot is discussed in Chapter 5.

(iii) Malalignments

This term is used to denote an abnormal relationship between the transverse plane of the forefoot and the sagittal plane of the hindfoot. Normally this is about a right angle. It can be due to a primary hindfoot problem, or to one in the forefoot, but these do not necessarily give rise to symptoms unless the foot as a whole cannot compensate. Failure to compensate occurs in two particular situations: when the foot is over-stressed, e.g. with severe athletic activity, or with increasing age, when the joints of the foot tend to stiffen. It is interesting to note that loss of joint mobility may also occur after prolonged immobilisation in a plaster cast, and this too can precipitate symptoms.

a Hindfoot varus (Fig. 4.13A). This situation arises, like persistent femoral anteversion, as a failure of development postnatally of an intrauterine position. The inversion of the hindfoot extends into the forefoot, and thus in order to bring the forefoot into a horizontal position, the foot has to pronate.

b. Forefoot varus, or supinated forefoot. Here the forefoot is inverted relative to the hindfoot with the result that in order for the forefoot to come into the transverse plane at foot flat during gait, the foot has to hyperpronate, stressing the posterior tibial tendon, once it has utilised all the available midtarsal rotation. It has been suggested that the fixed plantarflexed first metatarsal is a compensatory mechanism too, but there is no more evidence for this than for it being a primary cause of the the valgus (pronated) forefoot (Fig. 4.13B).

c. Forefoot valgus, or pronated forefoot. With the forefoot everted relative to the hindfoot, compensation following saturation of midtarsal joint movement occurs by the foot supinating. As there is almost always much more inversion available at the subtalar joint than eversion, there is more compensation available for this particular malalignment (Fig. 4.13C).

Treatment is orthotic, aiming to control subtalar movement, and compensating for (not correcting) the abnormal alignment.

(iv) Digital abnormalities

Children are frequently presented at an orthopaedic clinic with curly or otherwise slightly deformed toes. There are three elements to these deformities:

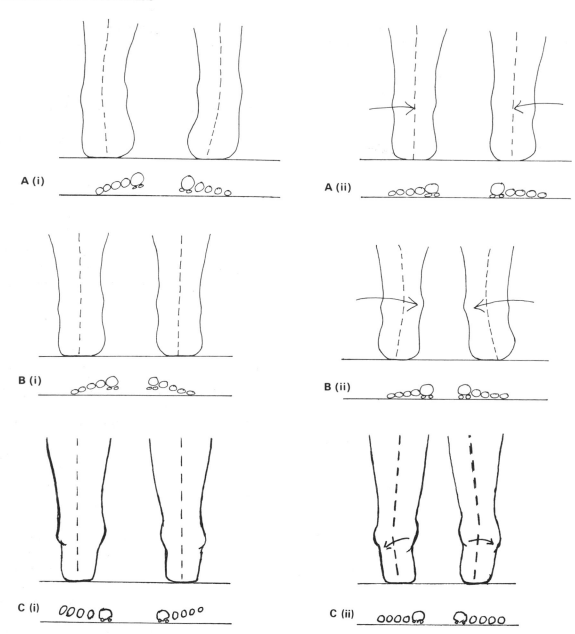

Fig. 4.13   Hindfoot/forefoot malalignments.
(A) Hindfoot varus. Hindfoot and forefoot both inverted. (i) Usually compensated by pronation to the vertical to bring both plantar surfaces to the horizontal (ii).
(B) Forefoot varus (supinated forefoot). Forefoot only inverted (i). Usually compensated by pronation of hindfoot to bring plantar surface of forefoot to the horizontal (ii). Alternatively compensated by hallux flexus.
(C) Forefoot valgus. (i) Forefoot everted. (ii) Usually compensated by supination of the foot to bring plantar surface of forefoot to the longitudinal.

1. medial or lateral deviation from the midline of the digit
2. axial rotation
3. interphalangeal joint flexion.

Those present from birth frequently correct with growth. They are uninfluenced by strapping, although this may be acceptable therapy to calm an anxious parent. If causing symptoms because of overlapping and rubbing in shoes, they are best treated with orthodigital splints. Surgery rarely has a place, but the curly overlapped fifth toe can be satisfactorily dealt with this way. Claw toes, too, can be corrected by a flexor to extensor tendon transfer.

(v) Juvenile hallux rigidus

Whilst not common, this condition causes much discomfort to its suffers, who are usually teenage males. It is now thought that the aetiology is recurrent minor trauma, or a single incident which produces a chondral injury. The resulting pain and muscle spasm results in loss of extension at the metatarsophalangeal joint. The patient walks on the outer border of the foot to avoid the painful area. Rest in a cast is recommended first-line treatment, with a proximal phalangeal osteotomy being reserved for those in whom symptoms persist.

(vi) Juvenile hallux valgus

Like many other foot problems, footwear has been universally blamed for the presence of this condition in teenagers. In almost all cases, a strong family history can be elicited. Footwear may aggravate an established tendency to valgus deformity, and may cause bunion formation by friction over the medial eminence of the metatarsal head, but does not *cause* hallux valgus. The valgus is often accompanied by a varus deformity of the first metatarsal. Up to 20° of valgus can be normal, but a useful guide to whether surgery is indicated is the position of the sesamoids on a profile X-ray: no subluxation, no operation. Surgery should not be carried out before the foot is skeletally mature at about the age of 14. Until then, the position of the hallux can be controlled with an orthodigital splint.

(vii) Hallux varus

While this is an extremely uncommon condition in the United Kingdom, it is not so elsewhere, e.g. in India. Commonly seen with metatarsus varus, it frequently corrects with growth. Occasionally surgery is necessary for the satisfactory fitting of footwear.

(viii) Sever's disease

Listed here for want of a better place, this condition was originally thought to be an osteochondritic lesion of the posterior calcaneus, associated with fragmenting apophyses. We now know that the X-ray appearances are normal, and believe that the condition is a traction apophysitis. It frequently responds to rest, but a cautionary warning must be given: forefoot malalignments may result in a varus or valgus calcaneus which may produce stress at the insertion of the tendo Achilles, and unless this primary problem is compensated, symptoms may not resolve, or may recur.

TRAUMA

(i) Freiberg's infraction

This condition, once thought to belong to the osteochondritides, is now regarded as being the result of an osteochondral fracture. How this equates with its recognised incidence mainly in girls around the age of 13, is difficult to explain. It may appear as an incidental finding in women with hallux valgus in the later years of life, with no recollection of ever having suffered symptoms. On the other hand, it can present as an acute arthritis of the second or third metatarsophalangeal joint with no X-ray signs being visible for several weeks. The metatarsal head flattens, and occasionally produces prolific osteophytes and it is these which are more likely to cause symptoms. Treatment in the growing foot is expectant, resting it when acutely painful, and relieving direct pressure on the metatarsal head by appropriate padding.

(ii) Fatigue fractures

These are most likely to occur in the athletic youngster, either in sport or in dance, and appear in the second and occasionally third metatarsal shafts. X-ray changes may not be visible until three weeks after the initial onset of symptoms.

Treatment is rest in a plaster of Paris slipper cast. Very rarely a fracture may occur towards the base of the fifth metatarsal (Jones fracture). It can be difficult to heal, but this may be due to the continuation of the precipitating forces, as would happen with a supinated forefoot, and thus the foot should always be examined closely for evidence of such abnormality.

THE RATIONALE OF TREATMENT

The first requirement is of course to make a diagnosis, and to this end it must be re-emphasized that the foot is at one end of a kinetic chain, and therefore responsive to variations in normal anatomy and pathological disorders above it. Before deciding that the foot is the primary seat of pathology, careful examination of the whole limb is required, and in a child this is particularly relevant. Identification of disorders, or even suspicion of disorders more proximal, require referral to an orthopaedic surgeon for evaluation.

Once these problems have been dealt with, or not, whichever is the case, attention can be turned to the foot. Surgery may or may not have been carried out in the meantime, and an understanding surgeon will always keep in mind what the orthotist and podiatrist can contribute, and tailor his surgery accordingly. This is surgico-orthotic integration and is a very important concept in the treatment not only of children, but of all patients. Conversely, the orthotist and the podiatrist must have some idea of what they can do to help the surgeon make the most of surgery. It is two-way teamwork.

The general requirement is to have a plantigrade, painless, mobile, foot. Developmental structural deformities such as juvenile hallux valgus are best not operated on until after skeletal maturity, and the conservative management with orthodigital orthoses is preferred until that time is reached. Preoperative care is here in the hands of the podiatrist. Similarly, where a forefoot malalignment is diagnosed, and where operation has no place, short- or long-term care may be required. Postoperatively, the podiatrist can offer much help in the treatment of residual symptoms and deformity.

FURTHER READING

Anderson E G 1990 Fatigue fractures of the foot. Injury (21) 275–279
Fixsen J, Lloyd-Roberts G 1988 The foot in childhood. Churchill Livingstone, Edinburgh
Gould J S 1988 The foot book. Williams and Wilkins, Baltimore

Hessinger R N 1987 The pediatric lower extremity. Orthopedic Clinics of North America 18: 4
Jahss M H 1982 Disorders of the foot, Vols I & II. Saunders, Philadelphia

5. The adult foot

Patricia M. Boyd   Donald Neale   George Rendall

The common structural and functional disorders of the adult foot arise mainly from developmental anomalies of childhood and adolescence. If these have been of marked or moderate severity they may well have been diagnosed at an early stage and subsequently supervised. They are rarely easily correctable, the effects of residual deformity and malfunction only becoming apparent fully as skeletal growth is completed. More minor degrees of developmental anomalies, previously unrecognised because they were asymptomatic, may come to light only under the functional stresses of adult life. Occupation, levels of activity and footwear factors also combine to increase the incidence of adult foot complaints.

The majority of such conditions manifest themselves in the forefoot and thus tend to be diagnosed incorrectly as local in origin. While impaction and constriction from unsuitable footwear contribute to many forefoot conditions, the chief reasons for their high incidence must be sought in the malfunctions of the rearfoot during the stance phase of the gait cycle, which distort the forefoot when at its most vulnerable, i.e. under maximum mechanical stress during the propulsive phase. The key to the successful mangement of adult foot disorders lies in the understanding of such malfunctions.

For the most part, adult foot disorders present clinically as established deformities, the end result of various aetiological factors. Similar deformities result from diverse causes and it is therefore more convenient to discuss them under headings which describe their clinical features rather than their aetiology. The precise aetiology of any case is of interest mainly to the clinician. The patient's primary concern, on the other hand, is to obtain relief from pain and disability. Many of the symptoms arise less from the underlying deformity than from the associated lesions of the skin and soft tissues which are a result of the deformity. Ligamentous and muscular strain, bursitis, ulcerations, helomata and callosities are the most common of these painful symptoms, and although they represent the last manifestations in the chain of cause and effect, they are often the first concern to the patient and practitioner.

The management of established adult conditions falls into various phases. The first is the provision of prompt relief of the immediately painful symptoms, and this may require considerable time and effort. Skilful operating, the use of appropriate medicaments and well-designed padding and strapping are the essential techniques in this first phase (Ch. 11).

The second phase is concerned with more durable methods of eliminating or at least minimising the abnormal stresses causing such symptoms and entails the effective management of the underlying deformity by the provision of orthoses designed for the particular case and, if necessary, the modification of footwear (Ch. 13).

Phase three is concerned with the possibility of surgical intervention to correct or reduce the basic deformity. Although surgery is sometimes indicated at an early stage, it is frequently delayed on medical grounds or for personal and domestic reasons. In the latter cases, there remains an essential role for conservative management (Ch. 18).

Phase four is concerned with postoperative supervision or the management of chronic deformity in inoperable cases. In a considerable number of such cases continued management by the provision of protective appliances and suitable footwear is essential for the patient's well-being, which can be greatly enhanced by close collaboration between surgeon and podiatrist.

In order to understand the development of pathologies which result from dysfunction it is necessary first to consider the movements, normal and abnormal, associated with them. The most important of these are subtalar pronation and supination.

PRONATION AND SUPINATION

Pronation and supination occur at the subtalar joint. These are normal movements provided they occur at the right times during the gait cycle and to the right magnitude (see Ch. 2).

The subtalar joint and the ankle joint together are the link between the leg and the foot. They can be considered as a universal joint or torque translator, allowing the foot to adapt to variations in walking surfaces and in body posture, and to act as a shock absorber, lessening the impact between the foot and the ground during the contact phase of gait. The subtalar joint is also the key to the foot becoming a rigid lever for propulsion. It is these same motions that allow the subtalar joint to compensate for deformities in the foot and lower limb.

This ability to compensate enables the individual to function with a plantargrade foot in what appears to be a smooth and efficient manner. However, motion used at the subtalar joint to compensate for deformity may limit the amount of motion available for normal locomotion and disrupt the normal timing of pronation and supination during the gait cycle. This abnormal compensatory pronation and supination may give rise to deformity and its associated symptoms.

PES PLANUS—FLAT FOOT

Abnormal compensatory pronation most commonly produces conditions for the podiatrist to treat, due to the functional effects of pronation within and outwith the foot. Feet which pronate excessively have tended to be classified as flat and, though there are a number of other causes, most

flat feet are a result of compensatory subtalar pronation.

Intrinsic effects of subtalar pronation

As pronation occurs normally in the contact phase, the talus plantarflexes and adducts and the calcaneus everts. Thus frontal plane motion is transmitted to the forefoot through the calcaneus, whilst sagittal and transverse plane motions are transmitted through the talus.

Eversion of the rearfoot with pronation twists the medial side of the foot against the ground. Medial ground reaction forces push up on the medial side of the forefoot, supinating the forefoot at the longitudinal axis of the midtarsal joint. The longitudinal axis lies close to the transverse and sagittal planes, so that most of its supinatory motion is inversion (i.e. frontal plane). This *unlocking* of the longitudinal axis can be seen as forefoot inversion.

Adduction and plantarflexion of the talus with subtalar joint pronation effects a change in the range and direction of midtarsal joint motion. The midtarsal joint consists of four bones: the *calcaneus*, which articulates anteriorly with the *cuboid* and the *talus*, which articulate anteriorly with the *navicular*. Manter (1941) suggested two axes of motion: a longitudinal axis, which allows, primarily, inversion and eversion, and an oblique axis which permits dorsiflexion with abduction and plantar flexion with adduction. The oblique axis has two component axes: the calcaneocuboid and the talonavicular, which on subtalar pronation become increasingly parallel or congruent. When parallel, they function as one increasing motion in the oblique axis of the midtarsal joint. Supination causes these axes to diverge so that they no longer act as one, opposing each other's action and restricting the range of movement (Elftmann 1960) (Fig. 5.1).

Adduction and plantarflexion of the talus lowers the axis of motion of the talonavicular joint so that it approximates more closely the plane of the calcaneocuboid axis. This effects an increase in the total range of motion available at the oblique axis of the midtarsal joint. Lowering the axis of motion of the midtarsal joint also has the effect of raising the inclination of the plane of

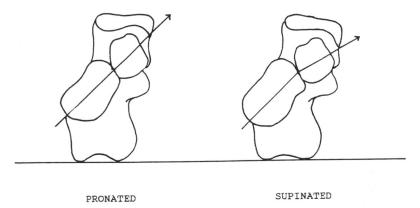

PRONATED   SUPINATED

Fig. 5.1   The oblique axis has two components: the calcaneocuboid axis and the talonavicular axis. During subtalar pronation, these become parallel, acting as one to increase midtarsal mobility. In the supinated foot they diverge and oppose each other, leading to restriction of movement.

motion of the joint, so that more of its motion occurs in the sagittal plane. Put simply, pronation of the subtalar joint increases the total range of motion and particularly the amount of dorsiflexion available in the oblique axis of the midtarsal joint. Subtalar joint pronation can be said to *unlock* the oblique axis of the midtarsal joint.

Plantarflexion of the talus also reduces the congruence of the talonavicular joint, destabilising it, so that the range of motion is increased medially. The navicular might be perceived as the hinge on which the first ray swings. Destabilising the navicular increases the motion and reduces the axial stability of the first ray. Subtalar joint pronation also flattens the line of action of the peroneus longus muscle across the plantar arch, reducing the plantarflexion function of the muscle. This destabilises the 1st ray so that, when subjected to sagittal plane ground reaction forces, it is readily dorsiflexed.

Increased ranges of motion enhance adaptability, thus are useful to the foot in the contact and early midstance phases. However, when pronation occurs late in the gait cycle, or to such an extent that the foot cannot recover, hypermobility renders the forefoot incapable of normal function. Reaction forces produce malalignment of the joints of the forefoot and midtarsus. Typical results of these malalignments are such common structural foot deformities as hallux abducto valgus, hallux rigidus, lesser toe deformities and

flat foot. These abnormal reaction forces can also be transmitted to the rearfoot and leg, causing problems outwith the foot.

Extrinsic effects of subtalar pronation

The talar trochlea is held between the tibia and fibula at the ankle joint. Motions of the calcaneus are transferred through the closed kinetic chain to the talus and the lower limb, which can be seen with normal pronation and supination of the subtalar joint during walking. As the calcaneus everts during pronation in the contact phase of the gait cycle, the talus adducts and plantarflexes, causing internal rotation and forward tilt of the tibia and fibula. At the same time this motion produces knee flexion. The medial condyle of the femur rolls more quickly than the lateral condyle, thus allowing the transverse plane rotation of the tibia to precede internal rotation of the femur. These movements form part of the normal shock absorbing mechanism of the lower limb. As the cycle progresses the opposite motion occurs; the limb rotates externally and the foot locks with supination into a firm propulsive lever.

However, when pronation becomes exaggerated or prolonged in abnormal compensatory motion, this motion is also transferred through the talus to the lower limb. Internal rotation of the tibia and fibula is more marked and knee flexion increases. The timing of return into supination is disrupted and external rotation of the limb, which is initiated by the pelvis and femur, is not followed as directly as it should be by the tibia, which lags behind, introducing a damaging torque within the knee joint. As it is unable to extend and lock for propulsion, the knee is now unstable and vulnerable to the stresses produced by propulsion, with its ligaments and muscles coming under strain. The limb as a whole remains internally rotated and impaired function continues into the trunk. The pelvis tilts forward and the lumbar spine increases its anterior curve giving rise to lumbar lordosis. The muscles supporting the lower spine and the sacroiliac joints also become strained. Under stress, these structures will become fatigued with walking and ordinary activities, giving rise to ankle, knee or low back pain.

Structural causes of abnormal subtalar pronation

The structural abnormalities of the foot and lower limb that require compensation at the subtalar joint are usually congenital, originating from abnormal foetal development. Many may be due to intra-uterine moulding, where a limb or a foot is compressed against the wall of the uterus, others to uneven epiphyseal growth which has led to asymmetry, or to genetic factors; malnutrition and trauma may also cause a few. However the majority of clinical presentations are idiopathic in nature.

The classification of these structural abnormalities (Table 5.1) is dependent on such variables as the cardinal body plane in which the deformity is found, the type of compensation necessary to cope with the abnormality, the intrinsic or extrinsic nature of the structural abnormality and the timing during the gait cycle of the necessary compensation.

This last category is significant in that it determines the amount of damage that can be inflicted on the foot or lower limb. An abnormality such as forefoot varus that requires abnormal compensatory pronation late in the gait cycle, when the foot is in propulsion, will be more damaging than an abnormality such as rearfoot varus, which requires a greater amount of pronation but at the correct time of the gait cycle: contact and early midstance phase.

The instability of the foot produced by late abnormal compensatory pronation makes it vulnerable to the greater ground reaction forces experienced during propulsion and to opposing torques occurring between the foot and the limb. Secondary deformity and pain associated with hyperkeratotic lesions are usually the result. In contrast, where increased pronation occurs at the contact phase of gait, the foot may well recover into supination prior to propulsion thereby minimising abnormal function. Some of the more common structural abnormalities are described in this chapter.

Structural abnormalities

Rearfoot varus (Fig. 5.2)

When the subtalar joint is in the neutral position the calcaneus is in a position of inversion and the foot shows a moderate to high arched form. The foot is inverted and may also be somewhat adducted, and if used habitually in that position, it would be overloaded along its lateral border. Lesions may develop at the base and at the head of the fifth metatarsal, and possibly externally on the fifth toe. In practice, under the influence of lateral ground reaction forces the foot usually pronates to bring the heel and the medial border of the forefoot into normal ground contact. It is thereby predisposed to strain, especially if factors of overuse apply. The symptoms are of pain and swelling from ligamentous and muscular strain affecting both the feet and legs, with possible low back pain. The plantar surface may show hyperkeratotic lesions under the second, third and fourth metatarsal heads and along the medial borders of the heel and the hallux.

Forefoot varus (Fig 5.3)

The forefoot lies in a fixed position of inversion, which is not usually maintained under load, but if it is, the leg and foot tend to abduct sharply at midstance (*abductory twist*), pivoting on the fifth metatarsal head where a plantar callosity develops. As the forefoot becomes weight-

Table 5.1   Classification of functional abnormalities.

Name	Definition and functional implications
Frontal plane	
Coxa vara	Increased angulation of the femoral shaft and neck; tends to precede development of tibial valgum.
Coxa valga	Decreased angulation of the femoral shaft and neck; tends to precede development of tibial varum.
Tibial varum/genu varum	Angulation of the tibia relative to the supporting surface, in which the distal end of the tibia is directed toward the mid-line of the body; tends to produce rearfoot varus.
Tibial valgum/genu valgum	Angulation of the tibia relative to the supporting surface, in which the distal end of the tibia is directed away from the mid-line of the body; tends to produce forefoot supinatus.
Rearfoot/hindfoot varus	Inversion of the heel relative to the supporting surface when the STJ is in neutral and the patient is in their normal angle and base of gait. Where sufficient motion is available, compensatory pronation of the STJ occurs.
Rearfoot/hindfoot valgus	Eversion of the heel relative to the supporting surface when the STJ is neutral and the patient is in their normal angle and base of gait. Where sufficient motion is available, compensatory supination of the MTJ (longitudinal axis) usually occurs, producing forefoot supinatus.
Subtalar varus	Inversion of the calcaneus relative to the tibia when the STJ is neutral; tends to produce rearfoot varus.
Forefoot varus	Inversion of the forefoot relative to the rearfoot when the STJ is neutral and the MTJ is locked in both axes. Where sufficient motion is available, compensatory pronation of the STJ usually occurs (see also forefoot supinatus).
Forefoot valgus	Eversion of the forefoot relative to the rearfoot when the STJ is neutral and the MTJ is locked in both axes. Where sufficient motion is available, compensatory supination of the MTJ (longitudinal axis), and also the STJ, usually occurs.
Sagittal plane	

Flexion contractures of the hip and knee are common in patients with neural pathology and are important functionally in that they tend to preclude normal muscle alignment and function.

Flexion of the knees	Often associated with tight hamstrings and may lead to gastrocnemius equinus.
Genu recurvatum	Hyperextension of the knee may produce or be a result of ankle equinus.
Ankle equinus	Limitation of ankle dorsiflexion to less than 10°. Pronatory compensation occurs in the STJ and MTJ (oblique axis). Alternatively, early heel lift and rapid, late abduction of the hip may be seen.
Ankle calcaneus	Excessive ankle dorsiflexion. Leads to prolonged heel loading and a propulsive gait.
Forefoot equinus	Plantarflexion of the forefoot relative to the hindfoot will tend to be compensated at the ankle joint. Using ankle dorsiflexion to enable heel contact often creates functional equinus of the ankle.
Plantarflexed 1st ray	Creates an everted forefoot to hindfoot relationship (i.e. forefoot valgus). When hypermobile, compensatory dorsiflexion of the 1st ray occurs.
Elevated 1st ray	Tends to produce restriction of 1st MPJ motion.
Transverse plane	
Internal torsion/rotation of the hip, femur or tibia	Produces lateral forefoot loading in propulsion, and therefore late STJ pronation.
External torsion/rotation of the hip, femur or tibia	Produces medial forefoot loading in propulsion and therefore late supination of the MTJ (longitudinal axis). May lead to development of forefoot supinatus.
Forefoot adductus	Fixed adduction of the forefoot relative to the rearfoot destabilises the intrinsic musculature and leads to toe deformities.
Miscellaneous factors	
Forefoot supinatus	Fixed supination of the longitudinal axis as a result of chronic calcaneal eversion in stance and gait. Functionally indistinguishable from forefoot varus.
Limb length differential	Leads to pelvic tilt and asymmetrical gait. Classically, pronation occurs in the longer limb and supination and ankle plantarflexion in the shorter (see also Ch. 10).
High activity levels	Will tend to lead to higher stress on joints and higher ranges of motion. Propulsive pronation can be a major source of problems in such cases (see also Ch. 10).

Abbreviations: MPJ—metatarsophalangeal joint; MTJ—midtarsal joint; STJ—subtalar joint.

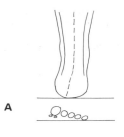

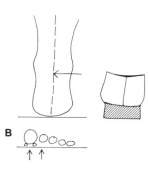

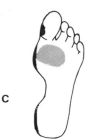

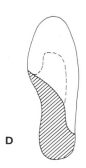

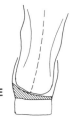

Fig. 5.2   Hindfoot varus: 'chronic foot strain'. Relative positions of hindfoot and metatarsal heads of right foot at rest (A) and under load (B), from rear.

A. Calcaneus inverted: moderate to high arch, tending to be rigid; foot also inverted, possibly mildly adducted.

B. Lateral border overloaded unless hindfoot pronates to vertical; symptoms of postural fatigue in foot, leg and lower back; possible retro-calcaneal bursitis from heel movement. Shoes worn from lateral heel to medial sole; bulging of medial heel counter.
(Arrows below line indicate abnormal pressures; arrow above line indicates movement.)

C. Plantar callosities possible at medial heel, second, third and fourth metatarsal heads and medial side of hallux.

D and E. Management options.
1. Supporting padding and strapping if foot strain symptoms are acute or severe.
2. Palliative valgus insole with medial heel wedge; metatarsal cushioning if required.
3. Functional orthosis with medial hindfoot posting to stabilise inversion.

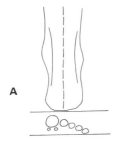

Fig. 5.3   Forefoot varus. Relative positions of hindfoot and metatarsal heads of right foot at rest (A) and under load (B), from rear.
A. Forefoot inverted on hindfoot; possibly also mildly adducted.

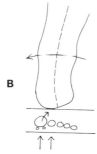

B. Marked compensatory pronation of hindfoot to enable forefoot to become horizontal; resultant hypermobility of forefoot; first metatarsal segment hypermobile and elevated; second metatarsal overloaded; hallux plantarflexed. Shoes worn from medial heel to medial sole; possible broken shank; bulging on medial side of uppers.
(Arrows below line indicate abnormal pressures; arrow above line indicates movement.)

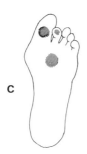

C. Variable symptoms of foot strain: flattening and elongation of medial arch, possible hallux flexus, probable hallux abductovalgus. Possible plantar fasciitis or heel spur syndrome. Plantar lesions under second metatarsal head and interphalangeal joint of hallux.

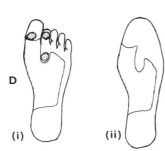

D and E. Management options.
1. Valgus and shaft padding to support medial border and to relieve overloading of second metatarsal head and interphalangeal joint.
2. Symptomatic treatment for forefoot lesions and pain in heel.
3. Palliative valgus and shaft insole.
4. Functional orthosis with medial forefoot posting.
5. Half Thomas heel and medial flare if shoe distortion severe.

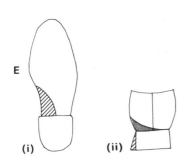

bearing during the stance phase of the walking cycle, the entire foot is forced into pronation in order to bring the medial border of the forefoot into ground contact, thus the foot is rendered hypermobile and various sequelae may ensue.

The hypermobility of the forefoot may cause the first metatarsal to elevate under load, with compensatory overloading of the more stable second metatarsal. Dorsal subluxation of the first metatarsal at the metatarsophalangeal joint may follow, eventually leading to a hallux limitus with overloading of the interphalangeal joint.

The hallux may be held firmly plantarflexed in a bid to stabilise the forefoot, thereby also limiting dorsiflexion at the metatarsophalangeal joint and overloading the interphalangeal joint, which may become extended. This represents a functional, though not fixed, hallux flexus deformity.

Alternatively, the hallux may become subluxated laterally at the metatarsophalangeal joint, particularly if the first alone or all the metatarsals are adducted, progressing to hallux abductovalgus. Impaction and constriction of the lesser toes secondary to the pronation and elongation of the foot is likely to cause medial deviation and clawing of these toes. This process is aggravated by the tension of the long flexor tendons becoming more oblique as the rearfoot tilts into pronation and the metatarsophalangeal articulations of these toes are deviated from their normally straight alignments. The hypermobility of the first metatarsal entails substantial overloading of the second, third and fourth metatarsal heads with the formation of helomata at these sites, and probably another also under the interphalangeal joint of the hallux.

In the young to middle-aged adult, the main complaints may be proximal to the foot, depending on activity. The patient may complain of low back pain, knee pain or ankle strain as the excessive prolonged pronation produces postural instability. (see Ch. 10).

Ankle equinus (Fig 5.4)

Ankle equinus is defined as a limitation of less than 10° of dorsiflexion at the ankle. It can be due to congenital shortness of the triceps surae muscles, bony malformation of the ankle mortice, acquired triceps surae muscle shortness due to footwear or activity, or as part of general ligamentous laxity. External torsion of the tibia or external rotation of the limb will also lead to inadequate sagittal plane motion at the ankle joint.

When ankle equinus is present the foot and lower limb compensate for it, either by adapting the gait or by using other joints to achieve the range of motion required. Some common compensations are shortening the length of the stride, keeping the knee slightly flexed through the gait cycle, raising the heel prematurely at heel lift (giving a bouncy or springy gait), using a prolonged pronation at the subtalar joint to unlock the midtarsal joint, allowing some dorsiflexion of the forefoot, and performing an abductory twist of the foot prior to heel lift.

The effect of some of these compensatory mechanisms can be damaging either to the foot or to parts of the lower limb, e.g. functioning with a permanently flexed knee can lead to increased pressures on the patellae giving rise to knee pain.

Prolonged pronation during the gait cycle can lead to subluxation of the tarsal and metatarsal joints, resulting in severe trauma in the foot. This leads to a rigid rocker-bottom foot with tarsal arthritis and plantar lesions. Early heel lift can lead to overloading of the forefoot with painful secondary lesions developing. From midstance to heel lift, normal gait requires the tibia to move forward over the foot to make an angle of 10° from the vertical. If, for whatever reason, the ankle is unable to produce this range of motion, the forward motion of the tibia is transferred to the foot, forcing the forefoot against the ground. This is a common cause of metatarsalgia, or metatarsal bursitis.

Patients with ankle equinus often complain that they cannot wear low-heeled shoes or go barefoot for very long without pain developing in the calf muscles. The compensatory pronation of the foot is accompanied by forced dorsiflexion of the forefoot in relation to the rearfoot, and this is thought to be a contributory factor in some cases of calcaneal spurs because of the added tension on the plantar fascia.

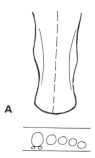

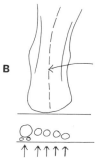

Fig. 5.4   Ankle equinus, short or tight tendo Achilles group. Relative positions of hindfoot and metatarsal heads of right foot at rest (A) and under load (B), from rear.
A. Limitation of dorsiflexion at ankle; foot usually well arched, tending to be rigid but may be flexible.

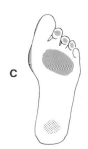

B. Compensatory pronation at subtalar joint to permit further dorsiflexion at midtarsal joint. Forefoot relatively elevated, supinated and hypermobile. Springy gait as heel lifts off prematurely.
(Arrows below line indicate abnormal pressures; arrow above line indicates movement.)

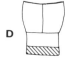

C. Possible symptoms of foot strain, plantarfasciitis or calcaneal spur. Secondary forefoot conditions may include metatarsalgia, hallux abductovalgus and clawed toes with associated dorsal and apical lesions. Midtarsal joint subluxation.

D. Management options, depending on cause:
1. Stretching for tight posterior muscle group.
2. If insufficient, raise heels to compensate for ankle equinus, or insert heel lifts in shoes; or consider tendon lengthening.
3. Palliative valgus and metatarsal insole if foot strain symptoms severe.
4.. Symptomatic treatment for possible plantar fasciitis or calcaneal spur.
5. Symptomatic treatment for secondary forefoot lesions.
6. Functional orthosis if indicated.

Ligamentous laxity

This describes a physical state which can be classed as being within the normal variation. It may range from being a very mild form of laxity manifesting as increased flexibility of the fingers and toes, to extreme laxity, where there is excessive hyperextension of elbows and knees, toes and fingers. If the lower jaw appears to protrude further than the upper, this can also be a sign of ligamentous laxity.

One paradoxical aspect of ligamentous laxity is a relative tightness of the triceps surae muscle group and tight hamstrings, as a result of the repeated protective muscle contraction needed to prevent hyperextension and instability of the knees. It produces an ankle equinus that is usually compensated by abnormal pronation at the subtalar joint, with consequent unlocking of the midtarsal joint seen particularly in females. Males tend to compensate with an early heel lift. With severe ligamentous laxity, the looseness of the ligaments can cause the foot to roll into excessive pronation and the tightness of the triceps surae group perpetuates this situation.

Another effect of ligamentous laxity is the exaggeration of movements, particularly those of pronation. In an otherwise structurally sound foot, it is possible to find excessive pronation with eversion of the calcaneus simply because ligamentous structures are too elastic to maintain the normal arch configuration.

Rearfoot valgus (syn. congenital pes plano valgus) (Fig. 5.5)

Rearfoot valgus has been described as *normal flat foot* since it is defined as flat foot without pronation or exceptional dysfunction. This condition was formerly thought to be an important and common cause of flat foot, but current thinking postulates that it is in fact a relatively rare cause, and that most flat foot is the result of abnormal subtalar pronation. Rearfoot valgus may originate in the subtalar joint but is more commonly associated with genu valgum. The tibia is usually splayed and the calcaneum tends to retain a position of eversion relative to the ground. The forefoot becomes plantargrade by inverting/

supinating at the longitudinal axis of the midtarsal joint so that development of a supinatus deformity is not uncommon. It is often associated with ligamentous laxity and obesity and where this is the case, knee pain and medial ankle instability are common sequelae. There may be also a problem with late pronation, particularly in the presence of supinatus. Foot problems vary, but substantial skin lesions are not the norm. Foot strain and pain and instability in the knees, hips and lower back may cause persistent problems which do not have straightforward solutions. Similarly, lax ligaments will exaggerate compensatory pronation for structural abnormality, giving marked features of abnormal pronation.

Management of flat foot

Since the underlying defects are of a permanent nature, durable managemental measures are required in the longer term to both accommodate the primary deformity and control the secondary symptoms. This necessitates the design of functional or accommodative orthoses, together with any necessary footwear modifications. Bearing in mind the different sources of the primary abnormal pronation, the following procedures may be indicated:

Rearfoot varus (Fig. 5.2, p.56)

a. medial heel wedging or heel cups to stabilise the inverted position of the rearfoot and to prevent abnormal pronation on weight-bearing;
b. valgus support to the medial border of the foot but without elevating the first metatarsal;
c. metatarsal padding to relieve possible plantar lesions and symptoms of metatarsalgia;
d. functional orthosis with medial rearfoot posting;
e. footwear with broad-based heels of average height.

Forefoot varus (Fig. 5.3, p.57)

a. medial forefoot wedging to prevent abnormal pronation;

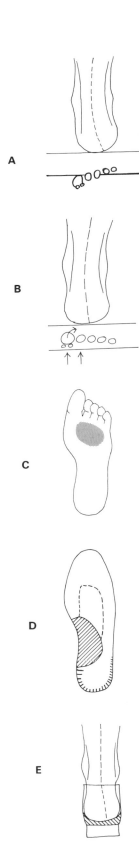

Fig. 5.5 Pes plano-valgus: hindfoot valgus, 'congenital flat foot'. Relative positions of hindfoot and metatarsal heads of right foot at rest (A) and under load (B), from rear.

A. Calcaneus everted; low convex medial arch; prominent medial malleolus; tarsus usually rigid; forefoot abducted on hindfoot and everted.

B. Fixed eversion of hindfoot; bowing of tendo Achilles (Helbing's sign); forefoot supinated to horizontal; first metatarsal hypermobile, elevated and inverted. 'Flat-footed' abducted angle of gait; shoes worn down at lateral heel and medial sole; shank flattened, possibly broken.
(Arrows below line indicate abnormal pressures; arrow above line indicates movement.)

C. Variable plantar lesions, depending on state of metatarsophalangeal joints; possibly diffuse callus; deformity may be asymptomatic or present symptoms of tarsal arthritis.

D and E. Management options.
1. Accommodative insole with heel cupped for fixed calcaneal eversion; resilient valgus support if symptomatic; additional metatarsal cushioning if necessary.
2. If foot mobile, valgus flange also.
3. Symptomatic treatment for forefoot lesions.
4. Wedge-soled shoes suitable, but not rigid shanks.

b. valgus support to the medial border of the foot;

c. shaft padding to the first metatarsal and proximal phalanx of the hallus;

d. metatarsal padding with a U-shaped cavity to relieve overloading of the second metatarsal head;

e. functional orthosis with medial forefoot posting;

f. in severe long-standing cases, an extended heel (a half Thomas heel) and a medial flare;

g. symptomatic treatment of forefoot lesions.

Ankle equinus (Fig. 5.4, p.59)

Treatment varies with the cause. In the bony form with congenital shortening of the triceps surae muscle group, heel lifts can be inserted into the shoes or a higher-heeled shoe can be worn. Where the deforming effects of equinus have been long-term and foot realignment is necessary, a functional orthotic device can be prescribed, in combination with the heel lifts.

In acquired ankle equinus, the first aim of management is to stretch the triceps surae muscle group, if this is possible, using a muscle stretching regime, after which a functional orthosis can be instituted to realign the foot if necessary. If prolonged pronation has been the mode of compensation used for the condition, functional orthoses will help to keep the muscle group stretched. Treatment for the abnormal pronation requires a regular regime of stretching to be carried out each day.

Ligamentous laxity

Treatment is to stretch the triceps surae muscle group in a suitable daily regime and to maintain the improvement. Functional orthoses with a high medial post will control the abnormal pronation, allowing the foot to function from its ideal position, and will help to sustain the muscle stretch.

Surgical treatment. Most patients with flat foot deformity may obtain adequate relief from orthotic devices. However, the clinician should not be misled into believing that pes plano valgus is a benign condition—the instability present in this type of foot may lead to other problems such as hallux valgus and hammer toes. Many patients assume that painful feet are the norm and are reluctant to express concern over these symptoms.

Surgical intervention should be considered in adult patients with symptomatic deformity which fails to respond to conservative measures, and in children with gross deformity and/or instability. Usually adults will undergo arthrodesing procedures while younger patients may obtain good results with reconstructive measures prior to osseous adaptation. Many patients undergoing surgical repair of the deformity will also require Achilles tendon lengthening or gastrocnemius recession.

Other forms of flat foot

Paralytic flat foot may occur rarely following injury or disease affecting the posterior tibial nerve, leading to paralysis of the invertor and flexor muscles and a flaccid flat foot. So-called *spastic flat foot*, on the other hand, is due to spasm of the peroneal muscles which hold the foot in an everted and abducted posture because of some painful focus in the tarsal joints. This is usually identified as a tarsal synostosis (see Ch. 4). *Foot drop*, in which dorsiflexion capacity is lost following poliomyelitis and paralysis of the anterior tibial nerve, is another flaccid condition requiring differentiation by examination and history. *Arthritic flat foot* is seen occasionally in advanced rheumatoid arthritis; the foot is held in eversion and abduction in consequence of the disease process in the tarsal joints. *Traumatic flat foot* may follow fractures of the ankle or of the calcaneus.

All of the foregoing represent cases of chronic deformity which require accommodation in appropriately modified footwear, together with supporting orthoses to relieve symptoms and to limit deformation of the foot on weight-bearing.

Foot strain

The degree of foot strain is related directly to the amount of excessive weight-bearing the foot may be undergoing and whether the onset of the strain is sudden or gradual.

Acute foot strain is rare and can be attributed most commonly to sudden or unusual overactivity which produces inflammation at the sites of ligamentous and muscular attachments, and at joints. The feet become hot, swollen and tender. Complete rest is indicated for a few days, with the symptoms being relieved by the use of contrast footbaths and supportive bandaging.

Chronic foot strain is more common among people whose occupation involves much standing, since static loading of the feet is more tiring than a similar load borne during walking, when muscular activity stimulates a higher metabolic rate in the tissues. The symptoms of chronic foot strain are pain and tenderness in the region of the tarsus with aching and tenderness of the leg muscles. Frequently, pain is experienced in the metatarsal area. Examination usually elicits tenderness at the sites mentioned and the feet are commonly hyperhidrotic and liable to be swollen after exertion. On weight-bearing, the change of shape and contour from normal becomes obvious as the feet pronate, flatten and elongate. The calcaneus is everted and the tendo Achilles is laterally deflected below the ankle showing a positive *Helbing's sign*.

Various secondary lesions are likely to be present in the forefoot, including deformity of the hallux and of the lesser toes, together with plantar and digital helomata and callosities. Footwear is likely to show a pattern of wear marks running from the lateral border of the heel to the medial border of the sole, possibly with bulging of the medial aspect of the heel counter.

Management of foot strain

Short-term relief of symptoms is best obtained by figure of eight strapping of the foot and ankle (see Ch.11), applied to ensure inversion of the calcaneus and plantarflexion of the first metatarsal. Depending on the degree of deformity of the foot on weight-bearing, valgus padding and tarsal strapping to support the medial border may also be incorporated into this dressing. Firm supportive footwear must be worn at all times with this dressing and the feet must not bear weight unless suitably shod. The strapping will give support and relief for up to 10 days at a time,

which is usually long enough to alleviate the symptoms.

PES CAVUS—THE HIGHLY ARCHED FOOT (Fig. 5.6)

Pes cavus is a general term which covers all types of abnormally highly arched feet and, like the term flat foot, it is descriptive but not specifically diagnostic. A more precise definition of the nature of the deformity in specific cases requires a clear distinction to be drawn between those which are secondary to a neurological disorder and those which arise from intrinsic structural anomalies. The former category is more likely to underlie the deformity, so that it may be the only presenting symptom of neuropathy, showing the necessity for a thorough neurological examination.

The neurological defects most responsible are spina bifida, poliomyelitis, cerebral palsy and Charcot-Marie-Tooth disease. Other neuropathies causing foot deformity include muscular dystrophy, cerebral vascular accidents and Friedreich's ataxia. The multiplicity of muscle imbalances resulting from such sources present many forms of foot deformity including pes cavus, drop-foot, paralytic flat-foot and talipes equinovarus. Management may require major surgery to secure optimum stability and function, combined with continuing after-care for chronic residual deformity with associated pressure lesions and tendencies to ulceration. Orthotic therapy in combination with appropriate footwear modifications represents the best long-term management.

The intrinsic structural variations associated with the highly arched foot are forefoot valgus, plantarflexed first ray, and rearfoot varus.

Forefoot valgus (Fig. 5.7)

Forefoot valgus is a structural abnormality in which the plantar aspect of the forefoot is everted relative to the plantar aspect of the rearfoot when the subtalar joint is in the neutral position and the midtarsal joint is pronated. Compensation for this deformity occurs in two forms producing two different foot types.

The first type of compensation is supination of the subtalar joint, which occurs when there is

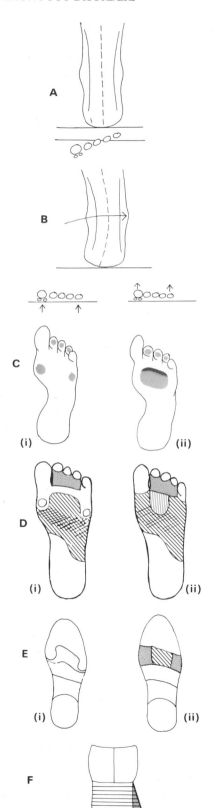

Fig. 5.6 Pes cavus: forefoot valgus, plantarflexed 1st ray, hindfoot varus. Relative positions of hindfoot and metatarsal heads of right foot at rest (A) and under load (B), seen from the rear.

A. High arch, mobile or rigid; forefoot everted on hindfoot; first ray plantarflexed, possibly fifth also; both commonly relatively fixed, but mobile in some cases. Tight plantar fascia, possibly some metatarsus adductus.

B. Postural instability from compensatory inversion of hindfoot; possibly chronic ankle sprain. Forefoot lesions variable, depending on behaviour under load of first and fifth rays. (Arrows below line indicate abnormal pressures; arrows above line indicate movement)

C. (i) If both first and fifth rays fixed, plantar helomata under both metatarsal heads, probably severe, often vascular. (ii) If both first and fifth rays hypermobile and elevating, diffuse callosity under middle metatarsal heads, usually heavy. A combination of such lesions is possible. Liability to ulceration in neuropathic states. Clawing of middle toes with apical and dorsal lesions.

D. First stage management. (i) Double-winged metatarsal padding extended posteriorly to load medial border. Alternatively, metatarsal padding only on foot with tarsal platforms in shoes. Orthodigital splints for toes. (ii) If metatarsophalangeal joints mobile, padding as above; if fixed, plantar cover extended posteriorly to lateral border with cavity (-ies) for 2, 3 and/or 4 as required. Maximum metatarsal bar effect required. Orthodigital splints for toes.

E. Long-term management.
(i) Insole with tarsal platform extended to metatarsals 2, 3 and 4; metatarsal bar effect accentuated. Orthodigital splints for toes.
(ii) Insole as above if metatarsophalangeal joints mobile; if fixed, plantar cushion for middle metatarsal heads with tarsal platform extended anteriorly into shafts under first and fifth. Maximum metatarsal bar effect required. Orthodigital splints for toes.

F. Buttressed heel if required to maintain lateral postural stability.

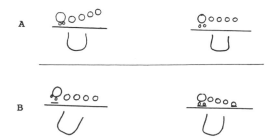

Fig. 5.7 A and B show the uncompensated and compensated forms of forefoot valgus and plantarflexed 1st ray. Skin lesions develop under the 1st MPJ in forefoot valgus, and under the 1st and 5th MPJs in a plantarflexed 1st ray deformity. (MPJ = metatarsophalangeal joint)

inadequate motion available at the midtarsal joint to parallel the forefoot to the rearfoot. This may result from limited midtarsal joint motion or because the forefoot valgus deformity is too large for the joint motion to absorb. Subtalar joint supination allows the lateral border of the foot to become weight-bearing. This has the effect of locking the foot into a rigid structure with little shock absorption and also leads to ankle instability on the lateral side. It causes the peroneus longus muscle to become pulled tight on the supinated foot, plantarflexing the first ray and perpetuating the deformity. The increased declination of the metatarsals and loss of function of the lumbricals results in clawing and retraction of the toes and tightening of the plantar fascia. The first and fifth metatarsal heads are overloaded so that plantar helomata and callosities occur at these sites.

In other cases forefoot valgus is compensated only at the midtarsal joint, which supinates around its longitudinal axis allowing the forefoot to become parallel to the rearfoot. The longitudinal twist that is now present in the foot leads to forefoot instability during propulsion and is responsible for abnormal action of the long and short extensors and flexors, resulting in clawing and inversion of the lateral toes. This foot looks highly arched when non-weight-bearing but flattens substantially when fully loaded.

Fixed plantarflexion of the first ray

This deformity differs from forefoot valgus in that the first metatarsal alone is in a plantarflexed

position relative to the other metatarsals. Compensation for this is the same as for forefoot valgus. It is common for the pattern of lesions to differ, with loading being principally on the first and fifth metatarsals because of the existence of a significant transverse arch across the metatarsal heads (see Fig. 5.6, p.64). Lateral instability of the ankle is also a common feature.

Rearfoot varus

In the neutral calcaneal stance position, the calcaneus is inverted and the foot shows a moderate to high-arched form. The forefoot is similarly inverted and may also be somewhat adducted. In some cases, there is a small range of subtalar joint motion which is insufficient to provide full compensation of the deformity by pronation. Active plantarflexion of the first metatarsal brings the medial border of the forefoot into ground contact. The foot has reduced capacity for shock absorption and is prone to arthritic changes in the tarsal region. It is also predisposed to foot strain, especially if factors such as obesity or occupational demands are present. The toes are clawed and the metatarsal heads become prominent; the plantar fibro-fatty pad tends to be moved distally, exposing the metatarsal heads to trauma and consequent heloma and callus formation.

Forefoot equinus

Forefoot equinus is present when the transverse plane of the forefoot is in a more plantarflexed position than that of the rearfoot, with the subtalar joint neutral and the midtarsal joint pronated, thus the foot appears to be highly-arched when not weight-bearing. In order that the transverse planes of both forefoot and rearfoot are on the same plane for locomotion, abnormal subtalar joint pronation is often required, with subsequent unlocking of the midtarsal joint. Without this form of compensation, ankle joint dorsiflexion required for normal gait is used up and an equinus attitude develops at the ankle.

The effect of the forefoot equinus is to cause subluxation of the forefoot, leading to secondary lesions. Stretching of the plantar muscles, and/or heel lifts are indicated to alleviate the situation.

Clinical features of pes cavus

The possible problems arising from pes cavus may be those of postural instability and strain as the body tries to function on a base which is rigid and unstable. Recurrent ankle sprains result from the varus inclination of the calcaneus and the lack of subtalar adaptability. Knee pain, whether medial or lateral, results from strain on the ligaments and uneven compression on the articular cartilage. Hip pain manifests from the lack of shock absorption in the foot and knee during the contact phase, causing shock to reverberate to the hip joint and, often, the sacroiliac joints.

The pain and disability which pes cavus causes in the adult patient often arise directly from the secondary effects on the skin and soft tissues. The abnormal architecture of the foot reduces its capacity for shock absorption while simultaneously increasing the compressive stresses under the heel and the metatarsal heads. Deep heel pain may arise from excessive tensile stress on the calcaneal attachment of the plantar fascia, particularly in athletes and patients of middle-age or above who are overweight.

The metatarsophalangeal area is often burdened additionally by the retraction and clawing of the toes, which may progress to cause subluxation of one or more of the metatarsophalangeal joints, thus increasing the excessive compressional stresses on the plantar tissues. The three central metatarsals are firmly articulated at their bases and have a limited range of dorsiflexion and plantarflexion. Their angle of declination to the surface is increased by any abnormal height of arch and this, combined with retraction of the middle toes and possibly subluxation of their metatarsophalangeal joints, causes the formation of heavy plantar callus beneath them (see Fig. 5.6C, p.64). This sometimes forms a particularly dense furrow running transversely across the distal margin of the callus, which is indicated by a hollowing-out of the insole of the shoe. This results in a transverse ridge of material forming anterior to the actual weight-bearing area, against which the plantar tissues impinge at each step.

In some cases, it is the first and fifth metatarsal heads which suffer from major overloading, and severe vascular and neurovascular plantar helomata may form in these areas (Fig. 5.6C, p.64). The first and fifth metatarsals are relatively plantarflexed in relation to the others—held by their tight fascial bands—and because the height of the arch shortens the distance between the heel and the metatarsal heads, they lie more posteriorly in the shoe, where it narrows into the waist. The first and fifth metatarsal heads overlie the side edges, and the uneven surfaces on which they rest contribute to the highly vascular and neurovascular nature of the plantar lesions. The first and fifth toes may be retracted, thereby pinning their respective metatarsal heads more firmly to the surface.

In some cases, all these factors may be involved. The hallux may show a *trigger toe* deformity, with possibly a dorsal heloma or bursitis over the interphalangeal joint. The fifth toe usually appears retracted, adducted and internally rotated, hence the term *digitus quintus varus*. These digital deformities all predispose to dorsal and apical helomata, which may be severe, as are the plantar lesions.

In some cases of neurological origin, both nutrition and sensation are deficient and the metabolism of the skin and soft tissues is impaired. The pressure lesions already described are thus more likely to ulcerate, with the possibility of secondary infections. On areas of concentrated pressure, as under the first and fifth metatarsal heads, the resultant necrosis may extend into the joint. This may occur gradually beneath a heavy plantar lesion or callus, the enucleation of which exposes a sinus from which may exude a seropurulent discharge and possibly synovial fluid from the joint cavity. This condition is termed a *perforating* or *penetrating ulcer* and depending on the degree of neurological deficiency, it may be relatively painless. Further destruction of the joint may ensue from the infective arthritis.

Management of pes cavus

Where there is postural instability, the aim in management is to try to restore the foot to a stable base, and by increasing the areas of weight-bearing, particularly the lateral border, this can be achieved to some extent. Functional orthoses will balance the foot, particularly in the case of compensatory subtalar supination, giving a degree of adaptability and shock absorption by balancing the forefoot with a lateral intrinsic forefoot post in mild cases, or supporting the rearfoot with a medial rearfoot post. Thus the foot can be prevented from twisting into a severely supinated position and some adaptability is restored.

In many cases the rearfoot varus deformity that accompanies pes cavus is compensated at the subtalar joint by pronation. This is often difficult to observe as the calcaneus may still be inverted and there will be no flattening of the longitudinal arch or medial bulging. The management is the same as for compensated rearfoot varus with or without the high arch configuration. A medial heel post will control the pronation and give the varus rearfoot a stable area for heel contact during gait. Flexible and shock absorbing materials should be used as the foot with pes cavus often lacks these qualities.

In severe and long standing cases the most pressing need in the management of pes cavus in adults is to control the various superficial lesions which are the immediate source of pain, disability and possibly infection. The enucleation and reduction of plantar helomata and callosities and the debridement and cleansing of ulcerated areas are of first importance in the restoration of comfort and the control of any infective processes. In the case of heavily nucleated plantar lesions, chemical cautery and exfoliation may be indicated, but care is necessary to avoid precipitating ulceration.

Relief of the plantar tissues from excessive weight-bearing is best secured initially by adhesive padding. Depending on the distribution of the plantar lesions, either a double-winged metatarsal pad or a plantar cover with cavity for one or more metatarsal heads is indicated (see Fig. 5.6 D, p.64). Each of these types of pad should be extended down the lateral border of the foot. Both patterns incorporate the principle of a weight relieving metatarsal bar just behind the metatarsal heads and also the principle of bringing the lateral border into weight-bearing. Additional digital

paddings of appropriate design may be required as a first stage measure.

Longer term conservative management has three aspects: first, to provide a durable method of relieving abnormal overloading of the plantar tissues by appropriate orthoses; secondly, to prevent excessive pressure on deformed digits; and thirdly, to provide footwear capable of accommodating both the foot and the necessary orthoses. Early in the management programme, protective insoles should be designed incorporating the following features (see Fig. 5.6E, p.64):

1. a resilient base to provide additional shock absorption.
2. a tarsal platform *filler pad*, designed to raise the insole surface sufficiently to ensure that the lateral border of the foot bears weight as in a normal foot. The tarsal platform provides additional postural stability and reduces any tendency towards lateral sprain of the ankle; it also reduces overloading of the heel and relieves any deep heel pain at the origin of the plantar fascia.
3. metatarsal padding designed to deflect the excessive compressional stresses on the metatarsal area should incorporate:
   (a) a metatarsal bar element shaped to the metatarsal formula of the foot
   (b) a double-winged metatarsal pad to protect metatarsals 1 and 5 or a plantar cover to provide cushioning for metatarsals 2, 3 or 4
   (c) a combination of all three.

The therapeutic objective of such insoles is to achieve the maximum possible redistribution of excessive compressional forces and to provide maximum shock absorption under areas which may continue to be overloaded. The thickness, shape and density of the materials used should be determined carefully in each case. An insole which is no more than a mirror image of the plantar surface of the foot is quite inadequate to reduce the damaging trauma to the soft tissues. The tarsal platform, the metatarsal bar element and the design of the metatarsal padding are all of crucial importance in obtaining good results.

With pain free weight-bearing restored, the

provision of a functional orthosis with lateral forefoot posting can be considered.

Digital correction and protection are also necessary. For the middle three toes orthodigital splints are indicated (Ch.11). These will provide correction of the digital deformities as well as protection for the vulnerable dorsal and apical areas (see Fig. 5.6 D, p.64). For the first and fifth toes, individual shields in silicone are most effective.

The required combination of insoles and digital appliances is unlikely to be accommodated without the provision of special shoes or modifications to conventional footwear. Provided both the insoles and the digital appliances have been well designed to give the maximum effect with the minimum bulk, and have proved to be effective, compromise should not be considered in order to reduce their volume to facilitate the wearing of inadequate shoes.

The footwear requires to be well fitting, with wide openings to allow ease of entry, and should have shock absorbent soles and heels. The frontal capacity can be enlarged by modifications to the footwear (Ch.13). The more severe forms of pes cavus require individually made footwear which must be designed to accommodate the necessary insoles and other appliances. Cooperation between the shoemaker, appliance maker, podiatrist and surgeon is highly desirable during the designing and fitting of such shoes. A lateral heel buttress (see Fig. 5.6 F, p.64) may be necessary to provide additional postural stability, and possibly a reverse Thomas heel extended forward on the lateral side if metatarsus adductus is evident.

Surgical treatment. Many patients with pes cavus deformity may benefit from surgical intervention. Digital arthrodesis is quite beneficial in alleviating lesions on the toes as well as protrusion of the metatarsal heads on the plantar surface due to buckling of the digits (Ch.18). Patients with flexible or mobile cavus deformity which produces symptoms may benefit from an osteotomy (e.g. Dwyers calcaneal osteotomy, dorsiflexory first metatarsal osteotomy). In cases of rigid or severe contracture or neuromuscular disease, triple arthrodesis is usually preferred. Such arthrodesing procedures are often combined with appropriate digital repair.

TARSAL ARTHRITIS

The subtalar, midtarsal and tarsometatarsal joints may become affected by osteoarthrosis or rheumatoid arthritis. The former condition is seen in middle-aged and elderly patients with some concomitant mechanical foot disorder, e.g. ankle equinus, which is the underlying cause of the abnormal wear and tear on the joints. Most commonly, the midtarsal joint is affected in patients of above average weight with highly-arched and rather rigid feet. The condition develops gradually, is usually mild to moderate in degree, and is marked by pain when the weight-bearing foot is inverted or everted.

In rheumatoid arthritis, pain may be severe during acute phases of the disease so that the patient is barely able to walk. In periods of remission from the condition weight-bearing may be possible, but painful. This disease affects the interphalangeal and metatarsophalangeal joints more than the tarsal joints and occurs in younger age groups (Ch. 22).

In addition to whatever medication or therapy is needed for the general condition, local treatment should consist of relative immobilisation of painful joints. This is best achieved by the provision of a tarsal cradle (the combination of a tarsal platform with a valgus support). This supports both the lateral and medial borders of the foot simultaneously and thus minimises movements of inversion and eversion. It is usually required as a permanent feature of a supporting insole. Temporarily, an elastic anklet may give some relief.

PAIN IN THE HEEL

At the moment of heel strike, there is compression of the extreme posterior fibro-fatty padding, which is followed by a progressive compression of the remainder of the plantar pad of the heel for a short phase, prior to the forward transmission of force and weight through the joints of the midfoot and forefoot. Considerable emphasis has been placed upon the significance of trauma and mechanical factors in the aetiology of pain in the rearfoot.

Posterior tuberosity (heel bump)

Pain arising from the posterior aspect of the heel may occur in young patients who develop a firm fibro-fatty swelling over the posterior aspect of the calcaneus. Pathologically, the swelling consists of hypertrophic subcutaneous tissue and there may be some prominence of the posterior superior angle of the calcaneus. The aetiology of the subcutaneous swelling is not clear, but there is often an association with recurrent chilblains and generally cold extremities, suggesting that trophic changes take place at the site of pressure and friction. General thickening of the subcutaneous tissue around the lower leg and ankle may often be found in the presence of heel bumps associated with erythrocyanosis.

This condition is not necessarily painful and does not always lead to clinical manifestations, but any which do occur are invariably due to pressure from the heel counter of the shoe.

The treatment of these lesions consists of shoe modifications, the most straightforward being the removal of the heel stiffening overlying the bump. In the short term, padding and strapping to re-distribute pressure away from the lesion is an adequate measure. If symptoms persist despite attention to footwear, the posterior-superior part of the calcaneus may be removed through an incision lateral to the tendo Achilles. Alterna-tively, a wedge of bone may be removed from the body of the calcaneus. This has the effect of slightly shortening the calcaneus and diminishing the prominence of the heel.

Calcaneal bursitis

Pain may arise at the posterior aspect of the heel due to inflammation of one of the bursae associ-ated with the tendo Achilles.

Superficial bursitis

Bursitis may occur due to the application of shearing stress to the tissue overlying the posterior aspect of the calcaneus near to the point of attach-ment of the tendo Achilles. Normal superficial bursae are present in most individuals and sometimes these may become inflamed. In others, an acquired bursa may develop in response to the shearing stresses produced between bone and tendon structures and the counter of the shoe, and any such bursa is subject to inflammation. This occurs commonly with rearfoot varus because the calcaneus constantly pronates to and supinates from the vertical. Occupational factors may be significant and inadequate or ill-designed footwear may also contribute.

Any of the three phases of bursitis may occur in a superficial bursa and treatment will depend upon the phase. In the acute phase, complete rest may be required, while in the chronic phase, in which no signs of inflammation are present, no treatment may be necessary. The most common manifestation is in the subacute phase when elimination of shearing stresses by the appli-cation of appropriate padding and strapping, and possibly some general rest, will normally be adequate. Heat therapy can be useful. Emphasis is placed upon the importance of identifying the causal factors and removing or preventing them. The case history and the examination of footwear will often identify the most significant factors.

Deep bursitis

The bursa deep to the tendo Achilles is a constant anatomical feature and lies over the upper third of the posterior surface of the calcaneus. It is rarely involved in pathological changes but can become inflamed due to mechanical irritation or infection.

The onset can be insidious or acute and there may be an association with occupational factors, sporting or unaccustomed activity, or inadequate footwear. The patient complains of pain which is particularly noticeable when the ankle joint is moved. Examination often reveals a swelling on both sides of the tendo Achilles, giving a bi-lobed appearance, with pain on extension and flexion of the ankle joint. When pressure is applied to one side of the swelling a fluctuation can be felt on the other side.

Treatment of mechanically induced bursitis is similar to that prescribed for other examples of aseptic inflammation, and varies with the severity of the symptoms. The removal of causative factors and rest, possibly with immobilisation achieved with suitable strappings, provide relief. The use of cold in acute cases, or the application of heat in subacute or chronic stages, is effective. A 1 cm heel raise is helpful when bursitis affects the posterior aspect of the heel. This reduces tensile stress on the area of insertion of the tendo Achilles and also compression of the inflamed bursa during walking.

In the case of infected bursitis, whether it is deep or superficial to the tendo Achilles, antibiotic therapy is indicated and surgical intervention may become necessary to drain the serous pus which can be produced. The inflammation tends to be acute and rapid in onset and is a prominent feature in infective bursitis. There may be an obvious route for spread of infection from an infected superficial lesion near to the bursa, or the spread may be from a site which is not obvious on examination.

Plantar heel pain

Pain in the plantar pad of the heel is a relatively common condition in some young patients, although it occurs more frequently in patients over 40 years of age, and its incidence increases steadily during the fifth and sixth decade of life. The plethora of names given to this condition implies, erroneously, a heterogeneous group of disorders. The terms *plantar fasciitis* and *periostitis of the calcaneus* are applied to a condition in which the main clinical features are deep pain in the plantar aspect of the heel, usually most severe on rising from bed or after resting in a chair for some time. The patient tends to complain somewhat vaguely of pain arising from the heel and careful questioning is necessary to locate the point of pain. Firm pressure with the thumb will elicit a deep tender spot, often over the medial tubercle of the calcaneus or sometimes centrally within the plantar aspect of the heel. These sites correspond to the attachments of deep ligamentous structures to the calcaneus and, in particular, the attachment of the central band of the plantar aponeurosis to the medial tubercle of the calcaneus. The importance of the examination to demonstrate the presence of a deep tender area cannot be over emphasised since there is a very clear syndrome in which the main features are simply those

described, and in which no other abnormality need be present. X-rays are of little value since, although it is true that in long-standing cases a spur can be detected on the calcaneus, such spurs are not uncommon: they may be found in about 10% of the population, most of whom will have had no history of pain.

The most likely explanation of this well-localised lesion is that the attachments of ligamentous structures to the calcaneus become inflamed and eroded. Ligamentous attachment to bone is effected by a sequence of modifications to the composition of the ligament. The collagen fibres initially become more dense, then associated with cartilaginous cells, then finally calcified and attached to the surface of bone by a cement line. The joining structure is termed an *enthesis*. Entheses have been shown to be metabolically active sites which can be infiltrated by inflammatory cells. The cause of inflammatory changes at attachment sites is unclear, although the changes noted take place along the route of numerous small vessels which pass through the enthesis.

The term *enthesopathy* has been applied to the rather striking condition which appears microscopically as a focal inflammatory lesion localised to ligamentous attachments. The result of these inflammatory changes is that the greater part of the affected attachment is destroyed, producing a small erosion or defect in the cortical bone. The connective tissue surrounding the attachment is infiltrated by a collection of inflammatory cells. As a response to the erosive inflammatory changes which take place at the enthesis, healing ultimately takes place by the laying down of new bone. Since the inflammatory process seems to be chronic, the laying down of bone proceeds over a period of time, which could account for the appearance of a spur of bone on the calcaneus in cases of long standing localised heel pain. The phenomenon of severe pain occurring on rising after rest may be accounted for by some degree of inflammatory oedema in a site where there is very limited space due to tight compartmentalisation of the tissues by strong connective tissue septae. Accumulation of fluid in such a site would be an obvious cause of pain, as increased pressure is put upon nerve endings within the tissue on weight-bearing. This would tend to occur after rest when inflammatory exudate will have had a chance to accumulate within the tissue. It is notable that the pain tends to diminish within half an hour of walking; this could be accounted for by simple improvement in lymphatic and venous drainage due to the mechanical effects of movement.

Treatment of deep localised heel pain

Treatment falls under three headings and, depending upon the degree of severity, a combination of these forms of treatment may be indicated. Techniques to cushion the heel and to redistribute pressure away from the most sensitive area are possible; secondly, techniques to improve the condition by the application of heat may be used; and thirdly, it is possible to inject a specific anti-inflammatory preparation, usually a corticosteroid, into the the area. The first two of these techniques are within the scope of practice of the podiatrist, while, at present, the injection of corticosteroids is not. Nevertheless this must be considered as part of the whole management of severe deep localised heel pain.

Padding and orthotic technique. Padding and orthoses used to relieve deep heel pain fall into two categories:

(a) those used simply to cushion the heel
(b) devices which will reduce tensile stress on the attachment of the plantar ligamentous structures and thereby relieve strain.

As would be expected from a consideration of the nature of the lesion, simple cushioning pads prove to be of relatively little value. The popularity of simple cushioning padding for the heel arose from the misconception that pain in the heel was simply due to contusion in virtually all cases, and that a cushion would allow the tissue to recover. In practice, this proved to be erroneous, although in cases in which simple contusion is a clear cause of diffuse heel pain, cushioning does play a useful part in management.

A device of any sort to reduce the tensile stress on the fascial attachments to the calcaneus will relieve some of the pain. The longer the condition has been present, the longer it will take to heal,

and in many chronic cases there will be some residual pain. Treatment should be sought before excessive degeneration of the attachment of the fascia has occurred.

A reinforced figure of eight strapping, which inverts the calcaneus and increases its angle of inclination, is helpful in the short term. The calcaneus may be tilted upward at its anterior end by a felt bar fitted into the shoe. A tarsal platform (*filler pad*) acts similarly by elevating the cuboid. Combined with sponge heel cushions, these forms of padding offer alternative possibilities of short-term treatment while an orthosis is being constructed and specific forms of treatment are undertaken. The combined valgus and filler insole (*tarsal cradle*) relieves part of the tensile stress on the calcaneal attachments. The provision of such appliances should be thought of as an adjunct to more active forms of treatment rather than as a complete treatment in itself.

A second, more active, form of treatment is that of ultra-high frequency sound (ultrasound) diathermy. This technique enables the practitioner to direct a localised beam of ultrasound energy on to the area, thereby producing a number of effects, which include increase in temperature and several other non-thermal effects. For complete description of technique and apparatus, see the relevant section in Chapter 14.

Normally a course of ultrasound diathermy extending over a period of four to six weeks, and comprising two treatments each week, will be sufficient; the dosage will be of the order of $1.0-1.5$ W/cm^2 for a period of five minutes for each treatment field. The total number of treatments would not normally exceed 8–10.

The third technique which may be applied in conjunction with ultrasound diathermy and the application of an orthotic is the injection of hydrocortisone or a similar corticosteroid. It is very important that the deep tender spot is well identified and marked. The injection of the appropriate steroid is made close to the attachment of the ligamentous structures to the calcaneus. It is essential that the procedure is carried out under strict aseptic conditions. The dosage of steroid varies according to the preparation chosen, with 15–20 mg of hydrocortisone acetate commonly used. Alternatively, preparations which have a longer duration of action may be employed and triamcinolone acetonide 40 mg is frequently used to suppress the inflammatory lesion and reduce symptoms. The steroid preparation is mixed usually with an equal volume of 1% plain lignocaine solution to reduce the pain which would otherwise occur on introducing extra fluid into an already tender and rather limited space.

The disadvantages of using the steroid injection technique are: first, that there is a certain amount of discomfort to the patient when the needle is introduced into the deeper tissue of the heel — even with the incorporation of 1% plain lignocaine solution; secondly, the long-term follow up does not indicate that there is continued improvement in the symptoms. In general, although the short-term results over three to four weeks following injection are very good, long-term monitoring over a period of three months indicates that there can be a considerable degree of relapse. These rather disappointing studies of patients receiving intralesional injections contrast unfavourably with the rather more encouraging studies of patients who have received ultrasound diathermy treatment, and in whom, after a period of three months, pain is much relieved or abolished altogether.

Surgical treatment. Although several operations have been devised for this condition there is no evidence that the results are superior to non-operative treatment, and they are best avoided.

DISORDERS OF THE FOREFOOT

Forefoot disorders constitute the most common source of complaint among adult patients. As the final element in the locomotive cycle, the forefoot sustains the total thrust of propulsion during the toeing-off phase while the opposite foot is swinging free or beginning the contact phase. As illustrated in the sections on pes planus and pes cavus, any intrinsic or extrinsic abnormality affecting the foot exerts its full effect at the moment of maximum load.

Once the structural integrity and functional efficiency of the forefoot become impaired, various manifestations follow which require attention as clinical entities because of the pain and disability they cause. In their aetiology and management, they have to be regarded as syndromes requiring a general assessment of the patient and should not be treated as purely local phenomena.

The predominant importance of the first metatarsal segment in the propulsive function is reflected in the high incidence of its various deformities and their major effects. The most important of these disorders are hallux abductovalgus, hallux limitus and hallux rigidus, and hallux flexus. Other common conditions of clinical importance are metatarsalgia, plantar digital neuritis, splaying of the metatarsals and digital deformities.

HALLUX ABDUCTOVALGUS

Definitions

Hallux abductovalgus (HAV) is a complex deformity of the medial column involving abduction and external rotation of the first toe and adduction and internal rotation of the first metatarsal. The displacement of the hallux occurs at the metatarsophalangeal joint, whilst the metatarsal is displaced mainly at the metatarsal/medial cuneiform joint. Deformity is said to exist when abduction of the hallux on the metatarsal is greater than 10–12°.

Incidence

With estimates in the population as high as 70%, this very common pathology is most prevalent in the mature female. Ninety per cent of all cases seeking surgery are women (Hardy & Clapman 1952), though no such gender related difference has been observed in children or adolescents (Johnston 1956). Both the degree and the frequency of HAV increase with age.

Clinical features

In an established case the clinical features include:

1. Abduction and valgus deviation of the hallux, adduction of the first metatarsal and lateral subluxation of the metatarsophalangeal joint. In extreme cases, the joint may be dislocated. The hallux impinges on the second toe which it may override or, more frequently, underlie. The second toe often develops into a hammer toe which may also eventually become dislocated at the metatarsophalangeal joint.

2. The central toes are usually abducted and clawed, while the fifth toe may be displaced medially and underlie the fourth. Their respective metatarsophalangeal joints may become subluxated, or even dislocated in some instances. Metatarsalgia is usually present and sometimes severe.

3. Secondary osteoarthrosis of the first metatarsophalangeal joint is a common feature, with peripheral osteophytic proliferation which may limit dorsiflexion of the hallux.

4. Numerous secondary lesions may occur where the skin and soft tissues are subjected to trauma. These include bursitis over the medial prominence of the metatarsal head, plantar helomata and callosities, dorsal, apical and interdigital helomata on the toes and deformities and other conditions of the nails.

The basic deformity ranges in degree from slight to very severe and the symptoms are highly variable. Pain in and around the joint may be experienced, probably from ligamentous strain or muscular spasm consequent upon the disordered function. In many cases, deformity itself is painless, having developed gradually from childhood. In some cases, the secondary osteoarthrosis may, however, give considerable pain. Symptoms may also result from ischaemia or neuritis in vessels and nerves as they are stretched around the medial eminence. The chief sources of pain are usually the superficial lesions.

Aetiology

A number of aetiological factors have been identified and strong associations have been described between hallux abductovalgus and constrictive footwear, hereditary factors and abnormal function — particularly abnormal subtalar pronation and degenerative disease.

Biomechanics/pathomechanics of hallux abductovalgus

Abnormal subtalar pronation is generally accepted by podiatrists as a dominant cause of hallux abductovalgus, although it is likely that this is most damaging when accompanied by constrictive footwear, heavy weight-bearing and/or adductus of the first ray.

Pronation of the subtalar joint increases first ray mobility by reducing both the stability of the navicular and the vertical/sagittal plane effect of peroneus longus, so that the first metatarsal is displaced more readily by sagittal plane ground reaction forces. These dorsiflex and invert the first ray on its axis, which runs approximately parallel to the transverse plane and at 45° to the frontal and sagittal. Inversion of the first ray rotates the transverse axis of motion of the first metatarsophalangeal joint out of the transverse plane so that sagittal plane ground reaction force on the toe affects transverse plane deviation. This means that the normal dorsiflexion seen in the propulsive phase is accompanied by abduction. Abduction occurring with propulsive phase dorsiflexion angulates the toe to the line of progression producing reaction forces which are more medial than normal. Any eversion occurring at this time will increase the abductory effect due to increased displacement of the metatarsal.

If pronation occurs during the propulsive phase, tibio/talar internal rotation, resisted by abductory ground reaction force applied through the first toe, will also tend to produce lateral deviation. In this case, the deviation occurs in the vertical axis of the metatarsophalangeal joint. This axis normally has only minimal transverse plane motion available. Subjected to repeated abduction the medial ligaments stretch, thus increasing available abduction. Eventually the first metatarsophalangeal joint may subluxate medially producing the hallux abductus deformity.

During late mid-stance and propulsion, the flexor hallucis longus and brevis fix the hallux to resist sagittal plane reaction forces. Fixation of the hallux by the flexors also maintains its position in the frontal plane so that it cannot invert with the unstable metatarsal. This establishes an evertory torque at the metatarsophalangeal joint, which rotates the toe relative to the metatarsal, creating the frontal plane (valgus) component of the deformity.

As the first toe becomes increasingly angulated relative to the metatarsal reaction forces (from the ground and from the extensor and flexor musculature), the force is no longer transmitted down the line of the metatarsal but at an angle to it. This creates an abductory moment at the metatarsophalangeal joint and also an adductory moment at the base of the first metatarsal. This moment around the already unstable first metatarsal encourages medial deviation at the first metatarsal cuneiform joint (i.e. metatarsus primus adductus).

Predisposing factors

Heredity

Sandelin (1922, quoted in Kelikian 1965) suggests that 54% of patients with HAV show a family history of HAV, while Edgar (in Klenerman 1982) suggests a factor of 58%–63%. This is significantly higher than in controls, but the very high prevalence of hallux abductovalgus and possible heightened awareness among those with the condition make such statistics vulnerable to scrutiny. To date, no accepted genetic trait has been identified for hallux abductovalgus, but it is possible that some other predisposing factors, e.g. forefoot adductus or ligamentous laxity, may be passed genetically or that familial behaviour patterns relating to footwear may predispose. Heredity is therefore generally accepted as a possible causative factor.

Muscle imbalance

McBride (1935) suggested that the mechanical advantage held by the adductor hallucis over the abductor hallucis, because of the angle of its pull, predisposed the foot to hallux abductovalgus. This seems an unlikely initiator of the pathological process but overpull of the adductor and loss of abductory function would exacerbate a developing hallux abductovalgus.

Ligamentous laxity

Associated with subtalar joint pronation, ligamentous laxity may lead to instability, a characteristic precursor of hallux abductovalgus.

Forefoot adductus

Adduction of the metatarsals or of the first metatarsal in isolation gives rise to increased pressure on the medial aspect of the foot, with digits becoming abducted relative to the long axis of their metatarsals. This allows the flexor and extensor tendons to produce a *bowstring* effect on the lateral side, and increases the mechanical advantage of the lateral intrinsic muscles. This may initiate hallux abductovalgus and will consolidate it, if it is developing.

Footwear

The debate over the importance of footwear continues but there can be little doubt that footwear affects the development of hallux abductovalgus. In comparative studies between shod and unshod populations in Nigeria (Barnicott & Hardy 1955), St Helena (Shine 1965) and Hong Kong (Sim Fook & Hodgson 1958) all researchers discovered a markedly higher prevalence of hallux abductovalgus in shod populations. In the latter case the ratio was 17:1. This may go some of the way to explaining gender influence on prevalence—women's fashion shoes being a possible factor. Current preferences for broader, less sexually definitive sports footwear may break this association.

Miscellaneous aetiological factors

Other factors such as obesity, overloading and rheumatoid arthritis may contribute to cause or development. Certain obscure factors such as iatrogenesis, trauma and forefoot adductus may produce hallux abductovalgus without other aetiologies.

Pathology

Authorities differ as to the precise mechanisms by

which the deformity becomes established, but the sequence of pathological processes may be summarised as follows:

1. In response to the aforementioned aetiological factors, the first toe becomes displaced laterally.

2. Due to reaction from the forces on the first toe and first metatarsal instability, the first ray is displaced medially. As a result of the transverse plane angle created at the first metatarsophalangeal joint, the hallux is no longer stable and is pulled laterally by the transverse head of the adductor hallucis. The abductor hallucis is working at a mechanical disadvantage because of the pronation of the foot, and is unable to balance the pull of the adductor sufficiently to prevent the initial angulation at the metatarsophalangeal joint becoming increased. This deformation is further exacerbated by the tension on the long extensor and flexor tendons across the joint: the bowstring effect.

3. The capsule and collateral ligaments of the joint adapt to the deformity, the medial ligament stretching and the lateral one shortening. Weight-bearing stresses force the metatarsal head medially and its sesamoidal ridge overrides the medial sesamoid and becomes gradually eroded. The sesamoids appear to be laterally displaced on X-ray, but the main movement has been that of the first metatarsal head medially as the metatarsal becomes progressively more adducted.

4. Osseous changes occur in response to the altered function of the joint. Osteophytic proliferation from constant irritation may accentuate the medial prominence. Additional bone may be laid down on the dorsolateral aspect of the metatarsal head to maintain an articulation with the base of the hallux. A similar adaptation may occur at the lateral plantar aspect to maintain articulation with the sesamoids. Persistence of the elevated position of the first metatarsal imposes a limitation of dorsiflexion on the hallux, so that a degree of hallux limitus is also present.

5. As the deformity progresses, the second toe tends to be displaced dorsally by the abduction of the hallux, developing a hammer-toe deformity, possibly with subluxation or even dislocation of its metatarsophalangeal joint. The third and fourth toes may become clawed and retracted and the fifth metatarsophalangeal joint becomes deformed, the fifth toe becoming adducted and the metatarsal abducted as splaying of the metatarsal occurs. In extreme cases, the hallux becomes completely dislocated and may lie at right angles to its metatarsal.

6. The skin and soft tissues overlying bony prominences are subjected to abnormal shearing and compressive stresses which cause various superficial lesions. Bursitis (*bunion*) is a common occurrence over the medial prominence of the metatarsal head and is often the chief source of pain, particularly if it should become infected. Even without infection, recurrent bursitis can be very debilitating. In addition to the painful swelling, a sinus may form from which the bursal contents exude to the surface and periodically dry up into a hard corneous plug. Sometimes a fistula develops from the bursa into the joint, provoking discharge of synovial fluid and exacerbating the risks of infection. Bursitis may also develop over the lateral aspect of the fifth metatarsal head (*tailor's bunion*), although this condition can also occur independently. Dorsal, interdigital and apical helomata result from deformities of the lesser toes; the dorsal lesions sometimes develop underlying bursitis. The overloading of the metatarsal heads, resulting from the disturbance of normal forefoot function, may cause the formation of plantar helomata and callus, notably under the second and third metatarsals. Metatarsalgia is a common complication. Involution, onychophosis and onychocryptosis are possible conditions affecting the nail of the hallux.

Management

First phase management in painful cases is essentially symptomatic. It includes, for example:

(a) protection and medication, including heat therapy where indicated for bursitis
(b) treatment of painful helomata and callosities
(c) padding and strapping to reduce the degree of the valgus deformity, provided this is still possible, and if not, to protect it and other vulnerable prominences from trauma.

The 'butterfly' or 'flask' strapping is the most

effective short-term measure. By reducing the deformation of the first metatarsophalangeal joint, it relieves strain on capsular tissues and ligaments and provides quick relief from pain. Protective padding for the medial prominence is incorporated in the dressing in the form of a crescent or oval cavity pad. Any necessary medication may either be applied as an ointment pack within the oval cavity pad and left for the duration of the dressing, or it may be applied in solution through an aperture left for this purpose in the pad. The latter method is useful in treating a sinus as it allows frequent application without disturbing the dressing, except for the uncovering and recovering of the aperture which is independently sealed with an adhesive cover.

An interdigital wedge between the first and second toes may reinforce the element of correction as well as eliminating the likely interdigital pressure between the interphalangeal joints, which is responsible for the formation of helomata in this area. Metatarsal padding and strapping complete the dressing which, properly applied, achieves the maximum possible correction of all forefoot alignments and maximum protection of points of pressure. Protective and corrective padding for the lesser digits should be included as necessary. Support or correction for the primary pronation is also required. This may be in the form of temporary heel wedges and/or valgus padding built into the shoes.

Such techniques should be applied at short intervals to achieve early and complete relief from painful symptoms.

Longer term management aims at:

(a) replacement of all adhesive forefoot dressings by replaceable and durable alternatives
(b) provision of permanent correction, or accommodation of the abnormal pronation
(c) provision of footwear to accommodate all necessary foot appliances.

Continuing protection for the forefoot deformities can best be provided by hallux shields and dorsoplantar digital splints (see Ch. 13). Hallux shields may be fabricated on casts from latex rubber or built up directly on the foot from silicone compounds (see Fig. 5.8). They are designed to protect the medial prominence, thus

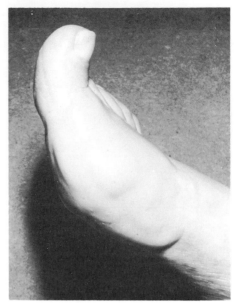

Fig 5.8   Silicone shield for hallux abductovalgus.

obviating recurrent bursitis. Protection for the plantar or dorsal aspects of the metatarsophalangeal and interphalangeal joints may be built into the shield if required. Similarly, interdigital wedging between the first and second toes can be included in order to prevent recurrent interdigital lesions, the wedges being shaped anatomically correctly to conform to the respective phalanges.

The deformities of the lesser toes may be well-controlled by orthodigital splints designed to conform precisely to the needs of the individual case. The variations possible on the basic design should ensure both adequate protection for traumatised areas and optimum correction of digital malalignments. The splints also provide a stable base under pressure of weight-bearing, from which an interdigital wedge may buttress the tendency of the hallux to abduct.

The ways and means of controlling abnormal pronation have been described in the section pes planovalgus.

The essential features of footwear suitable for adult hallux abductovalgus are:

1. extra width and depth of the forepart to accommodate the forefoot deformity together with the protective shields and splints;

2. rigid shanks to ensure a firm foundation for supporting valgus insoles;
3. a close fit round the heel and adjustable fastening to ensure the foot is held firmly back in the heel seat.

All these features may be found in particular brands of shoes. Alternatively, modifications to otherwise suitable footwear may be made by:

(a) replacing the front of the shoes with an enlarged version;
(b) balloon patches over the medial prominence;
(c) additional eyelets to improve ease of entry.

In severe cases specially made shoes may be required, but special care is necessary in the fitting in respect of the shape and depth of the forepart, the design of the upper to provide ease of entry when appliances are worn, and the weight, which should be kept to a minimum.

Surgical treatment

According to Giannestras, over 80 types of surgical procedure for hallux abductovalgus have been described. Many of these techniques are now obsolete and others are merely personalised modifications of standard techniques. Three types of approach are now commonly used (Fig. 5.9):

1. Osteotomy—to correct metatarsus primus adductus
2. Arthrodesis—fusion of the joint
3. Arthroplasty—removal of part of the joint leaving an intact, if altered, joint.

The main criterion for selection of procedure appears to be age. Osteotomies of the metatarsal are used in young patients with mild to moderate HAV. Keller's arthroplasties (resection of the proximal portion of the proximal phalanx) are used for mild to severe HAV in older patients. Arthodesis is used mainly in more severe cases and more commonly in the younger age group.

Two other approaches worthy of mention are the bunionectomy and the McBride procedure. Bunionectomy is a minimum trauma procedure used mainly on elderly patients to remove a painful medial eminence. The McBride procedure involves transferring the abductor hallucis tendon from the phalanx to the metatarsal in order to discourage adduction of the metatarsal. This is used in children and adolescents. In such cases the underlying cause of the deformity should always be sought and, where appropriate, a regime including functional orthoses instituted.

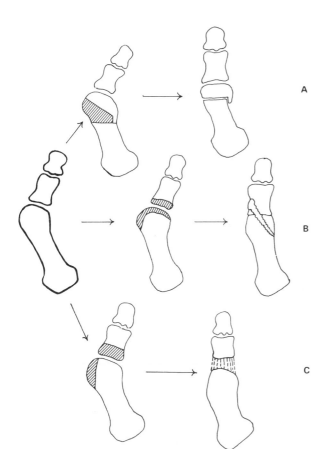

Fig. 5.9 Main operations for hallux abductovalgus: (A) Osteotomy of first metatarsal. (B) Arthrodesis of first metatarsophalangeal joint. (C) Keller's arthroplasty.

HALLUX LIMITUS: HALLUX RIGIDUS

These terms denote different degrees of loss of dorsiflexion at the first metatarsophalangeal joint. The normal range of dorsiflexion which is demonstrable in passive movement is 90°. This requires the first metatarsal to be plantarflexed so as to allow the proximal phalanx to glide dorsally without hindrance on the metatarsal head. If the metatarsal is manually dorsiflexed, the range of movement is seen to be markedly reduced. In standing tip-toe the hallux is horizontal and the metatarsal vertical—or nearly so (see Fig. 5.10). This extreme position of the joint is also reached in running and jumping, the metatarsal dorsiflexing on the fixed hallux as the heel rises. In walking, a smaller range of movement is sufficient and this decreases with age and less vigorous activity. Less than sufficient movement for the gait and activities of a particular individual becomes abnormal and probably symptomatic.

Significant limitation of dorsiflexion is termed *hallux limitus*. Total loss of dorsiflexion, which occurs in both acute and advanced cases, is termed *hallux rigidus*. This term is often used interchangeably with *hallux limitus*, but strictly speaking it should be reserved for total loss of movement in the joint, as the term implies.

Although an acute form may occasionally be seen in adolescents, the condition is most commonly a chronic disorder in adults. It is more common in men than women, usually bilateral and particularly affects tall people with long narrow feet. If unilateral, the relevant aetiological

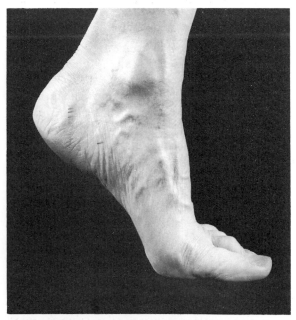

Fig. 5.10 Normal range of dorsiflexion of first metatarsophalangeal joint.

factors may be asymmetry of the two feet or unilateral injury.

Clinical features

The main feature is the loss or limitation of dorsiflexion, the degree of which should be carefully assessed. Since the joint is the most important constituent of the metatarsophalangeal hinge, on which the foot swings upward and forward as the heel is raised in locomotion, significant secondary effects result from its malfunction. Pain and stiffness in the joint may be partly compensated by the foot supinating and thereby overloading its lateral border. The resultant postural instability may strain the lateral ligaments of the ankle and recurrent ankle sprain may occur. The foot hinges abnormally on the axis of the second metatarsophalangeal joint and the interphalangeal joint of the hallux, which is usually hyperextended. The resultant imbalanced weight distribution is reflected in the formation of plantar callosities beneath these sites and also under the fifth metatarsal head because of the inverted attitude of the foot. This causes abnormal wear at the lateral sides of the heel and sole of the shoe and at the tip of the sole. The increased pressure on the distal phalanx may provoke various nail disorders such as painful nail grooves and onychocryptosis. Where there has been additional persistent pressure from the front of the shoe, as is often the case, onychogryphosis, subungual heloma, subungual haematoma and subungual exostosis are all possible complications.

Osteophytic ridging is commonly present on the dorsal margins of the joint, constituting a major factor in its loss of function (see Fig. 5.11). In some cases the dorsal prominence is so pronounced that it may be surmounted by an adventitious bursa. In other cases a tendinitis of the extensor hallucis longus may develop.

The degree of pain varies with the mode of onset and the extent of pathological changes within the joint. Except for the secondary plantar lesions, a slow insidious onset over many years may be virtually painless, whereas a more rapid progress may be extremely painful and crippling. In women, symptoms may be exacerbated by the

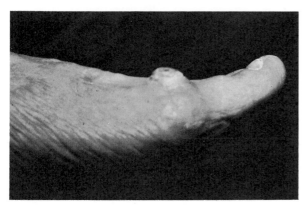

Fig. 5.11 Hallux rigidus showing dorsal exostosis.

wearing of high heels which force the joint into further dorsiflexion.

Aetiology and pathology

Excluding the small minority of cases caused by sudden direct trauma or inflammatory joint disease (rheumatoid arthritis, gout), the aetiological factors are essentially mechanical. The condition originates in a localised traumatic osteoarthrosis resulting from impaction of the joint, which becomes progressive and chronic as the underlying causative factors persist.

A number of factors predispose the joint to trauma. The long narrow foot is vulnerable to persistent impaction from footwear which is too short, or too loosely fitting to prevent the foot slipping forward at each step. A particularly long hallux poses a similar shoe fitting problem, as does a long first metatarsal, which also necessitates some adduction of the foot to bring the hinge axis of the metatarsophalangeal joints perpendicular to the angle of gait. Malformation of the epiphysis of the proximal phalanx may occur, resulting in some loss of congruity of the articular facets of the joint. Tightness of the medial band of the plantar fascia has a restraining effect on dorsiflexion of the joint. Congenital dorsiflexion of the first metatarsal (metatarsus primus elevatus) necessitates a compensatory plantarflexion of the hallux in standing and walking, which has to be maintained by over-action of its flexor muscles, which thereby limit dorsiflexion. Such an habitual attitude may induce adaptive contractures in the peri-articular

tissues which will perpetuate the relative rigidity of the joint. Congenital shortness of the first metatarsal has a similar effect, as has a forefoot varus deformity. (see also hallux flexus p. 81).

The most critical aetiological factor is hypermobility of the first metatarsal on weight-bearing. This may be a localised hypermobility of the first ray or part of a general hypermobility of the foot consequent upon persistent abnormal pronation of the rearfoot. Elevation of the metatarsal head which occurs under load for either of these reasons disrupts the normal function of the joint. To achieve the 65–70° of dorsiflexion needed for normal walking, the first metatarsal must plantarflex.

Ground reaction forces prevent this happening, and as the heel rises the upper margin of the convex metatarsal head impinges with considerable force against the dorsal rim of the concavity at the base of the proximal phalanx. Constant repetition of this process of compression and shearing induces a subacute arthritis with eventual erosion of the articular cartilage, narrowing of the joint space, increased density of sub-articular bone and proliferation of osteophytes on the dorsolateral margins of either or both of the two bones (Fig. 5.12).

In the earlier stages, this impaired function may be completely pain free and passive first metatarsophalangeal joint motion may be normal. This is termed *functional* hallux limitus, indicating that the limitation only occurs with gait as a secondary affect of abnormal pronation. At this stage, with control of abnormal pronation with functional orthoses, normal joint function can be restored. Occasionally, pain in and around the joint on movement may be severe and protective muscle spasm may hold it relatively immobile. Where pronation of the rearfoot is the primary cause of impaction of the joint, it pre-empts, to some extent, the normal reaction of inversion and adduction which would otherwise occur to protect the joint. Consequently, both injury to the joint and its resultant symptoms are more severe in such cases. The impaction is intensified by the elongation which occurs in the foot, and the leg muscles are subjected to additional strain in countering the pronation and protecting the joint.

In later stages, movement becomes more

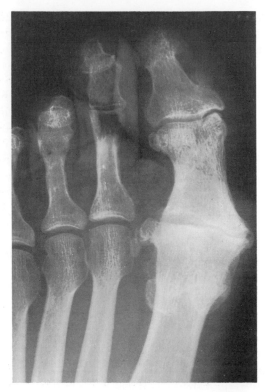

Fig. 5.12 Hallux rigidus: X-ray showing joint changes.

restricted because of the degeneration of the articular cartilages and the osteophytic formations.
Pain may then become less severe. Ultimately,
pain in the joint may cease altogether as all
movement is lost, but pain from the secondary
features such as plantar helomata may be considerable. The oblique thrust of weight-bearing
stresses through the foot consequent upon its
inversion and adduction may also cause some
compression and deformity of the lesser toes with
associated dorsal and interdigital lesions.

Management

Conservative management of the deformity in
adults is directed towards three objectives: to
relieve pain, to maintain maximum pain-free
movement and to compensate for the disturbance
of normal weight-bearing.

In the many cases where relief of pain is the first
consideration, immobilisation of the joint by
padding and strapping is indicated in the short
term. It can be effective, provided the design of

the padding and the application of the strapping
are correctly matched to the needs of the
individual case. An essential preliminary is to
ascertain the most tolerable position of the joint
and to design the padding accordingly.

When pain is acute, a shaft pad under the joint
gives immobilisation, particularly if combined
with immobilising strapping, extending from the
hallux to the metatarsal area. When pain is less
acute or receding, some gentle movement can be
tolerated and a single wing plantar metatarsal pad
with a wing cut deep to allow plantarflexion of the
first ray may help.

In some cases it is necessary to protect a painful
dorsal exostosis with an oval cavity pad, or the
plantar aspect of the interphalangeal joint with a
cavity pad shaped to the full size of the toe, so as
to transfer pressure from the joint to the full
extent of the proximal phalanx. Added depth in
the shoes is essential. Upper insertions, slit
releases or balloon patches may be needed.

In addition to such local measures hypermobility must be restrained as much as possible.
Normally, this stems from abnormal subtalar
pronation and must be controlled. Medial heel
wedges or a *cobra pad*, where the medial wedging
is extended distally to lie under the navicular in
the form of a 'D' pad, can be used with the initial
short term padding.

Heat therapy applied between re-application of
the preferred dressing at intervals of a week may
be beneficial in relieving pain.

All the foregoing measures are short term but
are useful when the patient must be kept
ambulant. They need to be used with discrimination to ensure the earliest possible relief from
pain. Easy fitting but stiff soled shoes are imperative at this stage, as is the abandonment of any
footwear likely to cause impaction of the hallux.
Attention is required to any plantar or digital
lesions.

When pain has subsided, manual traction and
circumduction of the hallux may be started.
These manipulations should be preceded by heat
therapy and the patient should be encouraged to
repeat the movements daily. Adhesive dressings
should be discontinued in favour of durable
orthoses incorporating such protective padding
previously found to have been necessary. Hallux

shields in latex or silicone may be necessary to shield the area of the joint, particularly if there are prominent exostoses.

For long-term conservative management, reliance must be placed on patient-specific orthoses. These should meet three criteria: to stabilise the foot by controlling abnormal pronation or supination, to keep movement in the joint as nearly as possible pain-free and to protect overloaded areas of the plantar surface.

Hypermobility within the foot secondary to abnormal pronation must be prevented by functional orthoses where arthritic joint changes are not severe, because there is no satisfactory method of stabilising a hypermobile first ray, which permits pronation. Stabilising the first metatarsal in its elevated position by placing shaft padding beneath it increases its load-bearing capacity despite its laxity, but may not wholly counter the pronatory influence. Medial heel wedging and valgus padding are additional requirements in all such cases.

Shaft padding also minimises the dorsiflexion of the joint, thereby contributing to the patient's comfort and it protects the interphalangeal joint from the effects of overloading.

Compensatory supination of the foot, which is effective in minimising joint symptoms, may lead to recurrent lateral ankle sprain and/or plantar lesions under the fifth metatarsal head. This effect can be well controlled by supporting the lateral tarsal area with a tarsal platform ('filler pad'), which simultaneously stabilises the ankle and relieves pressure on the fifth metatarsal head. For the latter purpose, it can be extended under the middle metatarsal heads to provide a wing. In cases such as the highly arched but flaccid foot, in which compensatory supination is inhibited by early pronation, the foot requires to be balanced in a neutral position which controls both the pronatory and the supinatory tendencies. This is achieved by a combination of both tarsal platform and valgus support which together stabilise both the medial and the lateral structures of the foot.

Appropriate metatarsal padding must also be incorporated into the insole design to relieve excessive pressure on the areas subject to plantar helomata and callosities. The choice of corrective and protective measures depends on the extent of the pathological changes and their aetiology. Some examples for possible applications are given in Figure 5.13.

Sufficient length and depth of footwear is essential to obviate any impaction of the hallux or pressure on an enlarged joint. A low heel is desirable for both men and women and the soles should be as stiff as possible so as to act as splints. An additional sole is often sufficient for this purpose. In heavy working boots a steel splint may be fitted from heel to toe, suitably curved and shaped to conform to the heel pitch, the toe spring and the shape of the sole. A rocker sole to enable the foot to rock over the stiff joint is a possible alternative. However, some of these devices are unsuitable for use in certain occupations such as those involving much climbing of stairs or ladders, and for many women's shoes. If conservative measures do not succeed in relieving symptoms, and if long-term reliance on appliances and footwear adjustments is unacceptable, surgical intervention is indicated.

Surgical treatment. Most cases of hallux limitus are caused by excessive joint tension. If severe degenerative changes are not evident then it may be possible to salvage the joint. Cheilectomy may remove osteophytic hypertrophy, but will not relax the periarticular tissues sufficiently to alter the long-term prognosis. A modified Watermann or Austin procedure, which shortens the first metatarsal, will assist in relieving joint tension. Plantarflexion of the capital fragment may be performed simultaneously to offset the functional loss of weight-bearing length.

If the joint is deemed non-functional, then arthroplasty with either a hemi- or total joint implant may be used. Adequate resection of bone is necessary to ensure that the implant is not subjected to the excessive tension which was present prior to surgery. A structural metatarsus primus elevatus may also lead to hallux limitus, and is best managed by plantarflexory osteotomy of the first metatarsal.

HALLUX FLEXUS

This term describes the abnormal position of the hallux which is plantarflexed from the first

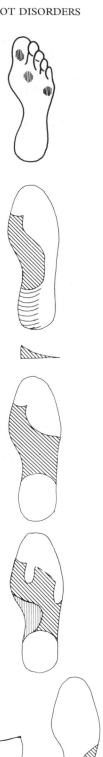

Fig. 5.13   Hallux rigidus.
A. Typical distribution of plantar lesions.

B. Medial heel wedging with valgus and shaft padding to control pronation, stabilise elevated first metatarsal, and minimise movement in 1st metatarsophalangeal joint.

C. Tarsal platform and shaft padding to stabilise compensatory supination, and minimise overloading and strain of lateral border and ankle. Metatarsal bar element may be added if required to aid rocker action and to reduce supination of forefoot.

D. Combination of tarsal platform, valgus, shaft and shaped metatarsal padding to balance foot medio-laterally and to protect 2nd and 5th metatarsal heads and interphalangeal joint of hallux from overloading. Metatarsal bar element and/or heel wedges added as necessary.

E. Flared heel and/or reverse Thomas heel if lateral ankle instability present.

metatarsophalangeal joint. The deformity is usually mobile, but may become fixed.

In the great majority of cases its only significance is as a secondary feature of one or other of the following syndromes: forefoot varus, a hypermobile or short first metatarsal, or a congenital metatarsus primus elevatus. In all such cases, the plantarflexion of the hallux occurs as a functional compensation to improve the stability and functional capacity of the forefoot in the presence of an unstable and relatively incompetent first metatarsal. The plantarflexion is initiated by the flexor muscles of the hallux, but secondary contractures in the joint capsule from persistence of the abnormal attitude result in some limitation of dorsiflexion even at rest. Eventually pathological changes in the joint similar to those in hallux limitus may ensue, further limiting dorsiflexion and consolidating the flexion deformity. The effect is to disturb the normal pattern of weight-bearing by overloading the interphalangeal joint and the second metatarsal head, with the probable result of painful lesions developing at these sites.

Hallux flexus may also develop temporarily in response to painful stimuli from the region of the plantar surface of the first and second metatarsal heads, e.g. from a verruca. The diagnosis and cure in these cases is usually obvious. Occasionally, hallux flexus may be the result of either direct trauma or indirect injury, e.g. paralysis of the anterior tibial nerve to the extensor muscles of the hallux.

The treatment of the deformity and its effect depends on the identification of the primary syndrome and the application of appropriate measures, as described in foregoing pages. Basically, these are designed to balance the foot posture with suitable orthoses which will also protect over-loaded areas of the plantar surface (see also hallux limitus, hallux rigidus pp. 72 & 77)

METATARSALGIA

Metatarsalgia is a general term denoting pain in the metatarsophalangeal area and it is symptomatic of many different conditions. A number of specific local conditions including stress fracture, plantar digital neuritis and arthritis are all sources of pain in this region and they are mentioned elsewhere. The term 'functional metatarsalgia' denotes pain in the area caused by abnormal mechanical stresses resulting from disordered function of the foot.

The differential diagnosis and management of functional metatarsalgia is obviously bound up with the underlying condition. Its association with pes planovalgus, pes cavus and hallux abductovalgus has already been mentioned, but it may also be symptomatic of other metatarsophalangeal abnormalities.

Metatarsophalangeal abnormalities

In stance, the five metatarsal heads lie in the same transverse plane on bearing weight and share the load equally, except that the first takes a double load through its two sesamoids. The middle three metatarsals are firmly articulated at their bases and have only a very limited range of dorsoplantar movement at their heads for purposes of shock absorption and adaptation to the surface. The first and fifth, however, have capacity for movement in all three planes, and this enables them, in locomotion, to adjust to varying attitudes of the forefoot to the ground and to varying and uneven surfaces.

Apart from the previously mentioned effects on the metatarsophalangeal area of hindfoot deformities and hallux abductovalgus, the position and functioning of the middle three metatarsal heads is usually disturbed only by malposition and malfunction of their respective digits as when they are pinned down by digital retraction or subluxation. The first and fifth metatarsals, on the other hand, may in some cases be either hypermobile or relatively dorsiflexed in relation to the others. In each case they are elevated excessively under load, are relatively incompetent as weight-bearing members and thereby overload their neighbours. In other cases they may be relatively plantar-flexed and held in that position by tight fascial bands so that they themselves are overloaded—an actual 'transverse metatarsal arch', which is pathological. Such disturbances of normal weight-bearing are reflected in the pattern of hyperkeratotic lesions seen on the plantar surface.

Medio-lateral stability of the metatarsophalangeal area is provided passively by the transverse metatarsal ligaments and actively by the tranverse head of the adductor hallucis, which together restrain the natural spread of the metatarsals under load. When the foot as a whole is hypermobile, as with persistent abnormal pronation, and also in hallux abductovalgus, these structures are often unable to prevent the metatarsals splaying apart because the adductor hallucis no longer has a stable anchorage at its medial insertion. The splaying is most marked in the case of the first and fifth metatarsals as they are less firmly articulated at their bases than the others. This not only increases the width of the forefoot, it also initiates or increases the tendency to abduction of their metatarsals. Both hallux abductovalgus and digitus quintus varus deformities are thereby precipitated or worsened. The splaying of the metatarsals together with the hypermobility of the foot causes shearing stresses on the first and fifth metatarsal heads from contract with the sides of the footwear, with resultant exostosis and bursal formation at these sites.

The plantar tissues of the forefoot undergo compression, shearing and tensile stresses in the normal course of standing and walking. The excessive stresses which provoke the pain responses comprised under the term metatarsalgia may be produced in various ways.

Abnormal compression

This occurs from undue rigidity of the foot (as in rigid pes cavus, ankle equinus and forefoot equinus); from fixation of one or more metatarsals or metatarsophalangeal joints, such as may occur from impaction and constriction of the toes or fixed plantarflexion of the first or fifth rays; from fixed retraction or clawing of the toes; or from subluxation or dislocation of any of the metatarsophalangeal joints. In hallux abductovalgus, for example, the second toe may become hammered and the metatarsophalangeal joint subluxated or dislocated.

Persistent abnormal compression of the plantar tissues results in contusion and inflammation of the soft tissues and in nucleated plantar keratosis.

Abnormal shearing

Abnormal shearing occurs most commonly form hypermobility of the whole foot (as with abnormal pronation); from hypermobility of the first and fifth rays; and also from forward movement of the foot in an ill-fitting shoe. Abnormal shearing results in inflammation of the plantar tissues, diffuse plantar keratosis and possibly in bursal formation beneath and anterior to the metatarsal heads.

Abnormal compression and shearing may occur concurrently in the same foot, as in a hypermobile foot with a subluxated hammer toe. Evidence of both types of stress is presented in the form of a diffuse plantar callus with a nucleus under the fixed metatarsal head.

Abnormal tensile stresses

These result from splaying of the metatarsals, and the resultant strain on the transverse ligaments and muscles, and the intrinsic muscle fatigue, contribute to the pain of metatarsalgia.

Other contributory factors include excessive weight-bearing (obesity, pregnancy, occupational factors) and unsuitable footwear (short and narrow shoes which impede toe function, incorrect heel-to-ball fitting, soles too thin to give adequate protection). Local ischaemia, however caused, may also be a factor. Atrophy or displacement of the plantar fibro-fatty pads under the metatarsal heads, with consequent loss of shock absorption, is seen in rheumatoid arthritis and in old age.

Persistent traumatisation of the plantar tissues induces *fibrosis* in the dermis as a functional adaptation, often accompanied by some corresponding diminution of adipose tissue. Fibrosis is clinically manifest as a toughening or induration of the integument into deep folds or craters underlying plantar helomata and callosities. After enucleation, these structural deformations in the dermis are clearly palpable as fixed corrugations or pits in the otherwise uniform and even texture of the plantar skin. Their shape and size are indicative of the types of abnormal stresses which have caused them and so are significant diagnostically. If the abnormal stresses are not adequately controlled such dermal deformations provide ready-made sites for continuing hyperkeratotic activity and add significantly to the chronicity of plantar lesions. The papillae at the crests or margins of these irregularities are often hypertrophied, the neurovascular elements within them providing an additional source of pain. In addition to whatever mechanical therapy is indicated, medication by astringents, caustics, exfoliants or emollients may be required for the local dermal fibrosis (Ch. 11).

Management

The successful management of metatarsalgia, as of other conditions, depends upon identifying the

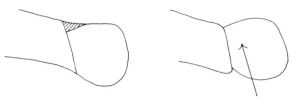

Fig. 5.15   Metatarsalgia: metatarsal osteotomy.

causes and eliminating or mitigating their ill-effects. In the cases where metatarsalgia is symptomatic of forefoot rather than hindfoot malfunction, the main consideration must be to ensure maximum function of the lesser toes and their metatarsophalangeal joints. Retraction and clawing of the toes, which impairs their normal function and pins down their respective metatarsal heads, needs to be corrected as far as possible by orthodigital splints which straighten the toes, improve their alignment with their metatarsals and promote better toe function. When necessary, metatarsal padding may be combined with them, the digital splints holding the metatarsal padding in place—with or without a metatarsal brace (Fig. 5.14). The same design is also effective as a palliative measure, when no improvement in digital function can be expected.

Passive and active exercises should be instituted to stretch the toes and improve the range of movement of the metatarsophalangeal joints. Re-education of the intrinsic muscles is assisted by the use of Faradic foot baths, which also relieve the metatarsalgia.

Various types of metatarsal padding are illustrated in Chapter 11. The metatarsal brace—with or without padding—controls transverse splaying of the metatarsals and is helpful in certain cases. Palliative metatarsal cushioning is indicated in cases of atrophy or displacement of the plantar fibro-fatty pads. In the majority of cases, symptoms are relieved completely by attention to the underlying foot fault and to shoe fitting problems.

When metatarsalgia is due to prominence of a single metatarsal head and symptoms are unrelieved by conservative measures, metatarsal osteotomy may be helpful. The cut is made obliquely through the neck of the metatarsal, allowing the head to ride up into a position in which it is no longer prominent (Fig. 5.15).

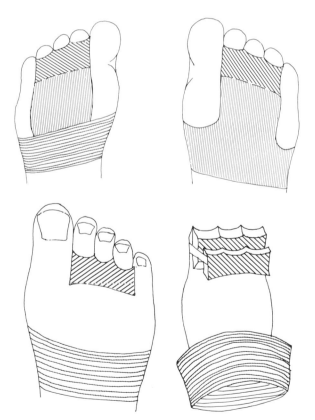

Fig. 5.14   Metatarsalgia: metatarsal brace combined with orthodigital splints.

PLANTAR DIGITAL NEURITIS (MORTON'S METATARSALGIA)

Plantar digital neuritis most frequently occurs in the nerve supplying the 3rd/4th interdigital space and occasionally in the nerve to the 2nd/3rd interdigital space (Fig. 5.16). It is almost always unilateral, typically affecting women between about 25 and 50 years of age. The symptoms vary in severity from an occasional pins and needles sensation to a sudden and acute pain around the metatarsal heads, which brings the sufferer to a halt. The pain frequently radiates forwards to one or both of the fourth and third toes and occasionally extends up the leg. A painful attack typically occurs suddenly after a period of walking or standing on a hard or possibly uneven surface. Shoes which unduly constrict the forefoot may precipitate or worsen the pain, and relief is often obtained by removing the shoe and massaging or squeezing the forefoot. If the foot is examined at

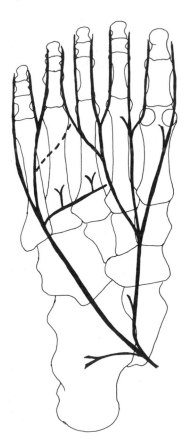

Fig. 5.16   Plantar digital neuritis: the plantar nerves.

the time, some congestion or cyanosis may be observed. On later examination no structural abnormality may be evident; however manual compression of the forefoot across the metatarsal heads together with upward pressure on the sole of the foot in the region of he 3rd/4th interspace may elicit a painful click (known as 'Mulder's click'). This is a reasonably certain diagnostic feature of an inter-metatarsal neuroma.

Aetiology and pathology

Although the symptoms of plantar digital neuritis are typical, the aetiology is uncertain and various explanations for the condition have been put forward.

Morton originally suggested that the pain arose from the pinching of a digital nerve by the metatarsal head, and this is generally thought to be the most common factor. Additional factors have subsequently been suggested and they are briefly summarised:

1. Referred pain from inflammation of the medial plantar nerve, as it was affected by adjacent arthritis of the second metatarso-cuneiform joint—the arthritis being induced by strain in this joint from overloading of the second metatarsal segment secondary to a short and incompetent first metatarsal. This view is not now widely held.

2. The presence of a neurofibroma, which has been frequently demonstrated, and excision of which has become standard surgical practice.

3. Occlusion of the plantar digital artery by weight-bearing pressure and fibrosis of the surrounding tissues, the resultant ischaemia inducing symptoms.

4. Fibrosis of the neurovascular bundles caused by abnormal shearing stresses in the area as the metatarsal heads move excessively to and fro because of abnormal pronation of the foot. The partial occlusion of blood vessels by fibrosis is compounded by constriction of the forefoot by footwear, which thus precipitates a painful attack.

It is difficult to escape the conclusion that the typical symptoms do not always arise from the same pathological features, but it seems likely that any circumstances which give rise to continuing abnormal compressional or shearing stresses in that area will bring about fibrosis and consequent ischaemia in the plantar neurovascular bundles.

Management

The foot should be carefully assessed for any structural or functional disorder which may underlie the complaint, particularly abnormal pronation and hypermobility which abducts the forefoot in relation to the hindfoot and thereby generates abnormal stresses in this particular area when the foot is weight-bearing and wearing shoes. Pronation should restrained by appropriately designed insoles. Any footwear suspected of unduly constricting the forefoot should be discarded, at least temporarily.

Padding should be applied to reduce the pressure of weight-bearing on the affected area and also to improve the functional alignment of the respective metatarsal segments. A plantar metatarsal pad with a cavity for the sensitive area is often effective, particularly if secured in place with full metatarsal strapping. Digital padding is also usually necessary (although often overlooked) in order to straighten toes which may be partially clawed or axially rotated. Alternative combinations of such padding may need to be undertaken in order to eliminate the particular juxtaposition of the bones and tissues which excite the painful attacks. When found effective, the padding should be supplied in durable form, as an insole, a metatarsal brace, a dorsoplantar digital splint, or a combination of the two latter appliances.

If necessary, the condition can be very satisfactorily dealt with surgically. The neuroma is excised through either a plantar or dorsal incision. No further treatement is neccessary after removal of the stitches. Although pain is relieved, there will be some numbness in the affected toe cleft (almost invariably the one between the third and fourth toes) and patients should be warned of this before operation.

MARCH FRACTURE (PIED FORCÉ)

Fracture of the neck of one of the lesser metatarsals, most often the second or third, may occur in circumstances involving abnormal stress in the particular bone (stress fracture). The fracture is the culmination of persistent abnormal stress, e.g. forced marching.

The site of the fracture is painful and swollen, tender to touch and to any movement of the metatarsal head. The swelling over the neck of the metatarsal is localised and firm. There is always a recent history of unusual overactivity. The diagnosis is confirmed by X-ray although the oblique hairline fracture may not be evident initially or for some days thereafter. The cortex of the bone is then irregular with marked callus formation (see Fig. 5.17).

Surgical supervision is required. Immobilisation of the part in a walking plaster and relief from weight-bearing are essential and union is usually uneventful. Pending setting in plaster, a weight relieving metatarsal pad cut out over the affected metatarsal head and applied with a full metatarsal strapping will give temporary relief from pain.

A similar type of fracture of the neck of a metatarsal may, of course, be precipitated by sudden trauma, as could occur when jumping off a bus.

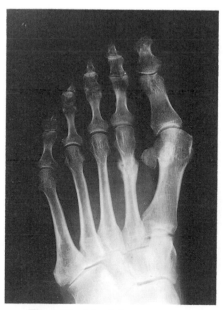

Fig. 5.17 March fracture.

FREIBERG'S INFRACTION

The late effect of Freiberg's infraction of the second metatarsal head (occasionally the third) is to leave flattened articular surfaces at the metatarsophalangeal joint (see Fig. 5.18). In later life this results in osteoarthrosis with limitation of dorsoplantar movement, periarticular osteophytic proliferation and pain. Pending possible surgical intervention, treatment is directed to relief of weight-bearing by protective padding, preferably by means of a well-designed insole, and possibly a rocker sole.

Operative treatment is indicated if pain is unrelieved by such measures. The procedures preferred are excision of the head of the affected metatarsal or excision of the proximal half of the proximal phalanx of the corresponding toe.

DIGITAL MALFUNCTIONS AND DEFORMITIES

Retracted toes

In this condition, the toes are drawn back into a dorsiflexed position and are therefore less effective in locomotion. They are subjected to shoe pressure on the dorsum of their interphalangeal joints with resultant dorsal lesions. The condition is one aspect of the ankle equinus syndrome, with limitation of dorsiflexion of the foot, tightness of the tendo Achilles group of muscles, relative inefficiency of the tibialis anterior and overaction of the digital extensors in assisting dorsiflexion of the foot. This is termed 'extensor substitution'.

The primary condition needs correction or accommodation as previously described. Additionally, exercises may be indicated to improve the muscle imbalance. Orthodigital splints are effective in improving the alignment and function of the toes and protecting their dorsal surfaces from shoe pressure. Surgical correction is discussed in Chapter 18.

Claw toes

In this condition, the interphalangeal joints are flexed and the toes are drawn into a claw-like position. They are usually extended at the metatarsophalangeal joints. They therefore suffer from greatly increased pressure on their apices and on the dorsum of their proximal interphalangeal joints. These areas are commonly the sites of painful and persistent apical and dorsal helomata and/or bursitis.

In some cases, the deformity is merely the end result of persistent impaction and constriction from ill-fitting footwear. More commonly it is symptomatic of various alternative aetiologies.

In abnormal pronation of the foot, the tibialis posterior and the long digital flexors may overact to maintain stability. In so doing, the long flexors overpower the interossei and lumbricals, thus buckling and clawing the toes. This process is termed 'flexor stabilisation'.

In *pes cavus* of neurological origin, notably Charcot-Marie-Tooth disease, wasting of the intrinsic muscles which normally keep the toes straight results in imbalanced flexor/extensor activity which contracts the toes into the typical clawed deformity. In other cases of pes cavus, where there is no neurological involvement, the forefoot is both adducted and plantarflexed at the midtarsal or tarsometatarsal joints. The toes are correspondingly abducted and dorsiflexed at their articulations with the metatarsals. Their lumbricals and interossei are mechanically at a disadvantage and the action of the long flexors and

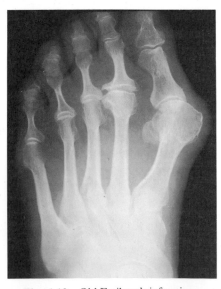

Fig. 5.18 Old Freiberg's infraction.

extensors on the terminal phalanges is therefore unrestrained. Without the moderating influence of the lumbricals and interossei on the interphalangeal joints, the toes are contracted into the clawed position.

Overaction of the long flexors may also occur to compensate for weakness of the tendo Achilles group in locomotion ('flexor substitution').

In *upper motor neurone lesions*, clawing of the toes occurs from spasmodic contraction of the long and short digital flexors. It may also be seen in *rheumatoid arthritis* as a result of the inflammatory process in the interphalangeal joints.

Clawing of the toes entails progressive subluxation of the metatarsophalangeal joints so that the metatarsal heads are more firmly pinned down in locomotion and thereby overloaded. This deformation of the metatarsal segments is clearly seen in clawing of the hallux. The first metatarsal is plantarflexed, the proximal phalanx extended and the distal phalanx flexed. This deformity is sometimes incorrectly called 'hallux flexus', but this term should be confined to flexion deformity of the whole toe, and not just of the terminal phalanx as in this case. Plantar hyperkeratosis develops under the first metatarsal head and possibly also under the distal phalanx, and a dorsal lesion appears over the interphalangeal joint. The latter may develop into a bursitis and an underlying exostosis. The lesser toes are subject to similar lesions on their dorsal surfaces and at their apices. Ulceration and infection may supervene at any of these sites.

Management

Conservative management of claw toes is directed to the treatment of their associated lesions and to protective padding. For the middle toes, orthodigital splints provide the most effective means of protection. For the first and fifth toes, individual shields in silicone rubber are generally more satisfactory.

Surgery is indicated if the deformities of the toes are too marked to allow symptoms to be adequately controlled by conservative means. Arthrodesis of the interphalangeal joints of the lesser toes may be carried out, and for the hallux,

transfer of the tendon of extensor hallucis longus to the neck of the first metatarsal (Ch. 18.).

Hammer toe

This is essentially a plantarflexion deformity of the proximal interphalangeal joint, the distal interphalangeal joint remaining normal or possibly dorsiflexed. It occurs in any of the three middle toes, the second being most commonly affected. The proximal phalanx is extended and the deformity therefore exposes the proximal interphalangeal joint to dorsal pressure and friction, and the apex of the toe to concentrated pressure as it bears weight. The abnormal joint positions become more or less fixed by adaptive contractures of the surrounding capsule and tendons, depending on how long the deformity has persisted.

In most early cases it is correctable by persistence with corrective splinting and manipulation. Ankylosis of the proximal interphalangeal joint may occur in long-standing cases.

The deformity is caused in various ways. It may be concomitant with a short first metatarsal segment, the abnormally short hallux exposing the second toe—and possibly also the third—to impaction from footwear fitted too short because the unusual digital formula has been overlooked. The second toe is also commonly deformed by pressure from an abducted hallux, which may more or less override the intermediate and distal phalanges. The fourth toe often becomes hammered because the fifth toe underrides it, elevating its proximal phalanx and causing shoe pressure on the dorsum of the proximal interphalangeal joint. The immediate cause of the deviation of the fifth toe is pressure from the lateral side of the shoe which may be too narrow or pointed, but hallux valgus and splaying of the metatarsals are the main factors, coupled with abduction of the forefoot where this occurs in pes plano valgus.

Where all three of the middle toes are affected, the primary cause may lie in failure of the lumbricals to keep the toes straight in locomotion, thus allowing the proximal phalanges to be excessively dorsiflexed on their respective metatarsal heads.

The digital flexors then act more powerfully on the intermediate and distal phalanges, flexing them into an attitude of deformity ('flexor stabilisation').

The chief effect of these deformities is to cause painful and persistent digital helomata. Adventitious bursitis also commonly occurs on the dorsal sites, particularly on the second and fourth toes, occasionally becoming secondarily infected. Ulceration may occur at the apices, more especially where the nutrition of the tissues is impaired by circulatory, neurological or metabolic deficiencies. Painful nail conditions may also arise from persistent trauma to the distal phalanges.

Management

Conservative management is therefore directed to correction of the deformities by splinting and manipulation where correction is still possible, or to provide maximum protection of both the dorsal and apical pressure points in chronic cases. Both of these objectives are best achieved by orthodigital splints covering all three middle toes. Padding for a single toe may be temporarily necessary to bring a particular lesion under control, but the maximum degree of correction or protection can be ensured only by controlling the position and alignment of all three toes simultaneously. This ensures that correction or protection of one toe is not obtained at the cost of displacing the others.

Surgery is indicated if conservative treatment does not resolve the problem of recurrent pressure

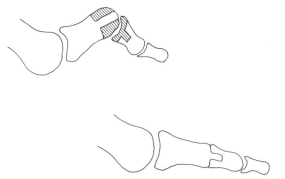

Fig. 5.19   Arthrodesis for hammer toe.

lesions. An arthrodesis of the proximal interphalangeal joint is performed, correcting any flexion deformity (Fig. 5.19). It may be necessary to divide capsule and tendon at the metatarsophalangeal joint to correct dorsiflexion of the proximal phalanx. In older patients, an alternative is to remove the proximal half of the proximal phalanx of the affected toe, making it slightly floppy and able to take up a position where there is no pressure upon it (Ch. 18).

Mallet toe

This is an abnormal plantarflexion of the distal phalanx only, most commonly of the second or third toes. It is not always symptomatic but may be the cause of persistent apical lesions.

It is amenable to the same treatment as hammer toes by means of orthodigital splints. If pressure on the apex is insufficiently relieved the toe may be straightened by arthrodesis of the terminal interphalangeal joint. Partial amputation of the toe is an effective alternative, although aesthetically not as acceptable.

Digitus quintus varus

This common deformity of the fifth toe is often congenital (see Ch. 4), but in the adult it is most commonly acquired. As with hallux abductovalgus, the persistent moulding effect of pointed footwear is a relevant factor, but the abduction of the forefoot secondary to pes plano valgus is probably more important. The toe is usually not only abducted but also axially rotated and flexed, indicating an oblique pull on the phalanges by the flexor tendons due to the abduction of the forefoot on the hindfoot.

The deformity is the immediate cause of painful pressure lesions dorsally, interdigitally and distally, which can best be relieved by latex or silicone rubber shields designed to provide optimum correction and protection. The abnormal pronation leading to the abduction of the forefoot must also be adequately controlled and any footwear faults eliminated as far as possible. Surgery may be indicated (Ch. 18).

FURTHER READING

Adams J C 1986 Outline of orthopaedics, 10th edn. Churchill Livingstone, Edinburgh

Ball J 1971 Enthesopathy of rheumatoid and ankylosing spondylitis. Annals of the Rheumatic Diseases 30: 3 (May) (The Heberden Oration)

Barnicott N A, Hardy R H 1955 The position of the hallux in West Africans. Journal of Anatomy 89: 355–361

Du Vries H L 1978 Surgery of the foot, 4th edn. Mosby, St Louis

Edgar 1982 In: Klenerman L (ed) The foot and its disorders, 2nd edn. Blackwell, Oxford

Elftmann H 1960 The transverse tarsal joint and its control. Clinical Orthopaedics 16: 41–45

Giannestras N J 1973 Foot disorders—medical and surgical management , 2nd edn. Lea and Febiger, Philadelphia

Haines R W, McDougall A 1954 The anatomy of hallux valgus. Journal of Bone and Joint Surgery 36-A: 272

Hardy R H, Clapham J C R 1952 Hallux valgus—predisposing anatomical causes. Lancet 1180–1183

Jahss M H 1982 Disorders of the foot, Vols I and II. Saunders, Philadelphia

Johnston O 1956 Further studies of the inheritance of hand and foot anomalies. Clinical Orthopaedics 8: 146–160

Klenerman L (ed) 1982 The foot and its disorders, 2nd edn. Blackwell, Oxford

Manter J T 1941 Movements of the subtalar and transverse tarsal joints. The Anatomical Record 80.4

Lake N C 1943 The foot, 3rd edn. Baillière Tindall & Cox, London

Morton D J 1935 The human foot. Columbia University Press, New York

Root M L, Orien W P, Weed J H 1977 Normal and abnormal function of the foot. Clinical Biomechanics, Vol II. Clinical Biomechanical Corporation, Los Angeles

Sandelin 1922 In: Kelekian 1965 Hallux valgus and allied deformities of the forefoot and metatarsalgia. Saunders, Phildelphia

Sandelin T 1923 Operative treatment of hallux valgus. Journal of Anatomy (Abstract from an original article in Fiinska 1922 Lakaresallskapets Handlingar, Hesingfors, 64: 543

Schuster R O 1975 Personal communication

Sgarlato T E 1981 A compendium of podiatric biomechanics. California College of Podiatric Medicine, San Francisco

Shine I 1965 Incidence of hallux valgus in a partially shoe wearing community. British Medical Journal 5461: 1648–1650

Siebel M O 1988 Foot function: A programmed text. Churchill Livingstone, Edinburgh

Sim Fook L, Hodgson A R 1958 A comparison of foot forms among non-shoe and shoe wearing Chinese populations. Journal of Bone and Joint Surgery 40: 1058–1062

Stamm T T 1958 A guide to orthopaedics. Blackwell, Oxford

6. Skin and subcutaneous tissues

Michael F. Whiting

CONDITIONS OF THE SKIN AND SUBCUTANEOUS TISSUES

The environment in which the foot functions predisposes to a range of disorders which arise from, or are related to, one or more of the special conditions which apply to the shod foot. Mechanical damage arises from interaction with the shoe or ground, and the role of the foot in weight-bearing and transmission results in the need for a high level of adaptation to meet demands placed upon it. The enclosed environment of the shoe is conducive to the development of extensive microbial flora which, combined with the possibility of mechanical abrasion, increases the risk of infection. These same environmental factors create conditions in which increased sweating easily takes place, with water retention in the skin due to non-evaporation associated with occlusion.

The foot is supplied by blood vessels which are at the periphery of the circulatory system and therefore more prone to damage from pathological processes and gravitational effects. Metabolic and neurological disease are both likely to involve the foot at some stage. Finally, the skin of the foot, which is encased for much of the time in footwear, may show a range of local disorders arising from the unique and somewhat hostile environment in which it is required to function. It may also demonstrate signs of general skin disease.

As a result of the interaction of these factors, the skin and subcutaneous tissues of the foot have associated with them a number of disorders, some of them specific to the foot, arising from different sources. It is possible to classify them into five groups:

1. *Conditions arising from mechanical stress.* Of these, the most common are helomata (corns) callosities (tyloma), bursitis and a range of complications which arise from them. Because of their frequency and ability to produce chronic disability, these conditions are discussed in some detail.

2. *Conditions arising from infection.* Bacterial infections of the foot mainly occur as complications of traumatic lesions or are associated with circulatory, neurological or metabolic disease and will be mentioned in these sections. Verrucae are caused by the human papilloma virus (HPV) and are the common virus infection of the foot. Tinea pedis or athlete's foot, is the most common mycotic infection and is caused by a number of pathogenic fungi. Each of these infections is discussed separately.

3. *Disorders of the sweat glands.* Hyperhidrosis, bromhidrosis and anhidrosis are states of altered function of the sweat glands and each has potential clinical significance.

4. *Deficiency states.* These arise from circulatory, neurological and metabolic disorders. Atherosclerosis affecting the arteries of the leg places the foot at risk of ischaemic ulceration and gangrene. Diabetes mellitus, both as a result of disordered metabolism and its associated macro- and microangiopathy, is prone to give rise to complications in the foot. Vasomotor dystrophy and vasospastic disorders which give rise to erythema pernio, Raynaud's disease, vascular spasm and trophic ulceration are included. The gravitational effects on circulation, giving rise to

varicose veins and varicose ulcers, are considered in relation to the tissues of the foot.

5. *Dermatological conditions* which affect the skin of the foot and have a wider significance, requiring recognition and possible referral, are reviewed. Included in this section are dermatitis, eczema and purpura.

CONDITIONS ARISING FROM MECHANICAL STRESSES

The mechanical stresses to which the skin and subcutaneous tissues of the foot are subjected are classified as compressional, tensile, shearing and torsional (Fig. 6.1). Understanding the way in which these stresses arise in the foot during movement and when standing is necessary in order to formulate effective treatment strategies.

Compressional stress arises from two convergent forces acting in opposite directions, e.g. the plantar tissues of the heel and forefoot undergo compression between superimposed bodyweight and the resistance of the ground beneath. Less obviously, the interdigital surfaces of the toes are compressed when the toes and forefoot are subjected to compression in the front of a tightly fitting shoe.

Tensile stress results in the stretching of tissues. It occurs when a force is applied in a single plane but is divergent, acting in opposite direction, e.g. the plantar ligaments and fascia are subjected to tensile stress on weight-bearing. Tensile stress is applied to the skin when the soft tissues are compressed under the heel and forefoot and the skin is stretched laterally during weight-bearing.

Shearing stress arises when forces act in different planes and in opposite directions. Shearing occurs commonly in the tissues of the feet because of

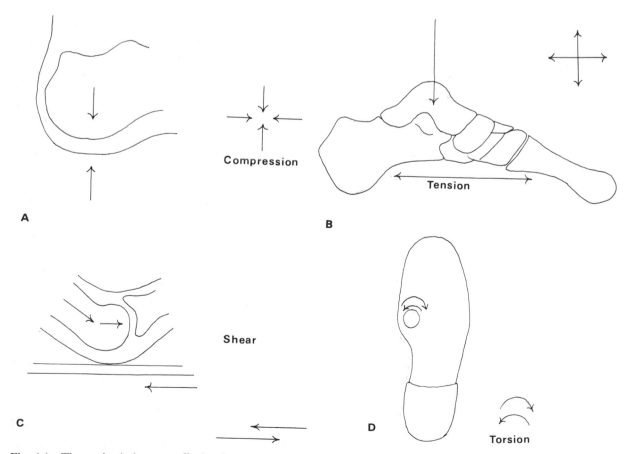

Fig. 6.1 The mechanical stresses affecting the structures of the feet. (A) Compression. (B) Tension. (C) Shear. (D) Torsion.

movements of the bony structures within the foot relative to the soft tissues, and movement between the foot and shoe during walking. It is potentially damaging to the tissues of the foot when one layer is forced violently over another.

Torsional stress is shearing combined with rotation. It occurs within the plantar tissues when the foot makes any pivoting motion.

Each of these mechanical stresses is normally well tolerated by the foot, but may give rise to pathological changes if the toleration threshold of the tissue is exceeded. The strength of tissues may be reduced in abnormal states and give rise to a reduced threshold of tolerance such that damage is more easily produced. For example, normal skin is strongly resistant to splitting from tensile stress (fissures) but skin which has been weakened by sweat retention and maceration, or is anhidrotic, splits easily.

When the tolerance of skin and subcutaneous tissue to mechanical stress has been exceeded, each produces its own characteristic effects which, if severe enough, result in tissue trauma and injury. Sustained mild injury to the skin and soft tissues of the foot may give rise to helomata, callosities, bursitis, blisters and small ulcerations. The nature of the lesion which is produced reflects the types of mechanical stress giving rise to it. Analysis of the mechanical cause of a lesion indicates the approach to remedial action which is likely to be most effective.

Hyperkeratosis

This is the name given to a state of thickening of the keratinised layers of the skin. It occurs in a wide range of skin disorders but in the foot is most commonly seen in the form of *callus*, which is a discrete area of thickened skin, or in *helomata*, which are small areas of callus containing a deep centre or nucleus of parakeratotic cells which press into the underlying dermis to cause pain.

The normal physiological process of keratinisation which maintains the stratum corneum as a horny protective cover, becomes stimulated to overactivity under the influence of intermittent compression. The resultant hypertrophy of the stratum corneum is thought to be the product of accelerated proliferation of epidermal cells, stimu- lated by reactive hyperaemia, and stronger cohesion of the surface cells which decreases the rate of desquamation. This process is termed *hyperkeratosis* and it is a normal protective response as seen, for example, in the hands of manual labourers. Any asymptomatic area of such physiological callus on the foot has a protective function and does not require to be removed. Hyperkeratosis becomes pathological only when it is so thick that it causes painful symptoms and significant deformation to the normal papillary stratification of the skin. Hyperkeratosis may also result from congenital, hormonal, occupational and infective factors, but in the present context only traumatic hyperkeratosis is considered.

Hyperkeratotic lesions

The size, shape, thickness and density of an area of traumatic hyperkeratosis is indicative of the stresses responsible for its development. A *callus* (*callosity* or *tyloma*) is a diffuse area of relatively even thickness. An *heloma* is an area of callus which is complicated by a deep central mass of cornified cells, called a *nucleus*, which presses into the underlying dermis. The nucleus is usually an inverted cone but varies in shape and size according to the location and the prevailing stresses.

Corns (Lat. *cornu*: a horn) or helomata (Grk. *helos*: a stone wedge) are classified as hard (*heloma durum*), soft (*heloma molle*), vascular (*heloma vasculare*) and neurovascular (*heloma neurovasculare*).

Helomata durum (Fig. 6.2) occur on the dorsum of the interphalangeal joints of the toes, on their apices and on the plantar surface of the foot beneath the metatarsal heads. Less frequently, they arise on the plantar medial aspect of the interphalangeal joint of the hallux. They also occur interdigitally, beneath a nail (*subungual heloma*), or in the nail sulcus (*onychophosis*).

Heloma durum is always indicative of concentrated, intermittent pressure affecting these sites, often as a result of deformity or dysfunction of the foot or the toes. On the plantar surfaces and the apices of the toes, pressure arises from the inter-

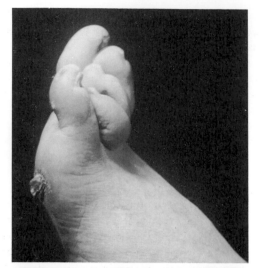

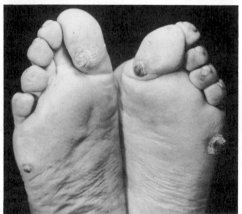

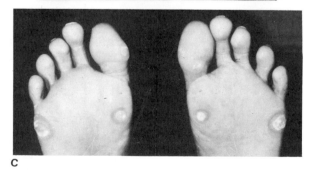

Fig. 6.2 (A, B and C) Plantar helomata.

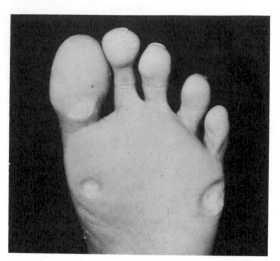

Fig. 6.3 Plantar helomata after enucleation.

Treatment involves the removal of overlying callus by minute dissection with a scalpel followed by the excision of the nucleus by partial or whole section. This can be achieved podiatrically without breaching the dermo-epidermal junction, although a small amount of bleeding can be regarded as acceptable if the thorough removal of an established, irregular nucleus is undertaken in a single treatment session. Keratolytic medication is sometimes used if it is not possible to remove the whole of nucleus (see Ch.11).

Protective padding, designed to deflect pressure from the site, should be applied to protect the area postoperatively. In the longer term, the causative mechanical factors should be identified and a management scheme developed to correct function or accommodate fixed deformity. Frequently, it is possible to design and fabricate an orthotic device which affords long term protection and correction. In most instances shoe advice is necessary and orthotic treatment should be delayed until there is compliance (see Ch. 13).

Complete cure is possible and depends upon the cooperation of the patient, who should be prepared to follow footwear advice and regularly use orthotics which have been prescribed to correct underlying mechanical dysfunction.

Helomata molle. These occur only interdigitally, commonly in the fourth cleft but also in

action of body weight and ground resistance. On other sites, pressure is generated between the weight-bearing foot and footwear, or between adjacent toes due to the constraining effect of tight shoes. The nuclei lie underneath a margin of surrounding callus (Fig. 6.3).

other interdigital spaces. There is usually no nucleus. The lesion is either wholly or partially ring-shaped with a central area of atrophy in which the skin is extremely thin, appearing almost denuded of normal stratum corneum. This general shape and appearance is determined by the moulding of the intervening skin between the opposing bony prominences of the inter-phalangeal joints. In the fourth web, however, the lesion usually arises between the lateral aspect of the proximal phalanx of the fourth toe and the medial aspect of the proximal interphalangeal joint of the fifth toe. Extreme deformity or dis-location of the fifth or fourth toes may cause exceptions to this general rule. Characteristically there is maceration of the ring-shaped hyperker-atosis. This is due to the retention of sweat, which the close proximity of the toes does not allow to evaporate.

The treatment is the careful removal of the rubbery hyperkeratosis by scalpel followed by the application of medication to dry the skin. Advice to keep the interdigital spaces dry by careful towelling and powdering after bathing may be sufficient. Alternatively the application of a 3% solution of salicylic acid in 70% alcohol once or twice daily for seven days will provide sufficient astringency. Relief of interdigital pressure is achieved with a soft silicone interdigital orthotic. Advice concerning footwear, aimed at achieving reduction in interdigital pressure, should be given.

Vascular and neurovascular helomata. In these lesions, small blood vessels and nerve endings arising from the dermis become caught up in the region of the dermo-epidermal junction at the nucleus, which has become complicated by secondary injury. In such instances, the dermo-epidermal junction is grossly disrupted and the dermal papillary structure is deformed by longstanding or repeated injury due, e.g. to a coterminus chilblain, inexpert self treatment with a razor blade or otherwise incompetent treatment. Hypertrophic dermal papillae project around the periphery of the lesion and often within the nucleus itself. These appear as an irregular pattern of capillary loops between a number of small concentrations of dense stratum corneum (micronuclei). Interspersed between these abnormal structures are white, grey or discoloured yellow specks and lines which arise from dense connective tissue containing nerve endings and dilated small blood vessels. Dermal elements disorganised in this way and pinched by hyperkeratotic skin give rise to intense pain and discomfort. Capillary haemorrhage is likely to result from unskilful operating, repeated attempts at which progressively worsen the deformation of the skin strata.

Treatment is complicated by the difficulty of enucleating multiple small nuclei and the presence of nerve endings and blood vessels which give rise to pain and bleeding during operative treatment. Skilful enucleation is possible in some instances and infiltrated local anaesthesia with a 1% solution of plain lignocaine enables the reduc-tion of overlying callus and a significant propor-tion of the nuclear elements, provided that bleeding can be controlled. The application of escharotic medication such as silver nitrate or the reducing agent pyrogallol in suitable strengths is effective but requires several treatments before the micronuclei are removed. Pyrogallol has the advantage of being analgesic and thus facilitates further operative reduction without the need for local anaesthetic infiltration for subsequent treat-ments.

Pyrogallol should not be used on more than three successive occasions because, at therapeutic concentrations, it is cumulative in effect and can produce a sudden and pain free tissue breakdown which can be difficult to resolve. Salicylic acid is not used because of the maceration and fogging of the epidermis, which prevent discrimination between nuclei and connective tissue elements. Electrosurgery, using recently developed apparatus, shows promising results (Ch. 11).

Helomata miliare. Unlike other helomata, these are not produced solely by mechanical injury, although they occur most frequently under the weight-bearing aspect of the foot. They are localised areas of parakeratotic stratum corneum cells, similar to the nucleus of heloma durum, without any surrounding callus. In common with the nucleus of heloma durum, it can be shown histologically that the granular layer of the epidermis is absent immediately beneath the funnel shaped cone of parakeratotic cells which form the lesion. Apart from the retention of cell nuclei in these stratum corneum cells, they are not otherwise remarkable. Histochemically, they do not contain significantly increased amounts of cholesterol, as has been suggested by some. Although usually found in relation to areas of increased pressure, they also occur on apparently non weight-bearing sites and are more common in dry skin conditions, such as anhidrosis.

The treatment is by the removal of symptom producing lesions by partial or whole section using a scalpel. The majority of lesions produce no symptoms and do not require treatment. However, the regular application of an emollient will improve the hydration of the skin and improvement in the texture of the skin is often associated with a reduction in the number of focal hyperkeratotic plugs. In more severe cases, the regular application of a keratoplastic topical medicine such as 10% urea will assist treatment.

Complications of hyperkeratotic lesions

If the pressure which gives rise to helomata becomes particularly intense, or if the intermittent pattern is replaced by continuous compression due, e.g. to the fixation of a deformity or intense pressure from ill-fitting footwear, then the soft tissue under the lesion may break down and become necrotic. Due to the tough nature of the overlying hyperkeratosis, this necrosis, which is associated with inflammation and exudation, is contained. Exudate subsequently macerates the overlying hyperkeratotic skin and it becomes weakened, allowing a route for colonisation for pathogens. Infection of the skin may follow and, dependent upon the colonising organism and state of the host defences, this either remains localised or spreads into the surrounding tissue (*cellulitis*).

Infection. Infection is a constant hazard because of the foot's confinement in a warm, humid environment. Such infections usually remain localised and resolve rapidly once treated with drainage and antiseptic dressings. In the foot, due to the potential for a reduced blood supply, the possibility of a spreading cellulitis—particularly if there is debility—should be considered. Stringent pre- and postoperative antiseptic procedures are always necessary in the practice of podiatry. Even minor infections of the skin of the foot should be speedily and effectively treated. A detailed account of the procedures to be followed is given in the section on bacterial infection (see also Chs 8 & 15).

Ulceration. Ulceration arises from the loss of continuity of the skin surface due to necrosis of skin cells. It is commonly associated with the following causative factors:

1. continuous trauma (in the foot, this is frequently compression)
2. loss or degeneration of subjacent adipose tissue
3. poor peripheral circulation, which results in trophic changes
4. neuropathy from any cause (diabetes is the most frequent).

An ulcer may exude clear uncontaminated tissue fluid or a purulent discharge; the latter indicates secondary infection (Fig. 6.4).

Ulceration associated with hyperkeratotic lesions usually heals well following the careful removal of the hyperkeratotic mass and deflection of pressure away from the site with appropriate

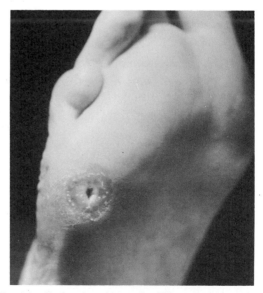

Fig. 6.4 Perforating ulcer under fifth metatarsal head. The sinus at the centre of the lesion may penetrate to the underlying metatarsal head and metatarsophalangeal joint.

padding. The ulcer is cleaned by irrigation with sterile saline and dressed with a sterile environmental dressing under which cell regeneration can take place rapidly. If there is cellulitis present, treatment with a suitable antibiotic is necessary.

Perforating ulcer. This form of deep ulceration may penetrate underlying structures such as joints or tendon sheaths. In this way, infection may be spread into deeper structures, even to the extent of entering bone (*osteomyelitis*). Ulceration which perforates into subjacent structures is consequently a serious complication of plantar hyperkeratosis and requires urgent treatment, possibly with simultaneous administration of antibiotics by mouth. This type of ulceration usually occurs underneath the metatarsophalangeal joints, particularly the first and fifth, although any may be affected.

In addition to the mechanical component, which is typically continuous pressure due to fixation or disordered function of the affected metatarsophalangeal joint, there is frequently coexistent neuropathy. This may be due to one of many neurological disorders, but most often will be found in association with diabetes. Neuropathy leads to reduced or absent pain sensation; injury is not sensed, nor is subsequent infection, so that the first manifestation noted by the patient is a discharge which may be profuse or slight and which smells with a characteristic musty odour. Alternatively, no outward signs are present and on reduction of a plantar callus a necrotic area is found, leading to a deep sinus which penetrates into the foot, possibly into the joint cavity. If only a small amount of clear discharge is present, there is no infection, while a copious discharge of pus is indicative of acute septic arthritis.

Following the complete removal of overlying hyperkeratosis, the cavity is drained and carefully cleaned and irrigated with sterile saline. The ulceration is dressed with a sterile dressing which may contain an antiseptic such as chlorhexidine. In some instances it is necessary to pack the cavity gently with a tulle dressing to maintain adequate drainage. It may be necessary to repeat the cleaning and debridement of the ulcer site and continue treatment with antiseptics until healing

from the base of the ulcer takes place (see Ch. 8). Antibiotics by mouth may also be necessary.

The maximum possible relief of weight-bearing should be provided by means of a well-designed orthotic. A metatarsal bar placed across the sole of the shoe to provide a rocking action may assist in preventing further damage. Reduction of weight may also be indicated if this is thought to be a factor in causing mechanical damage to the sole of the foot. If no apparent cause can be established for the ulceration, further investigation directed at determining potential neuropathy, circulatory deficit or metabolic disease should be undertaken.

Fibrosis (Fig. 6.5). Fibrosis (an increase of fibrous tissue) occurs in the dermal and subdermal tissues, most commonly on the plantar aspect of the foot, as a response to long standing mechanical stress and injury. It arises from repeated damage and chronicity of low grade inflammation with delayed healing, which results in the accumulation of scar tissue in the dermis. Subcutaneous fascia is often depleted with a consequent reduction in protective shock absorption locally. The surrounding soft tissues tend to become adapted to the presence of the lesion creating a *crater* which will rapidly fill with hyperkeratotic skin after it is removed unless the

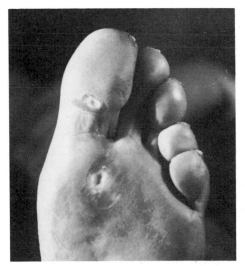

Fig. 6.5 Long-standing plantar helomata after enucleation. Their appearance resembles that of the perforating ulcer in Figure 6.4, but these cavities have bases and sides of tough fibrous tissue which tend to perpetuate their recurrence.

mechanical damage is reduced. Fibrosis is a major factor in the chronicity of many hyperkeratotic lesions.

Treatment depends on the repeated removal of overlying hyperkeratosis and effective deflection of pressure and shearing stress. Carefully designed and fitted orthotics associated with appropriate footwear advice, with good compliance on the part of the patient, are essential if progress is to be made in treating these resistant lesions. The use of escharotic caustic substances, such as pyrogallol and silver nitrate, assist in the reduction both of overlying hyperkeratosis and connective tissue elements in the dermis. Vitamin therapy, e.g. the use of fat soluble vitamins A and E, either alone or with pyrogallol, is effective in some instances. It is likely that fat soluble vitamins have a role to play in stimulating the activity of dermal cells, in particular the fibroblasts. Combined with effective mechanical therapy and regular reduction of the hyperkeratosis, the use of these topical medicines can be highly effective. Electrosurgery can also be employed in the management of such conditions (Ch. 11).

Synovial Sacs. These small sacs are cavities created in the tissues by persistent shearing stress. The tissue is damaged but with the result that semi-organised synovial structures develop in the connective tissue of the dermis. Such tissue damage is represented by a rupture occurring just below the dermo-epidermal junction, often beneath heloma durum at a site of intermittent pressure and shearing. Small superficial bursae formed in this way fill with synovial fluid which may exude on enucleation. Elimination of the incomplete bursae can be achieved by employing appropriate astringent topical medication, such as silver nitrate, or by electrosurgical removal. Protective padding, aimed at reducing the effects of shear, is necessary to avoid chronic recurrence. Such synovial structures occurring at a deeper level may form a sinus which communicates to the surface or with the underlying joint to form a fistula. The structure may become consolidated and fibrotic to create a chronic adventitious bursa with recurrent episodes of bursitis.

Dermal protrusions. Dermal protrusions are small herniations of the dermis beyond the level of the dermo-epidermal junction. Two common examples are those which occur at the apex of a lesser toe and those in association with plantar helomata.

The apex or pulp of a toe, most commonly the fifth as it underlies the fourth, may be affected by constant compression and pinching. This results in deformation and hypertrophy of the dermal papillae which protrude from the dermis like a small coxcomb. The epidermal covering is very thin and there may be fissuring of the surface and discolouration from extravasation of blood from the hypertrophied papillae.

In the case of longstanding plantar helomata beneath the metatarsal heads, excessive reduction by operating or exfoliation may denude the epidermal layer to such an extent that the underlying dermal elements come to protrude into the enucleated area. In both cases the excessive compression responsible for the dermal protrusions must be relieved before topical medication with astringents can have any effect in reducing the hypertrophic dermal papillae.

Furrowing. Furrowing is seen in plantar callus when it becomes pinched into a deep trough. This may occur between adjacent metatarsal heads, as in a splayed foot which has been constricted in narrow footwear, or immediately anterior to the metatarsophalangeal joints, as seen in mobile pes cavus. The margins of the furrow are often highly vascular and may contain fibrotic elements associated with enlarged hypertrophic dermal papillae. Like other cutaneous deformations, furrows are indicative of the causative mechanical stresses which effective treatment will aim to moderate.

Fissures. Fissures are splits in the epidermis consequent upon a loss of elasticity in the skin and when its texture and strength have been altered by changes in hydration. They occur interdigitally when the skin is macerated, and around the heel when the skin is excessively dry. Careful drying and astringent medication is required interdigitally for fissures associated with maceration, while emollients are indicated for dry heel fissures. The edges of heel fissures may be heavily calloused and need to be reduced operatively before medication is administered. Weight relieving padding will help to reduce the compression of the plantar heel tissues and consequently the tensile stress exerted on the epidermis as the skin bulges on weight-bearing.

Principles of treatment

All mechanically induced hyperkeratotic lesions and their associated complications require a comprehensive regime of treatment involving operative, medicinal and mechanical aspects of therapy. The objective is to restore the skin and subcutaneous tissues as nearly as possible to normal and to eliminate or mitigate the stresses responsible for the condition. This objective is usually attainable, provided a programme of treatment is planned and conducted over an adequate period of time. Treatment which is merely episodic and temporarily palliative is usually ineffectual and tends to become endlessly repetitive which is unsatisfactory both to the patient and practitioner.

The operative enucleation of helomata and the reduction of callosities can be achieved painlessly and without bleeding provided that the correct scalpel is chosen and a careful operating technique is employed. The maintenance of firm skin tension during operating is essential to a safe technique.

An important element in treatment is the relief of abnormal mechanical stresses which produce hyperkeratosis. For plantar lesions this entails the identification and correction, to the fullest extent possible, of underlying structural and functional defects (Ch. 5). Dorsal lesions and those on the lateral aspects of the feet require identification of the mechanical stresses occurring between the foot and its covering footwear. Mechanical protection is achieved with properly designed digital paddings. Initially, these may be adhesive, but subsequently should be detachable. The range of devices available includes corrective and protective orthodigital splints for the intermediate toes, shields for the hallux and fifth toe, and interdigital wedges. These may be fabricated from a variety of materials which are described in Chapters 11 & 13. When combined with suitable footwear and given satisfactory compliance on the part of the patient in following advice, such measures provide good clinical results.

Bursae

Bursae occur both naturally (anatomical) and adventitiously (developing in response to need, usually superficial) in the subcutaneous tissues. They are small connective tissue sacs which are lined with synovial cells and contain synovial fluid. Anatomical bursae are found at sites where there is a need to reduce both friction and shearing. They assist in achieving freedom and smoothness of movement at points of potential resistance to free movement. Adventitious bursae can develop beneath helomata, and at sites where the soft tissues are subjected to excessive shearing stresses, as in hallux abductovalgus (Fig. 6.6). Sites in the foot where bursae are liable to become inflamed due to mechanical trauma are:

(i)   on the medial aspect of the first metatarsal in hallux abductovalgus
(ii) on the posterior aspect of the heel, either superficially between the skin and the tendo Achilles, or retrocalcaneally between the calcaneus and the insertion of the tendo Achilles
(iii) under the plantar aspect of the calcaneus
(iv) over the lateral aspect of the cuboid in talipes equino varus
(v)   under an heloma over an interphalangeal joint.

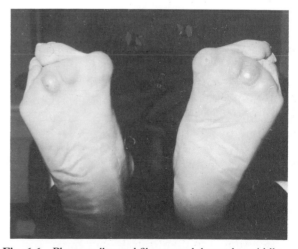

Fig. 6.6   Plantar callus and fibrous nodules under middle metatarsal heads, indicating overloading secondary to hallux abductovalgus deformity.

Inflamed bursae arise as a result of either trauma or infection.

Traumatic bursitis. This is occasioned by undue shearing stress at any one of the sites mentioned. The bursa first gives rise to the symptoms of pain and swelling. If there is continued irritation and injury, the condition may become chronic with further distention from the accumulation of fluid within the bursal sac. Synovial fluid may track either towards the surface, through a sinus, or inwards to the joint through a fistula. Both channels may develop, allowing synovial fluid from a joint to discharge onto the surface.

Infective bursitis. This may be established by spread of infection via a sinus or through the cavity left after enucleation of helomata. The inflammation is frequently widespread and may extend over a considerable area. The inflammation may resolve if the infecting organism is not virulent, but otherwise suppuration and further spread of the infection into the surrounding connective tissues may ensue.

Treatment of bursitis

Traumatic bursitis. If acute, with no sinus, the most effective treatment is to rest the area and reduce the hyperaemic phase of the inflammatory process by the use of cooling lotions such as a wet compress or the application of a cold gel bag. Subsequently, the reabsorption of the excess fluid within the bursal sac may be hastened by the application of heat and rubefacients. When bursitis occurs beneath an heloma, reduction of the hyperkeratosis often exposes a sinus. The sinus should be cleaned and then closed if possible by means of astringents (see Ch. 11). Any potential trauma to the area must be prevented by protective padding.

Infective bursitis. This must be treated promptly in order to avoid any possible spread of the infection. It is necessary to establish drainage if this is not already taking place naturally. Once the infection has been controlled, which may require the administration of antibiotics, treatment is similar to that for traumatic bursitis.

Rest is an important element in the treatment of bursitis, but this does not usually imply complete immobility, which is rarely practicable. Sufficient immobilization can be secured by the use of protective padding which protects the tissues from harmful mechanical injury. Subsequently, protective shields and footwear modifications should be prescribed to prevent recurrence. If conservative measures prove inadequate, surgical excision of the bursa together with surgical correction of the underlying deformity may be required.

Calcaneal bursitis is covered in Chapter 5.

Tenosynovitis

Tenosynovitis (inflammation of a tendon sheath) occurs infrequently in feet and almost invariably arises from mechanical strain. The extensor tendon sheaths in front of the ankle are sometimes affected. The Achilles tendon has no true sheath but may suffer strain with inflammation (tendonitis) from over use. Bursae around the Achilles tendon are subject to acute bursitis from the same cause. The symptoms of tenosynovitis are usually mild, with some swelling, stiffness, pain and crepitus on movement.

Treatment

Treatment is directed at immobilisation with padding and strapping, together with cold or heat therapy to resolve the inflammation. Tendonitis of the tendo Achilles may be caused by over-activity, such as athletic training, which should be suspended temporarily. If associated with an ankle equinus, however, the footwear should be suitably modified by a permanent increase in the height of the heel.

The tendon of the long extensor of the great toe is particularly prone to inflammation in cases where the hallux is hyperextended as, for example, in pes cavus. The tendon then stands out from the dorsum of the foot and is liable to be irritated by the crease in the upper of the shoe. A small heloma may develop first and enucleation may expose a sinus leading to the tendon sheath. This cavity may be repeatedly plugged by dried exudate, but infection may occur through the sinus.

It is not always easy to remove completely the source of irritation. The fault may be a shoe which is too loose or a deep fold in the upper, due to surplus material in an oversized shoe. A change to more suitable footwear or modifications to existing shoes may be indicated. Protection for the tendon is provided by appropriate padding. A permanent shield made from latex or silicone may be required.

Ganglion

A ganglion is a firm swelling protruding from a tendon sheath or joint capsule which has herniated, allowing synovial fluid to escape and form a rigidly encapsulated cyst. Ganglia are not inflammatory and the swelling may be hard or soft and fluctuant. They occur fairly commonly on the dorsum of the foot, around the lateral aspect of the ankle, over the calcaneocuboid joint and around the first metatarsophalangeal joint. At this latter site, pressure may cause the fluid contents to track anteriorly or posteriorly in relation to the joint. On examination, the swelling can be related to the underlying joint or tendon structures from which it derives. The skin can be moved over the ganglion easily but the cyst is usually tied firmly to its structure of origin so that it cannot be mobilised over the underlying bones and joints. A light passed into the cyst from a pocket torch causes the whole cyst to glow (transillumination) as the synovial contents of the ganglion readily transmit light.

Ganglia are often asymptomatic and may be left alone. If symptoms are produced, usually because of pressure from the shoe, then surgical removal is indicated. It is not possible to aspirate ganglia because they frequently prove to be internally divided into cavities by multiple connective tissue septae, and the aspiration needle cannot be directed to each minute locule of synovium. Occasionally, they prove to be attached extensively and surgical removal may not be straightfoward.

CONDITIONS ARISING FROM INFECTIONS

Bacterial infection

Severe infections of the foot are not common. Antibiotic treatment is efficient, so that bacterial infection is quickly treated in most instances, and spread of the organism from the initial location is limited. Most bacterial infections of the foot are relatively minor incidents, which can be resolved with simple measures and may not require antibiotic treatment.

Predisposing factors are extremely important when considering bacterial infections. Such infections are generally more prevalent in older people and in association with debility and systematic illness, poor hygiene, inadequate nutrition and anaemia. In some instances, medicines such as corticosteroids and immunosuppressive and cytotoxic drugs may contribute to reduced resistance. Some medical conditions are of importance since they are associated with an increase in the incidence and severity of bacterial infection. Amongst such disorders diabetes mellitus is the most frequent from the viewpoint of the podiatrist, with ischaemic disorders due to atherosclerosis representing the second most important group.

The skin of the human foot supports a relatively large microflora. This is due to the effect of occlusion in footwear and the associated moisture retention, particularly in the interdigital spaces and toe webbing. The specialised thick stratum corneum of the plantar skin acts as a barrier to the ingress of otherwise commensal organisms and pathogens. The relative absence of hair on the dorsal thin skinned areas of the foot reduces the possibility of bacteria gaining access via the hair follicle. Footwear is a relevant factor in the aetiology of many of the common lesions of bacterial origin occurring in the foot. Shoes create an environment which is high in humidity and temperature and therefore conducive to the establishment of large populations of bacteria.

Ill fitting footwear tends to produce abrasions and other mechanically induced lesions which represent a route of entry for bacteria. Occlusive footwear tends to produce increased numbers of organisms which would normally be present in smaller numbers. There are also factors such as the prolonged use of corticosteroids, antibiotics and immunosuppressive medicines which alter the immune response of the host to infection. These may also alter the normal relationship and therefore equilibrium of the skin flora, so that changes in populations of microorganism may become significant. This is the case when there is an overgrowth or increase in the number of potential pathogens due to an alteration in environmental conditions which favours proliferation. Some organisms which are a normal part of the skin flora (commensal) can, due to rapid colonisation, act as opportunistic pathogens.

Erythrasma

Erythrasma is the most common bacterial infection of the foot. It is a mild infection, affecting body folds as well as the toe webs. In those sites, usually intertriginous, in which colonisation by *Corynebacterium minutissimum* occurs, a well circumscribed dry lesion appears with discoloured brownish patches covered by a fine scaling. In toe webbing the picture is less clear and erythrasma appears simply as maceration and fissuring. Because of its rather nondescript appearance in the interdigital site, this most common bacterial infection may be misdiagnosed as simple intertrigo or as an interdigital dermatophyte infection. This infection may account for the large number of apparent fungal infections which prove to be negative on culture and in which no mycelia can be demonstrated.

Treatment consists of the application of broad spectrum antiseptics. If infection is persistent then erythromycin given as a daily dose of 1g for between 7–10 ten days is indicated, and is virtually always curative. The significance of erythrasma, which is a common bacterial infection of the foot, should not be underestimated since its differential diagnosis should be considered carefully in cases of apparent interdigital mycosis.

Important aetiological factors in erythrasma include occlusion and increased humidity. It is likely that a break or damage to the epidermis is necessary for increased colonisation by the multiple members of the diphtheroid group of bacteria, collectively referred to as *C. minutissimum*. Only then will clinical manifestations of the disease become apparent. These organisms are also noteworthy since they are fluorescent. When viewed under Wood's ultraviolet light, they fluoresce coral red.

Intertrigo

This is not principally a bacterial infection since it is due to the effects of mechanical forces on the skin surface, notably friction and environmental factors such as increased temperature and moisture. Lesions occur only on contiguous skin surfaces and this includes the toe webbings of the feet. The early signs are redness and maceration, but later there may be marked surrounding inflammation with a white centre and exudation. At this stage, numerous secondary bacteria may colonize the area and so aggravate the lesion and prolong its course. No single organism can be identified as the main colonizing agent, but a number of different bacteria, fungi and yeasts may be involved as secondary contaminants.

Treatment is designed to separate and dry the contiguous skin surfaces by the application of absorbents simultaneously with a disposable interdigital wedge. Specific treatment may be indicated to eradicate secondary infection if this is severe.

Staphylococcal infections

Staphylococcus pyogenes can be considered the most frequent cause of pyogenic infection of the foot. Infections involving *Staph. pyogenes* frequently follow puncture wounds, abrasion, surgical incision and indeed any trauma to the foot. They also occur as secondary infections in cases of dermatophytosis. Often, this organism is responsible for infections in helomata durum which, for one reason or another, become damaged, allowing the ingress of this colonising pathogen. Lesions are typified by localised inflammation, abscess formation or discharge. *Staphylococcus pyogenes* has an extremely wide distribution. Because organisms of this species are the commonest cause of pyogenic infection, and the majority of them involve the skin and its appendages, they are of considerable importance to the podiatrist. The species is typified by the ability of the organism to form an enzyme which produces clotting of citrated plasma. The enzyme is similar to thrombin and is called coagulase.

All those staphylococci which produce coagulase (coagulase positive) belong to the species *Staphylococcus pyogenes*. They may occur as commensals as well as in lesions but are regarded in that situation as potential pathogens. Coagulase negative staphylococci are commonly found on the skin but are either non-pathogenic or only low-grade pathogens.

Occasionally, infection with *Staph. pyogenes* may occur on the dorsum of the foot due to colonization of hair follicles. The resulting folliculitis may be superseded by the development of a furuncle (a boil or carbuncle). These lesions occur only in areas where there are hair follicles and are therefore confined to the dorsum of the foot. The clinical picture is typical, and the site tends to point to the diagnosis since there is an obvious association with one of the small areas of hair on the dorsum of the foot and toes. All the signs of inflammation are present, and a tender nodule appears which becomes a fluctuating swelling over a period of three to four days.

Treatment is by the administration of antibiotics of a penicillinase resistant type, e.g. flucloxacillin, in a dose of 1 g per day for 7–10 days. When there is outright suppuration and the swelling becomes fluctuant, carefully timed surgical incision may be indicated so that drainage of the lesion may be achieved.

The most common staphylococcal infection to present in the podiatrists' surgery is that of an infected heloma durum, the causes of which have already been considered. The treatment of this lesion serves to typify the approach which should be made to virtually any localised infected lesion of the foot. The principles, therefore, apply to infected lesions of types other than the infected heloma durum which may be accompanied by an underlying abscess.

Commonly, an aseptic necrosis, which occurs due to the continuous pressure exerted by the nucleus of an heloma, leads to maceration of the overlying hyperkeratosis. This produces an opportunity for *Staphylococcus pyogenes* to gain entry into the deeper layers of the skin and subsequently to produce an abscess underneath the lesion. Inadvertent injuries during treatment and abrasion are therefore not the sole causes of infection.

The principle steps in treatment are:

1. Clean the area surrounding the lesion and finally the lesion itself.

2. Establish drainage by removal of the overlying tissue or by incision.

3. Clean out the abscess cavity by irrigating with sterile saline solution.

4. If there is considerable inflammation or if it proves difficult to expel all the pus from the abscess, a hypertonic saline foot bath may be used. The foot is immersed in the solution which is maintained at 43°C for 10–15 minutes.

5. After the footbath, the lesion is again thoroughly irrigated with a sterile solution to ensure that the abscess cavity is clean.

6. Apply a sterile dressing. (See also Ch. 8.)

The use of topical antibiotics is never indicated. The narrow spectrum of activity provided by antibiotic preparations limits their value. If a local medication is used, a broad spectrum antiseptic such as chlorhexidine should be selected. Staphylococci have an outstanding ability to develop resistance to antibiotics, which provides a further good reason for avoiding topical application of otherwise effective drugs. Adverse reactions to topical antibiotics are also too frequent for their use to be indicated, except in unusual circumstances. This is not to say that antibiotics are never indicated in the treatment of staphylococcal infections. In the case of the old, debilitated, diabetic or immunosuppressed patient, or in individuals who have a history of recurrent infection for any reason, antibiotic therapy may be indicated, but this would usually be by parenteral administration.

7. Protective padding is required to distribute pressure away from the lesion, if this has been an antagonizing factor. Appropriate padding will depend upon the site of the infected lesion.

8. Follow-up should usually take place twice weekly until healing is complete.

The above procedures are repeated until the infection has cleared. A final check made two to three weeks after the inflammation has subsided is prudent.

Collections of pus due to staphylococcal infection close to the nail plate and associated with the sulci or proximal to the eponychium are fairly common and need to be differentiated from paronychia due to *Candida albicans*. The treatment of these superficial infections follows the above pattern. The secondary infection associated with onychocryptosis is usually due to *Staph. pyogenes*, although numerous organisms will colonise a longstanding onychocryptosis.

Mechanical factors may be significant, particularly in relation to lesions on the dorsum of the toes, over the first metatarsophalangeal joint and on the lateral aspect of the fifth metatarsophalangeal joint. In all dorsal, medial and lateral sites modifications of footwear may be useful. These range from simply cutting a hole in an old shoe to accommodate a deformed joint which has developed an infected lesion, to the provision of a balloon patch or some other more permanent adaptation to accommodate deformity.

Streptococcal infections

The group of commonly occurring streptococci, *streptococcus pyogenes*, which may be carried by healthy individuals in the throat, nose or on the skin surface, are potentially extremely pathogenic, although they may be found occasionally as harmless commensals.

The aerobic strains are classified according to their haemolytic activity on a blood agar plate. All strains of *streptococcus pyogenes* are β-haemolytic, i.e. they can lyse red cells and decolourise haemoglobin in culture. It is this group that concerns the podiatrist principally since although the throat is the most likely site for colonisation, infections of the skin may occur. Generalised skin infection by *Strep. pyogenes* includes impetigo and erysipelas. Hypersensitive reactions to infections with *Strep. pyogenes* have been implicated in acute rheumatic disease, which sometimes follows a short time after a throat infection.

Streptococcus pyogenes does not remain localised in the same way as *Staphylococcus pyogenes* since the streptococcus is able to produce a number of enzymes which facilitate its migration into the tissues. Of the six or so enzymes produced, the most important in relation to the spread of infection from the skin into the connective tissues and from there into the circulation are:

1. *Streptokinase*, which is capable of breaking down fibrin. It facilitates the spread of streptococci through the fibrin barrier laid down as part of the normal host defence mechanism.

2. *Hyaluronidase*, which also facilitates the spread of *Streptococcus pyogenes* by breaking down hyaluronic acid — the cementing substance of connective tissue.

3. *Streptodornase*, which reduces the viscosity of purulent exudate, thereby facilitating movement of the streptococcus to the periphery of a superficial lesion.

In consequence, infections with *streptococcus pyogenes* tend to spread rapidly into surrounding tissue. The action of several enzymes allows the organism to spread in this way from the primary lesion into the connective tissues and from there into the lymphatic system. If unchecked, the spread may continue into the bloodstream. The conditions which occur as this process of extension takes place are considered below.

The primary lesion. Due to rapid spread away from the site of initial infection, the primary lesion may be unremarkable and consist merely of a short lived localised inflammatory reaction which very soon gives way to the more dramatic clinical manifestation of a streptococcal infection.

Cellulitis. This presents with localised redness, heat, pain, and diffuse oedema of the skin. It represents a spreading of the infection into the connective tissue subjacent to the skin. The infection may be arrested and resolved at this point by the vigorous inflammatory response. Alternatively, the spread may continue from the connective tissue into the smaller lymphatic vessels of the greater or lesser saphenous systems, producing lymphangitis.

Lymphangitis. This is typified by the appearance of a red line which conforms closely to the route of the saphenous vessels. Because most of the foot and all of the forefoot is drained by the greater saphenous system, lymphangitis will usually occur along the system of vessels which passes in front of the medial malleolus and then up the anteromedial aspect of the leg. Infections occurring in a small area confined mainly to the lateral and posterior aspect of the heel may produce lymphangitis of the lesser saphenous vessels, which run posteriorly to the lateral malleolus and up to the popliteal fossa, where the short vessels terminate.

In patients suffering from cellulitis which does not rapidly resolve, and more particularly in those suffering from lymphangitis, systemic symptoms become quite marked with pyrexia and other signs of toxaemia. If the infection is not halted at this stage, spread of infection may occur into the lymph nodes producing lymphadenitis.

Lymphadenitis. The lymph nodes become inflamed and tender and ultimately, if the infection persists, these may deteriorate into a series of abscesses. This is more likely to occur in the greater saphenous system, thereby implicating the inguinal lymph nodes, but it may occasionally involve the popliteal lymph nodes. Spread beyond the lymph nodes results in the appearance of *Streptococcus pyogenes* in the blood stream (*bacter-aemia*), and its possible multiplication and spread via the blood stream (*septicaemia*).

In practice, it is extremely unusual for streptococcal infections to pass beyond the stage at which cellulitis is the clinical manifestation. Since β-haemolytic streptococci are sensitive to penicillin, either orally or parenterally administered, antibiotics of the penicillin group will quickly eradicate the infection. Following treatment, care should to be taken to identify the means whereby the organism gained entry and to prevent as far as possible, any further opportunity for *Streptococcus pyogenes* to find a similar route of entry.

Pseudomonas pyocyanea (Ps. aeruginosa) infections

This is a Gram negative bacillus which tends to be resistant to the commonly used antibiotics. For this reason, it may give rise to persistent infections and these may occur on the foot. It may invade accidental or surgical wounds and give rise to a characteristically discoloured blue-green pus, which is further characterised by its smell. Since this organism is a contaminant of abraded wounds it must be differentiated from staphylococcal infections. While both produce localised inflammation and pus, the blue-green discolouration of the discharge and the musty-sweet smell produced by *Pseudomonas pyocyanea* infections readily indicate its presence.

Treatment. Since *Pseudomonas pyocyanea* is resistant to a wide variety of antibiotics, this infection may be persistent. Treatment by the local application of dilute acetic acid may be sufficient to eradicate superficial infections. Broad spectrum antiseptics may be effective, provided adequate drainage and debridement are first carried out.

Pseudomonas pyocyanea commonly occurs as a secondary bacterial infection in nails affected by one of the dermatophytes, when it tends to discolour the nail plate blue to black.

Bacterial paronychia

While a number of different bacteria may be involved, including staphylococci, streptococci, *Escherichia coli* and *Pseudomonas pyocyanea*, the presence of *Candida albicans* is most likely to produce chronic paronychia. Secondary bacterial infection is the usual cause of acute inflammatory exacerbations which occur during the course of chronic paronychia.

Treatment consists of dealing first with the secondary bacterial infection and then with the Candida infection. Clotrimazole 1% cream or solution, and miconazole nitrate cream 2% are effective against fungi, including the yeasts, and are useful following treatment with broad spectrum antibacterial medicaments.

Verrucae

Warts, particularly affecting the hands and feet, represent one of the most common *virus* infections of the skin. The frequency of this lesion seems to be related to the provision of swimming baths, sports centres and gymnasia. Management of viral infection calls for an understanding of the causative organism and any attempt at treatment should take into account the natural history of the infection. It is important to consider the normal outcome of this infection in view of its frequency and the consequent costs in providing treatment.

Warts are caused by the human papilloma virus (HPV), which induces benign spontaneously regressing epithelial tumours in the skin and mucosa (Jablonska & Orth 1983). The virus is widely distributed in nature and it has been the subject of considerable study. It is an isometric virus with a constant 72 units in its capsid (outer coat). A number of HPV types are recognised and classified according to molecular differences of nucleotide sequencing. There appears to be a preferential association between given HPV types, lesion morphology and location. However, because there may be some plurality of lesion type associated with HPV infection, relating specific viral types to particular lesion morphologies may not be sound.

The deep endophytic plantar or palmar wart is associated with HPV 1. The common wart, effecting the dorsal or palmar surface of the hands and the face, and the mosaic wart, of the plantar surface, is associated with HPV 2. The small keratosis punctata like lesions of the plantar and palmar surfaces are associated with HPV 4. Histological features of each type of wart and variations in immunity and regression are associated with HPV type.

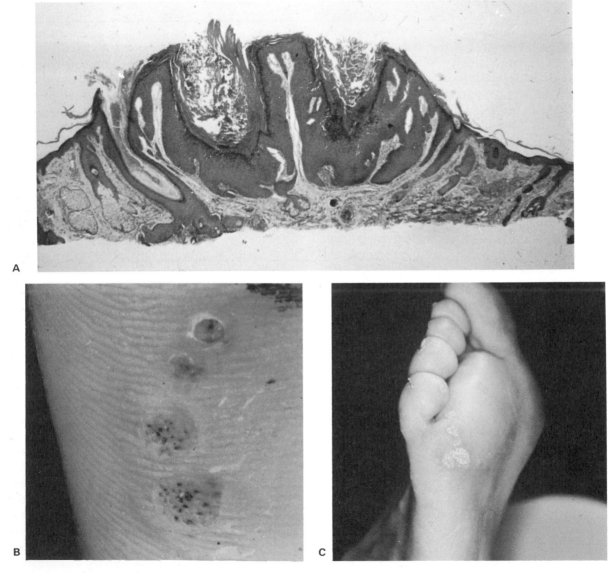

A

B

C

Fig. 6.7 (A) Transverse section of wart demonstrating acanthosis and hyperkeratosis. (B) Plantar warts—multiple. (C) Plantar warts—mosaic.

HPV is found in large numbers distributed throughout the cells of the prickle cell layer in infected tissue, and there is no difficulty in demonstrating its presence by electronmicrography, particularly in lesions of under 18 months' duration. The plantar wart occurs as a sharply circumscribed tumour with a hyperkeratotic covering which tends to obscure the typically papillomatous dermal component. The cells of the germinal layer appear normal. There is abnormal mitotic activity which leads to hyperplasia of the prickle cell layer (*acanthosis*). Additional notable features are the presence of vacuoles in affected cells and remarkable changes in the morphology of the dermo-epidermal junction, with gross enlargement and elongation of the rete pegs. The hypertrophic rete pegs converge in a characteristic centripetal fashion, i.e. they tend to become aligned between the superficial peripheral margin and a point deep in the centre of the lesion (Fig. 6.7A).

In the earliest stages, the lesion may be represented by minimal disturbance of the papillary structure, appearing not unlike a small vesicle, but characteristically the primary dermal ridge involved is sharply interrupted. Later there is a cessation of the normal pattern of dermal ridging at the periphery with a cloud-like or cauliflower pattern representing the papillomatous part of the lesion. Dilated capillaries may appear as red spots within the lesion and darker brown or black spots and streaks are seen in regressing lesions due to the presence of extensive intravascular thrombosis affecting the small vessels within the wart.

These changes are in no way neoplastic but represent an example of focal reactive hyperplasia of the epidermis. Warts due to HPV 1, HPV 2, and HPV 4 do not undergo malignant conversion.

Morphologically, there is considerable variation in the clinical appearance of warts. Weight-bearing sites on the plantar aspect of the foot modify the appearance of the lesion by forcing its mass into the dermis and leaving exposed only the hyperkeratotic overlay. For this reason, verrucae may be mistaken for helomata durum or discrete areas of callus, from which they may be differentiated by close examination of the papillary structure after removal of the overlying callus. Other differential factors are as follows:

Verrucae	Helomata
• Rapid onset	• Develop over months
• Occur at any site	• Sites of compression & friction
• Mainly affect the young	• Mainly affect middle aged & older
• Superficial capillaries which bleed readily	• Capillary bleeding is rare on removal of overlying hyperkeratosis

It is emphasised that these factors are only indicators and that diagnosis should be made on the basis of examination of the papillary structure of the skin using a 10× power magnifying glass if necessary. On non weight-bearing sites, the warty appearance of the papilloma which projects in a dome like fashion above the surface tends to be much more obvious and the differential diagnosis presents no problems.

Warts may occur as single or multiple tumours affecting any aspect of the foot. Not uncommonly, the lesion is shallow and covers a wide area. This so-called mosaic pattern is brought about by infection with HPV 2, whereas the deep endophytic type of plantar wart is caused by HPV 1. The mosaic wart tends to be shallow and pain-free while the deep plantar wart can be extremely painful (Fig. 6.7B & C).

HPV is probably inoculated mechanically through micro injury of the skin. This may take place during barefoot activities, especially when the skin has been wet for some time as in swimming, or due to sweating after intense exercise followed by showering. Such factors could well be associated reasons for the gently fluctuating endemic status of wart infections. These considerations will tend to suggest means for controlling local epidemics in schools and similar situations where it is feasible to isolate and treat the infected group, while regularly checking the others. However, it is almost impossible to apply this technique to a larger population and it is doubtful whether the practice of foot inspections at swimming baths achieves anything, since the virus will have spread quickly before a lesion becomes clinically obvious.

Since there is an immunological response to this infection, which confers some degree of protection after first infection, the anxiety which surrounds the appearance of this common foot lesion is not justified. It has been shown that humoral antibodies can be detected in the serum of individuals who have wart infection and that high levels of wart virus specific IgG are associated with regression of the lesion. The relationship between the appearance of humoral antibodies and the cell bound immune reactions which must occur prior to regression are not clear. However, there is abundant supportive evidence to show that regression is the normal outcome of infection and tumour development due to wart virus. Some patients with warts have been shown to have a defect of non-specific cell mediated immunity.

Regression takes place usually within six to eight months of onset and persistence beyond this time must be considered an indication that treatment may be necessary. Pain or disability for any reason constitute the main indication for active treatment. In the case of pain free lesions of recent onset in children and young adults, explanation of the expected outcome is preferable to immediate and possibly unnecessary treatment. Confusion can sometimes arise because the regressing wart tends to become painful or tender and may be inflamed for about two weeks prior to a sudden abatement of the discomfort. This painful phase may be misinterpreted and treatment begun. In fact, shortly after this phase there will be extensive intravascular thrombosis of the vessels running through the lesion so that they appear as black lines or streaks radiating from the centre, and the surrounding hyperkeratosis shows a yellow discolouration (Fig. 6.8).

Treatment. When treatment is indicated there are two potential avenues of approach:

1. to use anti-viral medicines
2. to destroy all the cells involved in the lesion and thereby ensure that virus infected cells do not survive.

In practice, the first of these has not proven to be effective. Clinical trials with anti-viral drugs idoxuridine in dimethylsulphoxide (DMSO), rimantadine hydrochloride and xenazoic acid have been disappointing. The most promising of these, idoxuridine, has been investigated in

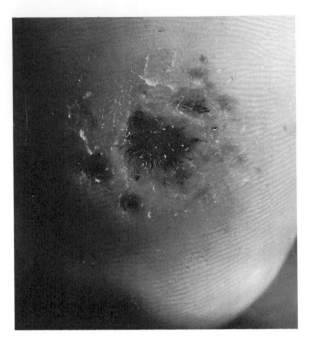

Fig. 6.8 Regressing wart: note the dilated vessels filled with coagulated blood. The thrombotic vessels appear to radiate from the centre.

clinical trials, but the results are no better than with existing treatment. There is a serious pharmacological drawback in that idoxuridine works by incorporation into the DNA of replicating virus, and in the case of an established wart there is not likely to be any increase in the number of virus particles, therefore no active replication takes place.

This leaves *destructive techniques* to eradicate the infected tissue and thus remove the cause of the lesion. All the techniques employed have in common one underlying principle: the wart, with a small margin of unaffected tissue, is destroyed and removed. Only the means of tissue destruction varies and the various techniques are described in Chapter 11.

Other skin infections

Scabies

Sarcoptes scabiei is the responsible organism and is just visible to the naked eye. It is transmitted by prolonged person to person contact. It burrows in the superficial layers of the skin. The commonest sites of infection are the hands and wrists but burrows are frequently seen on the sides of the feet and on the soles of young children. Other favoured sites are the elbows, buttocks and axillae, the breasts in the female and the male genitalia.

The burrow itself is the only diagnostic lesion and from it the female mite can be extracted with a needle. The patient becomes sensitised to the excretory products of the mites about a month after infestation. At this stage, an intensely itchy rash appears over the trunk and limbs. This may include blistering of the hands and feet, especially in children. The generalised rash may seem eczematous and it is always excoriated. Bacterial superinfection is common.

Treatment depends on the meticulous application of an effective scabiecide to all areas of skin below the neck. Gamma benzene hexachloride and benzyl benzoate are the most frequently used. Itch may persist for some weeks after the elimination of the parasite. It is absolutely essential to treat all close contacts, itching or not, to prevent reinfection.

Syphilis

The palms and soles are classically involved during the second stage of syphilitic infection. The patient may feel generally unwell, have a low grade fever and experience headaches and muscular discomfort. The eruption varies but on the soles it appears as bluish red spots developing into infiltrated papules. The overlying epidermis thickens before being shed, leaving a ring of scaling. Serological tests are always positive for syphilis at this stage and treatment with penicillin or an equivalent is curative.

AIDS

Clinical signs may take several years to develop after infection with the human immunodeficiency virus (HIV). Once the ability to cope with infection is impaired, the feet may be involved with florid tinea or viral warts. The onset of the acquired immunodeficiency syndrome (AIDS) may be revealed by the appearance of the irregular, indurated purple plaques of Kaposi's sarcoma anywhere on the skin.

Podiatrists, like all other health care professionals, should be constantly aware of the risk of transmission of HIV and other infections (e.g. hepatitis B) through blood and other body fluids. The best protection is the habitual use of safe techniques for all procedures with all patients.

Tinea pedis

The most common *fungal* infections of skin are those which occur on the feet. Footwear creates the necessary conditions of moisture and warmth between the toes and communal activity permits the spread of infection. Swimming baths and shared bathing facilities in schools, the services and other communal situations are often the most frequent locations of small scale epidemics. Tinea pedis in its chronic form is largely a disease of adults, while acute episodes of *athlete's foot* are more common in school age children. There are three common types:

1. Maceration and desquamation in the lateral toe spaces (Fig. 6.9). This is the commonest type and can be caused by any of three common organisms: *Trichophyton rubrum*, *Trichophyton interdigitale* and *Epidermophyton floccosum*.
2. Episodes of unilateral acute vesiculation on the soles, which are usually caused by *T. interdigitale* or *E. floccosum*.
3. Dry redness and diffuse scaling over the soles, the so-called moccasin type, is usually caused by *T. rubrum*.

Fungal hyphae are also capable of invading the nails (see Ch. 7). Acute tinea pedis may be followed by a vesicular eruption on the hands from which no fungus can be isolated. The term *trichophytide* is used to describe this reaction.

The clinical diagnosis of a fungal infection can be confirmed by microscopic examination of skin scrapings and the type of fungus can be identified by culture of the scales. A single species is usually grown, but mixed infections occasionally occur.

Clinical trials of topical treatments have not demonstrated any one to be greatly superior to the others. Well tried remedies include Castellani's

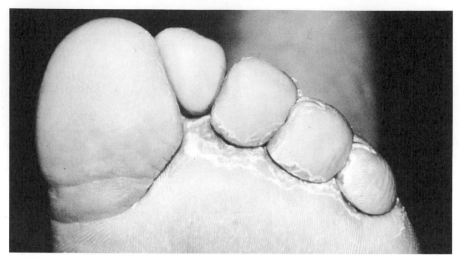

Fig. 6.9   Tinea pedis: interdigital maceration and desquamation.

paint and Whitfield's ointment. Newer topical agents include tolnaftate, clotrimazole and miconazole, which are more acceptable to the patient, and the latter two are also active against yeasts. These should be used twice daily. Widespread infections and those involving the nails are treated with systemic griseofulvin. Toenail infections may take more than 18 months to clear as the drug is incorporated only into newly formed nail. Griseofulvin is normally well tolerated and active against most dermatophyte infections.

Oral ketoconazole may be considered where griseofulvin causes an adverse reaction or the infection proves resistant to its use. It is now thought that long term ketoconazole for dermatophyte nail infection is unacceptable as a first line treatment because of the risk of hepatic toxicity. Ketoconazole is active against both yeasts and dermatophytes, but griseofulvin only against the latter. Until the infection has been cleared, patients should not go barefoot in places where they would expose others to the fungi, e.g. changing rooms and swimming baths. They should not allow anyone else to use their towels, shoes and socks. A non-absorbent bath mat, which can be cleaned with disinfectant, should be used. Anti-fungal powders may be used regularly inside the shoes as a prophylactic measure.

DISORDERS OF SWEATING

Hyperhidrosis

An excessive production of sweat from the palms and soles does not usually imply any disease process but is merely a physiological variant. Emotional disturbances, however, worsen the problem. Sweat may be produced continuously or intermittently, usually less in the winter than in summer.

Hyperhidrosis may affect either sex and often starts in childhood or adolescence. Young adult men are particularly prone to hyperhidrosis of the feet and there may be a family history of this condition. Clothing and shoes can become saturated and pools of sweat may form. The risk of developing pompholyx (q.v.) and contact eczema (q.v.) is increased by hyperhidrosis.

Treatment is far from satisfactory, but reassurance should be given that improvement will normally occur in the mid-twenties. Regular bathing of the feet in 3% formalin solution may help, as may the various commercial anti-perspirants and absorbent powders. Aluminium chloride hexahydrate in alcoholic solution may be effective, but often requires prolonged periods or overnight application; sometimes added polythene occlusion may be necessary. Iontophoresis with tap water or a solution of the anticholinergic drug glycopyrrhonium bromide may give a good response. The side effects of drugs that reduce sweating, such as propantheline, make them too troublesome for routine use. Sympathectomy, the surgical division of the nerve supply to the sweat glands controlling secretion, is rarely indicated.

Bromhidrosis

Malodour of the feet is usually the consequence of keratin decomposition in the presence of hyperhidrosis. Particularly around the toes and on the weight-bearing areas, this may be visible as multiple superficial pits—a 'worm eaten' appearance caused by corynebacterial overgrowth and known as *pitted keratolysis*. Fungal colonisation of the skin will worsen the situation. Measures to reduce sweat production and to control secondary infection will effect improvement. Talc, spray deodorants and absorbent insoles are simple remedies which the patient is likely to have tried before seeking advice. Regular washing and the avoidance of occlusive footwear are extremely important. Boric footbaths or 3% formalin soaks may also be tried.

Anhidrosis

When sweating does not occur the term anhidrosis is used. Unlike hyperhidrosis, it usually implies organic disease. It may occur as an isolated symptom or in association with other neurological defects.

Anhidrosis can originate at any of the levels involved in sweat production. Table 6.1 summarises some of the more important causes. Treatment will be directed towards the basic cause if possible. Failing this, the regular use of emollients such as lanolin or soft white paraffin may reduce discomfort.

Erythema pernio (chilblains)

Chilblains represent an abnormal vascular reaction to cold. They may be produced on rewarming by the more rapid dilatation of the constricted arterioles than of the draining venules. This is thought to lead to the exudation of fluid

Table 6.1   Some causes of anhidrosis.

Site	Causes
Brain	Hypothalamic disease
Spinal cord	Trauma, including surgery, syringomyelia
Peripheral nerve	Sympathectomy, drugs, leprosy, diabetes
Sweat glands	Absence, congenital ectodermal dysplasia, atrophy, scleroderma
Sweat ducts	Prickly heat, eczema, psoriasis

into the tissues. Chilblains occur at any age but are most common in children. They start in early winter, but outdoor workers may develop them in the spring.

Itching and erythema are followed by swelling of the subcutaneous tissues on the dorsum of the proximal phalanges of the toes, on the heels, the lower legs, the fingers, nose or ears. Chilblains may be single or multiple and usually subside in two to three weeks. Sometimes the reaction is more intense with ulceration and irreversible necrosis. Acrocyanosis or erythrocyanosis may be associated features (see Ch. 8).

Prevention by wearing warm clothing, avoiding cold and damp and taking adequate exercise and a good diet, is much more effective than any treatment used once the lesions have appeared. A local antipruritic such as menthol in aqueous cream may help. In the most severe cases, sympathectomy has been employed and there are recent reports of benefit from oral slow release preparations of nifedipine.

Trophic ulceration

Damage to the sensory nerves of the skin leads to anaesthesia and an increased liability to injury. Persistent painless ulceration may result on the pressure areas of the feet, under the metatarsal heads and the heels. This can be precipitated by ill fitting shoes or inexpert enucleation.

Some conditions predisposing to the formation of trophic ulcers are listed in Table 6.2. Similar, but usually painful, ulceration may be induced by vascular disease or X-rays.

The skin surrounding a trophic ulcer is hyperkeratotic and anhidrotic. Sinus formation and osteomyelitis of an underlying tarsal or metatarsal

Table 6.2 Some causes of trophic ulceration.

Diabetic peripheral neuropathy
Trauma to spinal cord or peripheral nerves
Spinal vascular disease
Syringomyelia
Poliomyelitis
Neurosyphilis (tabes dorsalis)
Polyneuropathy
Tuberculoid leprosy
Congenital absence of pain sensation

bone may follow the inadequate treatment of infections. Management depends on the relief of pressure, the correction if possible of the underlying disorder and the eradication of infection. Surgical intervention, e.g. the removal of a metatarsal head, may be required.

OTHER SKIN CONDITIONS AFFECTING THE FEET

Note: It is not possible to describe here all the other skin disorders which can involve the feet. Instead, only those that are common or particular to the feet are discussed. Only the clinical features will be detailed, as in most cases investigation and treatment will follow referral to a dermatologist.

Psoriasis and psoriasiform disorders

Psoriasis

Psoriasis is common, affecting approximately 1 person in 50. Onset is rare under 3 years of age, is most common between 15 and 40, but can occur at any age.

The cause of psoriasis is unknown but a predisposition to the disease can be inherited. Several factors are known to provoke attacks. Upper respiratory tract infections, especially streptococcal tonsillitis, can induce the guttate pattern with many tiny lesions on the trunk of older children. When psoriasis is in an active phase, new lesions may follow cuts or surgical wounds. This localization at the site of recent skin damage is known as the Koebner phenomenon, and it may also be found in lichen planus and viral warts. Most patients are helped by sunlight, but a few are made worse. A severe emotional upset can also precipitate a relapse.

Psoriasis varies greatly in its extent and appearance. It can be recognised by its clearly marginated red plaques with large silvery scales that are easily detached. On the soles, scaling may be thicker and more waxy. Thick fissured areas may mimic a hyperkeratotic eczema but the presence of lesions elsewhere assists in the diagnosis. The commonest sites are the elbows and knees. About 25% of patients show nail abnormalities, most commonly as tiny pits. Onycholysis commonly begins distally. Finally, the nail may become greatly thickened and turn a brownish yellow with much subungual hyperkeratosis. Psoriasis may be associated with an arthritis, usually of the distal interphalangeal joints of the fingers and toes. A distorted nail is usually present beyond the swollen painful joint. Patients with psoriasis can also develop coincidental rheumatoid arthritis or osteoarthrosis.

Psoriasis may subside spontaneously, and many patients respond to artificial or natural ultraviolet light. Coal tar preparations and dithranol remain the most common treatments for chronic plaques. Psoriasis is to some extent responsive to topical corticosteroids but their long term use may thin the skin or induce an eruptive phase. They are now less popular though they are still often used for lesions in the scalp and flexures.

Very severe cases may need systemic treatment with an antimitotic drug, e.g. methotrexate or the vitamin A derivative, Etretinate. Psoralens, naturally occurring photosensitisers, are used with long wave ultraviolet light (so-called PUVA therapy). This type of treatment needs expensive apparatus although small units are available for the local treatment of the feet or hands. The long term use of PUVA raises the risk of skin cancer and is therefore also confined to the more severe cases.

Palmo-plantar pustulosis

The soles and palms are particularly liable to develop this variant of psoriasis, in which sterile yellow pustules turn to yellow-brown surface flakes as they age, before being shed (Fig. 6.10). If pustules erupt without other manifestations of psoriasis, the differentiation from infected eczema of the palms and soles may be difficult. Pustular

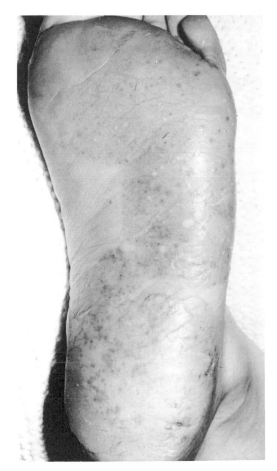

Fig. 6.10   Palmo-plantar pustulosis.

psoriasis is often chronic and responds poorly to treatment although Etretinate, a drug related to vitamin A, may help some but not all patients.

Reiter's disease

This disorder is a triad of urethritis, arthritis and conjunctivitis, but it may also include mucous membrane lesions and rarely an eruption on the soles (*keratoderma blenorrhagica*), which may resemble pustular psoriasis. Most cases follow a non-specific venereal infection but occasionally dysentery precedes its onset.

The fully developed skin lesions show irregular, heaped up yellowish masses of hyperkeratosis on the soles but pustulation is not always seen. The nails may also be involved, leading on occasion to their destruction. These changes subside over a period of months.

Pityriasis rubra pilaris

This rare disorder resembles psoriasis in some ways. It may affect much of the body surface with erythema and a fine granular scaling, although small areas are often spared. Characteristically the palms and soles are thickly hyperkeratotic and brown-orange. Diagnostic follicular papules surmounted by a horny plug are often best seen on the backs of the fingers. This is a chronic condition showing spontaneous remissions and relapses.

Eczema and dermatitis

The terms *eczema* and *dermatitis* are best regarded as being synonymous. Eczema is sometimes used to imply a constitutional process, and dermatitis a reaction to an external agent. Nevertheless, the distinction is by no means rigid and it is advisable to use the term eczema when speaking to patients as it does not carry the same industrial connotations to the lay person.

Acute eczema starts with erythema, vesiculation, oozing and crusting, whereas the skin in chronic eczema is dry, scaly and thickened.

Atopic eczema

The skin changes may or may not be accompanied by other manifestations of atopy, such as hay fever and asthma, and these disorders may also affect others in the family. This type of eczema often starts on the scalp or face as early as 3–4 months of age, and later spreads to involve the limb flexures and napkin areas. Itch is severe and, with constant rubbing, a dry scaly erythema develops in the flexures, with increase in skin markings known as *lichenification*. Lesions occur less frequently on the feet than on the hands but the ankle is commonly involved (Fig. 6.11). The skin elsewhere tends to be dry.

Fortunately, atopic eczema tends to remit spontaneously and a proportion will clear each year from the age of two upwards. Sometimes atopic eczema does not develop until puberty or even later and then it can pursue a very chronic course.

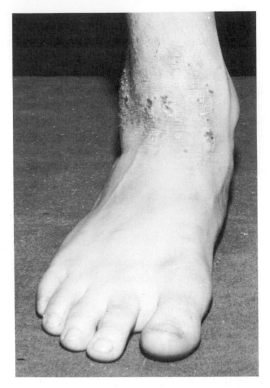

Fig. 6.11　Atopic eczema.

Eczema of the palms and soles

Some patients experience recurrent episodes of irritable vesiculation of the palms, soles and sides of the digits. These blisters may be larger than those usually seen in eczema and resemble sago grains. The term *pompholyx* is sometimes used to describe this pattern.

Another constitutional pattern of chronic eczema seen on the palms and soles is characterized by an initial microvesiculation and later by stubborn hyperkeratosis and fissuring (Fig. 6.12). In these cases, no precipitating cause can generally be found but allergic contact eczema and fungal infection must be excluded.

Irritant dermatitis

A single massive exposure, or more commonly recurrent exposure of the skin to mild acids, alkalis or degreasing agents, produces an irritant dermatitis. The mistaken regular bathing of the feet in antiseptics may give rise to this condition. Housewives' dermatitis of the hands is another well-known example.

Allergic contact dermatitis

True sensitisation of the skin can be produced by a wide variety of substances. Once this allergy is established, further exposure to the chemical will lead to an eczematous reaction. On the feet, chemicals added to rubber, chrome used to tan leather, nickel in shoe buckles or dyes in socks

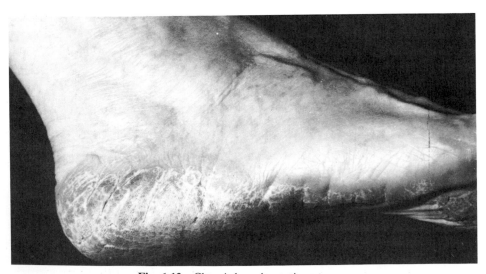

Fig. 6.12　Chronic hyperkeratotic eczema.

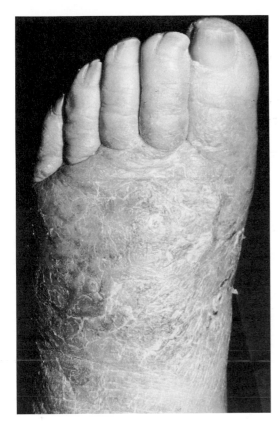

Fig. 6.13 Allergic contact dermatitis.

may be responsible (Fig. 6.13). The pattern of involvement, e.g. the weight-bearing area of the sole in rubber sensitivity, will assist in the diagnosis. Allergy to various components of medicaments, including preservatives and antibiotics, may exacerbate a pre-existing eczema.

The offending substance can be identified by the application of patch tests to normal skin on the patient's back. Positive reactions usually occur within 48 hours.

Varicose eczema

Impaired venous drainage leads to a variety of skin changes. Increased pigmentation and purpura appear along the lines of the veins and around the ankles. Eczematisation may follow and sudden exacerbations can lead to dissemination beyond the legs. In many chronic cases, white scarring (*atrophie blanche*) and ulceration ensue, the latter often beginning after a minor injury.

Lichen simplex

A localized area of dry thickened skin showing lichenification is referred to as *lichen simplex* or *circumscribed neurodermatitis*. Itch is always prominent and the thickening is due to repetitive, at times almost violent, scratching. As a result the surface may show fresh excoriations or haemorrhagic crusting. The lower leg and ankle are especially common sites.

Discoid eczema

The terms *discoid* or *nummular eczema* are used to describe the coin-like patches of erythema, vesiculation and crusting that are found most often on the limbs of adults. Individual lesions respond to treatment with topical steroid antiseptic mixtures but the general pattern is for most patients to go on to develop further patches.

Infective dermatitis

This is most commonly seen in those adolescent boys who pay little attention to hygiene and have a problem with hyperhidrosis. It starts on the dorsum of the foot near the toes and spreads towards the ankle. Bacterial infection plays an important part in its perpetuation.

Treatment of eczema

All eczemas are managed along broadly similar lines. Oozing acute eczemas are initially treated with soaks, e.g. potassium permanganate solution (1 in 10 000), or aqueous eosin paint may be applied. This is followed by the application of topical steroid creams, if the area is still moist, or ointments if dry, in order to suppress the eczema reaction. Tar preparations are used in chronic cases where lichenification is present. Systemic antihistamines are useful for their sedative and antipruritic qualities.

Infection commonly complicates eczema and a topical antibiotic is then applied with the steroid. Occasionally, systemic antibiotics are given if the patient becomes pyrexic or shows signs of cellulitis or lymphangitis related to the eczema.

Contact dermatitis responds partially to the

same therapy but the most important measure is to eliminate the offending allergen. The resolution of varicose eczema is assisted by elevation or support of the limb. Surgery to the underlying damaged veins may also be indicated. Local steroids should be kept to a minimum in the proximity of a varicose ulcer as they delay healing and promote secondary infection.

In cases of eczema of the feet, it is particularly important to exclude fungal infections by the examination of skin scrapings, since topical steroids will spread tinea pedis by suppressing resistance to the fungus.

Juvenile plantar dermatosis

This recently described condition affects the weight-bearing areas of children's forefeet. The involved parts of the sole and undersurfaces of the toes show a glazed, scaly, sometimes fissured erythema. The heels and insteps are less often involved (Fig. 6.14).

Its cause remains in some doubt, but the irritant effect of new synthetic materials in children's footwear may be important, though some think it is a localised manifestation of atopic

eczema. Treatment includes topical corticosteroids and is largely unsatisfactory. A change to cotton socks and open, sandal type footwear is usually recommended, while cork insoles may be helpful.

Palmoplantar keratoderma

Punctate or diffuse thickening of the palms and soles occurs in a variety of disorders. The term *tylosis* describes a diffuse dominantly inherited type. Keratoderma associated with structural and functional foot disorders has been described in an earlier section.

One common acquired pattern is *keratoderma climactericum*. This is seen in middle-aged, often obese women. The thickening is most marked on the sides of the heel and extends over the sole to the metatarsal heads (Fig. 6.15). Splitting and

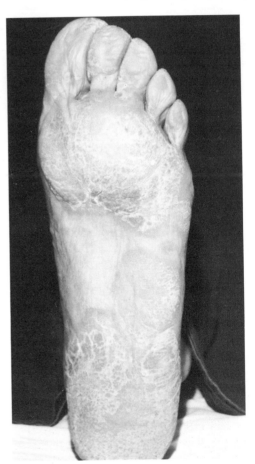

Fig. 6.15   Keratoderma climactericum.

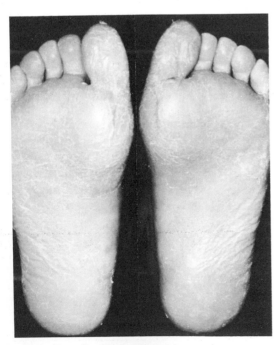

Fig. 6.14   Juvenile plantar dermatosis.

cracking of the keratin results in deep painful fissures. Associated hyperhidrosis may produce an unpleasant smell. Treatment is by removal of the thickened epidermis by regular reduction with a scalpel and the use of ointments containing salicylic acid. The thickening often recurs but acquired keratoderma may eventually improve.

Lichen planus

The cause of lichen planus is unknown. The common sites are the wrists, forearms, lower abdomen, back, legs and the mucous membranes. Both the dorsum of the foot and the soles may be affected. Individual lesions consist of itchy, flat, polygonal, violaceous papules that may be small and discrete, or fused to form larger plaques. The surface may show a network of fine white lines called *Wickham's striae*.

In about 10% of cases the nails are affected. The majority of these show only reversible longitudinal ridging, but cuticular hypertrophy may result in a triangular central projection, known as a pterygium, growing along the nail. This causes considerable deformity and occasionally permanent nail destruction ensues.

The eruption usually subsides spontaneously though only after months or even years. Brown macules often remain and take several months to fade. No fully effective treatment is known but topical corticosteroids often alleviate the itch and may partially suppress the rash.

Disorders of blood vessels

Urticaria

Urticaria, or nettle-rash, consists of short lived itchy weals which vary in diameter from a few millimetres to several centimetres. Individual lesions tend to fade after 8 to 24 hours, but purpura is occasionally left on dependent parts of the body. In chronic cases episodes recur at variable intervals.

Urticaria may be the result of an allergic reaction to a food substance or drug. Aspirin can exacerbate urticaria whatever its original cause. However, the precise cause in the majority of cases cannot be found.

The feet may be involved as part of a generalised eruption but are particularly affected by the rare pressure urticaria. Here, painful swelling of the soles occurs some hours after the repetitive pressure of walking or running. Manual labour may lead to the same appearance on the hands. The underlying mechanism of this and other physical urticarias is not known. It can be longlasting and disabling.

There is no really effective treatment for pressure urticaria other than avoidance of those activities which provoke it. Systemic antihistamines may alleviate, if not cure, other varieties. Non-sedative types such as terfenadine and astemizole allow the patient to continue with normal activities, such as driving, whilst under treatment.

Purpura

Purpura is the consequence of spontaneous bleeding into the skin. Small lesions a few millimetres in diameter are described as petechiae and larger lesions as bruises or ecchymoses. These areas are identified by their purplish colour when fresh and by failure to blanche on pressure.

A wide variety of disorders of the blood, blood vessels or the tissues supporting them may produce purpura. Elucidation of its cause depends on detailed medical investigation.

Purpura is particularly liable to develop on the lower limbs because of the effects of gravity and varicose veins — factors which increase the pressure exerted on vessel walls.

Talon noire (black heel)

In this condition, groups of bluish black specks appear on the heels, usually just above the thickened horny edge of the sole. It is believed to be due to the rupture of small capillaries by repetitive shearing stresses often exerted by a particular training shoe. It is most commonly seen in fit young persons and is entirely benign.

Tumours

The feet can be the site of birthmarks, e.g. linear naevi. These may appear as warty overgrowths of the epidermis, and can extend the whole length of a limb.

Pigmented moles

These are fairly common on the feet and although these have a very small chance of becoming malignant, the risk is increased on the sole, the toes and beneath the nails. The possibility of a *malignant melanoma* must be considered if a pre-existing mole grows rapidly, changes colour, begins to bleed or shows evidence of a surrounding inflammatory reaction (Fig. 6.16). Any suspect mole should be excised without delay and examined histologically.

Haemangiomas

Haemangiomas are vascular malformations. The familiar port wine stain or capillary haemangioma appears after a few weeks of life. An acquired haemangioma, called a *pyogenic granuloma*, may occur at the site of a trivial penetrating injury. The cherry red friable vascular tumour grows rapidly and requires removal under a local anaesthetic by curettage and cautery. Recurrence is not uncommon but the lesion is benign.

Small corn-like *keratoses* can appear on the palms and soles many years after the administration of arsenic which was used well into this century as a pharmacological agent. These patients also tend to develop multiple plaques of *intra-epidermal carcinoma*, often on the lower limbs. These areas are usually crusted, slightly raised and red.

Frank *squamous cell carcinomas* are less common on the legs than on the hands and face. They may, however, develop in areas of chronic inflammation as in the margin of a long-standing varicose ulcer. The tumour itself arises as a raised warty ulcerated nodule. Diagnosis is made by biopsy and treatment is by surgical removal or radiotherapy. Fortunately, squamous cell carcinomata of the skin spread less frequently than those derived from the other organs.

Other skin tumours occasionally appear on the feet but are not detailed here. However, one rare tumour of the sweat duct, the *eccrine poroma*, selectively grows on the sole or the palm. It forms a single skin coloured nodule up to 1 cm in diameter. This growth is not malignant.

Bullous disorders

Primarily blistering disorders are rare and do not selectively involve the feet, although these may be involved as part of a generalised eruption. Readers are referred to standard dermatological tests for further descriptions.

An exception to this is *epidermolysis bullosa*. The dominantly inherited variant may cause blistering only on the feet and this may first be noticed when the infant begins to crawl or walk. In mild forms, the onset may be delayed until adolescence. Trauma induces clear tense blisters which eventually heal without scarring. These may be pricked, drained and covered by a protective dressing. Recessively inherited forms of epidermolysis bullosa are much more severe with widespread involvement of the skin and mucous membranes. Considerable scarring ensues and lethal complications may eventually arise.

Granuloma annulare

Granuloma annulare consists of a group of small pink or skin coloured nodules, usually forming an arc or complete ring, varying from one to several

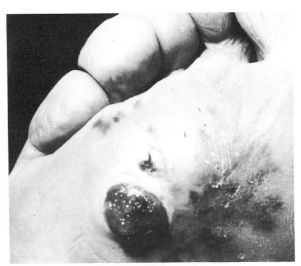

Fig. 6.16 Melanoma.

centimetres across. The lesions are asymptomatic and may be single or multiple.

Although the hands are the commonest site, the feet are affected in 20% of cases, usually in children. Granuloma annulare eventually fades but this may take some years. Its disappearance may be accelerated by freezing with liquid nitrogen or by intralesional injections of corticosteroids.

Drug eruptions

Adverse reactions to drugs are common and are frequently seen on the skin. The rashes vary considerably and may mimic common primary skin disorders. Very few drugs cause specific eruptions and a detailed history of medication is essential for diagnosis.

The feet are often involved as part of a widespread eruption. Occasionally, however, isolated lesions occur in the same places whenever a particular drug is taken. These *fixed drug eruptions* appear as a disc of erythema that fades on withdrawal of the drug, often leaving a patch of pigmentation.

FURTHER READING

Almeida J D, Goffe A P 1965 Antibody to wart virus in human sera, demonstrated by electron microscopy and precipitin tests. The Lancet II: 1205

Baran R, Dawber R P R 1984 Diseases of the nails and their management. Blackwell, Oxford

Bunney, M H 1982 Viral warts: their biology and treatment. Oxford University Press, Oxford

Gold S 1973 The enigma of viral warts. The Practitioner, Nov.

Jabonska S, Orth G 1983 Human papovaviruses. In: Champion R H (ed) Recent advances in dermatology. Churchill Livingstone, Edinburgh, pp 1–36

Johansson E, Pyrohonen S, Rostila T 1977 Warts and virus antibodies in patients with systemic lupus erythematosus. British Medical Journal I: 74–76

Le Rossignol J N 1980 An encyclopaedia of materia medica and therapeutics for chiropodists. Faber, London

Le Rossignol J N, Holliday C B 1963 A pharmacopoeia for chiropodists, 7th edn. Faber, London

Levene G M, Calnan C D 1974 A colour atlas of dermatology. Wolfe, London

Matthews R S, Shirodaria P Y 1973 Study of regressing warts by immunofluorescence. The Lancet, March

McMillan S A, Haire M 1975 Smooth muscles antibody in patients with warts. Clinical and Experimental Immunology 21: 339–344

Morrison W L 1976 Cell-mediated immune responses in patients with warts. British Journal of Dermatology 93: 553

Ogilvie M M 1970 Serological studies with human papova (wart) virus. Journal of Hygiene 68: 479

Pyrhonen S, Penttinen K 1972 Wart virus antibodies and the prognosis of wart disease. The Lancet Dec 23

Read P J 1972 An introduction to therapeutics for chiropodists, 2nd edn. Actinic Press, London

Reid T M S, Fraser N G, Kernohen I R 1976 Generalised warts and immune deficiency. British Journal of Dermatology 95: 559

Rook A, Wilkinson D S, Ebling F J G, Champion R H, Burton J L 1986 Textbook of dermatology, 4th edn. Vols I, II, III. Blackwell, Oxford

Shirodaria P V, Matthews R S 1975 An immunofluorescence study of warts. Clinical and Experimental Immunology 21: 329–338

Sneddon I B, Church R E 1983 Practical dermatology, 4th edn. Arnold, London

Solomons, Bethel 1983 Lecture notes on dermatology, 5th edn. Blackwell, Oxford

7. The human nail and its disorders

Margaret Johnson

The human nail is a hard plate of densely packed keratinised cells which protects the dorsal aspect of the digits and greatly enhances fine digital movements of the hand. Nails are descendants of claws, used for digging and fighting, but now only serve as a protection for the digit and to assist in basic behaviour, such as scratching and picking up small objects.

The nail is a flat, horny structure, roughly rectangular and transparent. It is the end product of the epithelial component of the nail unit, the *matrix*. The nail plate moves with the nail bed tissues to extend unattached as a free edge, growing past the distal tip of the finger or toe. The nail bed is normally seen through the plate as a pink area due to a rich vascular network. A paler cresent-shaped *lunula* is seen extending from the proximal nail fold of the hallux, thumb and some of the larger nails.

At the lunula, the nail is thin and the epidermis is thicker, so that the underlying capillaries cannot be seen. It is less firmly attached to the bed at this point and light is reflected from the interface between the nail and the bed, making the lunula appear white.

In profile, the nail plate emerges from the proximal nail fold at an angle to the surface of the dorsal digital skin. This angle is commonly called *Lovibond's angle* (Fig. 7.1A) and should be less than 180°. Only in abnormal circumstances, e.g. clubbing, is this angle greater (Fig. 7.1B).

The nail grooves mark the limit of the nail, are separated into proximal, distal and lateral grooves (sulci) and are best seen when the nail is avulsed. The distal groove at the hyponychium is covered by the nail plate; lying immediately proximal is a

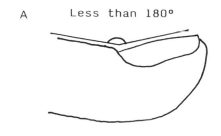

A   Less than 180°

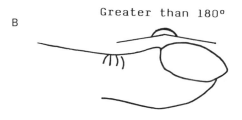

B   Greater than 180°

Fig. 7.1 (A) Lovibond's angle. (B) Clubbing.

thin pale translucent line known as *Terry's onycho-dermal band* (Fig. 7.2).

The proximal nail fold (PNF) is an extension of the skin of the surface of the digit and lies superficial to the matrix, which is deeper in tissues. It has a superficial and a deep epithelial border, the latter not being visible from the exterior. The PNF extends its stratum corneum onto the nail plate as a cuticle, which remains adhered for a short distance before being shed. The function of the cuticle is unclear—it may

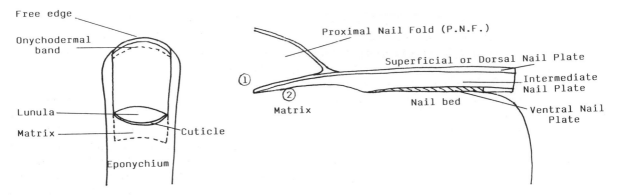

Fig. 7.2 Structure of the human nail. (1) Superficial layer of nail; (2) deep layer of nail.

prevent bacterial access to the thinner and more delicate tissues of the ventral PNF epidermis, or may help in forming a smooth nail surface.

The superficial skin of the PNF, extending from the distal interphalangeal joint to the nail plate, is devoid of hair follicles and is thinner than the dorsal skin of the digit. At the tip of the PNF adjacent to the cuticle, capillary loops can be seen and, if proliferative, can be associated with certain disease states, e.g. lupus erythematosus, dermato-myositis and phototoxic conditions.

The ventral PNF is thinner than the superficial PNF; it does not have epidermal ridges and may be the portal of entry for bacteria and/or irritating chemicals which produce *chronic paronychia*. It is continuous with the matrix epithelium but has a stratum granulosum which may be differentiated on staining.

Embryonic development and nail growth

The earliest anatomical sign of nail development occurs on the surface of the digit of the embryo at week 9, appearing as a flattened rectangular area. The primary nail field is outlined by grooves which are the forerunners of the proximal and distal grooves and lateral sulci (Zaias & Alvarez 1968). The nail field mesenchyme differentiates into the nail unit structures and the fully keratinised nail is complete in week 20 of gestation. Toe nail formation is usually 4 weeks later than that of the finger nail.

The theories proposed to explain the formation and growth of the human nail have polarised

between a single source of matrix production from the lunula (Zaias & Alvarez 1968; Norton 1971; Achten 1982) and a trilamellar structure where, in addition to the lunula, the nail bed and proximal nail fold contribute as the nail plate grows out (Lewis 1954; Lewin 1965; Hashimoto et al 1966; Jarrett & Spearman 1966; Samman 1986; Johnson et al 1991).

Zaias (1990) states that the nail plate is a uniform structure produced solely by the matrix, with onychocytes genetically directed diagonally and distally and not shaped or redirected by the PNF. The proximal portions of the matrix form the superficial nail plate and the distal matrix forms the deepest portion of the plate. As the nail produced from the lunula is in advance of that from the proximal matrix, this supports the theory that nail plate shape is related to lunula shape. Zaias shows also a direct relationship between nail plate thickness and the length of the matrix.

However, the exact structure of the nail plate is still disputed as Achten (1982) claims that nail embedded in paraffin and stained with the periodic acid shift method (PAS), toluidine blue and the sulphydryl groups, reveals three layers with differential staining. The most proximal cells of the matrix form the superficial layer of the nail, while the distal cells form the deeper nail layer which is thicker (see Fig. 7.2). As the nail grows distally and comes to rest on the nail bed distal to the lunula, a thin layer of keratin from the bed attaches to the under surface of the nail. Achten argues that this keratin does not form an integral part of the nail, but migrates with it and remains firmly attached to it even when the nail is surgically avulsed. Measurements of progressive thickness of the nail from the proximal lunula to the point of detachment at the onychodermal band have shown that about 19% of nail mass is formed by the nail bed as the nail grows out along it (Johnson et al 1991).

The nail bed has a surface with numerous parallel longitudinal ridges which fit closely into a similar pattern on the underside of the nail plate, thus ensuring a very strong cohesion between the two surfaces.

The three nail layers are often described as the dorsal, intermediate and ventral nail plates, and each is physicochemically different. Seen in transverse and longitudinal sections, the cells of the nail plate are arranged regularly and interlock like roof tiles, with the main axis horizontal. In the superficial layer, cells are flatter and closer together, and in the nail bed they are more polyhedral and less regularly arranged.

It is thought that the layers stain differently due to variations in the composition of the main polypeptide chains and the number of lateral bonds in the keratin molecule (Achten 1982). The more numerous the lateral bonds, the fewer free radicals are available to combine with different stains. In softer keratin, there is less bonding and therefore more staining (Fig. 7.3). Studies on the chemical composition of nails show moderately high concentrations of sulphur, selenium, calcium and potassium.

Blood supply and innervation

In the foot, the nail is supplied by two branches of the dorsal metatarsal artery and two branches of the plantar metatarsal artery, lying at the laterodorsal and lateroplantar areas of each toe. They form an anastomosis at the terminal phalanx, the plantar arteries supplying the pad of the toe and the nail bed.

Innervation of the proximo-dorsal area of the nail and bed is provided by two small branches from the dorsal nerves (superficial peroneal, deep peroneal and sural), while the medial and lateral plantar nerves provide a medial and lateral branch to each toe to supply the plantar skin, and extend to supply the anterodistal area of the nail bed and superficial skin.

Growth of the nail is continuous throughout life, the rate being greatest in the first two decades, when the nail plate is thin (Hamilton et al 1955). The rate of growth decreases with age and in the elderly, the nail plate loses its colour and may thicken and develop longitudinal ridges. The normal development of the nail depends on the matrix and nail bed having an adequate nerve and blood supply and interference with either will affect growth. Some systemic disorders may cause a reduction or an increase in the growth rate. Other factors which, directly or indirectly, have a detrimental effect on the development and growth of the nail are trauma, infection, nutritional deficiencies and some skin diseases. Congenital and inherited factors are not common.

As nail growth is continuous throughout life, periodic cutting is necessary and incorrect performance of this task may lead to onychocryptosis (ingrowing toe nail) — one of the most painful conditions to affect the nails. The free edge of a nail should be cut straight across or slighty convex with all rough and sharp edges smoothed; it should never be cut so short as to expose the nail

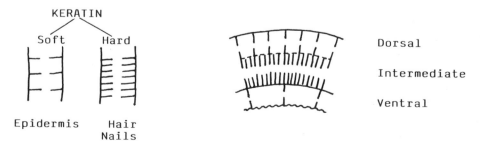

Fig. 7.3 Polypeptide chain composition in the human nail.

bed. The overall aim should be to ensure the nail complies with the shape of the toe.

INVOLUTION (PINCER, OMEGA NAIL)

This term describes a nail which increases in transverse curvature along the longitudinal axis of the nail, reaching its maximum at the distal part (Fig. 7.4). Three types of this condition exist (Fig. 7.5) and produce a variety of symptoms.

Tile-shaped nails often occur in association with yellow nail syndrome, affecting both finger and toe nails. The nail increases in transverse curvature, while the lateral edges of the nail remain parallel (Baran et al 1991). The condition rarely produces symptoms.

Plicatured nails occur where the surface of the plate remains flat while one or both edges of the nail form vertical parallel sides hidden by the sulcus tissue. Toe nails and finger nails are affected. Considerable pain may be caused in the

foot if the nail is thickened and subjected to shoe pressure, with the development of onychophosis.

Pincer (omega, trumpet) nail dystrophy shows longitudinal curvature, which ranges from a minimal asymptomatic incurving to involution so marked that the lateral edges of the nail practically meet, forming a cylinder or roll, hence the other names for this deformity. Lateral compression of the nail may result in strangulation of the soft nail bed tissues and the formation of subungual ulceration as the circulation to the nail bed and matrix is reduced. In all stages of the condition, the sulcus may become inflamed and may ulcerate, causing considerable pain.

Aetiology

Although the precise cause of involution is unknown, in toenails it is often associated with constriction from tight footwear or hosiery. In fingernails, an association with osteoarthritic changes in the distal interphalangeal joint has been shown (Zaias 1990) and heredity may play a part, particularly where all nails are affected (hidrotic ectodermal dysplasia, yellow nail syndrome). Some severe cases of involution have an underlying exostosis of the terminal phalanx which must be excised.

Treatment

In minor degrees, involution produces little or no discomfort and the main consideration is to ensure that the nail is cut to conform to the length and shape of the toe. The incurved edges should be reduced, if thickened, and advice given about correctly fitting footwear and hosiery.

More severe cases may be treated conservatively with careful clearing of the sulcus and the fitting of a nail brace. This is made from a short piece of 0.5 mm gauge stainless steel wire which applies a slight upward and outward tension to the nail edges to gradually correct them. The nail must be of adequate length to allow correct fitting of the side arms of the brace, and good contact of the nail plate with the nail bed is essential to allow effective tension for correction.

The brace is formed using a length of wire approximately 1.5 cm greater than the width of

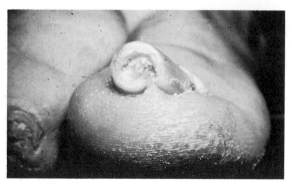

Fig. 7.4   Involution.

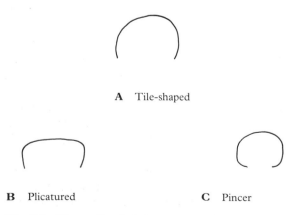

A   Tile-shaped

B   Plicatured

C   Pincer

Fig. 7.5   Types of involution.

the nail. At approximately the centre of the wire, a U-loop is formed in the horizontal plane so that the open end of the U faces towards the free edge of the nail. With round-nosed pliers, a small hook is made at each end of the wire, lying in the frontal plane and large enough to accept the thickness of the nail edges. The ends of the wire must be rounded and smoothed with a file before fitting. Finally, each arm of the brace from the hook to the central loop is shaped to conform to the actual curvature of the nail (Fig. 7.6).

The brace is applied by engaging each hook over the appropriate edge of the nail and tension is obtained by closing the long side of the loop as far as possible without applying so much tension that the nail splits. A light packing of cotton wool and suitable antiseptic may be inserted into each sulcus if necessary. The brace should be kept in

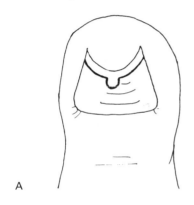

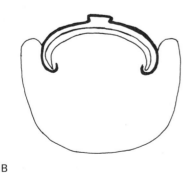

Fig. 7.6 Involution. (A) Nail brace in position, dorsal view. (B) Nail brace in position, transverse view.

position for at least one month and then reassessed for correction (calliper measurements) and tension which can be adjusted throughout the treatment.

Other derivatives of the nail brace are now available in plastic and are adhered to the nail, directly exerting upwards and outwards tension because of their performed shape or via rubber bands fitted to small plastic hooks. These are reported to be very successful where good adherence is achieved.

Severe and painful involution is likely to require a unilateral or bilateral partial nail avulsion with destruction of the matrix. Where lateral compression causes painful nail bed constriction and ulceration, a total nail avulsion with matrix destruction is the only means of providing relief.

If an underlying subungual exostosis is detected, this needs to be excised (see Ch. 18).

ONYCHOCRYPTOSIS (INGROWING TOE NAIL)

Onychocryptosis is a condition in which a spike, shoulder or serrated edge of the nail has pierced the epidermis of the sulcus and penetrated the dermal tissues. It occurs most frequently in the hallux of male adolescents and may be unilateral or bilateral. Initially, it causes little inconvenience but as the nail grows the offending portion penetrates further into the tissues and promotes an acute inflammation in the surrounding soft tissues which often becomes infected (paronychia).

The skin becomes red, shiny and tense and the toe appears swollen. There is throbbing pain, acute tenderness at the slightest pressure and a degree of localised hyperhidrosis. The continued penetration of the nail spike prevents normal healing by granulation of the wound and a prolific increase of granulation tissue is common (*hypergranulation*). This excess tissue, together with the swollen nail folds, overlaps the nail plate, sometimes to a considerable extent, partially obscuring it (Fig. 7.7).

Since infection is almost always present, pus may exude from the point of penetration in the sulcus and may be seen as a pocket lying beneath the sulcal epidermis or beneath the nail plate.

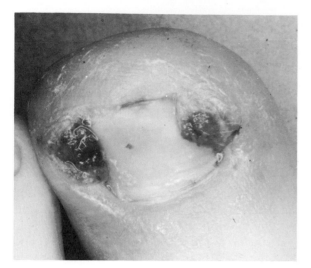

Fig. 7.7   Onychocryptosis with hypergranulation.

Zaias (1990) describes three stages of the condition with individual treatment regimes for each stage.

Stage I is the first sign of ingrowing, with minimal injury to the sulcus tissue but symptoms of pain, slight swelling, oedema, varying degrees of redness and hyperhidrosis. Elevation of the nail with non-absorbent cotton wool corrects the condition in 7–14 days after removal of the cause.

Stage II demonstrates acute pain, erythema, hyperhidrosis, granulation tissue from the ulcerated sulcus tissue, a seropurulent exudate and a foetid odour. The latter may be the result of Gram positive or colonic bacterial growth on the surface of the granulation tissue. Topical high potency steroids or intralesional corticosteroid injection of 2 mg/ml triamcinolone acetonide is reported to clear the granulating tissue, and the condition clears with further cotton wool packing as in stage I.

Stage III. The symptoms present at stage III are those described for stage II, with the addition of an epidermal overgrowth of the granulation tissue, thus making elevation of the nail out of the sulcus impossible. Surgical intervention with excision or cauterisation of the granulation is recommended (Fig. 7.8).

Aetiology

The most common predisposing factors are faulty

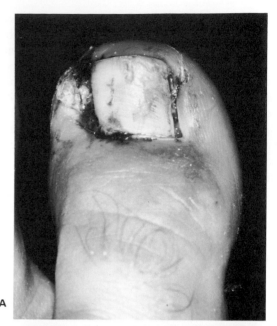

A

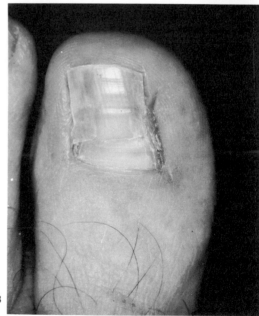

B

Fig. 7.8   (A) Onychocryptosis with hypergranulation. (B) Same case as (A) 8 weeks after partial nail avulsion. The nail plate is permanently flattened and narrowed after excision of the involuted nail edges.

nail cutting, hyperhidrosis, and pressure from ill-fitting footwear, although any disease state which causes an abnormal nail plate (e.g. onychomycosis or onychorrhexis) may promote piercing of the sulcus by the nail.

If a nail is cut too short, the corners cut obliquely, or is subjected to tearing, normal pressure on the underlying tissue is removed and without that resistance, the tissue begins to protrude. As the nail grows forward, it becomes embedded in the protruding tissue. All of the above are likely to result in a spike of nail being left deep in the sulcus, especially if the nail is involuted, increasing the risk of tissue penetration as the nail grows.

Maceration of the tissue of the sulcus is due commonly to hyperhidrosis in adolescent males, but may also arise from the overuse of hot footbaths by the young or elderly. Moist tissue is less resistant to lateral nail pressure caused by narrow footwear or abnormal weight-bearing forces, e.g. pronation or hallux limitus. As compression forces the lateral nail fold to roll over the edge of the nail plate, the sulcus deepens and the nail may penetrate the softened tissues.

Treatment

If onychocryptosis is uncomplicated by infection, the penetrating splinter may be located by careful probing and then removed with a small scalpel or fine nippers. Care must be taken to avoid further injury to the sulcus and to ensure that a spike of nail is not left deep in the sulcus. The edge of the nail can be smoothed with a Black's file although this should be avoided if the nail plate is extremely thin or shows signs of onychorrhexis. The area is then irrigated and dried thoroughly. It should be packed firmly with sterile cotton wool or gauze, making sure that this is inserted a little way under the nail plate to maintain elevation. An antiseptic astringent preparation should be applied to the packing and the toe covered with a non-adherent sterile dressing and tubegauze.

It is sometimes necessary to use an interdigital wedge to relieve pressure on the distal phalanx from the adjacent toe. In approximately 3–5 days, the nail should be inspected and re-packed, and then again at appropriate intervals until the nail has regained its normal length and shape. If there is associated hyperhidrosis, this requires an appropriate regime while the onychocryptosis is being treated.

When onychocryptosis is complicated by infection and suppuration is present, it is important to remove the splinter of nail, facilitating drainage and allowing healing to take place. Hot footbaths of magnesium sulphate solution or hypertonic saline solution may be used to reduce the inflammation and localise the sepsis before removal of the splinter is attempted.

Location and removal of the penetrating nail may cause considerable pain and if there are no contraindications, a local anaesthetic should be given. The injection should be made at the base of the toe, well away from the infected area. After the splinter is removed, the edge of the nail should be left smooth, the area irrigated thoroughly and dried carefully. A light packing of sterile gauze or cotton wool with a suitable broad-spectrum antiseptic agent can be applied and the toe covered with a sterile non-adherent dressing and tubegauze.

The patient should be advised to rest the foot and, if necessary, to cut away the upper of the slipper or shoe to remove all pressure from the toe. The patient should return the following day for renewal of dressings, and this must be repeated until the sepsis is cleared.

If hypergranulation tissue is present, it may be excised when the splinter of nail is removed, taking care to control the profuse bleeding which often results. Small amounts of granulation tissue may be reduced by applications of silver nitrate, avoiding introducing it into the sulcus.

Following this treatment the prognosis is good, but the patient must be given clear guidance on the predisposing factors to avoid recurrence. If the condition does not respond, it is likely that there is still a small nail splinter embedded in the sulcus and further careful investigation must be undertaken to locate the offending piece of nail. Where it is obvious that the onychocryptosis results from a minor involution of the nail, the application of a nail brace will flatten out the nail plate and reduce the involution. If conservative treatment of severe involution does not provide long term relief, nail surgery will invariably be necessary. This involves partial or complete avulsion of the nail and the destruction of part or the whole of the nail matrix. (see Ch. 18).

SUBUNGUAL EXOSTOSIS

Subungual exostosis (Fig. 7.9) is a small outgrowth of bone under the nail plate near its
free edge or immediately distal to it. Most
frequently, it occurs on the hallux in young
people, is slow growing and a source of considerable pain in the later stages. Trauma is a major
causative factor (Baran et al 1990), although this
is disputed by some authors (Cohen et al 1973).
Repeated trauma, though slight, from shoes
which are either too short, shallow or excessively
high heeled, is found by podiatrists to be a
common cause.

As the outgrowth increases, the nail becomes
elevated and displaced from the nail bed and
the tumour may emerge from the free edge or
destroy the nail plate. If the nail is eroded, the
nail bed tissue ulcerates and may become
infected. The protuberance offers a hard resistance to pressure and there is usually a clear line
of demarcation around the area. As the exostosis
increases, a fissure may develop at the edge of this
line of demarcation with a serous or purulent
exudate.

The epidermis covering the tumour becomes
stretched and thinned and takes on a bright red
colour which blanches on pressure. When the
exostosis protrudes distal to the free edge, the
bright red gives way to a more yellow colouration,
which must be differentiated from subungual
heloma and psoriasis. Accurate diagnosis of this
condition requires X-ray examination, which
shows trabeculated osseous growth, expansion of
the distal portion and a radiolucent fibrocartilage
cover.

Pathology

Following an injury to the periosteum of the distal
phalanx, a periostitis occurs. Initially, there is an
outgrowth of cartilage which later ossifies.

Treatment

Temporary relief may be given by means of
protective padding and advice on footwear, but
surgical excision is always the most satisfactory
treatment (see Ch. 18).

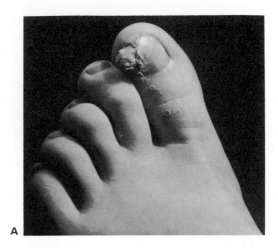

A

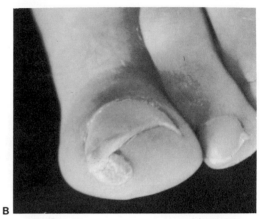

B

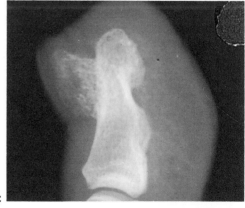

C

Fig. 7.9   (A) and (B) Subungual exostoses. (C) X-ray shows
elevation of nail plate by exostosis.

ONYCHAUXIS (HYPERTROPHIED NAIL)

This is an abnormal but uniform thickening of the
nail, increasing from the base to the free edge, and

is commonly seen in podiatric practice. It may be accompanied by slight brown colour changes in the nail plate and enlargement of the sulci due to the thickened lateral edges of the nail. Often, only the nail of the hallux is affected but the disorder may appear in other nails. The excessive growth makes nail cutting difficult and this is often neglected; subsequent shoe pressure may cause pain and discomfort. Unremitting pressure from footwear may lead to the development of sub-ungual aseptic necrosis, especially in the elderly. A differential diagnosis must be made from pachyonychia congenita, in which all the nails are affected and nail bed hypertrophy is a major feature.

Aetiology

Onychauxis occurs following damage to the nail matrix, for which there may be one or more causes:

1. single major trauma from a heavy blow or severe stubbing, or repeated minor trauma from shallow shoes or pressure from footwear on long and neglected nails
2. fungal infection of the nails and chronic skin diseases such as eczema, psoriasis and pityriasis rubra pilaris
3. poor peripheral circulation, especially in the elderly
4. some systemic disturbance, which may be suspected when several or all of the nails are affected, e.g. Darier's disease.

Pathology

Trauma to the nail matrix results in the excess production of onychocytes and the nail becomes progressively thicker as it grows along the nail bed. The reason for this permanent increase in production is unclear and as yet little research into it has been undertaken. Rayner (1973) reported that the proximal nail fold was shortened and everted and therefore unable to exert pressure on newly formed cells, but also that the nail matrix produced an epidermal type keratin which increased the thickness of the nail plate and

resulted in a thicker but softer intermediate nail layer.

Baran et al (1991) described hyperplasia of subungual tissues, seen in histological sections, as homogenous oval-shaped amorphous masses surrounded by normal squamous cells and separated from each other by empty spaces (+ve PAS stain).

Treatment

Irrespective of the cause, the nail should be reduced in size to as near normal as possible at each visit in order to relieve pain caused by pressure on the nail bed tissues. Footwear should be examined for correct fitting, but as the damage to the matrix is irreversible, regular treatment is necessary. In some cases, where the cause is linked to a skin disease such as eczema, stabilization of the skin condition results in a remarkable improvement in the nails of both the hands and feet.

If the patient is young and the condition confined to one toe nail, and if there are no other contraindications, avulsion of the nail and destruction of the matrix provides the most satisfactory treatment.

ONYCHOGRYPHOSIS (RAM'S HORN, OSTLER'S TOE)

Onychogryphosis is readily distinguishable from onychauxis since, as well as hypertrophy, there is also gross deformity of the nail which develops into a curved or 'ram's horn' shape (Figs 7.10 & 7.11). The nail is usually dark brown or yellowish in colour, with both longitudinal and transverse ridges on its surface. Commonly, the great toe is affected because its size and prominence makes it prone to injury, but the condition may also arise in other toes.

Aetiology

Any of the aetiological factors involved in the development of onychauxis may be the cause, but by far the most common cause is a single major trauma from a heavy blow or a severe stubbing of the toe. It is sometimes the result of neglect and

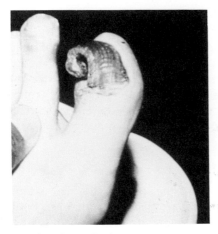

Fig. 7.10   Onychogryphosis.

the consequent increasing impaction from footwear against the lengthening nail. This may cause the nail's free edge to penetrate the soft tissues of the affected toe, and perhaps also of the adjacent toe, resulting in an area of ulceration.

Pathology

It is believed that the spiral like appearance of onychogryphosis is due to an uneven production of cells from the nail matrix, the damaged side of the matrix producing cells at a slower rate (Zaias 1990). However if the faster-growing side determines the direction of the deformity, it would be unlikely to find the same side damaged in each nail. The most common deviation in onychogryphosis is towards the median of each foot and the most likely explanation for this is shoe pressure.

Treatment

Palliative treatment consists of reduction of the hypertrophy by means of nail nippers and/or the nail drill, taking care to prevent haemorrhage from any nail bed tissue which has been caught up in the malformed nail. Throughout treatment, it is important to hold the toe firmly to avoid excessive pull on the underlying soft tissue. Footwear should be examined to ensure adequate fitting. This treatment, repeated at regular intervals, is usually sufficient to give the patient freedom from discomfort. In a young person, especially when only one toe is affected and when palliative measures have failed, avulsion with matrix destruction is the most satisfactory method of providing long-term relief.

ONYCHOPHOSIS

Onychophosis is a condition in which callus and/or the formation of an heloma occurs in the nail sulcus, possibly resulting in the sulcus becoming swollen and inflamed. In a mild case, the effect is little more than irritating, but it can develop to a degree where even slight pressure to the nail plate or the sulcus wall gives rise to acute, sharp pain. There may be associated hypertrophy of the shoulders of the nail plate.

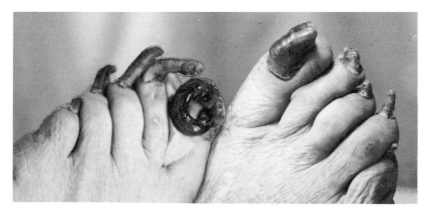

Fig. 7.11   Onychogryphosis.

Aetiology

1. Lateral pressure from constricting footwear or from an adjacent toe which has some structural abnormality, e.g. hallux abducto-valgus
2. Unskilled nail cutting, particularly if the lateral edges of the nail have been left rough or jagged, which may irritate the epithelium of the sulcus and give rise to callus and /or heloma
3. Unnecessarily harsh probing of the sulcus may lead to excessive thickening of the stratum corneum.

Treatment

It is sometimes necessary to soften onychophosis to facilitate its removal. This may be achieved by the application of a soak of hydrogen peroxide (3 vol) left in situ for several minutes; the callus can then be carefully cleared with a small scalpel and checked for the presence of helomata, which must be enucleated.

If removal is not possible after such a soak, it may be necessary to pack the sulcus with a keratolytic, such as 10–15% salicylic acid in WSP or collodion. This should be left in situ for no more than 7 days. Reduction of the callus and full enucleation can then be carried out, leaving a smooth edge to the nail plate. If the lateral edge of the nail is thickened this should be reduced with a Black's file or a pencil burr. Depending on skin texture, an antiseptic astringent or an emollient antiseptic should then be applied and a cotton wool packing inserted between the nail edge and the sulcus.

If it is necessary to reduce pressure from an adjacent toe, an interdigital wedge, made from semi-compressed felt or a long-lasting silicone material may be inserted. Footwear should always be examined to ensure adequate fitting and advice given on care of the nails.

SUBUNGUAL HELOMA

As the term implies, a subungual heloma is the development of a nucleated keratinised lesion under the nail plate. It may occur on any part of the nail bed. As the lesion develops, it detaches the nail from the nail bed and is seen as a small area of onycholysis which assumes a yellowish-grey colour. The colour does not change under pressure and this distinguishes a subungual heloma from a subungual exostosis. A further aid to diagnosis is that a subungual heloma will yield slightly to pressure, while the subungual exostosis presents hard resistance.

Aetiology

1. Trauma which may be slight but prolonged from shoes which are too short or too shallow, or sometimes from high-heeled shoes which produce abnormal pressure on the nail plate
2. Forefoot deformity, such as hallux limitus/rigidus with hyperextension of the hallux, or overlying toes in association with hallux abductovalgus. Each incurs increased pressure from the shoe onto the nail plate, resulting in keratinization of that particular part of the nail bed.

Treatment

If the heloma is near the free edge, an area of the nail plate can be removed to enable it to be enucleated. A suitable antiseptic emollient can then be applied together with protective padding, if necessary, and the dressing held with tubegauze.

Where the heloma is located towards the proximal half of the nail, it is necessary to reduce the nail overlying the lesion with a nail drill. Care must be taken not to drill into nail bed tissue. The remaining thin shell of nail can be removed with a scalpel and the area enucleated and dressed as before.

Treatment may require to be repeated, especially if the heloma forms proximally, and it is essential to eliminate the cause or provide permanent protection to prevent pain and the formation of an aseptic necrosis. Modification of footwear may accommodate the deformity but there are cases where surgery is indicated.

PARONYCHIA

Paronychia and onychia (see p. 135) frequently

occur together. The former is characterised by inflammation of the tissues surrounding the nail plate and the latter by inflammation of the matrix and the nail bed. Both conditions may be acute or chronic, and are always potentially serious as they most commonly arise from either a bacterial infection or a systemic disease. Acute paronychia begins with local redness, swelling and throbbing pain at the side of the nail; gentle lateral compression of the digit may produce a droplet of pus at the lateral or posterior fold. Chronic paronychia develops insidiously and may be unnoticed by the patient. Redness and mild swelling of the proximal nail fold is the earliest sign, which progresses slowly to resemble a semicircular cushion around the base of the nail (Fig. 7.12). The cuticle is detached and eventually the nail shows transverse ridging and becomes friable, which may cause shedding of the entire nail plate from the proximal margin.

Aetiology

Any traumatic incident which might facilitate the entry of bacteria or a foreign body into the tissues can predispose to paronychia. There are many causes, which include severe stubbing of the toe, slight injury to the periungual tissue, unskilled treatment with a scalpel and untreated ingrowing toe nail. The condition may be a manifestation of some systemic disease, such as diabetes mellitus, collagen vascular disease, sarcoidosis or vasculitis.

There is always the possibility that the infection will become widespread, therefore it is advisable to suggest that the patient should consult a physician. Spreading infection is particularly likely when more than one nail is affected. Chronic

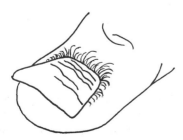

Fig. 7.12 Paronychia with swelling of the PNF and transverse ridging of the nail plate.

paronychia most often occurs in the finger nail, particularly among persons whose occupation entails regular immersion of their hands, e.g. barstaff, fishmongers and confectioners, thus rendering them more likely to infection, even after slight trauma. Young women are more susceptible to the condition.

Pathology

Once bacteria or some foreign body have gained access to the tissues, the natural defensive reaction of the body induces a local inflammatory response and the area becomes red, swollen and extremely painful. The oedema separates the nail fold from the proximal nail plate, allowing further access for bacteria, which are commonly of the staphylococcal or streptococcal type. Infection leads to the formation of pus, which may be expressed from the nail fold. The yeast *Candida Albicans* can also infect the tissue.

Treatment

Paronychia should always be regarded as potentially serious and it must be ascertained whether the condition is acute or chronic.

Acute paronychia is mainly the result of local trauma, and treatment is primarily directed towards the prevention of infection if this is not already present, and towards the reduction of inflammation and congestion. Cold compresses every 4 hours for 24 hours should be given to relieve congestion. This is followed by the application of an antiseptic and a suitable protective dressing. The treatment should be repeated at frequent intervals until the symptoms subside. It is important that the patient is advised to rest the foot as much as possible and to avoid the cause if practical to do so. Usually, if infection is not present, the condition resolves satisfactorily.

If infection is present, the first principle is to promote drainage of any pus by means of a hot antiseptic footbath, repeated at home every 4 hours, or by surgically removing the nail plate. Arrangements should be made for the patient to obtain appropriate systemic antibiotic therapy from the doctor while podiatric dressings continue at frequent intervals. Drainage, once established, must be maintained until all pus has been cleared. The insertion of a piece of sterile ribbon gauze will assist this process. Once complete drainage has been achieved, the lesion can be thoroughly cleansed with saline solution and dried. To promote healing, an antiseptic of wide antibacterial spectrum should be applied, covered by a sterile dressing. Such treatment is usually adequate but the condition may progress to become chronic when further medical advice should be sought.

ONYCHIA

Onychia is inflammation of the matrix and nail bed and frequently originates from paronychia. The clinical features of both conditions are similar and should always be regarded as serious. Local infection will cause suppuration, which produces a discolouration of the overlying nail plate (yellow, brown, black or green depending on the infecting organism). A throbbing pain, which increases in severity, is the common symptom, relief only being obtained by drainage of the pus.

Aetiology

1. Any traumatic incident which introduces bacteria or a foreign body into the tissues; the condition will probably be confined to one toe
2. Any one of a number of systemic diseases; it is likely that several of the toes will be affected.

Pathology

Onychia can, and often does, result from parony-chia (q.v.) and the pathology is similar. Bacterial invasion results in a purulent infection which collects beneath the nail plate, causing pressure and onycholysis (seen as separation of the nail from the nail bed).

Treatment

Immediate relief of acute pain will be obtained by removal of as much of the nail plate as necessary to provide drainage of the underlying pus. Once this is achieved, the further treatment is the same as for paronychia.

ONYCHOLYSIS

Onycholysis is separation of the nail from its bed at its distal end and/or its lateral margins (Baran et al 1991). It may be idiopathic or secondary to systemic and cutaneous diseases or may be the result of local causes. Air entering from the distal free edge gives a greyish-white appearance to the nail plate and forms variably shaped areas of detachment. If a sharp sculptured edge is present, it is likely to be self-induced by harsh manicuring. It is more common in finger nails than toe nails and affects women more frequently than men.

Aetiology

1. Idiopathic—Baran et al (1991) suggest that idiopathic onycholysis of women and sculptured onycholysis are probably the same condition
2. Systemic disease, such as poor peripheral circulation, thyrotoxicosis and iron deficiency anaemia
3. Cutaneous diseases, which include psoriasis, eczema and hyperhidrosis
4. Drug induced, due to the administration of bleomycin, retinoids, chlorpromazine, tetracyclines or thiazides
5. Local causes, such as trauma, where only one nail will be affected, or local infections, e.g. fungal, bacterial and viral. External irritants also result in onycholysis, the most common being prolonged immersion in hot water with added detergents or the use of solvents such as petrol and cosmetic nail polishes.

Pathology

Separation of the nail is usually symptomless but as the condition progresses, the space becomes filled with hard keratinous material from the exposed nail bed. The increased subungual pressure caused by this excess tissue may give rise to inflammation and very rarely becomes liable to infection.

Treatment

If a systemic cause is suspected, the patient should be advised to consult a physician. The single most important step in the treatment of onycholysis is to remove all of the detached nail at each visit. This prevents trauma from hosiery and bedclothes, allows possible mycotic material to be taken from the most proximal lytic area for culture, allows the nail bed to dry out where *Candida albicans* is the infecting organism, and permits application of a suitable antifungal preparation at the active edge of the disease. Within 3–4 months the nail should resume a normal, fully attached appearance (Zaias 1990).

ONYCHOMADESIS (ONYCHOPTOSIS, APLASTIC ANONYCHIA)

This condition involves spontaneous separation of the nail, beginning at the matrix area and quickly reaching the free edge. The separation is often accompanied by some transient arrest of nail growth, characterised by a Beau's line.

Aetiology

1. Trauma, resulting in a subungual haematoma, or from repeated minor trauma, e.g. sportsman's toe
2. Serious generalised diseases, e.g. bullous dermatoses, lichen planus or drug reactions
3. Local inflammation, e.g. paronychia or irradiation
4. Defective peripheral circulation or prolonged exposure to cold
5. It may be an inherited disorder (dominant) and shedding will occur periodically.

Treatment

If a newly formed subungual haematoma is present, treatment should be aimed at relieving pressure, which may necessitate puncturing the nail.

For those cases where trauma can be excluded, the podiatrist can protect the nail with simple tubegauze dressings or an acrylic resin plate, which prevents snagging on bedclothes and hosiery until the nail fully regrows.

ONYCHATROPHIA AND ANONYCHIA

Onychatrophia is used to describe a nail which has reached mature size and then undergoes partial or total regression. Anonychia is reserved to describe a nail which has failed to develop. However, the two conditions are difficult to differentiate.

Damage to the nail matrix resulting in onychatrophia is caused by lichen planus, cicatricial pemphigoid, severe paronychia, epidermolysis bullosa or severe psoriasis. Anonychia occurs with rare congenital disorders, e.g. nail-patella syndrome.

ONYCHORRHEXIS

This condition presents as a series of narrow, longitudinal, parallel superficial ridges. The nail is very brittle and splitting at the free edge is common. Ridging becomes more prominent with age but can be initiated by lichen planus, rheumatoid arthritis and peripheral circulatory disorders.

BEAU'S LINES

First described by Beau in 1846, these transverse ridges or grooves reflect a temporary retardation of the normal growth of the nail. They appear towards the proximal nail fold and move towards the free edge as the nail grows. The distance of the groove from the PNF indicates quite accurately the length of time since the onset of the event causing the growth retardation (nail growth being about 1 mm per week).

Aetiology

Any condition or disease which may temporarily arrest nail production from the matrix can be responsible. A single groove is usually the result of a severe febrile illness, although they have also been noted post-natally and after many other non-specific events. When the transverse ridges are due to paronychia or repeated minor trauma, they are often like rhythmic rippling.

Treatment

No specific treatment, other than reassurance, is necessary as the nail will resolve once the aetiological factor has been dealt with.

HIPPOCRATIC NAIL (CLUBBING)

Hippocratic nail is the term used to describe an exaggerated longitudinal curvature of the nail, sometimes extending over the apex of the toe, which gives the digit a *clubbed* appearance. The disorder is usually associated with some long-standing pulmonary or cardiac disorder and has been linked with thyroid disease, cirrhosis and ulcerative colitis (Fig. 7.13).

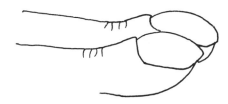

Fig. 7.13   Clubbing or hippocratic nail.

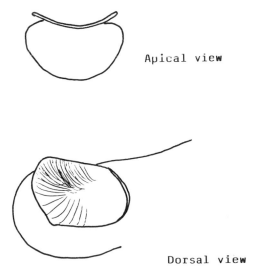

Apical view

Dorsal view

Fig. 7.14   Koilonychia (spoon-shaped nail).

KOILONYCHIA (SPOON-SHAPED NAIL)

This condition is more frequently met in finger nails than toe nails. The normal convex curvature is lost and instead it becomes slightly concave or spoon-shaped. In infancy, koilonychia is a temporary physiological condition, but after this stage there is a proven correlation between koilonychia and iron deficiency anaemia. Thin nails of any origin, occupational softening and congenital forms are all aetiological factors (Fig. 7.14).

ONYCHOMYCOSIS (TINEA UNGUIUM)

Onychomycosis is a fungal infection of the nail bed and nail plate. Fungi are microscopic vegetative organisms possessing no chlorophyll; they can only exist by utilising other organic matter for food. Certain groups of fungi, generally classified as *dermatophytes*, possess the ability to metabolise keratin and can thereby grow and proliferate in the presence of this protein. The human nail and its nail bed provide a suitable environment in which the dermatophytes can flourish, and once these fungi have established themselves in that situation the condition is known as onychomycosis. Since dermatophytes can utilize keratin as a source of food, it follows that any one or all of the nails will be liable to attack.

An infected nail plate becomes thickened and quite brittle and takes on a yellowish-brown colour, eventually developing a worm-eaten or *porous* appearance.

Aetiology

It is not always possible to pinpoint the actual source of the infection but one of the predisposing factors is failure to maintain a good standard of foot hygiene. Hyperhidrosis, communal showers, failure to dry the feet thoroughly following sporting activities and spread of an existing skin infection are all factors to be considered.

Pathology

Of the dermatophytes associated with onychomycosis, the most frequently identified in practice are *Trichophyton rubrum* and *T. interdigitale.*

Infection commonly commences at the distal edge of the nail and gradually spreads over the entire nail plate and nail bed. Eventually, the nail plate becomes onycholytic as subungual debris increases. White marks, indicating fissuring, may appear on the nail plate.

Treatment

To halt and perhaps ultimately to eradicate a fungal infection of the nail plate requires continuing careful treatment over many months. A full explanation of the treatment regime should be given to the patient as success will depend largely on patient compliance. Treatment involves the use of topical fungicides.

To facilitate their full potential, the nail should be thinned as far as it practicable, without causing pain, before the preparation is applied. Alternatively, the nail plate can be cut away so that the medicament can be applied directly to the active edge of the infection. The patient should repeat the treatment daily for one month or until new nail growth shows no signs of fungal infection. Thereafter, treatment should continue for up to three months to prevent reinfection.

Systemic fungal treatment with griseofulvin has been disappointing, with side effects which cause the patient to discontinue treatment after a short time. However, recent evidence suggests that terbinafine (Lamisil) will clear onychomycosis within twelve weeks with no reported side effects (Dykes et al 1990).

Advice on the spread of the infection via towels, hosiery and shoes must be emphasised, together with vigilant attention to drying and general personal hygiene.

LEUCONYCHIA

This term describes white markings on the nail in lines (*striata*), dots (*punctata*) or extending over the entire nail plate (*totalis*). They usually indicate minor trauma as a result of short shoes or sporting activities; more rarely, leuconychia may result from a systemic illness.

YELLOW NAIL SYNDROME

In this disorder, the rate of nail growth reduces greatly and sometimes almost ceases. All the nails becomes a yellowish-green colour; they also thicken and display an increased longitudinal curvature with some evidence of onycholysis. The condition is almost always associated with some underlying respiratory or lymphoedematous abnormality. Spontaneous recovery occurs in 30% of cases and the use of intravenous vitamin E is said to give beneficial results (Zaias 1990).

PTERYGIUM

Pterygium is adhesion of the eponychium to the nail bed following destruction of the matrix due to diminished circulation or some systemic disease. The entire nail plate is eventually shed.

FURTHER READING

Achten G 1982 In: Pierre, M (ed). The nail, Monograph 5. Churchill Livingstone, Edinburgh, ch 3 pp1–4
Baden H P 1987 Diseases of the hair and nails. Year Book Medical Publishers, Chicago, Illinois
Baran R, Dawber R P R 1984 Diseases of the nails and their management, 2nd edn. Blackwell Scientific Publications, Oxford
Baran R, Barth J H, Dawber R P R 1991 Nail disorders: common presenting signs, differential diagnosis and treatment. Martin Dunitz, London
Baran R, Dawber R P R, Levene G M 1991 A colour atlas of the hair, scalp and nails. Wolfe Publishing, London
Beaven D W, Brooks S E 1984 A colour atlas of the nail in clinical diagnosis. Wolfe Publishing, London
Burton J L 1990 Essentials of dermatology: student notes, 3rd edn. Churchill Livingstone, Edinburgh

Cohen H J, Franck S B, Minkin W, Gibbs R C 1973 Subungual exostosis. Archives of Dermatology (Chicago) 107: 431–432
Dykes P J, Thomas R, Finlay A Y 1990 Determination of terbinafine in nail samples during systemic treatment for onychomycosis. British Journal of Dermatology 123: 481–486
Gilman A G, Goodman L S, Rall T N, Murad F 1985 The pharmacological basis of therapeutics, 7th edn. Macmillan, Basingstoke
Hamilton J B, Terada H, Meistler G E 1955 Studies of growth throughout the lifespan in Japanese: growth and size of nails and relationships to age, sex, heredity and other factors. Journal of Gerontology 10: 401–415
Hashimoto K, Gross B G, Nelson R, Lever W F 1966 The ultrastructure of the skin of human embryos III. The

formation of the nail in 16–18 weeks old embryos. Journal of Investigative Dermatology 40: 143–145

Jarratt A, Spearman R I C 1966 The histochemistry of the human nail. Archives of Dermatology 94: 652–657

Johnson M, Comaish J S, Shuster S 1991 Nail is produced by the nail bed: a controversy resolved. British Journal of Dermatology 125: 27–29

Lewin K 1965 The normal finger nail. British Journal of Dermatology 77: 421–430

Lewis B L, 1954 Microscopic studies of fetal and mature nail and surrounding soft tissue. Archives of Dermatology 70: 732–747

Norton L A 1971 Incorporation of thymidine-methyl-H[3] and glycine-2-H[3] in the nail matrix and bed of humans. Journal of Investigative Dermatology 56: 61–68

Rayner V R 1973 An investigation into nail hypertrophy. The Chiropodist (Sept). 288–302

Samman P D, Fenton D A 1986 The nails in disease, 4th edn. William Heinemann, London

Zaias N 1967 The movement of the nail bed. Journal of Investigative Dermatology 45 (4): 402–403

Zaias N, Alvarez J 1968 The formation of the primate nail. An autoradiographic study in the squirrel monkey. Journal of Investigative Dermatology 51 (2): 120–136

Zaias N 1990 In: Zaias N (Ed) The nail in health and disease, 2nd edn. Appleton & Lange, Norwalk, Connecticut

8. Management of diabetic and other high risk patients

Barbara Wall

All patients should be regarded as being at risk of acquiring complications following podiatric treatment, the possibilities being minimised by employing adequate aseptic techniques before, during and after treatment. There are, however, several categories of patient who are deemed to be at high risk, meaning that they are more likely to have inadequate healing potential or an increased susceptibility to infection and/or predisposition to necrosis and ulceration. The patient group most frequently cited as being at high risk are diabetics, but it is important to realise that there are other systemic and local pathologies which place the affected patient in a high risk category (Table 8.1).

Diabetes mellitus affects approximately 1% of the population, although there is geographical and racial variation within this group. The podiatrist is frequently involved in the management of conditions secondary to the primary disease and these may be summarised, as shown in Table 8.2. There is debate whether it is the degree of control

Table 8.1 Sources of high risk categories.

1. *Vascular disorders*:
   Arterial, venous and lymphatic
   Macrovascular and microvascular, i.e. ischaemia
2. *Neurological disorders*:
   Peripheral and central nervous systems, i.e. sensory loss, deformity, alterations in gait
3. *Compromised immunity to infection*:
   Primary pathology, e.g. AIDS, diabetes mellitus
   Secondary to drug therapy, e.g. steroid therapy
4. *Arthritides*:
   e.g. rheumatoid arthritis
5. *Oedema*:
   e.g. in association with venous incompetence, chronic cardiac failure. Oedema prevents normal exchange of nutrients and metabolites between blood vessels and skin because the excess fluid compresses capillaries and increases the distance between the capillary and the superficial tissues.
6. *Metabolic disturbances*:
   e.g. diabetes mellitus
7. *Malnutrition*:
   This may occur more frequently than is supposed, particularly in the elderly of limited financial means or when cultural or religious conventions govern diet
8. *Psychological disturbances*:
   These can make it difficult for patients to care for themselves, e.g. depression. Patients with mental disability may require additional help in recognising and preventing foot problems

Table 8.2 Secondary disorders associated with diabetes mellitus that may affect the feet and lower limbs.

1. *Vascular*:
   Accelerated atherosclerosis
   Microvascular changes*
2. *Altered blood constituents*:
   Red blood cells become 'stiffer' and cannot flow easily through the capillaries; oxygen is not so readily given up by haemoglobin
   Abnormal white cells which are not so effective in phagocytosing and destroying pathogenic microorganisms
3. *Neuropathic*:
   Abnormal conduction in motor, sensory and autonomic nerves, resulting in deformity and alteration in appreciation of damaging stimuli. Autonomic neuropathy will lead to anhidrotic skin and alteration in blood flow to the foot as a result of sympathetic nerve damage
4. *Increased susceptibility to infection*:
   As a result of factors mentioned above.
5. *Impaired eyesight*:
   Diabetic retinopathy and cataracts may limit the patient in looking for signs of damage to their feet.
6. *Kidney disease*:
   This may result in oedema and increased susceptibility to infection.
7. *Abnormal non enzymatic glycosylation of various proteins*:
   This can include collagen, leading to abnormal wound healing and soft tissues

* There is much research being carried out at present looking at the inter-relationship between neuropathy, in particular autonomic neuropathy, and vascular disease in diabetes mellitus.

or the duration of the disease that is ultimately responsible for the severity of secondary complications. Recent studies suggest that the different aetiological factors responsible for producing Type I and Type II diabetes mellitus (also referred to as insulin dependent diabetes mellitus and non insulin dependent diabetes mellitus respectively) may be implicated in causing different effects on, e.g. blood vessels; thus secondary disorders resulting from Types I and II diabetes mellitus may be very different and so require different treatment.

AIMS IN TREATING HIGH RISK PATIENTS

The main aims when treating high risk patients, be they diabetic or not, can be summarised as follows:

1. Prevention of infection or injury
2. Effective management once there is an established open lesion or necrosis.

Carrying out these aims successfully can be difficult and demanding in many cases, and further consideration of what is involved is required.

Prevention of complications

Obtaining a detailed medical history is vital, with assessment of body systems including vascular, neurological and biomechanical examination. Any drug therapies being received by the patient should be explored; this would include non-prescription medication as well as that prescribed by medical practitioners.

Simple urinalysis and/or estimation of blood sugar using a correctly calibrated glucometer may be performed by the podiatrist, especially when there is a family history of diabetes mellitus, when there are episodes of infection, or when the patient shows signs and symptoms which suggest diabetes mellitus, such as repeated episodes of infection.

The use of forceplates (see Ch. 3) can be invaluable in locating areas of high pressure loading, particularly in the neuropathic foot. It should be noted that it is not only the very sophisticated systems that can be useful for this purpose, although if they are connected to a computerised system that calculates quantitative results, higher degrees of accuracy will be obtained for future reference.

Patient education regarding the relationship of the primary systemic pathology to their feet is important, but is frequently difficult; many educational and information packs are available, but they must be accompanied by explanations specific to the patient, bearing in mind intellectual, cultural and language differences.

Close attention to aseptic techniques must be stressed and the use of autoclaves is mandatory for instrument preparation. Skin preparation must be meticulous—probably the most important factor being thorough application of an alcohol based preparation; the added antiseptic element is probably less important than previously realised.

If caustic medicaments have to be applied in the treatment of lesions, they should be applied with care and their progress monitored closely. Minor surgical procedures should only be performed as a last resort and only after consultation with the patient's general practitioner.

Advice regarding suitable footwear and hose is essential and is considered in other chapters.

Management of established ulceration

An ulcer is an example of a wound which, for various reasons, will not heal. As most research concerning dressings is not restricted to *ulcer* treatments, the term *wound* is used in preference to ulcer in the following discussion.

In considering the management of wounds, the following three areas will be discussed:

- Examination of the wound
- The use of antiseptics and topical medicaments
- The use of dressings.

Examination of the wound

In order to assess the progress of a wound, a detailed history must be obtained on the initial consultation and observations recorded routinely at each treatment.

The initial history and examination should include vascular, neurological and biomechanical assessment, examination of footwear and hosiery, obtaining a specimen of any discharge for microscopy, culture and sensitivity of the organism to antibiotics, and obtaining a radiograph if necessary. Contact should be made with the patient's general practitioner in order to coordinate treatment.

The history should include the medical and surgical details. It is important to enquire about drug therapy as the underlying condition for which the medication is being administered may be of relevance, e.g. vitamin B injections for pernicious anaemia; or the drug itself may impair healing potential, e.g. corticosteroids. Some drugs may be responsible for producing adverse reactions in susceptible individuals, which could include drug eruptions. These may ulcerate and thus should be included in a differential diagnosis.

Points that should be explored when taking a history are shown in Table 8.3.

Observations that should be made by the podiatrist are shown in Table 8.4. If possible, photographs taken in a standardised manner should be obtained as these prove more accurate than a written account. However, if photographs cannot be taken, accurately labelled diagrams may suffice.

On subsequent visits, there should be full observation of the current status of the patient and wound and the recording of any subjective changes reported by the patient or their carers.

Swabs should be obtained from the wound and sent for microbiological examination (see Ch. 3). A request for identification of the

Table 8.3 History of the lesion.

1. The *duration* of the lesion
2. Any *changes in the size or appearance* of the lesion (note must be made of excessive bleeding, which may indicate malignant change, particularly in long standing ulcers)
3. Any changes in the *number* of lesions
4. Any *previous incidents* of similar ulceration
5. Any *pain or altered sensation* associated with the lesion
6. Are there any *other signs or symptoms* that the patient/podiatrist feels are related to the lesion?
7. Does the patient know the *cause* of the lesion?

Table 8.4 Observation of a wound/ulcer.

1. The precise anatomical *site* of the lesion
2. The *size* of the lesion. This should be measured accurately using one of the commercial measuring devices
3. The general appearance of the lesion and surrounding tissue, including the presence/absence of inflammation and signs of spreading infection (lymphangitis, lymphadenitis, cellulitis), the presence/absence of hyperkeratosis or maceration
4. The *sides* of the lesion; in particular, whether there is undermining of surrounding tissues. If so, the full extent of the lesion must be ascertained by judicious use of a sterile metal probe; this is particularly important in diabetic lesions as infection may spread rapidly if the full extent of the lesion is not revealed. The probe may also be used to estimate the *depth* of the lesion
5. The *base* of the lesion must be observed for the presence of slough or granulation tissue. Other deep structures that may have become involved, e.g. bone, joints or tendons, must be examined. It may be necessary to obtain a radiograph if deeper structures are thought to be involved or if osteomyelitis or septic arthropathy are suspected.
6. Any *discharge* should be noted and a specimen obtained for specialist microbiological examination. Specific points to be observed by the podiatrist are colour, odour and consistency. The quantity may be approximated by observing soiled dressings and enquiring from the patient how often the dressing is changed
7. Chronic lesions are often associated with the production of fibrous tissue that ties the base to deeper structures and hinders the healing process. By gentle manipulation of the lesion, the amount of fibrosis may be estimated

organism's sensitivity to antibiotic or other drugs should be made, as the increase in methycillin resistant *Staphyloccus aureus* (MRSA) and similar organisms makes proper identification of pathogens imperative before antimicrobial agents are prescribed.

It is important to remember that all wound surfaces will be populated by microorganisms, but not all such lesions are clinically *infected*, rather they may be described as *contaminated*. The degree of sepsis will depend on the type of infecting organism. Some authorities claim that many wounds can contain $10^6 - 10^8$ bacteria per gram of tissue without producing local sepsis (Lawrence 1991). Bacterial species which commonly contaminate open lesions are:

Staphylococcus aureus	33%
Other staphylococci	5%
Streptococcus faecalis	6%
Other streptococci	4%
Escherichia coli	19%

| Proteus spp | 10% |
| Bacteroides spp | 6% |

Taken from *The Journal of Hospital Medicine* 1981: 2 (Suppl).

Management of wounds

There has been much debate about the value of using surgical masks, hats and sterile gloves whilst treating wounds and open lesions. Current research suggests that the use of surgical masks plays no role in preventing air borne contamination of wounds (Report from an Infection Control Nurses Working Party 1984). The most suitable method of preventing contamination is to reduce conversation whilst treating the lesion and in effecting an efficient, well organised treatment. Hats may be useful, but this is questionable. Sterile surgical gloves may be used, but the use of clean non-sterile gloves is acceptable (see Ch. 15). A disposable plastic apron should be worn to protect the podiatrist as well as the patient against cross infection.

The use of pre-packed sterile instruments, medicaments and dressings is strongly recommended. It should be noted that they must be used in the correct manner otherwise cross infection may occur. Soiled dressings and swabs must be disposed of according to individual infection control policies.

The use of instruments on any open lesion and the amount of tissue debrided will depend on the aetiology and clinical appearance of the area at the time of treatment; it is important, as mentioned above (Table 8.4), to ensure full exploration of the lesion and to identify its extent.

Cleansing agents and desloughing agents

The wound will require cleansing and there is a wide variety of products available for this purpose. The removal of slough (a mixture of necrotic tissue, fibrin, leucocytes and bacteria), which can form a medium for further pathogenic activity, can be difficult. In an ischaemic ulcer, slough tends to be firmly adhered to its base, whereas in a neuropathic ulcer, slough may be less tightly bound and easier to remove. The intimate relationship between slough and healing granulation tissue must be remembered and the problems of disturbing the latter whilst removing the former taken into consideration.

The most commonly used wound cleansing agents include sterile isotonic saline, chlorhexidine gluconate, cetrimide and povidone iodine. Most cleansing products are available in a sterile form in single use sachets and the use of these is recommended. Solutions should be applied using sterile gauze or cotton wool; they may also be applied via a sterile syringe barrel without a needle attached.

Sterile aqueous solutions of chlorhexidine are suitable for irrigation of wounds. Chlorhexidine is effective against a wide range of Gram positive and Gram negative organisms, some fungi but not fungal spores. Chlorhexidine may be combined with cetrimide BP and this combination is available in a sterile single use sachet. Cetrimide has a wide range of bactericidal activities as well as detergent properties. The detergent properties and antiseptic properties make the combined product useful for cleansing *dirty* lesions. However the regular use of cetrimide, either by itself or in combination with other substances, is not recommended as it has been shown to have toxic effects on healthy tissue, even at low concentrations (Thomas 1990).

Povidone iodine is found in many products. It has a wide range of activity, however its effectiveness is reduced in the presence of pus. In order to retain its activity it must be applied at frequent intervals, short enough for the brown colour associated with the substance to remain. The brown colour indicates that the iodine is activated; when it is inactivated it converts to colourless iodides.

Other traditional cleansing agents, such as proflavine, are not recommended as their activity against certain pathogenic groups is limited. Hydrogen peroxide (10%) also has limited antibacterial properties and any beneficial effects are due to the mechanical bubbling resulting from the release of oxygen. Theoretically, liberated oxygen may enter the blood stream and cause an embolism, although this is unlikely to occur when used on the feet.

Agents used for removal of slough include hypochlorites and enzymes. Other methods include dextranomer beads and occlusive dressings which allow the enzymes and other products produced by leucocytes and other cells to debride the wound.

It should be noted that in experiments using solutions of isotonic saline, chlorhexidine, cetrimide and povidone iodine on open lesions, all agents with the exception of isotonic saline produced a transient closure of capillaries. Chlorhexidine's effect was virtually non toxic (Brennan et al 1986). In clinical practice, the reduction in capillary blood flow caused by closure of capillaries is short lived, but in most wounds the use of sterile isotonic saline for cleansing is suggested.

The hypochlorites have been used for many years and were introduced by Semmelweiss in the 19th century. The hypochlorites interact with protein and it is this reaction that imparts their antibacterial action. Sodium hypochlorite has a very high pH (alkaline); because of this there is a less irritant version which is known as Dakin's solution. Eusol (Edinburgh University Solution of Lime) is composed of calcium hypochlorite. The correct storage of hypochlorites is important and most hypochlorites are stable for no more than two weeks; however Milton (Richardson-Vick) is stable for a longer period, providing that it remains unopened. A sterile, single use product known as Chlorasol (Seton) is available and is claimed to be stable for over a year.

Hypochlorites have been used for dissolving thick necrotic slough, but are now used far less frequently as other substances are more effective and are without the potentially dangerous side effects of the hypochlorites. There have been several research papers in the last decade concluding that hypochlorites have serious deleterious effects on wounds (Brennan et al 1986); these effects include delayed production of collagen, irreversible shut down of nutritive capillaries and inhibition of neutrophil and macrophage activity. Serious systemic side effects have been reported after using large quantities of hypochlorites on large wounds—this is probably of no significance in routine podiatric practice.

Preparations containing enzymes can be used as desloughing agents, e.g. Varidase (Lederle). Enzymes such as streptokinase and streptodornase degrade fibrin and remove DNA from cell nuclei. DNA composes 30–70% of the solid part of purulent exudate (Hellgren & Vincent 1977). The enzyme agent is presented as a dry powder which must be kept refrigerated and is reconstituted with sterile isotonic sodium chloride solution (0.89% sodium chloride). The resultant solution can be injected under tough necrotic slough or held in contact with the slough via a film dressing and gauze.

Various organic acids held in substances such as propylene glycol, e.g. Aserbine, cause swelling of necrotic tissue, without affecting viable tissue, thus encouraging removal of slough from the wound base.

Agents such as Debrisan (Pharmacia) are composed of sterile beads of dextranomer 0.1–0.3 mm in diameter. They exert a hydrophilic action and act as absorbents and help remove debris and bacteria from the surface of wounds. They must be renewed twice a day. Some of the problems associated with their use have been overcome by the introduction of Debrisan paste, which contains dextranomer beads in polyethylene glycol and water. (It should be noted that if the bead form of Debrisan is spilled on to the floor the area will become extremely slippery.)

The use of occlusive dressings in wound debridement is described later.

Dressings

There has been an abundance of the so called *new breed* or *environmental* dressings in the last decade, with many more to come. Many of these are suitable for use by the podiatrist, but it must be stressed that they do not provide a universal panacea. In many long-standing wounds, the failure to produce effective healing is the result of underlying systemic pathologies and these, if not intractable, must be attended to before healing will take place, thus underlining the need for close cooperation with other health professionals. The dressings must also be used in strict accordance with the manufacturer's instructions otherwise they will prove ineffective. Many local factors can be affected by the podiatrist to maximise efficiency of these new products, e.g. local padding and attention to footwear.

Before considering the various types of wound dressings appropriate for podiatric practice, the frequently referred to *criteria for an ideal wound dressing*, as described by Turner (1979), will be considered, as these criteria form a suitable framework on which to base current concepts. Before considering these in detail, the following statement regarding the *characteristics necessary for optimum wound healing* (Turner 1979) forms an introduction; it should be noted that it takes into consideration the general status of the patient.

. . . those factors which will produce a micro-environment associated with the wound that will allow healing to proceed at a maximum possible rate commensurate with the age and physiological condition of the patient.

Criteria for the ideal wound dressing

The ability to remove excess exudate. The removal of excess exudate is important for three main reasons:

a. Exudate may be considered as a medium for growth of pathogens.
b. Exudate may cause maceration of the wound and its surrounding tissues.
c. If allowed to soak through a dressing, a concept known as *strike through*, exudate may allow entry of pathogens by capillary action through the dressing.

These points must be balanced by views which claim some positive points about exudate. Exudate contains substances derived from its cellular population (neutrophils, macrophages) which are used in the healing process. It has also been shown that by allowing a wound to dehydrate, re-epithelialisation is impaired—this is discussed below.

Thus it is a question of balance when considering a dressing's ability to absorb exudate.

The ability to maintain humidity at the wound/dressing interface. Until Winter's work in the 1950s, wounds were kept as dry as possible, e.g. using fans to maintain maximum dehydration. The rationale was that this regime was thought to discourage bacterial invasion. Winter (1962) questioned this approach, and showed that epithelial movement across a wound is compromised by thick scab formation. The epithelial cells have to seek a moist surface, hence in the case of a dry wound deep under the scab, re-epithelialisation is a slow and energy consuming process.

Permeability to gases. This may be considered a controversial point, but as will be seen from discussion below, the various arguments can be better understood if they are applied to wounds at different stages in the healing process.

For many years, an adequate source of oxygen was considered vital for successful wound healing; thus the early new breed dressings, e.g. Opsite (Smith & Nephew), were gas permeable. It was shown with these dressings that the neutrophil count in the exudate increased and that regeneration of epidermal cells was increased up to ten fold, particularly when exposed to an increased pO_2; both these observations show a beneficial effect to the wound. On the negative side of the argument, neo-angiogenesis (the production of new capillaries which form part of granulation tissue, which is vital in wound repair) is increased in a hypoxic (low pO_2) environment (Knighton 1981). This is thought to result from the effect of hypoxia on macrophages, which causes them to increase production of factors responsible for causing growth of new capillaries. The effect of hypoxia on other activities of macrophages is not thought to be important as they function in either aerobic or anaerobic conditions. Another suggested benefit of maintaining a hypoxic environment is that of pain relief: it is possible that the production of substances responsible for discomfort—e.g. prostaglandins (PGE_2)—may be hindered.

These two contradictory views are justified by Silver (1985), who puts forward the view that healing involves two types of tissue—connective and epithelial—and that each differs in its oxygen requirements. Connective tissue, in particular fibroblasts, requires some oxygen, but when exposed to increased oxygen tensions (pO_2 more than $30–40\,mmHg$), its activity is reduced. Epithelial cells require increased oxygen tensions to be effective.

The effect of carbon dioxide may be important; when carbon dioxide is lost from a wound the pH will increase and this may have local harmful effects; these are discussed below.

Maintenance of a suitable pH. Oxygen is released from haemoglobin most efficiently in an acidic environment (Bohr effect) or when there is an increased carbon dioxide tension (pCO_2); a high pH (alkaline condition) or low carbon dioxide tension will have the opposite effect on oxygen dissociation. It is also thought that a low pH (acid) environment may inhibit the growth of some pathogens and encourage natural removal of slough.

Maintenance of a suitable temperature. In a study of 420 patients, it has been shown that after routine wound cleansing, it takes 40 minutes for the surface of a wound to regain its original temperature and 3 hours before normal mitosis of cells returns (Myers 1982). The dissociation of oxygen from haemoglobin is reduced when the temperature is reduced by more than $10°C$. Thus dressings that allow strike through not only allow dehydration of the wound but may also cause a detrimental reduction in temperature by convection.

It is also relevant to bear these factors in mind when dressing lesions, and to leave wounds exposed for the minimum period of time (this also cuts down the risks of contamination and cross infection), and to avoid using cold solutions for cleansing.

Low adherence of the dressing to the surface of a wound. If a dressing adheres to a wound surface, it may have the effect of damaging granulation tissue and epithelium on removal, as these tissues may grow into the dressing, or it may become incorporated into the wound and produce foreign body reaction. Subjectively, there may be distress and pain to the patient at redressings if the material has become adhered to the wound.

It should be noted that some low or non-adherent dressings have been responsible for damage occurring around wounds due to autolysis of tissue by constituents of exudate that have been unable to travel through the pore structure of the dressing's plastic film interface. In these cases, exudate remains in contact with the wound and its surroundings, causing inflammation.

The ability to be free from contaminants. The dressing must be constructed of a material that can be rendered sterile and kept in that condition until use. It must not contain any substance that could cause a toxic reaction or which would adversely interact with the wound surface. It must not shed particles or fibres which could become incorporated into granulation tissue and cause chronic inflammatory changes, granuloma formation or hypertrophic scarring.

Impermeability to microorganisms. The dressing should not allow the ingress of pathogenic organisms; the situation where this is most likely to occur is when the dressing allows strike through. It has been shown that pseudomonas and proteus can pass through a moist dressing in hours (Colebrook 1948); thus a highly absorbent dressing is indicated. Suitable dressings allow *horizontal* spread of exudate as opposed to vertical spread (surgical gauze) and dressings should be changed before strike through has occurred.

Other factors. These include:

- *Patient comfort and acceptability.* Some of the earlier dressings (in particular the hydrogels— see below) were unacceptable because of malodour and fluid produced by the interaction of the active constituents of the product and exudate; new developments have remedied this and other problems.
- *Ease of application.* Some of the dressings are difficult to apply to the contours of the foot as they are designed for application to larger, flatter body surfaces. There may be problems in ensuring that dressings stay in situ, but with judicious use of adhesive strappings and bandages, some of these disadvantages may be overcome.
- *Cost.* This is of relevance to podiatrists as some dressings are packaged in uneconomical sizes, although smaller, more suitable sizes are becoming available.

Types of dressings

The introduction and availability of wound dressings is increasing at a prodigious rate, so much so that any description will be out of date within months; thus this section will not discuss the individual properties of dressings but rather describe the features of the groups of currently available products. *It should be stressed that before using any of these dressings, practitioners should make themselves fully aware of the indications and contraindications of the product, either by consulting the manufacturer or by referring to MIMS or the British National Formulary.*

Conventional dressings

Examples—Gauze swabs BP, Tulle gras

Most podiatrists will be using one or more of these dressings, often because of availability and cost. There are problems associated with them and these should be seriously considered when looking at the advantages and disadvantages of *conventional* versus *new breed/environmental* dressings, e.g. strike through and associated dehydration and heat loss, shedding of fibres (which become incorporated into the wound) and problems with the dressing adhering to the lesion at dressing changes. This latter problem may be encountered with tulle gras as granulation tissue may grow through the structure and actually incorporate the dressing into the wound. Discussion of autolysis under some non-adherent dressings has taken place above.

Some dressings, particularly those constructed from viscose and perhaps impregnated with medicaments, e.g. Inadine—a viscose dressing combined with povidone iodine (Johnson & Johnson)—may be more suitable, disregarding current debate concerning the use/non-use of topical antiseptics.

Semipermeable films

Examples — Bioclusive (Johnson & Johnson), Tegaderm (3M Healthcare), Ensure-It (Becton Dickinson UK)

The first available film dressing was Opsite, which was developed as adhesive incise drapes for general surgery. This type of dressing is composed of semi-permeable, hypoallergenic adhesive coated film; the actual constituents differ with each product.

These products are gas and water vapour permeable, tissue compatible and without any component that can be shed into a wound; they are transparent and therefore allow observation of the wound without removal and are generally acceptable to patients. They are not absorptive. It is claimed that Opsite reduces the number of pathogens, acting as a barrier to bacterial colonisation; this has not been found to be the case with similar products. Products from this group are suitable for lesions which are not heavily contaminated by pathogens, where there is some granulation tissue and where exudate is not excessive.

Some problems that may be experienced are the collecting of exudate under the film, which will simulate blister formation (which may be evacuated using a syringe) plus problems in the application of the product as it may stick to itself, causing uneven spread onto the wound surface. There may be some trauma when the product is removed.

This group of products may be used prophylactically, as they resist shear stress. A clinical situation where this property may prove useful is in protecting heels and other vulnerable areas from rubbing, particularly when the patient is bed-bound.

Semi-permeable hydrogels

Examples—Geliperm (Geistlich), Vigilon (Bard), Scherisorb (Smith & Nephew), Spenco Second Skin

Structurally, these products are hydrophilic polymers which contain a high percentage of water. There are two basic types of gel: the first group are presented in the form of a sheet (not dissimilar to a thin slice of table jelly); the second group are known as amorphous hydrogels (these may be compared to wallpaper paste in consistency). Both forms are absorptive, the first group swell but retain their form and the second group absorb fluid until their substance becomes dispersed in water.

The first group of hydrogels consist of products which contain approximately 96% water (some product variation), are transparent, flexible and easily moulded, with mechanical properties similar to that of soft tissues which protect the delicate granulation tissue. They are permeable to gas and impermeable to pathogens and can be used to carry and deliver various drugs to the wound—of particular interest is the possibility of delivering growth factors via hydrogels. The hydrogel will dehydrate and must be replaced or rehydrated with sterile isotonic saline or fragmentation may occur. They are kept in place using adhesive tape (e.g. Chirofix). They should not be used when anaerobic organisms have been isolated. Disadvantages to their use are their poor thermal insulation and high cost.

Within this first group of hydrogels are products with a lower water content, which renders them capable of greater absorption of exudate.

The second, or amorphous hydrogel group (e.g. Scherisorb gel), may be of use in desloughing lesions by rehydrating dry necrotic tissue. Members of this group are very effective at absorbing exudate and it has been suggested that this may help reduce local oedema. The amorphous hydrogels are kept in situ by the application of gauze or another secondary dressing over them.

Impermeable hydrocolloids

Examples — Granuflex (Convatec), Biofilm (CliniMed), Comfeel (Coloplast)

These are so called *interactive* dressings. In general terms, they are composed of hydrogels in combination with substances such as elastromeric compounds, adhesives, polysaccharides and proteins. These substances adhere and interact with the wound surface and are held on a water repellent flexible foam backing which should not require a secondary dressing over it. The hydrocolloid may also be presented as a paste, which is used in lesions covered by heavy slough and exudate. There are many other presentations, e.g. bandages coated with hydrocolloids; thus they are often referred to as *wound management systems*.

The interaction of the dressing with the wound produces a yellow semi-liquid product that caused problems in the early versions — it was malodorous and frequently was not contained within the dressing; newer products are much improved in this respect. The resultant interactive product is protective for the wound surface, absorptive and, as implied by the product title, impermeable. The advantages of producing a hypoxic and acidic environment on the production of neo-angiogenesis have been discussed above. The dressing also maintains a moist environment and provides thermal insulation and is reasonably easy to apply and remove. The hypoxic environment may be contraindicated if anaerobic pathogens are isolated from the surface of the wound. Hydrocolloids may also be used as desloughing agents. They are relatively inexpensive.

Alginate dressings

Examples — Kaltocarb (BritCair), Sorbsan (Steriseal)

These products are manufactured from alginates derived from various types of seaweed. In some respects, they represent a very old treatment: sailors used seaweed many years ago for dressing wounds and for effecting haemostasis.

When in contact with exudate or blood, the alginate fibres convert via a calcium/sodium ion exchange into a hydrophilic gel which is absorbent and provides a moist interface protective to underlying structures. It is relatively easy to remove after irrigating the area with isotonic saline solution. The fibres theoretically present no problem as they are biodegradable; however, this may not be as simple and complete a process as reported. Their use in dry wounds is contraindicated, as is their use in deep narrow wounds. There have been reports of patients experiencing a mild burning sensation when alginates are applied; this may be due to the intensely hydrophilic properties of the product causing rapid dehydration and can be minimised by moistening the dressing with sterile isotonic saline prior to application.

Foams

Examples — Lyofoam (Ultra Laboratories), Allevyn (Smith & Nephew)

The earliest foams used as wound dressings were probably marine sponges; in 1884, Joseph

Gamgee introduced an artificial antiseptic absorbent sponge.

Foams such as Lyofoam are indicated for wounds with reasonable amounts of exudate. The manufacturing process produces a dressing with a smooth, non-adherent hydrophilic inner layer and an outer layer of untreated hydrophobic foam. The outer layer helps prevent strike through, as it allows lateral spread of exudate, although a secondary dressing may be required. Foam dressings are very permeable to gas and allow adequate hydration of the wound surface. They also provide extremely effective thermal insulation.

Silastic Foam (Dow Corning) is a silicone based product composed of two components that are mixed at the time of treatment. An individual mixing device is produced. It can only be used easily on deep cavities with a fairly regular shape. It helps prevent premature closure of a wound, but can lead to foreign body reactions. Its use is contraindicated in dirty wounds and there have been reports of toxic effects from the product but at present it is still available.

Other dressings

Almost any substance imaginable has been used as a wound dressing at some point in history; some of the more ancient treatments are being reassessed in a truly scientific manner. One good example is that of honey and sucrose. Honey has a low pH (approximately 3.7) and this possibly renders it liable to kill some pathogenic organisms. Sugar may act in a similar way to dextranomer beads and aid in removing exudate and slough.

New approaches include the amalgamation of growth factors into a suitable vehicle which can be held in intimate contact with a wound. One problem may be availability of new dressings as it is not clear whether they will be regarded as drugs (liable to be prescribed) or dressings, which may be more easily available for the podiatrist. Other developments may include methods of seeding the patient's own epithelial cells onto a suitable culture medium and using the resultant skin on wounds (Shakespeare 1991).

Knowing which group of dressings to use for

Table 8.5   Guide to dressing choice.

State of wound	*Type of dressing*
Covered with thick slough with exudate	Polysaccharide beads
	Hydrogel paste
	Hydrocolloid paste
Covered with slough with little exudate	Hydrocolloid gel
Covered with black necrotic cap	Enzyme preparations
	Hydrocolloid sheet
	Hydrogel paste
Covered with granulation tissue with exudate	Hydrocolloid sheet
	Alginate dressing
	Polyurethane foam
Covered with new epithelium with little exudate	Semi permeable films
	Hydrocolloid sheet
Covered with new epithelium with exudate	Alginates
	Hydrocolloid sheet
	Polyurethane foam
	Knitted viscose

NB *Clinically infected wounds should be treated with an appropriate dressing in conjunction with systemic antibiotics.*

what type of wound is not easy, and *every patient must be treated individually with a treatment plan specific to them.* See Table 8.5, but this should only be used as a *guide* to management.

Other aspects of treatment

The use of antiseptics on wounds is disputed. Most antiseptics can be shown to have a negative effect on the microenvironment of a wound (see the discussion of cleansing agents as most of these can be used as postoperative antiseptics). The vehicle holding the antiseptic may cause sensitivity reactions or prevent drainage of exudate. The advent of the dressings described makes the use of antiseptics unnecessary and may, in fact, alter their properties. The use of topical antibiotics is unwarranted — antibiotics must be given systemically and only after sensitivity of the organism to the appropriate drug is ascertained.

The use of padding and orthotics to protect open lesions may be indicated but each patient will require a specific prescription, therefore only general comments can be made.

In general terms, soft cushioning padding will be indicated rather than firmer redistributive materials; very firm products may compress nutritive blood vessels and compromise blood flow to the area. Accurate positioning of padding is vital, and is not always an easy task, particularly when large sheet dressings have been used. As little adhesive as practically possible should be placed on the skin, the use of conforming bandages or plastic sprays may be used to protect surrounding skin.

When areas of high pressure are identified, casted insoles constructed from Plastazote, which lies on top of Poron or Cleron supported on a base of Birkocork or a similar material, can be very helpful as a preventative measure as well as in the treatment of established lesions.

Footwear and hosiery must be carefully selected, and, if necessary, modifications such as balloon patching may be executed. Plastazote bootees may be constructed, although they are probably not suitable for an active patient. Bespoke or semi-bespoke shoes may be the answer for long term problems or as a preventative measure, however the availability of such footwear may be limited by the patient's means or the availability of Health Service facilities. Enquiries should be made as to the type of footwear worn around the house. Slippers, often a popular choice, are not ideal unless well fitting, as they cause shearing stresses and cause dressings to move.

Rest and elevation of the limb can be advised, but the danger of the patient developing a deep vein thrombosis if they become immobile should not be overlooked. Other problems associated with immobility are the development of pressure sores and, if the limb is not sufficiently elevated, oedema may ensue.

Other health professionals should be enlisted in the care of the patient if pertinent; these may include the general practitioner, district nursing service, physiotherapy departments and social services. Every opportunity should be taken to help the patient and their carers. The nature of the problem and how carers can involve themselves in the treatment programme, requires clear explanation to ensure effective cooperation.

Other approaches to treatment

Scotchcast boots

This method of treating neuropathic ulceration is being practised in various centres throughout the United Kingdom. The healing rates are very promising. The boot is in intimate contact with the whole foot and ulcer and can be constructed so that it can either be removed or remain on the foot. For full details, see several specialist references which are available (Burden 1989).

Summary

The high risk patient can be a challenge to the podiatrist; the adage of prevention being better than cure holds true with this group of patients. The importance of keeping accurate and up to date records of the patient's medical/surgical status cannot be over stressed, neither can the importance of keeping channels of communication open with others involved in the care of the patient. Advice and education are important, but only if the patient understands the aims and is prepared to comply—the responsibility for this lies in the main with the podiatrist.

If wounds do develop they must be treated on an individual basis; an understanding of the wound healing process will help in utilising the new breed dressings to maximum effect. The development of dressings is rapid, and frequent inspection of the medical and nursing press for contemporary views can help in finding suitable treatments for patients.

Other areas of current interest in the treatment of wounds are the use of laser, ultrasound and electromagnetic forces.

FURTHER READING

Brennan S, Leaper D J 1985 The effect of antiseptics on a healing wound: a study using the rabbit ear chamber. British Journal of Surgery 72: 780–782

Brennan S, Foster M E, Leaper D J 1986 Antiseptic toxicity in wounds healing by secondary intention. Journal of Hospital Medicine 8: 263–267

Burden A C 1989 Modification of the 'Leicester' (Scotchcast) boot. Practical Diabetes 6 (3): 118–119

Colebrook L, Hood A M 1948 Infection through soaked dressings. Lancet 2: 682–683

Hellgren L, Vincent J 1977 Degradation and liquefaction effect of streptokinase and streptodornase and stabilised trypsin on necroses, crusts of fibrinoid purulent exudate and clotted blood from leg ulcers. Journal of Internal Medical Research 5: 334–337

Knighton D 1981 Regulation of wound healing angiogenesis: effect of oxygen gradient and inspired oxygen. Surgery 90: 262–270

Lawrence C 1991 Bacterial infection of wounds. Wound Management 1: 14

Myers J A 1982 Modern plastic surgical dressings. Health and Social Services Journal 336–337

Report of an Infection Control Nurses Association Working Party on Ward Preventive Clothing 1984. Infection Control Nurses Association

Shakespeare P 1991 Cultured human skin epithelium for wound repair. Journal of Tissue Viability 1: 19–20

Silver I A 1985 Oxygen and tissue repair in an environment for healing: the role of occlusion. In: Ryan T J (ed) International Congress and Symposium Series No. 88. Royal Society of Medicine, London 15–19

Thomas S 1990 Wound management and dressings. Pharmaceutical Press, Royal Pharmaceutical Society of Great Britain, London p 79

Turner T D 1979 Products and their development in wound management. Symposium, on Wound Healing, Espoo, Finland 1–3 Nov 1979

Winter G D 1962 Formation of the scab and the rate of epithelialisation of superficial wounds in the skin of the young domestic pig. Nature 193: 293–294

9. The ageing foot

Gwen French   Sue J. Braid   Alison M. Barlow

The last two decades have seen a great increase in the volume of literature published about the elderly. This has included surveys to determine the medical and social needs of this section of the population, and has also described the effects of ageing on body systems. The process of ageing is no longer considered to be anything other than a normal phenomenon. However, ageing is often accompanied by more severe degenerative changes which may manifest as specific diseases.

One omission from the literature has been an attempt to define the term ageing itself. It appears to be generally accepted that the term *elderly* is associated with age in terms of years, and that the retirement age, i.e. 60–65 years, is the age at which one makes the transition from middle age to elderly. Hamdy (1984) states, 'Any population can be divided into three main groups; a financially productive working population, which supports a young dependent population, and an elderly population which has retired from active wage-earning employment'.

The elderly population is continuing to increase, although it is expected that the balance of different age groups will change. 'Those aged 65–74 are projected to make up 53% of the population aged 65 and over in the year 2001, and there will be a dramatic increase among those aged 85 or over, who are projected to make up 11% of the elderly in 2001 compared with just over 8% in 1984' (OPCS 1986). It is also interesting to note that 64% of disabled people in Britain are over the age of 75.

Podiatry has a key role to play in this scenario. The most expensive patient is the one who occupies a hospital bed. The independent mobile person, who can attend local health facilities, requires only minimal public expenditure. Adequate appraisal today of the determinants of this dependency spectrum will lower the costly manpower requirements of tomorrow.

Resistance to health threatening factors diminishes progressively through life and the function of the podiatrist in the geriatric field can become progressively demanding. Broadly, the task is to maintain mobility, and to delay the semi-mobile from becoming the expensively nursed immobile. Old age must not be considered as being synonymous with disease and disability. Many elderly people differ from the young only by being somewhat slower and having a reduced fatigue threshold.

Age can also influence a person's willingness to accept treatment. Anxiety about the procedures which are (often wrongly) imagined to be painful can delay the timely removal of onychogryphosis and cutaneous lesions, which again can be precursors of ulcerative and infective states. Reassurance by the podiatrist is needed, together with the willingness to spend extra time, especially when some of the more bizarre looking hypertrophies require attention. Patient confidence may need to be captured by spreading treatments over a series of attendances in much the same manner as is sometimes necessary with children.

SKIN AND NAIL CHANGES

Both Gilchrist (1979) and Gibbs (1975) stated that the most common signs of ageing skin are dryness, scaling and atrophy, and the most common change in pedal skin as a result of ageing is hyperkeratosis.

Structural and functional alterations caused by

intrinsic ageing and independent of environmental insults are now recognised in the skin of elderly individuals. Structurally, the aged epidermis becomes thinner, the keratinocytes become less adherent to one another, and there is flattening of the dermo-epidermal interface. The number of melanocytes and Langerhans cells is decreased. The dermis becomes atrophic and it is relatively acellular and avascular. Dermal collagen, elastin and glycosaminoglycans are altered. The subcutaneous tissue is diminished in some areas, especially the face, shins, hands and feet, while in others, particularly the abdomen in men and the thighs in women, it is increased.

Due to the loss of elasticity, the atrophic skin and the subcutaneous tissues take longer to regain their normal configuration when pinched between thumb and forefinger. The number of eccrine glands is reduced and both the eccrine and apocrine glands undergo attenuation. Sebaceous glands tend to increase in size, but paradoxically their secretory output is lessened. The nail plate is generally thinned, the surface ridged and lustreless, and the lunula decreased in size. Functional alterations noted in the skin of elderly persons include a decreased growth rate of the epidermis, hair and nails, delayed wound healing, reduced dermal clearance of fluids and foreign materials, and compromised vascular responsiveness. Eccrine and apocrine secretions are diminished. The cutaneous immune and inflammatory responses are impaired (Fenske & Lober 1986).

Skin atrophy can take the form of insidious thinning which requires nothing more than woollen hosiery, fleece-lined shoes or slippers, or — occasionally — polyurethane foam pads to cushion and protect potential decubital lesions.

Where vascular insufficiency is an added feature, the slow erosion of terminal phalanges through digital apices, or the prominence of the styloid process of either of the malleoli through the overlying skin can be encountered. These states normally tend to be painful at night.

A further type of skin atrophy is associated with steroid therapy, usually systemic but occasionally topical. Thick plantar skin does not usually succumb to steroid abuse, but drugs prescribed for a non-infective itch-scratch-itch cycle, such as neurodermatitis, may be misapplied to abrasions and other trivial lesions on the dorsal or lateral areas of the foot. Persistent mistreatment of such a nature causes skin atrophy in association with telangiectasis, ecchymosis and cyanosis or pigmentation. Recovery of skin texture is poor and telangiectasis continues, but the cyanosis may fade if bland antiseptic barrier cream is used under a non-occlusive, ventilated dressing.

Fungal infection of the skin in the elderly does not usually present as an urgent problem but may be encountered as a chronic recurring condition in those who have previously been infected in early life. In contrast, fungal infections of the nails appear to be more common. English (1976) found that over 40% of elderly patients attending a chiropody (sic) clinic with thickened nails were microscopically positive for onychomycosis. Cartwright & Henderson (1986) observed thickened nails in over 40% of cases. This was consistent with the findings of Barlow (1987) (Table 9.1).

Both onychauxis and onychogryphosis are common in the elderly and may become more severe when neglected (Fig. 9.1). Shires (1988) examined 26 elderly patients and discovered 31

Table 9.1   Frequency of first nail conditions by sex (535 patients). From *Clinical Rehabilitation* 4: 217–222 (1990).

	Onychauxis	Onychogryphosis	Onychomycosis	Involution
Female	80	40	57	61
	(20.8%)	(10.4%)	(14.8%)	(15.9%)
Male	17	20	35	27
	(11.3%)	(13.2%)	(23.2%)	(17.9%)
Total	97	60	92	88
	(18.1%)	(11.2%)	(17.2%)	(16.4%)
	6.01	0.63	4.78	0.20
Significance	$p < 0.05$	NS	$p < 0.05$	NS

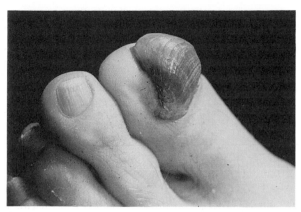

Fig. 9.1 Onychogryphosis typical of those which reveal subungual ulceration.

dermatitis. Generally, eczema is said to be rare in the elderly. However, the localised form of neuro-dermatitis described as nummular or discoid eczema is not unknown and may also be associated with anxiety states. This condition is frequently accompanied by intense itching.

Itching without any obvious lesions is a symptom often complained of by the elderly. This condition, known as senile pruritis, is thought to be affected by air conditioning and central heating with the hot or cold dry air demoisturising the already atrophic skin. Pseudokeratoses or stuccokeratosis, in which plugs or plaques of keratinised skin develop, are benign conditions easily removed or relieved by the application of mild emollients and moisturisers.

Verrucae are rare in the elderly and, unless they cause undue discomfort, are probably best left untreated. They should always be monitored carefully as occasionally they mask malignancy.

FOOT DEFORMITY IN THE ELDERLY

There is a high incidence of foot deformity among the elderly, females being almost twice as likely to have foot deformity than males. The commonest deformities found among the elderly are hallux abductovalgus (Table 9.2) and lesser toe deformities, (Figs 9.2 & 9.3), both of which have been found to be significantly more prevalent in females than males (Braid 1987). These findings are consistent with the random survey of the elderly carried out by Cartwright & Henderson (1986).

Foot deformity in the elderly is often fixed by osteo-arthritic joint change, and further complicated by an inability to accommodate the feet in suitable footwear. Fixed deformities of the toes can lead to soreness and heloma formation interdigitally, and moist fissures may develop either

ulcerated nails, 23 of which were pain-free, so that patients were unaware of their existence. These ulcers occur as a result of pressure and may be described as sterile subungual pressure necrosis. When the nail is cut at the free edge, or reduced in thickness by the drill, a serous or watery discharge occurs. Occasionally this may be spontaneous, when it gives rise to alarm on the part of the patient or carers. The fluid pressure does cause discomfort in some cases, but release of the fluid gives immediate relief. Provided that the nail is reduced in thickness and the appropriate measures are taken to avoid infection, these cases resolve satisfactorily but those patients who have vascular or sensory impairment need to be monitored very carefully.

The onset of psoriasis is rare in the elderly although exacerbation of the disease occurs with emotional stress and occasionally a mild localised psoriatic patch will become rapidly generalised as a result of the stresses encountered by such events as the loss of a marriage partner or the need to move into a different home. Extreme forms of the disease may present as an acute exfoliative

Table 9.2 Prevalence of deformities. From *Clinical Rehabilitation* 4: 217–222 (1990).

	Hallux abductovalgus	Hallux rigidus	Hammer 2nd toes	Clawed/retracted toes	More than one deformity
Female	238(61.8%)	52(13.5%)	91(23.6%)	139(36.1%)	198(51.4%)
Male	47(31.1%)	32(21.1%)	13(8.6%)	42(27.8%)	47(27.8%)
Total	285(53.2%)	84(15.7%)	104(19.4%)	181(33.8%)	245(45.7%)
Significance	$\chi^2 = 40.22$	$\chi^2 = 4.23$	$\chi^2 = 14.81$	$\chi^2 = 2.67$	$\chi^2 = 17.2$
	$p < 0.001$	$p < 0.05$	$p < 0.001$	NS	$p < 0.001$

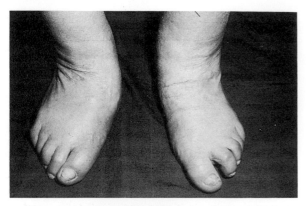

Fig. 9.2 Generalised osteo-arthritic changes and deformity in the feet of an elderly female patient.

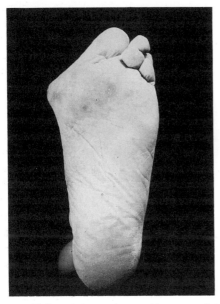

Fig. 9.3 Hallux abductovalgus and lesser toe deformities typical of those found in the elderly.

because the toes are fixed or because the elderly person is physically unable to dry between the toes after bathing. Pressure points and heloma formation commonly occur over the interphalangeal joints of the toes and may develop over the medial exostosis in hallux abductovalgus. An associated bursa develops infrequently, and bursitis and sinus formation over the medial exostosis are uncommon findings among this age group.

Plantar callosities and helomata develop as a result of incompetence of the first metatarso-phalangeal (MTP) joint in hallux abducto-valgus, and where subluxation of the toes occurs localised lesions may develop over the corresponding metatarsal head. Braid (1987) also compared the incidence of foot deformity between the sexes and found that whilst hallux abductovalgus was significantly more common in females, hallux rigidus was found to be significantly more common in males (Table 9.2). The condition may result in development of callosities and helomata over the interphalangeal joint of the hallux on the plantar surface of the foot, or over the fifth metatarsophalangeal joint (Fig. 9.4). This is consistent with the findings of Barlow (1987), who found that significantly more males than females had helomata formation over the 5th MTP joint. Where deformity is so severe as to render it impossible for patients to accommodate their feet in standard footwear, advice on extra-depth footwear or referral for orthopaedic/ surgical footwear may be required.

Mobility

Mobility is of prime importance in the elderly. Senile ataxia, falls and fatigue can lead to a marked diminution of a person's self-confidence in their ability to walk. Careful attention to the feet is essential in this type of patient in order to ensure that the foot is not used as an excuse to avoid beneficial exercise. Footwear must be light-weight, supportive, well fitting and should hold the heel back into the heel cup. The number of

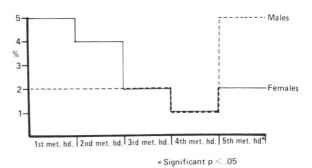

* Significant $p < .05$

Fig.9.4 Frequency of plantar helomata. From *Clinical Rehabilitation* 4: 217–222 (1990).

elderly people whose mobility is impaired *solely* as a result of foot problems appears to be relatively small. Braid (1987) found that of 536 elderly aged 75+ interviewed/examined, only 31 (5.8%) said that they felt that foot problems hindered their mobility. However, foot problems may arise as a result of hindered mobility due to generalised systemic disease, e.g. vascular disease, rheumatoid arthritis, etc., and the podiatrist has a vital role to play in maintaining the feet in as healthy a condition as possible in these circumstances, such that mobility is not further impeded.

Accurate assessment of ranges of joint motion is often difficult to carry out in the elderly patient. They may be unable to relax the foot significantly to allow an accurate assessment to be made and many resist passive motion of the foot. Osteoarthritic changes may result in slight to severe limitation of joint motion. Orthoses may be beneficial to the elderly patient. On the whole, these tend to be protective cushioning type devices, constructed from materials which are not likely to cause tissue irritation or to lead to possible necrosis. Lightweight walking frames and a trolley to carry small articles such as a tea tray will also provide the physical as well as psychological support for the housebound old person. Walking sticks with a non-skid ferrule and elbow and axillary crutches also have a place for some.

GENERAL PHYSICAL/MENTAL INFLUENCES

Obvious *physical disabilities*, such as arthritis, amputation, stroke, respiratory disease or colostomy, will all impose burdens on mobility as well as upon general personality. Gross obesity, which may be related to bad dietary habits, lack of exercise, endocrine disturbances, or genetic factors affecting general metabolism, will adversely affect all weight-bearing structures, not least the feet. Conversely, the grossly emaciated and the cachectic patients will be poor risks with impaired healing processes and vulnerability to infection and hypothermia.

Although each of the above states must remain the responsibility of the physician, the podiatrist

should not automatically assume that the GP is aware of the condition. Some old people are proud of the fact that they have not troubled a doctor for years. Health and religious eccentrics as well as immigrants with language problems can be difficult to persuade that further medical help will benefit the local foot lesion.

Old people living alone understandably can be liable to neglect good *nutrition* — even where Meals on Wheels are provided. A combination of apathy and poverty can lead to low-grade vitamin deficiency: this state should be considered when delayed healing in the absence of other pathological processes is found.

Public awareness of *hypothermia* is greater today than in the recent past and it should be borne in mind when visiting the poorer sections of the community. Social services should be alerted as well as the GP when subjective appreciation of low skin temperature is impaired together with a low oral temperature, pulse and respiratory rate.

Mental health can affect the podiatric management of the aged. The chronically depressed and withdrawn patients are usually easy to treat since they tend to be submissive and to accept clinical attention almost with a sense of fatalism. However, such patients will not comply well with instructions concerning hygiene or routine medication; lay or professional aid will probably be needed for patients with ulcerative or infective lesions requiring simple dressing changes or saline baths.

Although they are few in number, the elderly hyperactive and manic patients can be a very serious risk both to themselves and to the operator. No treatment should be commenced until the podiatrist is satisfied that the previously requested sedative has been given by the patient's doctor— and that it is really effective.

Drug and alcohol abuse are not the exclusive prerogatives of the young, and the chronically addicted should be regarded with the same caution as the hyperactive and the athetotic, although many can be calmed and soothed by a carefully chosen approach. Applied psychology and the art of communication, especially where deafness or a language barrier is a feature, are skills which are usually acquired by practice and experience, and may be supported where necessary by a chaperon or an interpreter. The construction of questions in taking the history may need to be tailored to the mental capacity of the patient. Some will be able to cope with open-ended enquiries, others will need the more closely-filtered questions which require only a yes/no response. The podiatrist should liaise with relatives or carers of the elderly in order that effective treatment may be provided.

SYSTEMIC MEDICATION

It is necessary for the podiatrist to ascertain the nature of any regular medication which the patient is taking. Questions put to patients should always be phrased in an easily understandable form and this is perhaps even more important when taking a case history from the elderly patient. Weekly injections, e.g. vitamin B_{12} (Cytamen), may not be thought of necessarily as medication because it is neither drunk as medicine nor swallowed as tablets. The elderly respond better to individual questions, e.g. 'Do you take any tablets for anything?', 'Do you take any medicine for anything?', rather than to a blanket question covering all three of the above: 'Are you taking any medicines at all?' The response may reveal:

1. A general systemic disease, e.g. diabetes, collagen disorder, anaemia, heart disease, infection, pulmonary disorder
2. Drugs which have the potential to modify or mask signs and symptoms which could be present in the feet. Anti-inflammatory drugs (steroidal and non-steroidal) can suppress an inflammatory response which may precede ulceration/infection. Diuretics may mask oedema, either totally or in degree of severity.

Prolonged antibiotic therapy reduces the numbers of commensal bacteria present on the skin surface. This, therefore, can create the right conditions for fungal infections to flourish, although they are seldom seen in the skin of the elderly.

Steroids

This group of drugs can be particularly important in podiatry. Although prolonged medication is undesirable, there are some life-threatening conditions, such as leukaemia, which leave little alternative. They are also used long-term where pain is an intractable feature and where the sedative effects of powerful analgesics are unacceptable, as in rheumatoid arthritis. Cushing-type mooning of the face, often with telangiectasis, should be a warning sign of the need for care. Skin thinning and atrophy commonly present on the lower leg and foot, and demand scrupulous bland antiseptic therapy. Antibacterial drugs should be a first line of attack, but liaison with the physician may paradoxically require an increased dosage of the steroid together with antibiotic reinforcement. Patients in this category are usually issued with a blue card to warn other practitioners, such as dentists and podiatrists, that this is an 'at risk' patient. A few, those treated at home for example, may not receive this warning card.

Although as a general maxim steroids — because they potentiate infection—should not be used in infected states, sometimes there are agonising decisions to be taken which involve a balance of risks. The podiatrist in this situation should be fully aware of infection risks and meticulous in ensuring that he or she does not contribute to them. No one can be expected to carry the details of every drug in memory, but it is reasonable to check in MIMS for details of toxicity, side-effects and contra-indications for drugs commonly encountered in general practice. The podiatrist can sometimes assist the general practitioner by reporting any unexpected clinical findings if these are of significance, so that the drug may be changed; or perhaps the current 'yellow card' system of reporting to the Committee on Safety of Medicines may be used.

VASCULAR IMPAIRMENT

Geriatric vascular insufficiencies range through a broad spectrum, with mild chilling and acrocyanosis at one end and gangrene at the other. They include:

Drainage defects	Venous incompetence:	varicosity phlebitis thrombosis
	Lymphatic blockage	

Combinations of the above, all exhibiting oedema, can be associated with back pressure arising from congestive heart failure.

Supply defects	Vasospastic:	Raynaud's phenomenon
	Arterial occlusion:	Atheroma Arteriosclerosis Thrombosis

Drainage

Very few of the lymphatic and venous states encountered in podiatry pose threats to the survival of the foot. Many, however, do degenerate into eczematoid conditions which create difficulties with adhesive dressings. Gross *oedema* arising from venous back pressure or the presence of lymphatic failure can result in serous leakage through the skin, sometimes preceded by bulla formation. Although the leaks occur more commonly on the lower leg, they can, especially in those who wear only loose, low-cut slippers, appear over the dorsal metatarsus.

Infection is not a common feature of these leaks because, although the fine breach in the skin continuity is a potential portal of entry, the high serous pressure maintains continuous drainage.

Supply defects

Mild arteriolar insufficiencies in the aged, such as complaints of coldness and chilblains, are treated exactly as in younger age groups. The principle is to promote internal heat production and to minimise external heat loss. Although other disabilities may prohibit vigorous exercise, this should not preclude the encouragement of extra movement. Tactful enquiries may need to be made about the adequacy of diet in the elderly housebound who live alone and cannot be bothered to look after themselves. These are the people who drift into the hypothermic risk category. Insulation involves not only the foot but the person as a whole and their living quarters. Liaison with the GP and district nurse is neces-

sary in these cases. Plastazote insoles are thermally beneficial and man made materials can be better insulators than traditional wool and leather footwear.

More serious vascular insufficiency is evidenced in the foot by skin which is smooth, shiny inelastic and hairless and by nail dystrophy. The long term establishment of a collateral circulation may reduce the importance of pulse impalpability. Blanching of the skin by limb elevation followed by observation of the speed and pattern of dependent rubor can indicate the presence of ischaemia (Fig. 9.5). Engorged veins are evidence that blood is reaching the foot. Routine testing of digital capillary reflux time is a useful method of monitoring the adequacy of the circulation. Light digital pressure on the pulp or apex of each toe will cause blanching. In the elderly the reflux of blood upon release of pressure is approximately 3–4 seconds, although individual variations may be noted.

Before carrying out digital capillary reflux tests it is useful to ensure that the feet have acclimatised to ambient room temperature, since a false impression of the circulatory state will be obtained if the test is undertaken on a patient entering the clinic from outside, particularly in winter. The use of the ankle/brachial index test is a valuable means of obtaining a more accurate estimate of peripheral blood flow and should be used whenever the podiatrist feels that there is cause for concern.

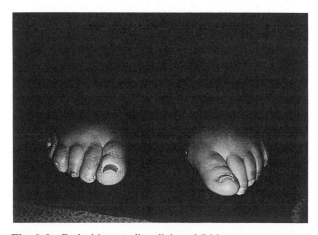

Fig. 9.5 Red, shiny, swollen digits exhibiting severe ischaemia.

Supporting the above signs will be a history of classical *intermittent claudication* affecting the calf muscles, the less well recognised cramp of plantar intrinsic muscles (rather akin to plantar digital neuritis, except that it does not possess a lancinating, electric shock character) and the significant complaint of night pain, insomnia and the need for nocturnal foot cooling.

Night pains

Night pains arise when the metabolic demands of the tissues of the foot exceed the competence of the available blood supply. Sufferers frequently discover for themselves that the metabolic demand rises when the foot becomes warm in bed. Metabolites accumulate from the higher level of cellular activity and, because of the vascular incompetence, they cannot be drained away fast enough. Since the metabolites are themselves cytoirritant or even cytotoxic, they promote a greater (unsatisfied) demand for blood and thus a vicious circle is established. Advanced cases of this type are helped by sleeping with the feet uncovered and exposed to the draught of an electric fan. Cold compresses and ice packs can damp down metabolic demands to a tolerable level but the prognosis is not good.

General vasodilators are of doubtful value in peripheral ischaemia and for some patients they could pose a hypotensive threat. Empirically, a regular 'nightcap' of an alcoholic beverage promotes peripheral vasodilation, thereby relieving night pains and inducing sleep, but the cost is prohibitive to many. Apart from its well-documented property as an anti-inflammatory, phenylbutazone is occasionally prescribed for its less well reported side effect of enhancing blood flow. Normally, one would advocate that cigarette smoking should be discontinued because of its known role in the pathogenicity of small vessel disease. Whether this would be humane counselling for a 90 year old, confined to bed with very few pleasures in life, is a matter for the individual to decide.

Prolonged ischaemia is a pregangrenous state. It is characterized by toxaemia, which provokes weakness, incontinence, mental confusion and the destruction of morale. No podiatrist should witness these changes without summoning medical aid urgently (Figs 9.6 & 9.7). The sequel is gangrene, which will be either dry and painful or moist and infected.

ULCERATION

Ulceration in the elderly is a condition which can have limb or life-threatening consequences. Counsel of perfection is to treat the cause but this is not always possible. Progressive obliterative vascular disease is irreversible, but careful assessment of the causation will assist in creating optimum management conditions and diminish

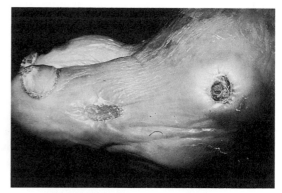

Fig. 9.6   Ischaemic ulceration in the elderly patient.

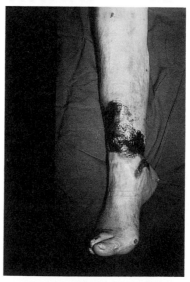

Fig. 9.7   Onset of gangrene in the same patient following injudicious handling of the limb at risk.

the risk of avoidable tissue damage. The comprehension of the patient is important in securing patient compliance and cooperation. This will obviously vary across the whole spectrum of age and conditions. The alert and active insomniac receiving heavy nocturnal sedation who develops a lateral malleolar ulcer is likely to be more cooperative and helpful than the senile alcoholic with advanced peripheral neuropathy. The latter, together with the senile demented patients, represent something of a challenge.

Aetiology

Listed below are conditions conducive to ulceration.

1. Ischaemia
   a. Atheroma
   b. Arteriosclerosis
   c. Raynaud's phenomenon
   d. Diabetes
2. Neuropathy
   a. Diabetes
   b. Leprosy
   c. Syphilis
   d. Subacute combined degeneration of the cord
   e. Psychotropic drug abuse (including alcohol)
   f. Iatrogenic
3. Metabolic disorders
   a. Sequestration of gouty tophi
   b. Malnutrition
4. Intrinsic trauma
   a. Rheumatoid nodular and bursal erosions
   b. Bony sequestration
   c. Arthritic hyperostoses
   d. Postural overload (secondary to obesity, surgery, etc.)
5. Extrinsic trauma
   a. Footwear
   b. Appliances (including splints)
   c. Dressings
   d. Bedsores
   e. Physical, chemical injury
6. Neoplasia
   Very uncommon but should be considered when all other factors have been excluded.

In all these conditions, infection may be a superimposed problem.

The evaluation of the quality of lower limb innervation in the elderly demands a recognition that degenerative processes will modify clinical responses which are demonstrable in the young. Some proprioceptive loss is normal. Diminution of the appreciation of vibration which would be significant in a 30 year old may be compatible with normal ageing. The significance of motor fatigue has to be judged in relation to the patient as a whole person. Is it the harbinger of multiple sclerosis or attributable to a small cerebrovascular accident needing referral?

Ataxia and loss of confidence after a fall may be attributable to a foot lesion, but consideration should be given to defects arising in other systems. Apart from such obvious neurological possibilities as subacute combined degeneration of the cord, abnormalities affecting the eyes, ears or nutrition (avitaminosis) can all co-exist with a foot problem which is regarded by the patient as the major cause of complaint. The physician will have a valuable ally if sensible early referrals arise from a judicious assessment of areas above the malleoli. It is unlikely that the podiatrist will be the first to be consulted for stocking and glove anaesthesia, but he may be the first to recognize early sensory loss which will degenerate into the potentially ulcerative neuropathy of diabetes. (Fig. 9.8). Leprosy, which was once very rare in

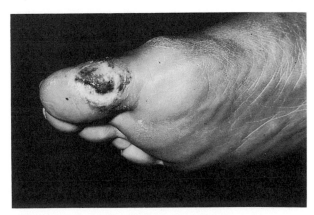

Fig. 9.8 Neuropathic ulceration of diabetes.

the UK, is now seen more frequently among recent Afro-Asian immigrants.

NEOPLASIA

Malignant lesions

Malignancy affecting the foot is rare and of those lesions which do occur the commonest are *melanoma* and *basal cell tumours*. Less common is *squamous cell carcinoma*.

Although melanoma may be a conversion from a formerly benign to a malignant state, it should be remembered that it can arise spontaneously. All moles on the foot should be regarded with suspicion and prompt surgical referral is required whenever there is a change in the character of hitherto benign lesion. Such changes would include serous leakage, splitting, extension of the edge, bleeding, pitting or thickening. In the elderly, one sees an occasional melanoma which can simulate subungual haematoma. The tumour will present as a small filament, with no history of trauma, and will increase slowly in length and width. An intra-epidermal haematoma can also mimic a melanoma, which is best examined by diascopy—the demonstration of melanotic grains seen through a microscope slide which is used to blanch the lesion and surrounding skin. Long term steroid therapy can induce cutaneous skin fragility which sometimes causes laking of blood and a pseudohaematoma. These sharply circumscribed, often slightly elevated lakes, are seen on the lower leg and dorsum of the foot. The lakes are slightly fluctuant when newly formed, but can become consolidated by fibrosis or they can ulcerate spontaneously.

Basal cell epithelioma may arise in a setting of traumatic hyperkeratosis, which acts as a mask (Fig. 9.9). It needs to be distinguished from mechanical extravasation arising as a sequel to faulty weight transmission through the skin. This semi-necrotic extravasation is slightly 'mushy' in texture when the overlying hyperkeratosis has been removed and it may look like dull velvet with variable moisture. The basal cell lesion differs postoperatively by being startlingly red, very smooth and highly light reflective. Lesions located within plantar callus can be complicated by the

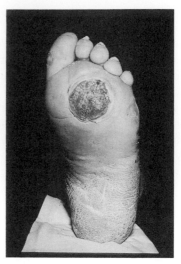

Fig. 9.9   Basal cell epithelioma after reduction of plantar callosity.

presence of white, shiny, fibrous material. Careful tissue reduction will reveal a sharply delineated edge which is sometimes rolled.

Squamous cell carcinoma rarely develops in areas of normal appearing unexposed skin. However, it may develop from burns, ulcers and osteomyelitic sinuses. Initially it may be seen as a small erythematous nodule. The surface may be smooth or rough and may or may not be ulcerated/bleeding. Metastases occur more readily from areas that have been previously damaged; the frequency can be up to 50%.

Bowen's disease is a lesion of squamous cell carcinoma. It appears as plaques of reddish papules or nodules. A very low percentage of these areas metastasise.

Kaposi's sarcoma most commonly affects men in their 60s, although it is now becoming more common in younger men affected by HIV. It is a disease of multicentric origin which primarily affects the skin and often begins with non-pitting oedema of one ankle, which later becomes bilateral. This is then followed by irregular reddish-blue, purple or reddish-brown macules. These macules may grow into nodules and even become verrucous. A coalescence of lesions gives rise to irregular patches and plaques that most commonly affect the feet or thighs.

Neoplasia arising in any area may be moderated by immunosuppressive medication which heightens the risk of infection. Operative procedures should be cautiously designed to produce minimal tissue damage compatible with the therapeutic aim. In such circumstances the hazard of creating a potential portal of entry for pathogenic organisms must be weighed against the risk of neglecting a lesion which may deteriorate to a threatening level. Faced with such a dilemma, a prudent podiatrist would seek the opinion of the prescribing physician.

Non-malignant lesions

A non-malignant tumour which does afflict the aged, especially in association with posterior nail folds, is *angiokeratoma*. This is a normal skin-coloured papilloma with a keratinized cap. The nail borders are equally the site of non-keratinized papillomata and skin tags. None of these lesions is dangerous, but some patients are concerned because they catch in hosiery as well as being cosmetically unacceptable. All can be treated by freezing with liquid nitrogen after a K-Y jelly thermocouple. When frozen solid, they are snipped off at the skin line with nail nippers and dressed with a non-adherent cover such as Micropad. If this is applied with moderate firmness before basal thawing has occurred, bleeding will not be a problem. They normally heal uneventfully in a few days.

PODIATRY PROVISION FOR ELDERLY PATIENTS

All health authorities provide podiatry for their elderly patients. There is a difference between authorities as to when a person becomes elderly: some may receive treatment at the age of 60, and some 65. Many elderly patients prefer to attend for private treatment.

The treatment may take place in a health centre near to the patient's home, in the patient's home —whether it be a nursing home or their own house—or, in some areas, in hospital out-patient clinics, especially if the patient has a condition such as diabetes or rheumatoid arthritis. These latter clinics will be connected to relevant departments and treat patients of all ages.

In recent years, the hospital podiatrist has become an essential part of the team working especially alongside rheumatologists and diabetologists in the management of the high risk patient, and in the facilitation of the multi-disciplinary approach to patient care. It is important that community podiatrists and private practitioners maintain liaison with general practitioners, community nurses and social services in order that the patient derives the best possible care in the community. Equally, effective liaison must exist between hospital based and community practitioners.

Domiciliary care

The treatment of patients in their own homes affords an ideal means of assessing the patient as a whole and their ability to cope with their condition and environment. For many old people, treatment at a clinic has a double value: not only does it provide care for the foot problem, it is a psychological stimulus which boosts motivation. The effect is that the treatment is regarded as a trip or a day out. Extra care with personal grooming and dress can disguise a patient's true life style. The cheerful little old lady who brightly agrees to the suggestion in the clinic to have saline baths twice daily may, when visited because of intervening acute illness, be found to be housed in a single top-floor room with no adequate facilities for the regime prescribed.

Even without intentional snooping, it is difficult not to perceive likely sources of threats to general and foot health. If the basic requirements of food, warmth, dryness, shelter and sleep cannot be met, then the podiatrist should be familiar with the location of the agencies concerned with social welfare. Health and social workers are spread patchily over the country, and rural and urban communities will differ quite markedly in their allocation of resources. Local knowledge will guide and influence one in requesting aid from GPs, district nurses, health visitors, social services, Home Help departments and Meals on Wheels organizers. Contact with voluntary agencies such as Age Concern, WRVS or the Red Cross may well be useful. Basically, the GP should be the lynch-pin in the overall care of the patient and some will prefer the podiatrist to route calls for aid through them. Others will welcome the independent initiative of the podiatrist who solicits the aid of other public services—but a copy note to the GP is a courtesy as well as a helpful protective memorandum in the event of any later misunderstanding. Even in the best ordered communities, personality clashes with eccentric old people can lead to inter-professional criticism.

Unlike any other podiatry practice, domiciliary work demands a number of working compromises which involve a safe and comfortable operating position for the operator and the patient, and cleanliness of the patient, the immediate environment and the operator's hands. No compromise should ever increase the risk to the patient. Two questions are helpful:

1. What are the consequences of undertaking treatment in this environment?
2. What are the consequences of *not* giving treatment?

As far as the consequences are predictable, they will be within an assessable time scale. For example, treatment is requested for an 80-year-old lady complaining of painful overgrown nails. On arrival, she is found to have moderate and uncomplicated bilateral onychauxis and one foot which is pale, painful and pulseless. The operating conditions are poor. It might just be possible to give treatment. It would be better, though, to recognise that the lady is suffering an acute obliterative arterial crisis and to telephone her GP as a matter of urgency. Such treatment as is possible should be provided and the patient should be reassured pending the arrival of the doctor. Obviously, the visiting podiatrist must make strenuous efforts to ensure such cases are followed up by the appropriate agencies.

It is especially in the domiciliary situation that the use of Foot Care Assistants (FCA) has given rise to great controversy. The majority of domiciliary calls may be of a more routine nature but the elderly are subject to multiple foot pathologies which require surveillance by a State Registered Chiropodist. Morris et al (1978) revealed that the majority of geriatric and psychiatric hospital patients had three or more podiatric conditions. 2% of patients were deemed to require no foot care and only a further 2% to be suitable for routine care by ward staff. Pelc (1979) surveyed 465 patients in clinics, surgeries and their own homes, of whom 423 were over the age of 65. Of the total, 82% were reported as having one or more general conditions which made it difficult or dangerous for them to attend to their own feet. These general conditions included poor peripheral circulation (46%) and diabetes (8%). However, in this study clinic patients accounted for 199 of the total and 58% of these who were free from such conditions were said to be suitable for care by FCAs. A further study revealing multiple pathologies in the elderly was conducted by Ebrahim et al (1981) and the undetected presence of subungual ulceration has been demonstrated by Shires (1988).

Calls for first aid figure slightly more frequently in domiciliary work with the aged. This is not just first aid for feet. The dropped frying pan and splash burns and contused and fractured toes will be met, but heads, hands and knees—all areas commonly damaged in falls by the ataxic and partially-slighted— will also be presented. Simple dressings should be given as an act of humanity, especially where exposure to infection is a hazard. Clinical judgement will dictate whether further help should be summoned.

The advent of prepacked sterile dressings and small dispensers for medicaments has made the adoption of sterile procedures more easy to accomplish in the domiciliary situation. Instrument packs are somewhat heavy on the domiciliary round and the introduction of portable sterilisers is a step forward.

The choice of items to be carried should be left to the individual practitioner but it is possible in some cases that appropriate drugs and dressings may be supplied on prescription by the GP and left in the patient's home as a 'working pool' for visiting health care professionals.

Institutional care

Visiting old people in a non-domestic environment is much less taxing than domiciliary work. Some will be in well-appointed nursing homes and others in poorly equipped psychogeriatric units, public or private. The great majority will be nursed and housed in conditions falling between these two extremes. Whatever the establishment, it is necessary to become familiar with the hierarchy of the institution. The matron, ward sister or warden—whoever is responsible for the nursing needs of the patient—should always know of the podiatrist's presence and the reason for calling. This opening courtesy is the passport to later cooperation if there should be a need to delegate dressing changes, footbaths or the routine application of external medication.

It will ensure that an anglepoise lamp, towels, receivers, nursing help with turning a patient in bed and sundry other services will be made available when possible. The podiatrist will also learn when is not an appropriate time to call. Ward rounds, cleaning, bed baths and similar activities which would be mutually exclusive and time-wasting are avoided. Some homes will be able to accept advice about nursing decubital lesions on autoclavable polyurethane sheets, gutter splints or heel cups. Although such items are the mutual province of nursing and podiatry, not all nursing establishments, especially the smaller, private ones, are always conversant with new products.

Pressure sores occur not only on the feet, but also on the sacrum and elbows. If good podiatry secures the resolution of a heel or a malleolar lesion one may be asked to apply those skills to other areas. It is a matter of assessing other calls upon available time which will determine the nature of what help can be given. At the very least, one can give general therapeutic advice about the merits of ripple beds, the advantages and disadvantages of water-repellent silicone creams for macerated lesions, or enzyme debriding agents where adherent necrotic slough is impairing resolution.

Apart from maintaining one's own record of the patient's progress, it is helpful to add a note of the foot condition and its treatment to the general ward notes and to avoid the use of podiatric jargon. This is particularly necessary if adhesive dressings should be left undisturbed during blanket baths, etc. or if routine simple dressing changes and medication are required. Access to the patient's general notes can save valuable time in taking a case history and even if a clear diagnosis is not immediately apparent, a look at the medication regime can be informative.

The rest, repair and convalescence of the post-surgical patient can be much disturbed by uncomfortable nails. Nail pain to lay and nursing attendants can seem to be out of all proportion to the apparent signs. To an hitherto ambulant elderly person, the enforced bedridden state can focus attention almost to an obsessive degree upon overgrown nails with impacted sulci. Although plate length and dystrophy together, perhaps, with hyperkeratotic sulci and subungual helomata can be a source of much discomfort, a fair proportion of cases of onychauxis exhibit a sterile subungual pressure necrosis.

When surgery has affected weight distribution (such as in hip arthroplasty, amputation, spinal fusion, etc.) there is much to be said for early assessment of foot function before the patient returns home. Podiatrists and physiotherapists have an overlapping interest in this field. Whilst walking exercises and postural re-education are best supervised by physiotherapists, it should be remembered that their efforts will be undermined if foot support and padding needs are not fully recognised and met. The elderly amputee, particularly, can benefit by having good stabilising filler insoles for the surviving foot. In the early days when the stump is becoming reconciled to its new home in the pylon socket, the podiatrist can alleviate discomfort by adding padding to the prosthesis if necessary.

MANAGEMENT

The management of foot pathologies in the elderly is based upon the general principles of clinical management of any age group. Attention should always be given to the patient's medical and social status, since these factors may influence the selection of particular treatment regimes. Liaison with medical practitioners, district nurses and social services departments is often important when, e.g. dressings need to be changed frequently, infection monitored and when patients are recommended to rest. Elderly patients with limited mobility and poor eyesight may have the greatest difficulty in replacing even a sterile prepacked dressing in appropriate conditions. They may need antibiotics when control of infection is difficult to obtain by other means and they may need additional help in the home, or for basic shopping needs if they live alone and have been advised to rest.

It should also be borne in mind that although most elderly patients will be cooperative and sensible in their attitude, some may be in the early stages of dementia and unable to recollect simple instructions concerning their foot problems. The more overt symptoms of senility are more easily recognised but bring their own problems of management. Apart from the socio-medical aspects of care, the management of foot problems in the elderly may be said to require:

1. maintenance of sterility
2. maintenance of tissue viability and/or promotion of tissue regeneration
3. protection from pressure and compensation for tissue atrophy.

Maintenance of sterility

Standard measures of preoperative and postoperative swabbing with a non-irritant antibacterial agent are sufficient in most cases, with 'no-touch' techniques used in the application of sterile dressings to ulcerated areas. Persistent infection which does not respond to treatment must be regarded with suspicion and every care taken to avoid cross-infection.

Antiseptic medicaments should be selected with care, bearing in mind that the skin is often denatured and atrophic. The continued use of medicaments to promote wound healing has recently been called into question. It has been suggested that many antiseptics are actually toxic to healing tissues (Leaper 1986) (Anthony 1987). Traditional dressing materials, such as gauze and other dry dressings, may also be contra-indicated since current thinking favours the maintenance of a moist environment which nonetheless allows uptake and absorption of exudate and cell debris (Turner 1979) (Harding 1987). An extensive list of wound management products including modern environmental dressings was published by Morgan (1988) and a further review of their relative merits by Turner (1991) and Fotherby et al (1991) (see also Ch. 8).

The greater difficulty in achieving wound healing on the feet is probably caused by impaction of the dressing upon weight-bearing and by pressure from the footwear. In selecting appropriate forms of padding to relieve pressure, careful judgement must be applied in weighing up the merits of the accurate positioning of adhesive pads against the greater versatility of the replaceable variety (see also Chs 11 & 13).

It must always be borne in mind that the treatment of the elderly involves consideration of sociological, biological and physiological factors which may influence not only the podiatric management but the overall health and well-being of the patient. Modern geriatric specialists regard their role as being more rehabilitative than custodial. Podiatry mirrors that philosophy. The maintenance and restoration of tissue function will contribute to remobilisation and the delay of immobility. Towards the end of life, comfort and protection are required; feet require the same considerations. The most appropriate care is ensured by the motivation of the patient as well as by the motivation of the podiatrist engaged in this clinically rewarding field. The ultimate aim is to add years to the life and life to the years.

FURTHER READING

Anthony D 1987 Pointers to good care. Nursing Times 83 (34): 27–29
Barlow A M 1987 Skin and nail deformity in the elderly foot aged 75 years and over. MSc thesis, University of Manchester
Bond J, Bond S 1988 Sociology and health care, 2nd edn. Churchill Livingstone, Edinburgh
Braid S J 1987 The prevalence of foot deformity in the elderly aged 75 years and over. MSc thesis, University of Manchester

Cartwright A, Henderson G 1986 More trouble with feet. HMSO, London
Ebrahim S B J, Sainsbury R, Watson S 1981 Foot problems of the elderly: a hospital survey. British Medical Journal 283: 949–950
English M P 1976 Nails and fungi—an interdisciplinary collaboration. The Chiropodist 31 (9): 234–239
Fenske N A, Lober C W 1986 Structural and functional changes of normal ageing skin. Journal of American Dermatology 15(4): 571–583

Fotherby et al 1991 Effect of various dressings on wound healing. Journal of Tissue Viability 1 (3): 68–70

Gibbs R C 1975 Skin and nail changes in the elderly foot. Journal of the American Podiatry Association 65: 471–474

Gilchrist A K 1979 Common foot problems in the elderly. Geriatrics, November: 67–70

Hamdy R C 1984 Geriatric medicine. Baillière Tindall, London

Harding K 1987 Wound healing. The Chiropodist 43(10): 195–197

Leaper D 1986 Antiseptics and their effect on healing tissue. Nursing Times, May 28: 45–47

Morgan D 1988 Formulary of wound management products. Care Science and Practice 6: 4

Morris J B, Brash L F, Hird M D 1978 Chiropodial survey of geriatric and psychiatric hospital in-patients—Angus district. Health Bulletin, September. Scottish Home and Health Department

OPCS Mid-1986 Population estimates, London

Pelc E 1979 Footcare assistants—how much would they help? Public Health, London 93: 306–310

Shires J 1988 Subungual ulceration . . . is there a need for health education? The Chiropodist 43: 29–32

Smiler I 1979 Geriatric foot care: an ageing challenge. Pennsylvania Podiatry Association

Turner T D 1979 A look at wound dressings. Health & Social Service Journal, 4 May: 529–531

Turner T 1991 Surgical dressings in the drug tariff. Wound Management 1: 1

10. Sports injuries

Patricia M. Boyd   Richard J. Bogdan

'There is a crack in everything God made', said Ralph Waldo Emerson. Nowhere does this concept manifest itself to a greater extent than in the athlete. The 'athlete' today is the average man and woman engaging in activities that were formerly called 'minor sports'. Running, cycling, racquet-ball, aerobic dancing and tennis are all examples of sports that many people pursue with determination to improve their physical and mental health.

It is this documented improvement in physical wellbeing that has been mainly responsible for the increased participation in sports. These athletes rarely pretend to be of world class or to have professional aspirations. They just enjoy athletics for the fun and competitiveness of sports, and especially for the physical fitness it bestows upon them. Athletes in these sports require medical care that allows them to continue training while alleviating any specific injury or problem at the same time. 'Sports Medicine' as it is now called, is concerned with structural integrity, muscle balance and posture, rarely orthopaedic surgery.

The majority of athletic injuries are due to overuse syndromes arising from innumerable repetitions of some physical activity. The best treatment plan requires a knowledge of the particular sport, and of the anatomical areas and the mechanics involved. In addition to these areas of treatment determination, the practitioner must know the athlete. The training regimen and environment of the athlete are critical in determining a treatment plan, and the quantity and quality of the training are critical to evaluation of an injury. The athlete's environment includes such factors as shoe gear, running surfaces, diet and sleep, and they are all vital to correct diagnosis and treatment of the athlete's problem. For example, it is important to know which terrains produce which symptoms if the patient is a runner, or which shoes provide adequate support if the patient is a basketball player. Evaluation of an athletic problem must also include proper evaluation of any relevant medical factors.

The following is an example of a special history questionnaire for athletes written by Kevin Kirby, DPM.

Runner-patient history

Training history

1. How long have you been running (in years)?
2. How many miles /day do you average?
3. How many miles /week do you run?
4. What's your longest run during the week?
5. What pace (in mins /mile) do you average in your workouts?
6. Do you do intervals, long slow distance and/ or long fast distance in your workouts?
7. What type of terrain do you usually run on (grass, dirt, concrete, asphalt, sand , hilly, flat, etc.)?
8. Do you run on any canted surfaces (on one side of the road, on beaches, or always around the track in the same direction)?
9. What time of day do you normally run (a.m., p.m., or mid-day)?

Racing history

10. How often do you race?
11. What distances do you normally race at?

Running shoe history

12. What model(s) of running shoes do you train in and/or race in?
13. How long have you had your present pair(s) of shoes?
14. Do you wear any orthotics, special arch supports, etc., in your shoes?
15. Do any of your pairs of shoes make the problem better or worse?
16. Do you 'build up' your running shoes to keep the soles from wearing out too quickly?
17. Where does the most outsole wear occur on your running shoes?
18. How do your shoes fit (too long, short, narrow, wide)?
19. Do you wear socks when you run? How many pairs?

Pre/post run activities

20. Do you stretch before and/or after your run and for how long?
21. What type of stretching do you do (describe it precisely)?
22. Do you warm-up/warm-down for your runs and for how long?
23. Do you do any muscle strengthening exercises (describe them)?
24. Do you participate in any other sports or any other physical activities?

Injury related history

25. Did you modify your training/racing schedule prior to your injury?
26. Did you run a particularly hard race or have a hard workout immediately prior to your injury?
27. Did you switch to another pair of running shoes prior to your injury?
28. Did you modify your shoe gear prior to your injury?
29. Was there any direct trauma associated with your injury?
30. Did you have another injury or any discomfort in your feet or legs prior to your injury that you tried to train through?
31. Have you cut back on your mileage or pace since your injury? Any results?

Past treatment

This is essential information. With acute injuries, it is necessary to know what the patient may have done for it already. Many patients do not know the concept of RICE (Rest, ice, Compression and Elevation) and their self-treatment may have altered the condition. It is very important that their return to activity should be gradual.

With chronic injuries, the question arises as to why a condition has not healed properly, even if the patient has rested for a long period. Often it is because the patient has never properly restrengthened the muscles. Atrophy occurs quickly and if the muscle is not re-strengthened, it will be susceptible to injury. Scar tissue adhesions will also make swelling and stiffness prominent. Biomechanical problems, e.g. leg length discrepancies which are not treated, may also contribute to chronic, recurrent injuries. Tight muscles are also a factor.

Functional instability often requires bracing, without which recurrent injury occurs.

Current limitations

This is what the patient can or cannot do. In treatment, the patient must not attempt anything that causes pain. Temporarily, an alternative sport may be required to keep up fitness levels.

Patient constraints

The treatment plan must be realistic so that the patient can complete the treatment in the time available.

A sensible diet is necessary. Many patients will not rest.

To summarise: following a diagnosis, a treatment plan is started, possibly with a follow-up programme, and a prognosis is formulated. Then after the patient's return, there are four possibilities for the patient's condition:

1. No improvement or worse
2. Somewhat improved
3. Greatly improved
4. Completely better.

If the patient is completely better a gradual return to activity is essential (see Fig. 10.1).

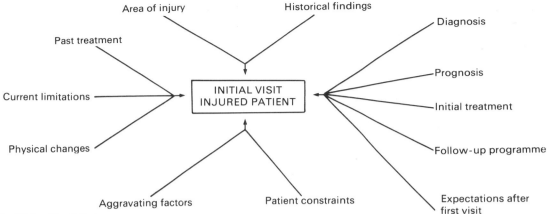

Fig. 10.1   The full picture.

Treatment list

Activity modification

1. Hard walk programme
2. Walk/run programme
3. Daily activity only (walking only)
4. Reduction of stair/hill walking
5. Reduce running partially
6. Discontinue speed work
7. Discontinue hills
8. Prolonged rest
9. Bike/swim alternative
10. Wheelchair or bed rest
11. Crutches or cane

Ice/heat

12. Contrast baths
13. Ice pack after activity
14. Ice massage
15. Hot water soaks/heat packs
16. Deep heat lotion massage

Shoes

17. Change shoes to more anti-pronation
18. Change shoes to more shock absorption
19. Modify shoes with built-in changes
20. Special shoes
21. Stay with same shoes
22. Biven shoe, wooden sole shoe

Taping/wraps

23. Rest strapping for midtarsal joint
24. Rest strapping for ankle
25. Combination of both
26. Figure 8 strapping
27. Special area taping (digits, etc.)
28. Removable ankle wrap
29. Removable knee wrap
30. Knee immobiliser
31. Tubigrip only
32. Tubigrip with horseshoes
33. Orthoplast or air casts
34. Lateral ankle splints

Foot inserts/orthoses

36. Spenco padding only
37. Sorbothane padding for heel
38. Foot accommodation (Korex)
39. Felt arch pad
40. Metatarsal support
41. Metatarsal bar
42. Runner's varus heel wedge
43. Heel cup
44. Forefoot/rearfoot wedge
45. Spenco or arch support
46. Cuboid padding
47. Heel lifts
48. Morton's extension
49. Latex shields
50. Bunion splints/digital splints

51. Biomechanical examination and casting for orthoses
52. Dispense orthoses
53. Modification of orthoses

Stretching

54. Static stretching home programme
55. Contract/relax home programme
56. Contract/relax therapy programme
57. Spray and stretch techniques
58. 45 min heat/ice stretch
59. Cryostretch programme; stretching after cold application

Strengthening/range of movement

60. Isometric strengthening
61. Theraband or elastic rubber tubing
62. Isotonic strengthening
63. Isokinetic strengthening
64. Upperbody isotonic programme
65. Range of motion exercises
66. Muscle stimulator (home use)

Physical therapy modalities

67. Ultrasound therapy
68. Electro-galvanic stimulation
69. Electro-acupuncture probe therapy
70. Dynamometer muscle test
71. Deep friction massage
72. Electro-accuscope therapy
73. Transcutaneous nerve stimulation

Medication

74. Aspirin
75. Strong anti-inflammatory medication
76. Oral steroid × 6 days
77. Vitamins
78. Oral calcium supplements
79. Iron supplements
80. Vitamin B_{12} injection
81. Short-acting cortisone injection
82. Long-acting cortisone injection
83. Hyaluronidase injection
84. Local anaesthesia diagnostic injection

85. Local anaesthesia therapeutic injection
86. Diet evaluation

Special tests

87. X-rays
88. Bone scan
89. Computerised tomography scan
90. Xerogram—reverse X-ray for soft tissues
91. Arthrogram
92. Nuclear magnetic resonance—electromagnetic X-ray without exposure

Surgery

93. Surgical discussion
94. Surgical intervention

Casts

95. Standard below knee cast
96. Removable below knee cast
97. Above knee cast
98. Unaboot soft cast—calamine lotion compressive bandage

Miscellaneous

99. Foot manipulation techniques
100. Orthopaedist referral
101. Neurologist referral
102. Internist referral
103. Chiropractic referral
104. Dietician referral
195. Rheumatologist referral
106. Vascular specialist referral
107. Evaluation

SUBUNGUAL HAEMATOMA

This painful injury is common to tennis players and runners and is due to impaction of the great toe against the upper of the shoe. Blood from ruptured capillaries collects beneath the great toe nail plate, causing pressure and tension (Fig. 10.2).

The impaction may be the fault of footwear being too short, narrow or shallow, or may be due to elongation of the foot from abnormal pronation.

Treatment is required to allow the blood to

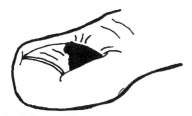

Fig. 10.2   Subungual haematoma.

escape and so relieve the pain. This is usually easily done by a small incision midway along the sulcus or, if necessary, by either piercing the nail or removing it. Control with an orthotic device may be needed to stop any excessive pronation.

BLISTERS

Blisters are a result of shearing stresses within the layers of the skin and can be produced by irritation from several sources: stones or foreign bodies within the shoes; running shoes that are too loose or ill fitting; improper shoes for the activity; or a biomechanical problem causing excessive pronation and hypermobility within the foot.

In the acute stage, the fluid within the blisters should be drained, using sterile techniques, and leaving a skin flap for protection. Additional protection can be given with shock absorbing materials such as Evazote and PPT insoles, and lubricating materials, examples of which can be bought at sports shops and can be applied directly to the foot. These materials are silicone gels that come in sheets (Spenco). They can be used in the treatment or prevention of blisters.

Examination of the footwear is important to ensure its adequacy for the particular sport; the foot should be examined as well, as biomechanical faults may be responsible for the excessive movement and friction. Examples are plantar flexed first ray and forefoot varus.

PAIN IN THE FOREFOOT

Pain in the ball of the foot can be very disabling for any athlete. Many sportsmen place a large proportion of the stress on the ball of the foot, and pain is usually due to unsupported loading of the area. The following list summarises the usual differential diagnostic considerations of a mechanical origin:

1. Sesamoiditis
2. Capsulitis
3. Bursitis
4. Neuroma
5. Stress fracture.

It is helpful to compartmentalise the forefoot into medial, central and lateral sections to aid differentiation. The medial section is the first ray, the central encompasses the second, third and fourth metatarsals, and the lateral is denoted by the fifth ray.

The most common complaints of the medial compartment are capsulitis of the first metatarsophalangeal joint, sesamoiditis, fracture of the sesamoid, and osteochondritis dissecans of the first metatarsal head. Mechanical disability of the first metatarsophalangeal joint, as occurs in hallux abducto valgus, plantarflexed first ray, and improper shoe gear, results in significant stress overload on this area. Proper treatment to eliminate inflammation and instability is necessary to return the athlete to his or her sport. Usually a supportive pad and strappings will ensure rest of the area while allowing for minimal function. Changes of terrain and shoes will also contribute to the success of this treatment.

A history of burning, numbness or radiating pain in this area would be unusual and might suggest some neurological involvement. Very rarely, neuromas have been found close to the fibular sesamoid in a ballet dancer, footballer and hurdler.

The central compartment provides more clinical entities and diagnostic challenges because of its participation in the stability of the foot during propulsion. In some foot types, the metatarsals move excessively in both the sagittal and transverse planes. This movement contributes to compression of the intermetatarsal nerves and bursae. With tight shoes, or thin soles, and with unshod feet, extreme forces may create pain and swelling sufficient to cause the athlete to limp.

Most commonly, the third intermetatarsal nerve develops such symptoms. The joining of the branches of the medial and lateral plantar nerves give rise to a larger nerve about the fourth toe which can easily be traumatised. This is the classical Morton's neuroma. Its symptoms can be very debilitating to the sprinter, tennis player, ballet dancer or runner. Cushioning of the forefoot by means of metatarsal supports and orthotics is necessary. Anti-inflammatory agents, such as ice, ultrasound, cortisone injection or vitamin B_{12}, may be necessary as intermediate stages during the four to eight weeks of treatment. If all else fails, surgical excision may be necessary. However, even after surgery, treatment for the lack of stability is of the utmost importance to prevent further complications.

Metatarsal stress fracture is an equally debilitating condition. This occurs most commonly in the central portion of the forefoot. The fracturing of the bone is due to the stress of continual pounding and vibration through the tissues during a repetitive sport. Cracks result in the crystalline meshwork, which the bone consistently attempts to remodel, but remodelling is never properly achieved, and a fracture is precipitated. The symptoms of a stress fracture differ from those of other forefoot conditions in that they are more intense, come about more quickly, and demonstrate significant swelling.

X-rays are essential in the evaluation of the stress fracture but it may take up to two weeks for the fracture line to show. It may also be necessary to go one stage further and to arrange for a bone scan.

The best treatment for the stress fracture is avoidance of any activity that causes pain. Many can be treated with a change in activity, rest, stiff supportive shoe gear, and plenty of ice treatment. However, at times, plaster casting and crutches may be the only therapy to resolve the immobilisation of the sportsman. Returning to activity should be delayed until further X-rays and a simple jump test prove negative.

Evaluation of the dynamics of the forefoot overload and how it may be reduced is essential for complete control of the clinical problem. The key to success is prevention of the overload.

FRACTURED SESAMOID

Pain in the first metatarsophalangeal joint can be experienced where the athlete is required to remain on the balls of the feet for given periods of time. Ballet dancers, aerobics and calisthenics dancers, hurdlers and runners are examples of this.

The main complaint of a fractured sesamoid is an aching pain that comes on with exercise and with dorsiflexion of the hallux. The symptoms are due to the irritation to the sesamoidal joint cartilage and plantar cartilage of the first metatarsal head. Symptoms are like those of osteoarthritis or gout of this joint. X-rays (medial oblique and axials) are required for the differential diagnosis. Appropriate lateral X-rays should also be obtained. They will show either of the sesamoids to be in pieces.

The forefoot valgus foot types and plantar flexed first ray deformities predispose to sesamoid fracture.

Treatment is with some type of immobilisation. Rest with accommodative padding should be the first line of treatment .

Persistent symptoms may require referral to an orthopaedic surgeon for a below-knee walking cast. Surgical removal of the sesamoids can lead to hallux abductovalgus or trigger toe deformities. The sesamoids act as mechanical fulcrums and are responsible for giving the intrinsic muscles of the foot stability as they function round the first metatarsophalangeal joint.

SUBLUXATION OF THE CUBOID

Subluxation of the cuboid is an irritating injury because although the athlete is not put out of action, it is nevertheless painful.

It occurs most commonly in those individuals with a cavus foot type who are prone to inversion sprains. The movement of inversion during a sprain pushes the cuboid out of alignment either dorsally or laterally. There are no outward signs of subluxation and no swelling. There is pain on the lateral aspect of the foot distal to the lateral malleolus. Pain occurs on running, when turning to the right and left, and on walking upstairs. Clicking and popping may be felt when putting the mid-tarsal joint through its range of motion. Swelling may be noted on the lateral aspect of the foot.

The fault is easily remedied by manipulation

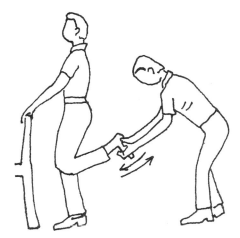

Fig. 10.3   Manipulation for subluxated cuboid.

HEEL SPUR SYNDROME

This is the most common disorder found in the heel and ankle area. It makes up about 12% of injuries in the foot and is found mostly in race walkers, runners and basketball players. It is a debilitating problem for any individual. The causes may be mechanical or systemic.

Pain is located in the region of the plantar surface of the medial tubercle of the calcaneus. The pain can be described as being deep and aching, or burning. It is due to an over-use traction of the thick medial band of the plantar fascia, which originates at the medial tubercle of the calcaneus. It may also be associated with the bursa found in this area.

On X-ray, in many cases, a spur of bone will be seen arising from the origin of the fascia. This is not diagnostic and is merely a sign of pronation of the subtalar joint. Table 10.2 shows the differential diagnosis, which is important as there are several possible medical reasons for the symptoms of mechanical spur syndrome.

Nerve entrapment syndrome can produce pain in the heel area, entrapment being of the tibial nerve or either of the medial or lateral plantar nerves, producing neuritis.

Enthesopathy is a term which describes an inflammation and cystic degeneration that occurs at the junctions between a muscle tendon or

(Fig. 10.3). The patient stands, holding the back of a chair. The manipulator grasps the affected foot firmly round the tarsus with both hands and with a whip-like action, quickly adducts and plantarflexes the foot, at the same time pressing the cuboid into its correct position. A rest strapping with a cuboid pad is then placed on the athlete's foot to maintain the manipulated position. Patients usually have immediate reduction of symptoms and will be able to return to sport in a few days. Chronic or unstable foot types require orthotic therapy to maintain the manipulated cuboid in place. See also Table 10.1.

Table 10.1   Treatment flow chart: cuboid subluxation.

Initial visit	*Second visit*	*Third visit*
Midtarsal strapping to increase stability of lateral arch	Initiate series—daily or every other day—of cuboid manipulation at this time	Try functional foot orthoses even if cuboid bone does not appear to be in proper alignment but if taping has helped
Ice massage for five minutes, five times daily to any tender areas	Consider functional foot orthoses only when cuboid bone is in the correct position	
Evaluation of 5th ray range of motion; consider a functional foot orthosis if 5th ray is dorsiflexed	Continue all forms of therapy of first visit, especially midtarsal taping	
X-ray evaluation for calcifications in peroneal tendon. Test for peroneal tendinitis. Start on peroneal stretching and strengthening programme as indicated	Correct any abnormalities of shoe gear or foot plant which overload lateral column of foot	
Initiate cuboid manipulation therapy	Continue physical therapy of ultrasound if any peroneal tendinitis is present	
	Consider bone scan if severe tenderness in one area is present	
If not significantly improving	If not significantly improving or reflare with activity	

Table 10.2 Differential diagnosis for mechanical heel spur syndrome.

1. Arthritis
2. Neuritis
3. Enthesopathy
4. Insufficient fat pad
5. Osteoid osteoma
6. Poor shoe gear
7. Calcaneal stress fracture

ligament and the periosteum to which the tendon or ligament attaches. Excessive strain and traction on that insertion gives rise to degeneration and pain. This can occur at any junction, and is commonly found in the knee and ankle.

Insufficient fat pad on the plantar surface of the heel can produce pain. The fat pad should be approximately 1 cm in thickness on weight-bearing and is built to absorb up to 12% of shock that the heel receives. Reduced subcutaneous fat allows the heel to become bruised and inflamed, giving rise to pain and discomfort. Icing and anti-inflammatory therapy should resolve this problem combined with a heel cup orthosis, which concentrates the remaining fat pad beneath the heel and provides extra shock absorption.

Injury from a direct blow or a traumatic bursitis or fracture are all possible causes of pain in the heel region. Rheumatoid arthritis and other systemic diseases should be ruled out before finalising diagnosis. Referral to the patient's GP for laboratory tests may be necessary.

Mechanical heel spur syndrome is produced by excessive pronation at the subtalar joint and subsequent supination of the midtarsal joint round its longitudinal axis. Because of its attachments, the plantar fascia is elongated with pronation and shortened with supination. In a foot that abnormally pronates through the gait cycle, no resupination can occur at toe off and the plantar fascia remains stretched and undergoes strain.

Football, rugby, baseball and cricket players require good support for the medial column and shock absorption in the heel. Most have a very flexible shoe which may require stiffening in the shank to support this area of the foot to prevent the mechanical heel spur syndrome.

Basketball is a traumatic sport with a lot of jumping and landing flat on the foot. Sudden deceleration also adds to the pull on the plantar fascia. Side-to-side sports such as tennis cause traction on the plantar fascia; as the player reaches and lunges, the foot is required to flatten along the medial column.

A hypermobile forefoot valgus foot type most commonly predisposes to the heel spur syndrome, particularly with women who have a high degree of genu valgum.

Initial therapy requires the RICE method, RICE being the mnemonic for treatment. R is for rest, with padding and strapping or reduction of the activity; I is for injection therapy under the auspices of a general practitioner. Injections of cortisone have proven useful in these heel pain cases; C is for cold to reduce inflammation; and E is for emotional support. It may be that the patient will have to give up that particular sport, and he or she won't be pleased!

Long-term therapy. Prevention from recurrence is important and steps can be taken to ensure this. Evaluate the surface the sport is being played on. It may be hard and non-forgiving. Footwear may be inadequate and non-shock absorbing and may not give enough stability to the foot. An orthosis is necessary if a mechanical anomaly is present in the foot to stabilise the medial column. This stabilisation of foot function may need augmentation with shock absorbing materials such as heel pads and other devices for the shoes. See also Table 10.3.

THE EQUINUS STATE

Equinus is defined as limitation of ankle dorsiflexion to less than 10°. 10° of dorsiflexion is necessary for normal gait and without it the function of the foot and structures within the lower limb are radically altered.

Equinus can be caused by several entities. These include congenital shortness of the gastrocnemius muscle; obliquity of the ankle joint; or a congenital osseous block. Dorsal lipping may occur at the neck of the talus, preventing free movement within the ankle mortice in sports that require jumping, such as football, basketball and ballet. Other possibilities are: injuries to the posterior muscle group or myositis resulting in fibrosis and contracture of the muscle belly;

Table 10.3 Treatment flow chart: heel spur syndrome.

Initial visit

3 positional Achilles stretch
Ice massage × 10 minutes × 3 daily
Self-tape midtarsal strapping
Anti-pronation shoes if patient runs
Heel accommodation if plantar pain
Contrast baths if swelling × 2 daily
If not improving significantly
↓
Second visit

Orthotic evaluation and casting
2 weeks anti-inflammatory medication
2 weeks ultrasound if chronic or EGS if acute
Cut activity to painfree only
If not improving significantly
↓
Third visit

Dispense orthosis
Continue therapy
If bursae—consider cortisone injection
X-rays
If not improving significantly or reflare occurs as activity is increased
↓
Fourth visit

Cortisone injections
Check orthotic control
Bone scan
BK cast × 4 weeks
If not helped
↓
Fifth visit

Surgical discussion

athletic hypertonicity due to overuse in a new training programme, causing metabolite build-up and contracture of the muscle; growth spurts in children where long bones outgrow the muscles; adaptive shortening of the muscle in women who wear high heeled shoes; and gastrocnemius muscle tightness and relative shortness in association with generalised ligamentous laxity.

Clinical features of ankle equinus

Equinus compensation can manifest in many ways. Because the required 10° of dorsiflexion is absent at the ankle joint, this motion is obtained by adaptations from other parts of the lower limb, particularly the midtarsal joints. Gait adaptations are: abducted feet with the hips functioning in an externally rotated position; short stride; early heel lift; knee flexion throughout the gait cycle; an abductory twist of the foot and forefoot subluxation, giving a break in the medial column. Footwear shows minimal lateral wear with excessive wear at the ball of the shoe.

The patient complains of leg cramps, digital deformities and hindfoot pain. There may be knee subluxation which also gives rise to pain.

The ankle joint must be tested for range of motion with the knee in the flexed and extended positions to determine whether the equinus is of a bony or soft tissue nature.

Treatment for osseous deformity is with heel lifts. Soft tissue deformity can be helped with heel lifts and stretching exercises. With athletic hypertonicity, various forms of heat will stimulate the circulation and flush away metabolites.

TENDO ACHILLES INJURIES

The area of the Achilles tendon that causes most complaints is the zone 8–10 cm proximal to the top of the posterior aspect of the calcaneus. There is an increase in calcaneal tendon disorders in individuals over the age of 35 years. The circulation in this area decreases by about 40% at this time.

The tendon comprises two muscles that are the main decelerators of the leg, in all activities. It is also a supinator of the subtalar joint and plantar flexor of the ankle. In activities such as ballet, the muscle group is also involved in sustaining various positions and movements.

Pain is usually the main complaint, either at the insertion, along the tendon or at the myotendinous junction, and is due to a strain of these structures.

Aetiological factors are many and varied. Variations in the surfaces on which the sport or activity is carried out, or inclination of running surfaces, can alter the torque applied to the Achilles tendon. Running uphill or downhill, or on canted roads, can alter the direction of the torque; low or negative heels can cause excessive torque on the tendon. Flexibility of the shoe at the metatarsal break is very important and inflexibility can cause increased strain. Hamstring and ilio-psoas muscle tightness should be evaluated to ensure that they are not contributing to the condition.

The tendo Achilles (TA) has a poor circulation and requires special warm-up and stretching. In side-to-side sports such as tennis, lungeing forward is an important factor in rupturing the TA where there has been inadequate warm-up. Tennis shoe soles are made of soft material and on weight-bearing can give the same effect as a negative heel, and a greater range of motion for the TA.

In 'contact' sports like basketball and rugby, a direct blow can cause a tendinitis. Basketball also requires spurt running and rapid deceleration and the triceps surae group is put under strain. A full study of the sport and playing surface is necessary to establish the aetiological factor.

TENDINITIS

Any of the above aetiologies may be responsible for an inflammation of the tendo Achilles.

Clinical features

Presentation is usually unilateral. The affected tendon is two or three times the normal size and there is crepitus, soft swelling and a torpidity on movement. Examine for any nodules above the insertion, the presence of which indicates rupture of some of the fibres. An X-ray with soft tissue density will show that the tendon is affected. The area will be hot and painful.

Treatment (Table 10.4)

Acute stage

Apply ice to the affected part 3–4 times per day for 10 minutes duration. Apply strapping to the foot and ankle to prevent movement and put a heel lift in the shoe to rest the part. Once the swelling is down, start mild stretching with ultrasound therapy 2–3 times per week for 3 weeks. Rest from the athletic activity will be necessary for 4–6 weeks, then it can be restarted gradually.

Table 10.4   Achilles tendinitis: treatment.

Initial visit

Check flexibility hamstrings:
  gastroc, soleus stretches, heel lifts
Check shoes: heel to ball ratio, not worn excessively;
  check especially heel counter; stable or new shoes
Check for swelling, tenderness: EGS and ice
Ice massage at home
Check training habits, eliminate hill running and speed work
Gait observation, excessive torque, instability: varus wedge

Second visit

Recheck swelling, tenderness: ultrasound 3×/wk for 2 wks
Recheck flexibility: hot water bath, hot/cold stretch routine
Orthotic casting
Alternate activity, no propulsion, bicycling, swimming
Continue stretches, ice massage
Check new shoes
Anti-inflammatory × 2 wks
X-rays if suspect bony block (stretching only gently) or
  insertional tendonitis

Third visit

Dispense orthotic: check for control
Continue ultrasound and ice massage if helpful
Consider tendinosis, tenosynovitis, partial rupture,
  retrocalcaneal bursitis, gout, plantaris rupture, posterior
  ankle capsulitis, os trigonum, fracture of posterior lateral
  process talus

Subsequent visits

Consider immobilising using a cast
Last resort: surgery

Chronic stage

This is generally the stage at which patients present themselves, having previously attempted to treat the acute stage themselves, but without taking adequate rest. They may even have applied heat. Significant changes will have taken place in the tendon and there will be some evidence of cystic degeneration. If patients continue with athletic activity, they will risk rupturing the tendon. At this stage, referral to an orthopaedic surgeon will be necessary for application of a below-knee plaster of Paris cast with the foot in plantar flexion for complete rest. If rupture has occurred, the surgeon may consider surgical intervention.

RETROCALCANEAL EXOSTOSIS (HAGLUND'S BUMP)

This is a hypertrophy of the posterior-lateral shelf

of the calcaneus, with or without a bursa. It is due to mechanical irritation during the gait cycle. The triceps surae muscles act as decelerators of the body as it moves forward over the foot. During the propulsive phase of the cycle, the heel is in constant contact with the counter of the shoe and it is this stress that gives rise to the exostosis. Other factors that influence the formation of the exostosis are: the inclination angle of the calcaneus—this can vary from heel to heel and cause the exostosis to cover a large area of the posterior aspect of the calcaneus; the pitch or degree of adduction of the calcaneus, which may cause the exostosis to be situated more laterally; and the amount of hindfoot varus, which will also influence the area and extent of the exostosis.

These bumps are difficult to deal with. Control with orthoses or lifting the heel with a lift in the shoe should be tried. Low counters or soft counters are also helpful. Excision may be necessary.

Such bumps are common on skiers and skaters and they may require orthotic control of the midstance or propulsive phase of gait. They are also produced in sports that require the plantar-flexed attitude of the ankle and rapid changes of direction; these include ballet, football, rugby and American football. They are often associated with inversion sprains (Fig. 10.4).

ANKLE SPRAINS

Ankle sprains, especially sprains of the lateral ligaments, are very common injuries. They are also the most missed and maltreated of the acute injuries in the casualty department. Ankle sprains require a lot of care and rehabilitation if the individual is not to be left with an unstable, weak ankle. Medial ankle sprains are much rarer than lateral sprains as the medial ligaments are thicker and stronger.

The lateral ankle ligaments are: the calcaneofibular, the posterior talofibular and the anterior talofibular; in 20% of the population the anterior talofibular ligament is missing, which leads to instability and constant sprain of the lateral structures (Fig. 10.5).

The position of the foot at the time of sprain will determine which ligament will be damaged. In the supinated position, the calcaneofibular ligament lies parallel with the ankle and subtalar joint axes and therefore has no counter action to the motion of supination. In this situation, the anterior talofibular ligament is the one that is strained. In the dorsiflexed position, the calcaneofibular ligament is the greatest restrainer of inversion and will be the structure that is damaged in this situation.

Identification of the damaged ligament is important if treatment is to be correct. Palpation will localise the pain, but pain and swelling will limit manipulation of the joint. X-ray is undoubtedly the best method of evaluation if rupture and fracture are to be ruled out.

Most lateral sprains occur in side-to-side sports like tennis and football, as the peroneals quickly fatigue and no longer control the ankle. A hindfoot varus of 5°–10° or a plantarflexed first ray deformity will predispose to lateral sprains.

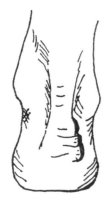

Fig. 10.4 Retrocalcaneal exostosis (Haglund's bump).

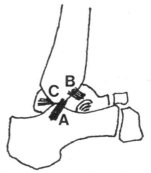

Fig. 10.5 The lateral ligaments: A. calcaneofibular; B. anterior talofibular; C. posterior talofibular.

Sometimes just stepping on something uneven, pivoting, trauma or running will result in a sprain.

Residual pain after about one month of the sprain may be due to an inflammation of the internal interosseous ligaments. Palpation of the area over the sinus tarsi elicits pain and inversion of the subtalar joint is also painful. The internal ligaments may have been ruptured during the sprain and may have healed poorly, resulting in malalignment and some capsular inflammation and fibrosis. It is a difficult injury to treat and may require referral for manipulation under local or general anaesthetic.

Treatment of any sprain depends very much on the severity. When total rupture or fracture has occurred, referral to an orthopaedic surgeon is necessary. Sprains short of rupture can be treated by the podiatrist.

For the first 36–48 hours, icing to reduce swelling should be carried out as often as possible. Strapping to prevent movement in the frontal plane should be applied and the limb elevated as high as can be tolerated. Once the acute stage has passed, weight-bearing can be resumed with supporting strapping, which should be such as to allow the patient, *however slowly*, to use a normal walking action. The importance of this should be stressed to patients so that they maintain as normal a gait as is possible. This is to be preferred to limping, even though the patient may move more quickly thereby. Strengthening of the muscles should begin, particularly the lateral muscles. Apply heat to the area to stimulate circulation, using heat, ice or ultrasound. Rehabilitate with exercises such as drawing with the toes, and use a wobble board or isometrics (15 repetitions three times per day with weights). Stabilise the foot with orthotic therapy using flat posts. For lateral instability, use a higher heel cup and lateral flare up to 1–2 cm. See Figure 10.6 for ankle sprain rehabilitation.

SHIN SPLINTS

This is a vague term describing many possible anomalies that arise as a stress reaction in the lower leg. Bone, muscle, tendon or insertion may be the source of pain.

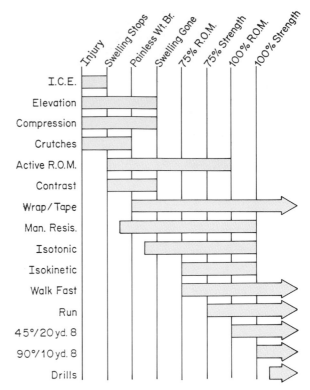

Fig. 10.6   Ankle sprain rehabilitation.

To determine which structure is involved, it will probably be necessary for the podiatrist to go out and watch that person perform the sport, or at least go and see how that sport is normally performed. This may give a clue as to which structures become fatigued.

Soft tissue aspects

Shin splints can be categorised according to the compartments of the lower limb (Fig. 10.7).

1. Anterior compartment

Pain is normally felt along the inner distal two-thirds of the tibial shaft. There is inflammation and stiffness and an ache, which is present at the beginning of the activity. Pain may be present with no activity, as swelling may be causing increased pressure on nerve endings. On examination, the patient may limp or walk with a stiff-legged gait.

The most commonly involved anterior muscles

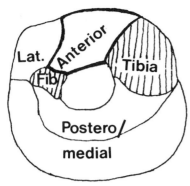

Fig. 10.7   Compartments of the lower leg.

are the extensor hallucis longus and the anterior tibial muscles. These are decelerators of the foot at heel strike and can be overused in situations such as downhill running, running on hard surfaces, or over-striding. They decelerate foot slap. These muscles also decelerate pronatory motion. They can become overworked or fatigued with exaggerated limb varus or foot types such as forefoot varus or supinatus, or forefoot equinus.

2. Lateral compartment

The peroneus longus and brevis muscles are those overworked with lateral compartment shin splints. They become fatigued in side-to-side sports, classically tennis, but also aerobic dance with much hopping from one foot to the other. A hypermobile first ray can also cause fatigue of the peroneus longus. Pain is experienced around the lateral malleolus and the distal one-third of the fibula.

3. Medial and posterior compartment

The posterior tibial is the muscle most commonly affected of all the posterior/medial muscles. Its main actions are to decelerate pronation around the oblique axis of the midtarsal joint, and also decelerate the internal rotation and forward momentum of the tibia; it also tries to accelerate re-supination of the subtalar joint. The stress on this muscle in a sport depends on the amount of utilisation of the mid-foot.

A runner can stress this muscle because running prolongs the amount of pronation in the gait cycle. More pronation requires more supinatory effort by the posterior tibial muscle.

Pain is frequently felt at the lower one-third of the tibia with posterior/medial shin splints. This is

Table 10.5   Ankle sprains: treatment.

Initial visit	*Third visit*	*Subsequent visits*
Determine severity, mechanism: X-rays if suspect fracture 5th metatars. base, beak of calcaneus, fibular neck	Begin ankle strengthening (progressive programme)	Test ankle strength
EGS with ice if acute swelling	Increase range of motion	If chronic resprain, consider stabilisation
Contrast baths; ultrasound if chronic swelling	Continue contrast baths	
Compression stocking with horsehoe pads on malleoli	Start toe raises, comparing affected and unaffected sides	
Weight-bearing as tolerated with crutches		
	Fourth visit	
	Progressive ankle strengthening, especially peroneals	
Second visit	Continue contrast baths, stretching range of motion	
Continue contrast baths, compression wrap	Teach strapping (Fig. 10.7)	
Increase range of motion (draw alphabet in warm water)	Encourage high top shoes, ankle brace, ankle strapping	
Begin stretching, especially Achilles	Consider orthotics if foot type a factor	
Observe gait for compensation (*stop* any compensation)	Begin BAPS or straight line running: progress to cutting drills (side-to-side agility running)	
If swelling is down, test for ankle instability and ankle strength		

Table 10.6   Treatment flow sheet: shin splints.

Initial visit	*Third visit*	*Fifth visit*
Ankle strapping, strengthening exercises for ankle invertors	Functional foot orthoses dispensed	Consider test for compartment syndrome and, if positive, consider surgical intervention with fascial stripping
Ice massage to painful areas of shins	Continue physical therapy to remove any residual swelling and as much tenderness as possible	
Neoprene shin sleeve		If bone scan negative, consider prolonged rest
Varus heel wedges		
Change of shoes to anti-pronation if a runner	Re-test muscle strength and consider manual resistance exercises, isotonic to increase strength if this is problem	Continue to treat any physical signs of swelling and tenderness with therapy
X-ray if chronic swelling		Question about any alternative exercises patient can participate in to maintain cardiovascular fitness
Activity modification to avoid pain	Consider bone scan if question of stress fracture still present	
If not improving significantly	If not improving significantly or if there is reflare as return to activity	
↓	↓	
Second visit	*Fourth visit*	
Two weeks of physical therapy with ultrasound	Question heavily about type of pain and consider compartment syndrome	
X-ray evaluation if stress fracture expected	Bone scan indicated to see radioactive uptake pattern	
Continue all home treatments	Check to ensure functional foot orthoses are properly controlling motion with the present shoes	
Consider functional foot orthoses if excessive subtalar joint pronation noted	If not improving significantly or if there is reflare as return to activity	
Strict guidelines on activity based on any pain		
Consider strong anti-inflammatory medication		
If not improving significantly		

almost certainly an enthesopathy, and pain is due to periostitis at the muscle attachment. There is a fibrocartilage break-down and a cyclic reaction is set up.

If the shin splint syndrome is due to a mechanical disorder producing abnormal pronation, fatigue of the muscle leads to less shock-absorption. Shock waves passing up the leg destroy bone cells and prevent the remodelling of the damaged bone. Stress fracture may occur. Therapy is aimed at preventing the excess pronation, thus lessening the shock and allowing muscle and bone to recover.

A subtalar varum or tibial varum predisposes to this syndrome. The available amount of eversion at the subtalar joint may be entirely used up with compensation for the subtalar varum or tibial varum, and there will thus be none left for shock absorption in normal gait. The posterior tibial muscle is the one that gets fatigued as it tries to maintain the function of shock absorption of the subtalar joint.

Treatment (Table 10.6)

Sporting activity should be stopped until the patient has spent two days being able to walk without pain. Patients can then restart the activity until a feeling of tightness arises. The muscle should then be iced and stretched. Limit the activity to a walk/run cycle. Allow patients to run only 10% of their normal distance, then gradually build up. Restrict activity to even terrain and ensure footwear is adequate and shock absorbing. Orthotic therapy to reposition the subtalar joint will be necessary.

ACUTE ANTERIOR COMPARTMENT SYNDROME

From Figure 10.7 it can be seen that the nerves, blood vessels and muscles are enclosed in a compartment surrounded by virtually non-stretchable structures.

Any ordinary activity, such as walking or

running, will result in increased capillary filtration to nourish the muscles and they will expand by 20–25% of their normal resting volume. Anteriorly, the crural fascia can expand to allow for this increase in bulk.

However, an activity such as running down a steep incline for too long can cause fatigue to the anterior muscle group as it tries to prevent foot slap. The muscles become less efficient, foot slap increases and shock waves reverberate up the leg. An inflammatory tendinitis or myositis sets up, increasing the extracellular fluid within the compartment.

Acute anterior compartment syndrome can result. This is an emergency situation which can lead to drastic complications. Increased pressure against the vascular bundles causes ischaemic pain and discomfort. Continuation of the activity increases the damage occurring within that compartment. Following the pain, there will be numbness and tingling on the dorsum of the foot which spreads proximally. The foot feels cold, and numbness on the dorsum makes the shoe feel loose. Motor control is lost and the foot is dragged.

On removal of the shoe, the foot and toes appear white and cool. The shin will be throb-bing. These are symptoms of a 'shut-down' syndrome.

Emergency treatment in a hospital is required to save the foot. Slitting of the crural fascia is the only remaining action. Permanent damage may have been caused, paralysing the anterior tibial or extensor hallucis longus muscles.

Chronic or recurrent anterior compartment syndrome is less severe and has no drastic results. It can be prevented with the use of orthotic therapy to avoid foot slap and by warning the athlete about the potential dangers of downhill running and excessive fatigue. Orthoses may be necessary to control the foot at heel strike right through to propulsion in cases of limb varus or hindfoot varus. Shock-absorbing materials are useful, and even limiting the amount of activity may be necessary to avoid symptoms. Ultimately, surgical fasciotomy may be the only treatment when all else fails.

TIBIAL / FIBULAR STRESS FRACTURES

The main aetiological factor in these conditions is poor shock absorption, whether of the limb with a mechanical disorder, where the foot is excessively pronated or supinated and rigid, or where muscle

Table 10.7 Treatment flow sheet: tibial stress fractures.

Initial visit	*Second visit*	*Third visit*
X-ray evaluation if pain present for 2–3 weeks at least Bone scan evaluation if X-rays are inconclusive or pain present less than 2 weeks 2–3 month rest period to allow fracture to heal Local physical therapy modalities to help remove swelling and muscle soreness during rest Make another appointment when patient has been pain-free for 2 weeks to re-evaluate the situation and analyse possible biomechanical problems causing inadequate shock absorption	Check for poor mechanics with inadequate shock absorption Recommend shoes with better shock absorption and consider Sorbothane or spenco padding for shoes Outline gradual return to activity programme at this time Have patient stay off downhills and poor shoes If pain return with activity	Re-X-ray to see if there is a non-healing fracture: 'dreaded black line' Consider pain elsewhere, e.g. coming from possible compartment syndrome or shin splints Treat the localised tenderness and swelling and when pain-free, place on a very gradual walk/run programme If still painful with return to activity

Fourth visit

Consider compartment testing for compartment syndrome
Consider low-back referred pain to area of leg
If X-ray evaluation inconclusive, consider bone scan if not previously taken; also consider prolonged period of rest

fatigue can no longer work the shock-absorbing mechanisms of joints, such as in downhill running.

Inadequate footwear may cause stress in that it may be worn down, non-shock absorptive or inadequate for the particular activity. The athlete may be unfit for prolonged activity or it may be the start of a new training programme.

Clinical features

There will be pain in the area of fracture which can be of sudden or gradual onset. Pain may be sharp or a deep ache. Swelling will be present if the bone fracture is near the skin surface. An X-ray or bone scan will be diagnostic.

Symptoms can be confused with shin splints or deep myositis.

Treatment (Table 10.7)

Rest is necessary for 6–8 weeks and occasionally 12 weeks to allow the fracture to heal. Rest in a plaster cast may be the answer in keen athletes. Determine the aetiology of the stress and take steps to prevent recurrence. Suggest swimming or cycling to maintain fitness.

THE KNEE

The knee is a complex joint and it is not within the scope of this chapter to describe the anatomy or the mechanics of the joint. Neither is it within the scope of practice of chiropodists and podiatrists to treat the knee as such. However, in many situations when the foot is treated, a beneficial effect is exerted on the knee. It is therefore necessary to understand the mechanics of the knee. The following section briefly explains several disorders that athletes may encounter and with which chiropodists and podiatrists may be able to help.

The patella

This is the sesamoid of the knee (Fig. 10.8) It works in a pulley-like groove on the femur and is a fulcrum for the action of the quadriceps muscles. It can adapt to forces that act upon it and it is an

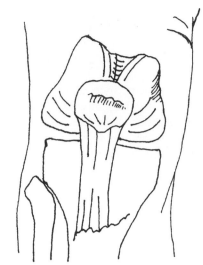

Fig. 10.8   The patella and trochlear groove.

external braking mechanism, producing a dynamic balance between hamstrings and quadriceps. It has a full $1\frac{1}{2}$cm of cartilage on the posterior surface to deal with the forces it endures.

The 'Q' angle (quadriceps angle)

This is an angle between a line drawn from the anterior superior iliac spine to the dorsal surface of the ipsilateral patella and a line bisecting the patellar-ligament (Fig. 10.9). It indicates the relationship between the pull of the quadriceps muscles and the position within its normal limits at about 15°. Any more than this and the change in direction of the pull of the quadriceps will cause the patella to be dislocated from the femoral groove. Uneven vectral forces prevent the vastus medialis from balancing the pull from the lateral muscles. A lateral shearing stress is set up on the posterior surface of the patella. Any sport that requires running will intensify these detrimental forces.

Runner's knee syndrome

This is a mild lateral subluxation of the patella and is *not* chondromalacia, for which it is commonly mistaken. It can be caused by an excessive 'Q' angle or excessive pronation of the foot. Lateral stress causing subluxation over a

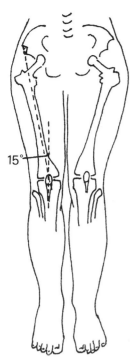

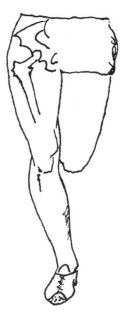

Fig. 10.10   Limb varus while running.

Fig. 10.9   The 'Q' angle.

period of years establishes a new position for the patella, creating an uneven pressure on the lateral surface. The shape of the patella changes as it adapts to these stresses and new position. Abnormal pronation causes internal rotation of the tibia; this produces pain.

The syndrome is frequently experienced by runners; the running motion and limb varus produced by running exacerbates the patellar dislocation (Fig. 10.10). Women, in particular, suffer with this problem because of their anatomical disadvantage, i.e. wider hips and higher 'Q' angle.

Orthotic therapy can realign the foot and prevent the changes that occur at the knee.

Chondromalacia patellae

This condition is commonly associated with vastus medialis tendinitis. It is described as a blistering, cystic change of the patellar cartilage and it usually affects the medial facet of the patella.

It is caused by the combination of several factors which ultimately push the patella out of its groove on the femur. These factors include: weakness of the vastus medialis muscle; a high 'Q' angle, which causes vastus imbalance and over-action of the lateral vasti; malalignment produced by pathomechanics of the foot, leading to abnormal excessive pronation and internal rotation of the tibia. Finally, aberrations of the anatomy can lead to malfunction, such as irregular shaped facets on the patella or an abnormally high vastus medialis insertion.

On examination, the patient will complain of a generalised, deep knee pain. The knee may be swollen with a chronic effusion of synovial fluid and there will be a positive patello-femoral grinding test when the condition is severe. The patella will appear out of alignment and there may well be a high 'Q' angle. The vastus medialis will be weak. X-rays will occasionally show spurring and the patient will be unable to do squats.

Before diagnosing chondromalacia patellae, several other anomalies should first be eliminated. These include chronic synovitis, causing swelling, chronic meniscal injuries, plica syndrome and sprain of the retinaculum.

Treatment involves ice and ultrasound, massage of the painful areas and realignment of the maltracking of the patella. This may be achieved with orthotic therapy, otherwise referral to an orthopaedic surgeon may be necessary for surgical management (Table 10.8).

Ankle equinus and knee pain

A short posterior muscle compartment or a bony block at the ankle producing ankle equinus can be responsible for knee pain. 10° of ankle dorsiflexion is necessary for normal gait. When this is reduced, one of the body's compensations is to lift the heel early during the walking cycle. The heel lifts slightly at mid-stance and the knee functions in an excessively flexed position.

The more the knee is flexed, the greater are the forces at the articulating facets of the patella. In joggers and long-distance runners this mechanism produces aching and discomfort during and after running. This is a satisfactory condition to treat as it responds well to heel lifts fitted in the running shoes combined with posterior muscle group stretching. Occasionally, flexed knee position is due to tight hamstrings or iliopsoas muscles.

Plica

This commonly occurs in individuals, causing no symptoms whatsoever, though it can also in some cases cause a great deal of pain and discomfort. In the embryo, the knee cap is surrounded by a large bursa which differentiates into the prepatellar, the suprapatellar and the infrapatellar bursae (Fig. 10.11). These can resorb completely in the adult and fall into folds laterally, superiorly and medially. With trauma, overuse or running, the structure can become inflamed, thickened and

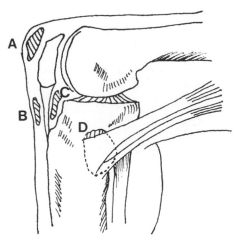

Fig. 10.11 The bursae of the knee:
A. Suprapatellar
B. Prepatellar
C. Infrapatellar
D. Pes anserinas.

fibrosed, and become almost ligamentous in nature. This can fold under the patella and displace it laterally. The vastus medialis is not powerful enough to pull the patella into its ideal situation and it subluxates. It can cause pain and clicking in the knee and can mimic other knee disorders.

Ilio-tibial band friction syndrome (ITBFS)

This is a painful, debilitating condition affecting a significant number of runners, especially the endurance runner. It is caused by friction of the ilio-tibial band as it passes back and forth over the lateral femoral epicondyle during flexion and extension of the knee (Fig. 10.12). The condition tends to occur mainly from overuse.

Table 10.8 Treatment flow sheet: chondromalacia patellae.

Initial visit	Second visit	Third visit
Ice pack to knee	Consider functional foot orthoses if excessive pronation is present	Consider gastrocnemius and soleus stretching programme and heel lifts
Activity modification to decrease any painful activities	Decrease activities further	Check function of foot orthoses and increase subtalar joint control if necessary
EGS and ice if swelling present on knee	Review all 1st visit recommendations and increase any not fully done	Continue to work on knee swelling if still present
Quadriceps stretching programme, five times daily	X-ray evaluation including sunrise view, and lateral knee to look for spurring and degeneration of posterior aspect of patella	If not significantly improving ↓
Neoprene knee brace with lateral patellar buttressing	If knee pain still persists	*Fourth visit*
		Orthopaedic consulation with view to possible surgery

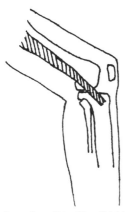

Fig. 10.12   Insertion of the ilio-tibial band.

The ilio-tibial band is a thickening of the fascia lata that extends from the iliac crest to insert into the lateral tibial condyle. The band receives insertions from the tensor fascia lata and gluteus maximus muscles. Excessive amounts of friction occurring during flexion and extension movements of the knee may produce mechanical irritation leading to inflammatory reactions within the iliotibial band, the underlying anatomical bursa, if present, and/or the periosteum of the lateral femoral condyle.

Clinical presentation is of pain on the lateral aspect of the knee close to the lateral femoral epicondyle and it may extend along the ilio-tibial band. On occasion, soft tissue swelling is present at this site. The pain is usually aggravated by repetitive knee movements in running but not with walking. Running downhill and over-striding also induces pain as the ilio-tibial band is compressed by the lateral femoral condyle. Side-to-side sports such as tennis and basketball do not aggravate the condition. The area is tender.

The diagnosis can be confirmed by the use of the compression test. With the knee flexed at 90°, pressure is applied over the lateral femoral epicondyle or just proximal to it. The knee is then extended slowly. At approximately 30° of flexion, a severe pain should be elicited which patients will describe as the same pain as they get when running.

Thorough examination of the knee should be performed to rule out other pathology which could include cysts, meniscal tears and chondromalacia.

Treatment emphasises a decrease in the amount of distance the patient is running. To stop completely is best but most runners will not do this. Running on flat soft surfaces, reducing speed and running to tolerance without pain should reduce symptoms. Ice massage, ultrasound and stretching will help (Table 10.9).

If the patient cannot run without pain, other training programmes should be instituted such as swimming and weight training. The muscles to be strengthened are the quadriceps, hamstrings and abductors. Reintroduction to running should be slow and gradual.

HAMSTRING TENDINITIS

Strain of a hamstring is a common injury as it is one of the flexor muscle groups and hence a group prone to shortening. It should be carefully stretched before any sport but particularly sprinting or running.

Table 10.9   Treatment flow sheet: ilio-tibial band syndrome.

Initial visit	*Second visit*	*Third visit*
Ilio-tibial band stretching programme	Physical therapy, usually ultrasound, followed by ice massage	At this time consider possible lateral meniscus and orthopaedic referral
Quadriceps strengthening programme with adductor strengthening programme	Consider testing excessive rotation factor with ankle taping	Use of knee arthrogram to check for possible tear in lateral meniscus is unsatisfactory on
Ice massage to injured area	If consider excessive varus stress, exclude such possible causes as short limb, worn out shoes, etc.	lateral side due to the position of the apopoteus ligament and its shadowing
Rule out meniscal disease and others in differential diagnosis		
Check for excessive rotation or varus stress situation in biomechanics	If reflare with return to activity	
If not significantly improving or reflare with activity		

It is possible for a muscle or a tendon of this group to be damaged at any part along its length, whether at the muscle belly or its tendon attachment at the ischial tuberosity.

A strain is normally caused by the sudden over-extension of a tight hamstring, whether at the hip or knee, with over-striding or sprinting. A hamstring that has previously been injured is never as strong again and predisposes to further damage.

On examination the hamstring will appear to be tight; there will be swelling and bruising only if some fibres have been ruptured. Pain will be present at the site of the sprain, e.g. at the ischial tuberosity but most commonly mid-thigh. Pain will increase if the muscle is contracted against resistance. The individual may have to walk with a fixed-knee position.

Treatment (Table 10.10)

The key factor is to stretch the hamstring muscles to ensure no further injuries. Ice should be used directly after the injury to keep down swelling and inflammation. After the acute stage, ultrasound and heat followed by massage will stimulate healing.

Finally, it may be necessary to change the style of running to avoid sprinting or over-striding and downhill running. Daily exercises and stretching should be part of the warm up routine to prevent injury recurring.

LEG LENGTH DISCREPANCY

During running, forces of up to three times body weight are transmitted through the feet and the lower limb. When a sport involves leaping and jumping, these forces can reach seven or eight times body weight.

A limb length difference starts to be significant at around 3 mm. With a leg length difference of 6 mm, the mere shifting from one side of the body to another, plus the added stress of a sport, can cause the equivalent of 2 cm difference. Given this difference, a sport such as cycling, skiing, rugby or basketball will produce a significant difference in function on one side of the body compared to the other, resulting in fatigue.

Leg length difference can be anatomical or physiological:

1. Anatomical leg length difference describes a true anatomical difference that exists between two legs. It is measurable without variation. The difference is found in both neutral calcaneal stance position and relaxed calcaneal stance position. The height of the femoral heads on X-ray is diagnostic.

2. Physiological leg length difference results when some other body structure or aberration affects the leg length measurement. This may include scoliosis, muscle imbalance, abnormal biomechanics of the foot, and may originate above the pelvis or below the malleoli.

Table 10.10 Treatment flow sheet: hamstring tendinitis.

Initial visit	Second visit	Third visit
Hamstring stretching programme done five times daily	Quadriceps and hamstring dynamometer testing for strength and ratios ·	Consider prolonged rest
Ice packs to injured area three times daily but especially after activity	Do not allow return to activity until flexibility and strength are normal	
Activity modification to decrease painful activity (especially hill work and speed work)	Consider functional foot orthoses if rotation is a significant problem	
If extremely tender, EGS and ice treatments three times a week until symptoms resolve	Check for history of sciatica and low back problems, possibly causing hyperinnervation of hamstring muscles and chronic tightness	
If rupture suspected or chronic problems, initiate hamstring strengthening exercise	Heel lifts to take some pressure off tendo Achilles and hamstrings	
If reflare with return to activity	Evaluate for short leg syndrome with hamstring tendonitis on side of long leg	
	If reflare with return to activity	

Functional leg length difference may occur in unilateral sports where over-development of one-half of the body produces a significant discrepancy.

Symptoms produced by leg length differences are: snapping of the ilio-tibial band, bursitis on the lateral aspect of the knee and low back complaints. There may also be unilateral knee pain and asymmetrical function of the feet. Below the knee, medial shin splints, Achilles tendon pain and ankle pain are also problems.

These symptoms are usually unilateral and should suggest some asymmetry of the body. It is necessary to carry out a full biomechanical examination to determine where the asymmetry lies.

A biomechanical examination should include measurements of the limbs (Fig.10.13) in order to quantify the difference. The measurement is taken from the anterior superior iliac spine to the medial or lateral malleolus. The femoral component should be measured at the joint line of the femur and tibia. Measuring can be difficult if bony landmarks are hard to find.

The examination should include the comparison of ranges of motion of the joints, their flexibility and quality of motion, both weight-bearing and non weight-bearing. Measurements of limb and limb segments, neutral and relaxed stance measurements, will eliminate the foot as a cause of discrepancy. Examine forefoot to hindfoot position. Look at the ankle axes and the subtalar joint axes. Determine whether there has been soft tissue injury or surgical intervention which might cause asymmetry.

One of the simplest forms of examination is to examine the patient `standing (Fig. 10.14) and walking in a swimsuit so that body proportions and attitudes can be observed. Look at the head, the neck and the back. Shoulders may tilt on the shorter side. In adults, the head will not tilt; it will straighten so that the eyes are parallel to the horizon, but look to see if the neck is curved. If a double scoliosis is present, the shoulders will level out. These are compensations which occur in the body and can give rise to pain. Elbow and hand position may appear lower on the shorter side and indentations and folds on the back will also appear on this side. On the posterior aspect, muscle compartments may be bulkier or even in spasm. Draw a line down the spins of the vertebrae and using a goniometer, measure

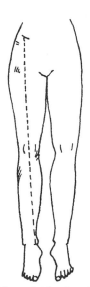

Fig. 10.13   Measuring leg length.

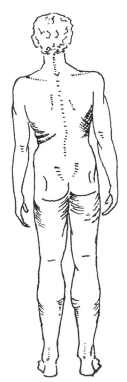

Fig. 10.14   Examination of the patient standing.

the degree of deviation. Look at the scapulae and sacral dimples.

Twists and rotations my be in the transverse plane; women are more prone to scoliosis than men. Arm swing can show up an asymmetry of the pelvis — the opposing arm will swing more with the shorter leg.

Compensations for leg length difference can take place in the feet. On the short side, the foot will supinate and maintain weight-bearing on the outside of the foot in an attempt to lengthen the limb. It may also function in an equinus position to prevent too much dorsiflexion and shortening occurring. The opposite will happen on the long limb. There will be excess wear on the inside of the shoe as the foot pronates and shortens that limb. 4–6 mm of shortening can occur with pronation at the subtalar joint.

Finally, go and watch the patient in action; watching the patients and the sport they are involved in may be a vital clue to diagnosis.

Typical case history

A 36-year-old male runs 30–50 km a week at a rate of 6 minutes per km. He complains of pain on the medial aspect of his left knee which started after an especially long run. The pain is present during the day, when activity is low, and becomes quite sharp when he changes direction. He warms up well, stretches well and warms down after his run. He finds the pain gets worse when he runs on harder surfaces. He has tried changing his running shoes; various shock-absorbing materials in the shoes, icing and ultrasound have all been to no avail.

He has noticed that the right leg of his trousers is a bit longer on that leg and recently has noticed some stiffness and discomfort in the right back and shoulder and in the lower back. On examination of his shoes, there is asymmetrical wear. They are worn out laterally on the right shoe and medially on the left shoe.

A runner complaining of unilateral knee pain should immediately suggest a leg length discrepancy. There are, of course, other aetiological factors for unilateral knee pain and these should be eliminated. Examples are: strain of the medial collateral ligaments of the knee; strain of the pes anserinus muscles insertion, i.e. gracilis, semitendinosus, sartorius; bruising from a traumatic injury; patellar subluxation and strained vastus medialis muscle; the plica syndrome.

Once these have been eliminated, then the reason for the leg length difference must be determined. The knee pain in this situation is a result of the pronated position of the foot on the longer leg. Pronation causes internal rotation of the tibia, increased flexion of the knee and more stress on the posterior aspect of the patella. The shorter leg is also prone to stress fracture because of the lack of shock absorption in the supinated foot and the position of the acetabulum directly over the femoral head.

Treatment of leg length discrepancies

1. Anatomical leg length discrepancy, once it has been determined, is reduced by a simple shoe lift or heel lift. It may be necessary to have some manipulative therapy to aid the readaption of body structures to the new position.

2. Physiological leg length difference may require an orthosis as well as a heel lift if poor foot mechanics are the aetiological factor.

Special exercises may be necessary to strengthen or stretch certain muscle groups that are unbalanced. The individual should be reassessed regularly to ensure the deforming force does not cause the condition to recur.

Care should be taken to avoid over correction of leg length discrepancy and it may be necessary to refer the patient to a manipulative therapist or physiotherapist for their expertise.

FOOTWEAR

Many of the current shoe evaluations in runners' magazines are not as practical as they are represented. The following practical suggestions should enable patients to find the right shoe for their particular needs.

Qualities

Select a toe box with adequate height over the toes and 2 cm length from the ends of the toes. Width of shoes varies according to the manufacturers' concept of the average foot. The correct width is necessary to avoid excessive squeezing of the forefoot. A loose shoe, however, will create fatigue problems of the forefoot. A 2 cm pinching of the material over the ball of the foot is necessary for a good fit. Some manufacturers have been producing varied widths and shoes with variable lace eyelets will help to adjust to individual needs.

Balance, or equilibrium, in the shoe is necessary to avoid excessive stresses and forces on the normal motion of the foot and limb during running. If the shoe tilts inwards, most of the foot motion will be in that direction, causing an overuse syndrome. Always check the heel counter on a flat surface to see if it is straight up and down, perpendicular to the supporting surface.

Flexibility of the ball of the shoe is important to avoid fatigue of the lower legs and muscle and tendon strains. If the shoe does not flex in the correct position, arch fatigue or foot strain can result. A shoe should bend easily with one finger at the ball or widest area of the shoe (Fig. 10.15).

Heel counter placement and rigidity are quite important for controlling the direction of forces on the foot during its heel contact phase in the gait cycle. If the heel counter is too soft or misplaced, the heel will wobble during the heel contact phase of the running gait. Close inspection and evaluation is necessary especially for the flat foot.

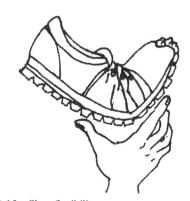

Fig. 10.15   Shoe flexibility.

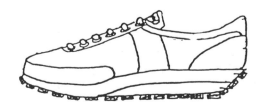

Fig. 10.16   The running shoe.

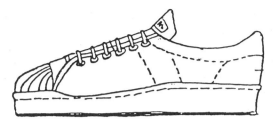

Fig. 10.17   The court sports shoe.

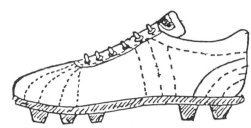

Fig. 10.18   The field sports shoe.

Weight and softness of the shoe seem to go hand in hand, for most light shoes have soft midsole materials. For a light person who has good foot structure and hits the ground hard, these shoes are adequate, but they fatigue and warp in 300–400 kilometers. Insoles of a soft and resilient material are needed, especially in the forefoot area, due to less midsole protection.

Last, and most important, is comfort, so that training for improved health and athletic achievement can be comfortable. Figures 10.16, 10.17 and 10.18 illustrate various shoe types.

The most important assessment is that of the biomechanical foot type. The two extremes are the flat foot and the highly arched foot. The types in between are even more common and more difficult to evaluate. The subtleties of feet involve the amount of motion, the angle and the flexibility or stiffness of the running feet during their application to the ground. These subtleties may result in excessive motion or shock of the foot joints during running. This excessive motion is transmitted to the limb increasing stress to the ankle, knee and hip.

Feet that pronate excessively require more control and support by the shoe at the heel and a harder firmer midsole. The supinating foot tends to be less flexible and shock absorbing and requires compensatory properties to be available within the shoe.

A runner's specific needs are different from a walker's. A runner places three to five times body weight on the heel and forefoot during each cycle of foot placement on the ground. The runner may land hard or soft, depending on his form, style and body weight.

Terrain can create abnormal demands on the lower extremities and the feet. Harder surfaces require a shock-absorbing sole and midsole. Softer surfaces, such as dirt and grass, require a more stable shoe for a consistently stable foot plant.

The number of miles run per day or week is a significant consideration—with increased mileage, some shoes will wear faster than others. Also, the dynamics of feet and legs change due to increased tightness or strength in the leg muscles. Greater speeds demand more shock absorption in the forefoot of the shoe.

Basic anatomy (Fig. 10.19)

There are special shoes for running, tennis, bicycling, skateboarding and even for javelin throwing and polevaulting. The specifications differ widely, but the basic make-up is still the same.

Outersole

The outersole is that part of the shoes that is in contact with the ground or the outermost covering on the plantar surface of the shoe. It can be made of a variety of different materials depending on the sport, ranging from the thick, high density rubber soles for hiking boots to the lightweight, flexible gum rubber soled shoes for volleyball. As there are many different kinds of soles, the patterns of the outersoles may vary considerably.

Four basic factors are involved in the design of outersoles: traction, flexibility, durability and weight. Not all sports shoes need to utilise all four factors. Traction is the material's ability to grip the supporting surface. Flexibility is the quality of being able to bend without breaking. Durability is the ability to exist for a long time while retaining the original qualities or capabilities. Weight is the final factor that has to be considered.

Midsole

Some shoes utilise a midsole to aid in further support and for shock absorption. This is seen as a layer of material that is placed on top of the outersole and holds the rest of the shoe up. One

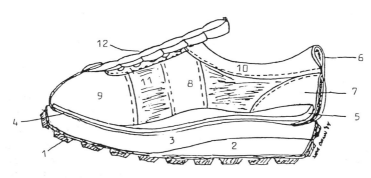

1 Outer sole	7 Heel counter
2 Wedge	8 Arch bandage
3 Midsole	9 Toe Box (with lining)
4 Insole board	10 Collar
5 Sockliner	11 Eyestay
6 Achilles Tendon Protector (pull tab)	12 Tongue

Fig. 10.19 Parts of the sports shoe.

can think of the midsole as being like the shock absorbers and leaf springs in a car. The ideal midsole would take up as much of the shock as possible, but not lose control of the foot during the process.

Those shoes that do not have a midsole, but require shock absorption, utilise another method: the single unit outersole. The single unit outersole has large cells or chambers which makes the outersoles more resilient to take up the shock.

Regular street shoes achieve midsole support by using steel or wood bars in the shank of the shoe to prevent uncontrolled hindfoot torque. Shock absorption comes from a multilayered heel and a good insole, but, as a rule, street shoes lack the capability to absorb shock as well as athletic shoes.

A wedge is sometimes placed in conjunction with the midsole to add to heel height and decrease stress. This reduces the amount of stretch required of the gastrocnemius-soleus complex and cushions the heel strike. Ski boots have some wedging to give a better frontal plane tilt and better 'edge' control.

Insole board

The insole board is the inner part of the shoe that runs the entire length of the shoe. The basic purpose of this is to give stability in the shoe to prevent twisting of the foot. This firm platform allows the manufacturers better quality control since, during the process of making the shoe, adjustments can be made more easily.

The insole board usually rests on top of the edges of the uppers, thereby adding more stability to the union between the uppers and the midsole/outersole. In most quality insole boards, the material is treated to resist moisture deterioration and micro-organism growth.

Sock liner

The sock liner is what the foot rests on inside the shoe. It can be removable and/or washable. The comfort of modern athletic shoes is largely attributable to the fact that current sock liners conform better with continual wear, thus causing fewer complications in terms of blisters or calluses. In addition, sock liners can contribute to the padding of the shoe, but it is only minimal.

The removable sock liners allow more room for the insertion of devices like orthotics or heel lifts, or, if toe space is required, more toe box room to allow for motion or splaying of the toes. Sock liners can be made out of a variety of different materials and also have different properties.

Uppers

The uppers consist of three basic parts. The area covering the forefoot is the vamp and the areas covering the midfoot and hindfoot are the inside (medial) and outside (lateral) quarters. The vamp can be two-piece, with the seam down the middle of the front of the shoe, or, more commonly, one piece, with no seams. The edge around the shoe where the upper meets the sole is called the featherline.

Uppers are generally of four basic patterns. The lace-to-lace design has the laces abutting the toe box with ten eyelets up to the ankle. This is found in high-top shoes and in basketball shoes. The circular vamp has stitching just on the sides and is curved round over the instep and to just below the laces. This is a common design in women's shoes. U-throat lacing seems to sit in a squared-off box of its own. Tennis shoes commonly employ this style, because it helps to keep the shoe material from bunching up. The saddle type of upper consists of two strips which support either side of the instep. In theory, this gives better support and accommodates for different widths.

In nylon uppers, leather is utilised to reinforce key points. Decorative stripes are also utilised in quality shoes to lend additional support. The foxing is the covering at the back and sides of the shoe. The front edge of the vamp forms the area of the toe box, which may have a leather overlay called the wing tip. A stiffener is sometimes placed underneath the wing tip. If the leather tip only covers the rim of the toe box and does not go up to joint the throat, it is called a mudguard tip or a moccasin toe box. The single unit outersole type of shoe will include this as part of the unit.

A padded area just below the ankle is known as the collar, with a projection above the heel which is known as a pull tab or Achilles tendon protector. The heel counter sits in the pocket in the back of the shoe. At the centre of the longitudinal arch is additional reinforcement. If it is on the outside, it is called a saddle; if on the inside, it is called an arch bandage.

The heel counter is an essential part of the athletic shoe because it holds the heel on the heel seat. Good heel counter will minimise the amount of hindfoot motion when the foot hits the ground. In a poor quality shoe, cardboard-like material is used which may feel hard at first but a quick run will reduce it to mush. Most good quality shoes have nylon counters which are premoulded and will keep their shape. It is important to ensure that the heel counter is firmly anchored.

The tongue is to protect the top of the foot from irritation due to the laces. This should be sewn into the shoe and not glued in. Many shoes now have tongues with a double slit three-quarters the way up from the attachment of the tongue through which the laces run and keep the tongue centred in the shoe.

The area of reinforced leather or suede around the instep is called the eyestay, and this is punched through to form eyelets for the laces. Some eyestays do not have eyelets but utilise plastic to form what is called the Ghilly speed lacing system. This is to allow faster, more even distribution of pressure when lacing the shoes. Finally, some shoes do not use laces at all, but strips of velcro for applying the same tension across the instep that lacing would do.

THERAPEUTIC MODALITIES

The use of heat and cold as therapy for sports injuries can prevent potentially debilitating and chronic conditions from arising. Once their action on blood vessels, skin and other structures is understood, their application can speed rehabilitation, lessen scarring and fibrosis and prevent sprains and strains. Heat and cold can be applied in various forms and they are easy to apply either at home or at the surgery. The details of theory and practice of these and other physical therapies are discussed in Ch. 14.

Cold

Cold can be used on acute injuries, such as sprains and strains, to reduce inflammation, suppress fluid build-up and swelling in the tissues and prevent scarring and adhesions. It can also be used as a mild analgesic in painful conditions.

Acute injuries, sprains and strains require immediate application of cold to prevent swelling. Cold in the form of an ice pack, for example, should be applied for the first 36 to 48 hours after injury.

Cold, if applied for 3 to 6 minutes, can also be used to give vasodilatation (Hunting response or reaction). This can be applied and combined with massage to produce stimulation of the circulation locally.

Heat

Heat should not be applied until 48 hours after an injury, and should not be used on areas which are oedematous. It can be used combined with cold in the form of contrast baths to produce the Hunting effect, which stimulates venous pumping and the removal of excess tissue fluid. Contrast baths should be followed by compressional strapping and elevation of the part to above the level of the heart. This procedure should be followed several times during the day.

Ultrasound

Ultrasound has a mild analgesic effect. It disrupts fibrous tissue which has formed after injury and so breaks up adhesions. It can be used to disrupt and break down a haematoma that has congealed. Its analgesic and heat-producing effect can also be used to relax muscle spasm. Details are discussed in Chapter 14.

Contra-indications

Ultrasound should not be used in the eye area, with heart or vascular disease, where there is embolism or haemorrhages, on anaesthetised skin, on the epiphyseal area in children or on bony prominences such as the spine.

For best effects it should be used once or twice

a day, 3–4 times per week. It must be used at least 6–8 times before it is discarded as being ineffective. 1 W/cm² for 10 minutes is required to produce an effect. The time period should be gradually increased. Some individuals are more sensitive than others to its effects.

Medical diathermy

This is an electromagnetic wave force generated between two pads applied one on either side of the injured part; it produces a deep heat. It can be used to treat deep bruising or tendonitis.

It especially stimulates the lymphatics and the collateral circulation, and is a good method of treatment for traumatic inflammatory processes: myalgia, neuralgia, muscle spasms, adhesions and chronic infections.

Contra-indications

Diathermy should not be used on haemorrhages, acute inflammatory processes, malignant tumours or burns.

Treatment

Application should be for 20–30 minutes, 3 times daily for 3–4 days. The patient will feel a deep warm 'glow' at the site of application. Fibrotic lesions may need longer treatment.

Homoeopathic arnica 30c

This is a relatively new therapy. Arnica is an excellent remedy for inflammation; it helps prevent excess fluid accumulating in the tissues and leads to less scarring and fibrous tissue formation. It is also known for its pain-relieving properties. It should be taken 3 times daily as required.

ADVICE TO ATHLETES

Stretching exercises

Before an individual attempts any form of sport, he or she must warm up with a series of stretches and exercises beforehand. Many injuries such as tears, sprains and strains can be avoided by taking time to stretch muscle groups, to set the circulation going and to prepare the body for action.

In modern life, the human body is curled into a sitting position for many hours of the day: at work behind a desk, in the car and watching TV. The muscles on the flexor surfaces shorten and require lengthening while those on the extensor surfaces require strengthening.

The reason for stretching exercises is to stimulate blood flow through the muscles, which function best when stretched to 110% of their resting length, and also to get the synovial fluid in the joints flowing. Exercises also increase flexibility if carried out over several months, improving function and the ability to carry out the sport.

Exercises can be devised for a general warm-up and for specific sports. A sound knowledge of anatomy and of the origins and insertions of muscle groups will be required if the exercises devised are to be effective in stretching particular muscles. There are many exercise books on the market which are easy to follow and can be used as the basis for a warm-up programme.

When following an exercise plan, start distally and work proximally. Probably the most important muscle group to stretch is the triceps surae, followed by the hamstrings.

Adductors and abductors need stretching in long-distance runners, and adductors in cyclists, skaters and hurdlers. These muscles are stabilisers of the hip.

When stretching a muscle it is important not to bounce the muscle. This stimulates the stretch receptors in the muscle to fire off and the muscle will contract rather than stretch. Go into the stretch slowly and hold for 10–15 seconds. Repeat this 15 times.

Warming up the muscle beforehand makes the stretch easier. A warm bath or spa bath for ten minutes is a good preparation before starting on a new activity or sport. Heat can be applied locally by heat pad on areas that have been injured in the past or on a tendo Achilles injury where some fibrosis has formed. Ice for 3–6 minutes also stimulates the circulation to a specific area.

Yoga and ballet are excellent activities for

maintaining strength and suppleness and it may be beneficial for a runner to take up one of these as an extra activity to maintain flexibility.

A common complaint from runners who have recently taken up the sport is pain in the calf muscles. Metabolites build up in these muscles and the muscles go into contraction, causing a false equinus. Heat and stretching exercises can overcome this problem.

Strengthening exercises

Strengthening exercises for the muscular system play an essential role in podiatric therapy. All types of exercise must be used in the correct proportion in athletics. The focal points should vary according to the individual athlete's constitution and condition, and the types of sport.

Types of strengthening methods

1. Isometric
2. Isotonic
3. Isokinetic

Isometric exercise from the first part of active therapeutic treatment after athletic injuries, such as sprains, tears, dislocations or fractures which are conservatively treated.

1. Isometric means 'same length'. Isometric contraction is an active contraction which produces no motion of the part. There is no work accomplished, but power is exerted against a fixed resistance.

The advantages of isometric exercise are as follows:

1. No cost for equipment
2. No equipment space required
3. It does not put a muscle or joint through a range of motion. It will allow particular strength only at a specific angle. This is good for rehabilitative runner's knee or athletes in a cast
4. It helps stabilise a joint.

The disadvantages of isometric exercise are:

1. Not so good for older patients: it raises the blood pressure so may put strain on the cardiovascular system
2. Does not develop or strengthen muscle power throughout the range of motion.

2. Isotonic conditioning is a type of exercise in which the muscle goes through a range of motion with a fixed weight. This is a dynamic exercise. There are two sub-categories of isotonic exercise:

A. *Concentric* stengthening—where a weight is lifted with the force of muscle contraction
B. *Eccentric* strengthening—where the contraction force of the muscle is against an overpowering weight resistance.

Concentric exercise is the best means of

Table 10.11   Muscle testing about the ankle and foot. Break hand resistance = 4 to 0 scale

Important muscle groups	Position of foot	Function in foot
1. Extensors		
A. Extensor digitorum longus	Dorsiflex ankle and toes	Decelerates foot
B. Extensor hallucis longus	Dorsiflex foot and hallux	to
C. Anterior tibialis	Invert foot and dorsiflex	ground (running)
2. Plantarflexors		
A. Gastrocnemius	Plantarflexed at ankle and knee extended	Decelerates foot pronation; stabilises knee, ankle and lateral column of the
B. Soleus	Plantarflexed at ankle and knee flexed	foot; decelerates body in forward motion
C. Tibialis posterior	Inverted foot and plantarflexed	Decelerates pronation and supports midtarsal joint
D. Flexor hallucis and digitorum longus	Plantarflexed at ankle	Decelerates pronation and forward leg motion
E. Peroneus longus	Plantarflexed and everted	Stabilises first ray, cuboid and ankle
F. Peroneus brevis	Plantarflexed and abducted	Stabilises lateral aspect of foot and ankle

producing strength with safety. During rehabilitation, the correct formula of repetitions to sets and repetitions to weight must be determined. The determination of endurance versus hypertrophy of the muscle is essential. The athlete's injury and sport will dictate this.

Eccentric exercise is the best means of producing strength but it is very dangerous. It can be termed dynamic negative work; however, during this form of exercise, muscular tension two or three times greater than normal can be created. This is very important for the sports podiatrist as much of the extrinsic musculature to the foot and ankle apply decelerating forces on poorly stabilised fulcrums.

3. Isokinetic or 'same speed' strengthening is exercise where the speed is set so that a specific range of motion is moved through per unit time. The speed of some of the machines can be set from 0–300 degrees (Cybex or Orthotron). The machine also pushes back against the operator as hard as he or she is pushing against it. It matches the user's strength through the muscle/joint range of motion.

The settings of the machine can be adjusted according to the type of strength the user wishes to develop. If hypertrophying of muscle is desired, slow speeds (0–100 degrees) are utilised. To increase speed and power, speeds above 120 degrees are set.

Many of the isokinetic machines have instructions to demonstrate range of motion and strengths in that range of motion. Universal and Nautilus machines are less sophisticated but attempt to accomplish a similar goal or resistative exercise throughout the range of motion.

The following is a suitable regime for starting a rehabilitative strengthening programme:

1. Electromuscular stimulation (EMS) to maintain tone in the injured musculature (see Ch.14)
2. Isometric exercise programme involving all muscles about the joint
3. Isotonic exercises of the above muscles
4. Ultimately, isokinetic training while the athlete returns to athletic activity. This may require 3–4 months of follow-up

FURTHER READING

Cavanagh P R 1980 The running shoe book. Anderson World Inc, Mountain View, California

Frankel V H 1980 Biomechanics of the skeletal system. Lea and Febiger, Philadelphia

Helfet A J, Gruebel Lee D M 1980 Disorders of the foot. Lippincott, Philadelphia

Hlavac H F 1977 The joints of the ankle. Williams and Wilkins, Baltimore

Inman V T, Ralston H J, Frank T 1981 Human walking. Williams and Wilkins, Baltimore

Jahss M A 1982 Disorders of the foot. Saunders, Philadelphia

Kirby K A, Valmassey R L 1983 The runner-patient history, Journal of American Podiatry Association 73 (1)

Lea R B, Smith L 1972 Non-surgical treatment of tendo Achilles rupture. Journal of Bone and Joint Surgery 41B

Mann R A 1982 Biomechanics of running: the foot and leg in running sports. Symposium of American Academy of Orthopedic Surgeons. Mosby, St Louis

Perry J, Antonelli D, Ford W 1975 Analysis of knee joint forces during flexed knee stance. Journal of Bone & Joint Surgery 57A (7): 961–67

Root J L, Orien W P, Weed J H 1977 Clinical biomechanics, Vol II. Normal and abnormal functions of the foot. Clinical Biomechanics Corp, Los Angeles

Subotnick S I 1975 Podiatric sports medicine. Futura Publishing, New York

Sgarlato T E 1978 Compendium of podiatric biomechanics. California College of Podiatric Medicine, San Francisco

Williams P L, Warwick R (eds) 1989 Grays's Anatomy, 37th edn. Churchill Livingstone, Edinburgh

11. Clinical therapeutics

Donald L. Lorimer   Donald Neale

THE THERAPEUTIC MANAGEMENT OF SUPERFICIAL LESIONS

The superficial lesions of the feet are the immediate source of much pain and disability in adult patients. They are unique to the feet and deserve particular consideration as clinical entities in their own right. Their effective treatment must always be a first priority in management, whether or not the underlying deformity or dsyfunction of which they may be symptoms is amenable to correction. The patient's first concern is to obtain relief from pain. The podiatrist's ability to treat such conditions successfully may well determine the patient's willingness to co-operate in further measures, such as changes of footwear, which may be necessary to deal with the underlying problem.

The range of therapeutic measures available include careful operating, discriminatory medication, applications of heat and cold, and protective dressings and padding. The use of such measures in a number of common conditions is discussed to exemplify effective management, it being presumed that any underlying pathology will also be appropriately treated.

Padding and strapping, in most cases an integral part of clinical therapies, may also be used as the sole therapeutic method. The principles upon which it is based provide the rationale for orthoses in the continuing management.

Operating

Nothing is more important for the quick relief of pain than skilful operating. Pain during operating and tenderness afterwards are proportional to the degree of trauma inflicted on sensitive tissues in the course of treatment. Essential elements in painless operating are therefore maximum immobilisation of the part by applied skin tension, and the correct type and size of instrument. In most cases, operating on superficial lesions, skilfully done, should be entirely painless. When this is impossible because of the nature of the condition, as in heloma vasculare and verruca pedis, operating should be reduced to the minimum with recourse to caustics and exfoliants to facilitate the desired result and protective padding to relieve pain. As an alternative, pre-operative anaesthesia or analgesia may be achieved, either by topical application or by injection, to allow complete enucleation.

Medicaments

With the exception of local anaesthetics, medicaments in podiatry are used as topical applications. They may have a specific function, as in the case of chemical caustics, antifungal agents and antiseptics, but they generally have a palliative effect. Topical therapy can be said to provide relief of symptoms and protection while the skin heals itself. Many of the agents used lack scientific explanation of their mode of action and are used because they are known to have been effective in the past. The fact that suitable agents may be selected and used empirically should not detract from their credibility but should encourage the practitioner to establish links which may add to the understanding of the mode of action. The form in which the agent is used, its mode of application, the state of the skin, the site of the lesion, and the patient's state of health are all factors to be considered in selection. The paramount concern should be to treat the lesion quickly and to use the minimum quantity of medicament. Long-term usage of medicaments should be avoided as some agents may cause allergic contact eczema. Where long-term application is unavoidable, as in the case of emollients in hyperkeratosis, the practitioner should be aware of this possibility and should minimise the risk by suggesting alternatives at regular intervals. In the treatment of specific conditions, such as fungal infections and verrucae, the patient should be advised to follow the recommended method and not to supplement or vary the treatment.

Dressings

Dressings give protection from infection and, in conjunction with padding, may contain a medicament and enhance its action. A number of preparations of sterile dry dressings, such as Melolin XA, are available in sterile packs. In this form they can be used for a wide variety of conditions and they simplify the 'no touch' technique. Tubular gauze dressings are effective for retaining dressings and also limit the need to touch any open lesion.

Padding and strapping

Most foot problems are mechanical in origin and mechanical therapy therefore has a vital role in their management, whether or not surgery also is required. Mechanical therapy includes both short-term treatment by adhesive dressings and long-term management by appliances and footwear modifications. There is nothing better than adhesive padding properly designed and applied to give immediate relief from pain following any necessary treatment of superficial lesions. There is nothing *worse* than relying on adhesive dressings as a continuing policy when more durable and hygienic alternatives are readily available. The combination of both methods affords the most effective, comprehensive and economical means of controlling mechanical foot disorders. Most of these require management which progresses from temporary palliation with adhesive dressings to optimum control and possible cure by the appropriate appliances and footwear modifications.

Though necessarily short lived, adhesive padding and strapping have both corrective and protective functions. Correction padding and strapping corrects or improves anatomical alignments and thereby reduces or eliminates abnormal stresses. When used in a corrective role, strapping is applied with sufficient tension to effect the required result without being intolerably firm or tight. Protective padding and strapping do not substantially affect the underlying deformity but they reduce to tolerable limits any abnormal stresses arising therefrom. The role of strapping is then only to secure padding closely to the foot in its correct position.

Padding may be applied directly to the foot in either an adhesive or replaceable form, it may be fitted into the footwear as an insert, or built into a corrective or protective appliance. The wide range of materials available provides a choice of densities from the very firm to the very soft, the choice depending on the therapeutic objective. Firm materials are needed to apply correction, to provide a firm base for bearing weight and to redistribute stresses from one area to another. Soft materials are required to provide shock absorption and cushioning for tissues subject to abnormal stresses, particularly if they are debilitated by disease and subject to ulceration and infection. Combinations of high and low density materials are often required for optimum effectiveness and good tolerance by the patient.

Review periods

Review periods are an important factor in good clinical practice. The management of conditions depends on the practitioner's ability to assess progress and to change or modify therapeutic measures as required. The choice of medicament, of its concentration, and of padding materials all depend on the patient's ability to attend for treatment. Review periods are variable depending upon a number of factors and they need to be considered in any strategic plan for treatment. The review of progress is facilitated by accurate case records which may be supplemented, in some instances, by photographs or accurate charting (see also Ch. 8).

CONTROL AND TREATMENT OF THE HYPERKERATOSES

Pathological callus

This common symptom of malfunction should be carefully removed with a suitable scalpel so that the area is clear of thickened skin. Callus which is present for some functional reason and produces no discomfort should not be removed. The choice of medicament to be applied postoperatively depends on the state of the patient's skin, whether moist or dry. Postoperative antiseptic agents are indicated, such as Savlon 0.1% in spirit, povidone-iodine or tincture of benzoin compound. The latter is said to prevent loss of moisture from the tissues but painting with collodion flex is better for that purpose. Applications of adhesive plaster in the form of fleecy web have a similar effect.

In moist skin, astringent agents should be used to improve its condition. Mild astringents are 3% salicylic acid in spirit and limited applications of 3% formaldehyde solution. Depending on the moistness of the skin, more astringent applications of silver nitrate solution at strengths of 25% or 50% may be used. The eschar so formed produces a protective film and it is suggested that it may inhibit the process of keratinization, but there is little evidence to support this view.

In dry skin, the best method is to use emollients to soften the skin and retain moisture. To be effective, the agent needs to be applied by the patient at least twice a day. The proprietary emollients used in the control of anhidrosis may be used.

Helomata durum

These commonly occur on the dorsum and apices of the middle toes and on the lateral aspect of the fifth toe. It is essential to eradicate the nucleus with a scalpel at the earliest stage possible. Enucleation should remove all the parakeratinised epidermal cells so that the underlying tissue can be restored to better condition. Enucleation can usually be accomplished without difficulty at the first visit, but if the toe is inflamed and tender, it may be advisable to apply a cooling lotion which can be left in place for 5–10 minutes prior to enucleation.

In long-standing cases, enucleation may need to be followed by cauterisation of the resultant cavity in order to minimise the possibilities of recurrence. With little underlying tissue, the choice of caustic agents is limited, but 30% salicylic acid ointment in white soft paraffin is one such agent. This should be applied with a masking plaster as for a verruca. It can be left in place for five to seven days and the resultant macerated tissue removed with a scalpel. This treatment may be necessary two or three times at weekly intervals followed by one or two applications of 25% silver nitrate solution. Thereafter, patients should be encouraged to restore elasticity to the area by the regular use of emollients applied with a deep kneading action to break down any subdermal adhesions. This is done by applying firm pressure while moving the superficial tissues to and fro over the underlying bone.

The presence of vascular insufficiency or peripheral neuropathy may make the use of caustics undesirable, but a mild exfoliant such as 12% or 20% salicylic acid in collodion can be used to facilitate enucleation. If any caustics are used, they should be monitored carefully to ensure that ulceration does not occur. On dorsal helomata the combination of 50% silver nitrate solution and an ointment buffer can produce a satisfactory result provided the eschar is removed after two weeks. Electrosurgery (described later) can also produce good results in carefully selected cases.

Interdigital helomata

These are evidence of abnormal compression of the interdigital tissue due to deformities such as hallux abductovalgus and claw toes, exacerbated in some cases by hypermobility and lengthening of the feet through excessive pronation and consequent constriction of the toes from footwear. Their complete cure depends on the elimination of such stresses, which is not always possible.

They may also be associated with hyperhidrosis, which determines their consistency as hard (helomata durum) or soft (helomata molle), and which, if present, needs to be controlled. Their enucleation requires skilful operating, especially when they are situated in the fourth web.

Helomata molle respond well to application of silver nitrate solution 20% following enucleation. This procedure should be repeated at intervals of two weeks. After two or three such applications it is possible to change to daily applications of 3% salicylic acid in spirit. Silicone orthodigital splints or interdigital wedges are the most effective forms of padding.

Vascular and neurovascular helomata

Lesions of this type are found over interphalangeal joints and beneath metatarsal heads. They are characterised by the protrusion of dermal structures into the overlying hyperkeratosis and the objective of treatment is to destroy these elements by cauterisation. The presence of nerve filaments and capillaries close to the surface makes these lesions highly sensitive and liable to bleed, so operating should be limited to removal of superficial callus without causing haemorrhage. Should haemorrhage occur, treatment with caustics must be delayed until the wound has healed. Any essential operating may be assisted by the preoperative application for some five minutes of 5% solution of potassium hydroxide to soften the overlying callus. Rarely, a local anaesthetic by nerve block or infiltration may be indicated if extensive excision of a part or the whole of the lesion is contemplated, but progressive cauterisation is the less traumatic treatment of choice.

In vascular lesions, applications of 50% solution of silver nitrate weekly over several visits are effective, but using this method for neurovascular corns could cause intense pain and is not recommended. An alternative is to apply pyrogallic acid 25% in white soft paraffin, suitably masked and padded as for the treatment of verruca. After seven days the eschar is removed and the treatment repeated. It is important to avoid breakdown of the tissue and the caustic should not be used on areas with little subdermal tissue if the local circulation is impaired. After the fourth treatment, the area should be treated with 50% silver nitrate solution and the resultant eschar removed after 14 days. It should then be possible to start the application of emollients and deep massage to restore the tissues to better condition.

If there is an impaired blood supply, milder caustics should be used such as salicylic acid 20% or 12% in collodion flex. If the patient is fair skinned, it may be better to use 30% salicylic acid in white soft paraffin instead of 25% pyrogallic acid ointment.

Electrocautery may also be used in the treatment of such lesions. Local impairment of circulation may make its use more problematical and, while early results seem encouraging, longer-term evaluation needs to be made. Vascular and neurovascular corns are often associated with a loss of subdermal tissue and it may be that any long-term improvement may need to be coupled with implants.

Digital padding for the lesser toes

The application of medicaments to digital lesions necessitates appropriate padding, either to redistribute the pressure on the lesion and thus to enhance the effect of the medicament, or to correct toe function.

The common deformities of the lesser toes are hammer toes, mallet toes, clawed and retracted toes, and digiti quinti varus. They may be purely local, or secondary to pes plano-valgus, pes cavus or hallux abductovalgus. They are all compounded of specific deformities of the individual phalanges, namely excessive extension or flexion, axial rotation, and medial or lateral deviation. Digital padding should be designed to exert maximum correction on such malalignments since they are only rarely fixed and some degree of correction is almost always possible. It is usually quite inadequate to pad merely to protect a particular lesion. Moreover, although single digit padding may be necessary as a short-term measure to bring a lesion under control, more positive control and correction is obtained in most cases by regarding the middle three toes as one functional unit and, where necessary, correcting and protecting all three simultaneously through one device.

Orthodigital splints (Fig. 11.1)

The common and major element in most digital deformities is excessive extension or flexion of the phalanges and it is logical first to control that element by combined dorsoplantar padding, which exerts reciprocal corrective pressure on the deformity. In a full orthodigital splint for the middle three toes, the dorsal pad exactly covers the proximal phalanges and controls any excessive extension of them. The plantar pad underlies the intermediate and distal phalanges and controls any excessive flexion of them. Before the advent and general use of silicone materials, the pads used to be constructed from felt and required to have their inner surfaces shaped to hold the toes in the corrected position. The silicones mould themselves into retaining grooves but require the digits to be held in the degree of correction until the material sets. Extension/flexion deformity is controlled by the dorsoplantar pads exerting reciprocal correction. Axial rotation and medial/lateral deviation are controlled by the combined effects of the grooving coupled with the bulk of the padding, which denies any space in the toebox for the phalanges to lie anywhere but in their corrected alignment. Adjacent toes, in fact, act as mediolateral splints to their neighbours.

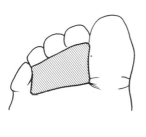

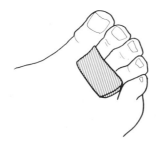

Fig. 11.1 Orthodigital splints—dimensions and positions of plantar prop and dorsal pad.

Bodyweight immobilises the plantar pad against the sole of the shoe, and the dorsal pad is held comfortably firm by pressure from the upper. The whole splint is thus securely in contact with the toes correcting unwanted deviations in the interphalangeal joints, while the metatarsophalangeal joints are left untrammelled to function normally.

The shape, thickness and density of each pad is determined by the needs of each case, as also is the relative degree of correction or protection required. In mobile digital deformities in children, the splints should be sufficiently firm and slightly oversize to ensure maximum correction. With fixed deformities in older patients, the splints may be almost wholly protective in function, while possibly restraining further deterioration. Many gradations between these two extremes are possible, but active correction should always be given priority over passive protection.

As a temporary measure, the splints can be constructed from adhesive felt and strapping, but they are more effective for long-term use when fabricated in a durable form. Silicone materials have the advantage of being durable, washable and, if necessary, adjustable. (see Digital appliances, p.248).

Orthodigital splints are the most effective method of controlling multiple deformities of the middle three toes and their associated dorsal, apical and interdigital lesions. The basic design can be varied to meet all contingencies. Where necessary, the dorsal pad can be extended into an oval cavity to afford greater protection to an interphalangeal prominence. The plantar pad can be extended as a prop under the fifth toe, or under the proximal phalanx of the hallux in hallux rigidus. The splint also affords a firm anchorage for an interdigital wedge, and may add considerably to the effectiveness of a metatarsal brace, of which it can form an integral part.

Partial splints are sufficient in certain cases and various alternative designs are possible. The padding may be confined only to the digit or digits most affected, sufficient bulk being provided to ensure the desired corrective or protective effect and also the necessary stability of the splint in wear. This usually entails the splint embracing at least two toes, but single digit partial splints are sometimes sufficient, particularly for the fifth toe and for a single hammer toe. When all three middle toes are clawed and a long plantar prop is required, the dorsal padding may be reduced to no more than retaining lugs.

Because of the need for precision in the sizing and fitting of orthodigital splints, several important points need to be observed when this technique is used:

1. The full thickness of the dorsal pad must not extend any further posteriorly than the base of the proximal phalanges, nor any further anteriorly than the proximal interphalangeal joints (except when a protective oval cavity pad is required).

2. The posterior edge of the plantar pad should conform to the plantar fatty pad of the foot. The full thickness of the pad should fit behind the pulp of the toes.

3. The pads must be thick enough to engage the pressure of the sole of the shoe on the plantar prop and the pressure of the shoe upper on the dorsal shield in order to maintain correction of the digits.

4. The medial and lateral edges of the pads should not overlap on to the first and fifth toes when all the toes are in a normally constricted position inside the footwear.

5. Good positional control for the plantar prop is maintained by allowing a concavity in each side of the pad to accommodate the pulp of the first and fifth toes.

For all interdigital lesions, correction of phalangeal malalignments is essential and this is best achieved by full or partial orthodigital splints. With severe digital deformities which are not suitable for surgical treatment, the required additional room in the front of the shoe is obtained by means of balloon patches, upper insertions or slit releases, or by complete replacement of the vamp.

Single digit padding

For the reasons previously given, collective padding for the three middle toes is generally more effective than single digit padding. On occasion, however, any of the lesser toes may require individual padding for dorsal, apical or interdigital lesions and, particularly in the case of the fifth toe, for its lateral aspect. While impaction and constriction from shoe pressure obviously contribute to such lesions, digital deformity is almost always the essential factor and one which is correctable either by padding or by surgery. The combination of dorsal and plantar padding is more effective than either alone and the same principle of reciprocal dorsoplantar correction should be applied for single digits as previously described for all three middle toes.

A combination of plantar prop with dorsal crescent or oval cavity pad is used to provided tolerable corrective splinting for the deformity as well as adequate protection for any lesions; temporarily, this splinting may be adhesive, utilising adhesive felt. Silicone rubber splints are the method of choice and are more durable. Properly designed, they ensure complete protection to vulnerable areas while also exerting maximum correction. The silicone technique has the great advantage that the material is directly moulded to the foot and this obviates any need for casting. Silicone shield and splints are also readily adjustable, if necessary, after being worn and are completely hygienic.

Any necessary footwear modifications to relieve harmful shoe pressure should of course be undertaken.

Helomata durum on the plantar metatarsal area

These are usually chronic in nature and they may be associated with pes cavus (under the first and fifth metatarsal heads), with hallux rigidus (under the second metatarsal head and the interphalangeal joint of the hallux), and with hallux abductovalgus (under the second and third metatarsal heads). Such chronicity results from fibrosis of the area surrounding the nucleus because of traumatic inflammation over a long period caused by faulty weight-bearing. Such lesions may prove difficult to eradicate successfully because the tissues at the weight-bearing area have lost their elasticity. They will respond to a certain extent to attempts to increase pliability but the main emphasis in management must be on deflective and protective padding and orthoses.

The use of pyrogallic acid 20% with 20% wheat germ oil in white soft paraffin is said to be effective in inhibiting the formation of fibrous tissue. There is no objective evidence to support this view but it may be that the increased frequency of treatment which is necessary for the application of pyrogallic acid ensures that the nucleus is brought under control giving the appearance of a cure. The use of wheat germ and pyrogallic acid should be limited in the same way as for applications of pyrogallic acid alone. If used, it can be alternated with plain buffering ointments. However, where there have been large 'fibrous' lesions, the plantar tissues never seem to regain their elasticity fully. Electrosurgery used on single lesions has produced significant improvement in selected cases, particularly those where blood supply is not impaired significantly. It requires the use of a tibial block.

Implants of silicone or bovine collagen do not seem to have been successful in replacing fibrofatty padding due to the difficulty in maintaining their location.

The treatment of plantar lesions located under the metatarsophalangeal joints involves the use of various forms of plantar metatarsal padding (PMP). Where, as in most cases, the forefoot derangement giving rise to such lesions is secondary to some malfunction of the hindfoot, the plantar metatarsal padding must be combined with the measures required to control the hindfoot.

Plantar metatarsal padding (PMP) (Fig. 11.2)

The range of movement in the metatarsophalangeal joints is crucial in determining the therapeutic objective and consequently the type and consistency of any padding required. In the presence of chronic fixation, subluxation or dislocation of these joints, plantar metatarsal padding is designed to palliate the consequential overloading of particular metatarsal heads by redistributing the excessive load. In cases of mobile clawed or retracted toes in which the metatarsal heads are pinned down by the retracted phalanges, metatarsal padding assists in correcting the alignment of the affected metatarsal segment, particularly if combined with the use of

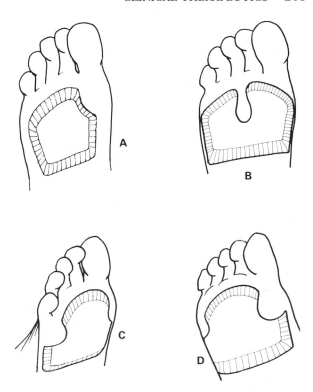

Fig. 11.2 Plantar metatarsal padding: (A) Basic PMP; (B) Broad U-section PMP; (C) Single-wing PMP for 5th metatarsal head; (D) Double-wing PMP for 1st and 5th metatarsal heads.

orthodigital splints. When used to assist in the correction of retraction of the toes, it is essential that the footwear worn by the patient will accommodate the increased length of the foot which results.

Initially, plantar metatarsal padding is most frequently used in its adhesive form, but it is readily convertible for long-term use into the form of metatarsal braces, with or without digital splints, or as one component of an insole (Valgus/PMP, Filler/PMP, etc).

The basic PMP (Fig. 11.2A) is shaped to cover the heads and part of the shafts of the three middle metatarsals so that on weight-bearing they are relatively elevated, provided they are sufficiently mobile. The shape conforms closely to that of the underlying metatarsals, avoiding impinging on the head of the first, and taking into account variations in the metatarsal formula. The full thickness of the pad lies beneath the metatarsal heads and it is bevelled off from there in all directions, being carefully graduated on its anterior and posterior edges to ensure that it is securely adhered without any irregularities to cause discomfort under load. In addition to improving the alignment of the middle three metatarsals, it relieves symptoms of metatarsalgia. The improvement in the line of the clawed or retracted toes needs to be maintained with orthodigital splints.

In conjunction with plantar padding, metatarsal strapping is used to control excessive splaying of the forefoot. The strapping encircles the metatarsus immediately behind the first and fifth metatarsal heads, non-stretch material normally being preferable. A 'half-met' strapping may often be sufficient. This leaves the dorsum free, the ends terminating on the dorsum of the first and fifth shafts after traversing the plantar surface. Two or three 2.5 cm or 3.75 cm wide straps half-overlapping each other are usually sufficient, their ends being sealed off with retention straps.

For the longer-term management of forefoot derangements, recourse must be made to replaceable metatarsal braces, accommodative insoles or functional orthoses, as appropriate.

Variations from the basic PMP include single-wing pads (PMP/SW) (Fig. 11.2C), double-wing pads (PMP/DW) (Fig. 11.2D) and U-section cut outs (PMPU) (Fig. 11.2B).

Winged pads are designed to protect either or both of the first and fifth metatarsal heads from overloading. When adhered to the foot, the wing is reverse bevelled, the thickness of the wing fitting immediately around and behind the metatarsal head or heads concerned. With a medial wing, the overall width of the pad must conform closely to the medial curve of the footwear so that no overlap of full thickness material on to the upper of the shoe is permitted, as this would unnecessarily tighten the vamp. The extra width required for anchorage is well bevelled and moulded around the metatarsal shaft. Full thickness will normally be provided under the middle metatarsal heads. The effect of the wings is to exert pressure on the metatarsal shafts on weight-bearing, thereby relieving pressure on the heads and relatively elevating them if mobile. This effect is akin to that of a metatarsal bar worn in the shoe, and if required, the same effect can be accentuated by the addition of a bar of material to a basic PMP immediately posterior to the metatarsal heads.

The U-section pad is similar to the basic PMP except that a U-shaped section is cut away anteriorly with reverse bevel to encircle and protect any one of the middle metatarsal heads as may be required.

Helomata miliare

These often present difficulties in treatment. If they do not cause pain, it is best to attempt control by the application of emollients, ranging from lanolin to the urea-containing compounds such as urea 10% cream, which affects the keratin linkages and increases the moisture content. This type of ointment may occasionally cause pruritic irritation. If the lesions are painful, it is necessary to enucleate them. As a preoperative preparation, the application of 5% potassium hydroxide solution is valuable if given about 15 minutes to soak. After enucleation, emollients can be applied.

If the nuclei are very close together, an application of 40% salicylic acid plaster for five to seven days will macerate them sufficiently for easy removal. Alternatively, an application of 20% salicylic acid in collodion is useful if the nuclei are not so close together.

Palmoplantar hyperkeratosis

This condition and its associated punctate form present problems in management. It is described by Thomson & Cotton as follows:

Palmoplantar hyperkeratosis is a minor feature of several more generalised genetic disorders as in Darier's disease, recessive ichthyosis and congenital ectodermal dysplasia. There is also a group of genetic diseases in which palmoplantar hyperkeratosis is the major presenting feature.

These conditions produce keratotic thickenings which can cause severe discomfort and interfere with the gait cycle. Much research into the genetic influence on autosomal dominant ichthyosis vulgaris has not yet revealed causative factors. When it appears in large plaques surrounded by an inflamed ring, its operative removal is often limited by the discomfort, which may be minimised by prior application of potassium hydroxide 5% solution. This also helps when reducing the punctate form by scalpel, but it is seldom possible to remove all the hypertrophic material. Painting the area each day with 20% salicylic acid in spirit helps to keep it softer. Applications of emollients such as urea-based creams help to retain water.

A preparation which seems effective in the control of this form of hyperkeratosis is magnesium sulphate paste BPC. Applied liberally, covered with gauze, secured occlusively and left for five days, it leaves the area well hydrated. It is useful if the area tends to fissure and it must be followed by regular applications of emollients. This treatment will have to be repeated from time to time.

The management of this condition is usually simple palliation.

VERRUCA PEDIS

Verrucae are known to regress naturally after some months, thereby reducing the case for active treatment if they are not painful. Active treatment is indicated when pain is acute, when the risk of cross-infection is high, as for other members of the same family, and when non-treatment would entail unacceptable limitations on activities such as swimming, games and athletics. Plastic waterproof socks are available for such activities to guard against cross-infection but are of little value in keeping dressings dry.

If treatment is to be commenced, it should be carried out quickly and effectively. The longer the time taken to reach a satisfactory conclusion, the greater the risk of producing a verruca resistant to treatment and causing pain to the patient. Although one foot only may be affected, both feet should be kept under observation during treatment as a check against cross-infection.

Measures for the treatment of verrucae are centred on cell destruction techniques. Efforts to employ antiviral agents have not been successful. Existing methods include chemical cautery, cryotherapy and electrosurgery. A growing number of practitioners are using actual cautery or curettage with promising results.

Chemical cautery

This retains an important place in the treatment of verrucae and, properly employed, it produces rapid results with little discomfort to the patient. The principal substances in use are salicylic acid, pyrogallic acid and monochloroacetic acid, their caustic actions being strictly confined to the verrucous tissue. The choice of agent depends on a number of factors, as follows:

Site. A lesion on a non weight-bearing area is usually superficial, so liquid caustics are useful, e.g. a saturated solution of monochloroacetic acid. A verruca on a weight-bearing area is relatively deeper and both liquid and ointment preparations are suitable. However, care must be exercised in the use of caustics where there is little underlying adipose tissue in order to avoid causing a severe breakdown or producing an inflammatory reaction in an underlying joint. In such a situation, milder caustics or strong astringents are indicated.

Number and size. Large verrucae respond well to ointment preparations. However, when numerous growths are present, masking is difficult and pyrogallic acid may produce tissue toxicity if used in large quantities. A large growth surrounded by smaller satellites may be treated with pyrogallic or salicylic acid ointments, and the satellites with either monochloroacetic or trichloroacetic acid solutions, or with toughened silver nitrate alone or together with trichloroacetic acid.

In general, over a series of treatments, caustic ointments or solutions are indicated for one or more large growths, while multiple small verrucae are more easily treated with solutions or silver nitrate stick. Cryotherapy or electrotherapy offer alternative single treatments for any type of verruca.

Skin texture. If moist, solutions of caustics are preferable; if dry, ointment preparations are indicated. Fair-skinned people seem to be less tolerant to the action of acids and often react adversely to pyrogallic acid.

Circulation. When the arterial supply is reduced, as with a diabetic or atherosclerotic patient, ulceration of the infected area must be avoided since healing would be delayed and bacterial infection could supervene. For the same reasons, similar care must be taken to avoid ulceration in the case of impaired venous circulation which results in the tissues being oedematous. In such instances, mild caustics or astringents are indicated. 20% salicylic acid plaster, Thuja occidentalis and weak solutions of formaldehyde are examples of such preparations.

Neuropathy. Where there is some degree of sensory loss, mild caustics or astringents are again indicated for the same reasons as for circulatory deficiency.

Availability of patient. When powerful acid caustics are used, it is essential to ensure that the patient is able to return within seven to fourteen days. Otherwise, an alternative form of treatment, such as cryotherapy or alkali treatment, would be advisable. Home treatment is another possibility.

Age. Very young children are often nervous as well as seeming to have low pain thresholds, so mild caustics are more suitable.

Caustic ointments or pastes tend to spread and this must be prevented by careful masking of the adjacent healthy tissue. The surrounding skin is first masked by thick adhesive stockinette through which a hole has been cut slightly smaller than the surface area of the verruca. (A light application of silver nitrate to the periphery of the lesion by means of the 70% silver nitrate pencil gives added protection against spreading.) The ointment is then applied through the hole to the verruca and sealed in with waterproof strapping to ensure its close contact. A cavity pad is applied over the dressing to relieve any pain on weight-bearing and to help to extrude the verruca. The padding is then totally covered with zinc oxide plaster, left in position for up to seven days and kept dry (Fig. 11.3).

At the second visit, the necrosed tissue is removed under strict aseptic conditions. If the verruca has not been totally destroyed, another application of the caustic should be made and repeated as necessary until necrosis is complete. If ulceration has occurred, an astringent antiseptic should be applied with a sterile dressing.

The objective of treatment with acids is to produce an *aseptic necrosis* and resultant sloughing of the verrucous tissue. With carefully controlled dosages and spacing of treatments, this is

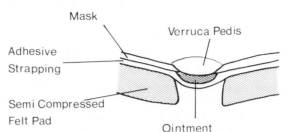

Fig. 11.3 Occlusive dressing and padding for the application of acids in ointment form for the treatment of verrucae.

normally a painless process. A simple healing ulcer is left which requires only an antiseptic protective dressing to ensure normal healing. In some cases, however, where monochloroacetic or pyrogallic acids have been used, some residual action of the agent may temporarily continue in the immediately adjacent tissues which produces some mild inflammation and discomfort. This can be controlled by antiseptic and astringent cooling lotions such as chlorhexidine gluconate 0.1% in spirit, or by a hot hypertonic footbath (45°C) using magnesium sulphate crystals. This assists by inducing a wider hyperaemia and by cleansing the ulcer by osmosis. As a general rule, in cases where ulceration is accompanied by inflammation, it is recommended that a hypertonic footbath be used.

Therapeutic agents

Salicylic acid is the main agent and it is usually applied in strengths of 60% to 70% in white soft paraffin; it may be combined with 5% chloral hydrate for its analgesic effect. The action of salicylic acid can be enhanced by combining it with a small amount of saturated solution of mono-chloroacetic acid, which should be applied first.

Monochloroacetic acid. The most effective way of using monochloroacetic acid is on its own as a freshly prepared saturated solution. It is best applied on a fine-pointed applicator stick so that its rate of absorption can be observed and controlled. Small amounts worked slowly into the surface render it translucent as the verruca gradually becomes slightly spongy. Care should be taken not to flood the surface with the solution nor to allow it to run over on to the surrounding skin. This eliminates any need for the use of petroleum jelly as a masking material. A light application of 70% silver nitrate pencil to the immediate periphery of the verruca provides an effective barrier.

Opinions differ about the extent to which any overlying callus should be removed before the acid is applied. Complete removal allows precise application of the acid but this may cause unnecessary pain as the acid is brought into immediate contact with sensory nerve endings in the hypertrophied papillae. If only just sufficient callus is removed to disclose the margins of the verruca (and in practice this may mean little or none), the remaining bulk of callus acts as a buffer to retain a larger dosage than could otherwise be applied, while making possible its gradual penetration with little or no pain. In this technique, the surface is merely scarified to assist absorption of the acid. In either case, protective padding is advisable to minimise pressure on the area and ensure maximum comfort, and if the site of the verruca so permits, cavity or aperture padding will assist extrusion of the verruca.

Monochloroacetic acid should not be used on areas which do not have much subcutaneous tissue or over joints. Used in conjunction with salicylic acid its action is very rapid and may cause some pain. The patient should be seen in about seven days when both acids are used together, but if used alone, up to fourteen days may be allowed for review. When tissue breakdown occurs, the ulceration should be treated as previously described.

Pyrogallic acid ointment is also a commonly used preparation which, because of limitations on manufacture imposed by the Medicines Act 1968, is becoming less readily available. Its most common concentrations are 25% and 50% in white soft paraffin. It should be applied in the same way as salicylic acid. Pyrogallic acid should be limited to four consecutive applications as it has a cumulative effect on the tissues and can become toxic. This effect can be limited by carefully removing the resultant eschar and cauterised tissue.

Single treatment techniques

In circumstances where patients may be unable to attend for a series of treatments, it may be necessary to employ a technique to destroy the verruca in a single treatment. Means for doing this are:

a. by potassium hydroxide
b. by cryotherapy, utilising carbon dioxide snow, liquid nitrogen, or nitrous oxide
c. by electrosurgery, using coagulation, desiccation or fulguration, by 'hot-wire' cautery, or with electrosurgical units
d. by curettage.

Potassium hydroxide

Potassium hydroxide in pellet form is a very effective but painful single treatment. The skin should be prepared by soaking in water and then dried before the pellet is applied by means of a plastic holder. The application may prove painful but should be maintained for two minutes. The foot should then be immersed in lukewarm water for about five minutes after which the area will have a white macerated appearance. The verruca can then be removed with a scalpel and the area examined with a magnifying glass to establish that total clearance has been achieved. If there is any remaining verrucous tissue, a small reapplication of potassium hydroxide will remove it. After satisfactory examination of the area, glacial acetic acid should be applied to neutralise any remaining potassium hydroxide.

It is claimed that as this treatment is clearly seen to leave normal tissue at its conclusion, it is not necessary to see the patient again, but in the interests of good management, it is recommended that a dry sterile dressing be applied after the treatment and the patient seen again in from three to seven days. A final review should be carried out after one month.

Cryotherapy

Cryotherapy is a method of treatment which, with recent advances in apparatus, has become more effective. It is necessary to cool the tissues to $-20°C$ to ensure tissue necrosis. Rapid cooling causes the formation of large ice crystals in the cellular and interstitial fluids with resultant cellular rupture. Slower cooling rates do not necessarily do this but they increase the quantity of tissue fluid, which causes cell wall rupture by electrolytic imbalance.

Rapid cooling coupled with low temperatures shortens the treatment time and also allows more accurate destruction of the lesion with much less pain and less destruction of peripheral tissue.

There are three methods available to produce localised freezing of tissue:

1. Carbon dioxide snow, which has a working temperature of −78.5°C. Its use in podiatry is not nowadays so great, but the apparatus which makes the snow into a useable stick is simple and effective and reasonably inexpensive to use and, with the use of plastic tweezers, its application to the site is relatively simple.

If used with a coupling medium, it is very effective and it succeeds in producing tissue temperatures down to −50°C. If the lesion is elevated to its fullest extent after the carbon dioxide snow has frozen the 'bridge' which it produces between itself and the lesion, it is possible to limit the freeze to the desired area. Formerly, it tended to be used without a coupling medium and this usually produced excessive pain and extensive necrosis.

2. Nitrous oxide, with a release temperature of −88.5°C, which is employed in sophisticated apparatus, using the Joule-Thompson principle. The probes available allow great accuracy in application and safety in use but they also lose a significant temperature advantage. (Studies of over a hundred applications show an average probe temperature of −52.4°C). The refinement of the apparatus enables it to be used with great accuracy although it is useful to be aware of this significant loss of capacity.

3. Liquid nitrogen, which has an operating temperature of −196°C. The apparatus available for its use is similar to the type of equipment available for nitrous oxide and recent advances in manufacturing have made this technique more easily used.

All techniques are potentially painful in their application but this can be minimised by the use of coupling gel and elevating the lesion when the source of cold is attached to the lesion. This localises the area to be frozen and also removes the source away from the body's blood supply, which can make a significant contribution towards failure to reduce the tissues to below −20°C. If the tissues do not reach this temperature, success in treatment is unlikely.

The minimum time for freezing using carbon dioxide snow or nitrous oxide equipment should be 30 seconds but in practice it is better to apply the source of cold for one minute. The operator should observe a purple halo around the probe and on its removal ice formation should be seen. Most single verrucae would require three applications with sufficient time allowed between each for the tissues to thaw. At the conclusion, there will be a hyperaemic reaction which will develop into a blister in about two days. This may be haemorrhagic. When using liquid nitrogen apparatus, with its much greater ability to freeze, the time should be reduced to 15 seconds for each freeze. Care must also be taken to elevate the lesion during the freeze. The number of applications may be reduced.

If it is on a weight-bearing area, the lesion should be protected with a suitable pad and it should be reviewed after a week. The blister should not be ruptured and within a few weeks it will dry and peel away with the verruca. A final review period should be made six to eight weeks after treatment. Superficial verrucae may respond to a single application of one minute.

There are few dangers associated with cryosurgical techniques other than spillage of liquid nitrogen or accidental contact with therapeutic probes. The use of nitrous oxide equipment produces large volumes of the gas which should be vented outside the building. The risk of some genetic irregularities has been noted in anaesthetists of child-bearing age, due to prolonged exposure to nitrous oxide.

Electrosurgery

Electrosurgery is also a single treatment technique but in this case it is necessary to use local anaesthesia. For verrucae on the digits, a digital nerve block is required but local infiltration should suffice for any on the dorsum of the foot or on the non weight-bearing plantar areas. The weight-bearing area where most verrucae occur is difficult to anaesthetise using local infiltration techniques and it is usually better to employ a tibial nerve block to anaesthetise most of the plantar surface. If the verruca is on the lateral aspect of the heel, it may be necessary to block conduction in the sural nerve.

The apparatus currently available is designed to convert domestic electrical supply into low voltage, high amperage current. There are a number of types of apparatus and these should be checked to see if they conform to local safety regulations. The use of such equipment is contra-indicated where pacemaker apparatus (particularly demand type pacemakers) are implanted in persons who are in the immediate vicinity of the electrosurgical appliance.

Most forms of electrosurgical apparatus depend on the patient being a part of the electrical circuit and great care must be taken to ensure good contact of the electrode attached to the patient, to avoid burning. The therapeutic probe electrode has a very high current density which creates the heat which destroys the tissue, but does not itself become hot and remains sterile. There are four techniques of administration:

1. Fulguration—in this technique, the therapeutic probe is passed over the lesion to be treated at a distance of about 2 mm so that the current arcs between the probe and the patient. This mode requires a higher voltage setting and produces wide sparks which result in superficial necroses which have an appearance of an eschar produced by silver nitrate. The necrosed area can be removed using a scalpel, thus making it possible to check the result and re-apply the treatment. The lesion should be left as a necrosed surface, which need not be covered with a dressing, for two to three weeks and the result checked. This method of application is particularly suitable for superficial mosaic verrucae.

2. Desiccation—the probe is in contact with the lesion and the sparks produced are much less evident. It produces a deeper necrosis which is still confined to the epidermis and still has the appearance of an eschar produced by silver

nitrate. This area can be removed with a scalpel and the procedure re-applied. It should be reviewed as above and is mainly used for the removal of mosaic and superficial verrucae.

3. Coagulation (Fig. 11.4)—this method uses a lower voltage current and the probe is inserted into the lesion where it produces heat which destroys the tissue, producing ulceration. It also combines elements of desiccation and fulguration and the surface area may have the appearance of an eschar. After treatment the area should be padded and covered with a dry sterile dressing with a review period of up to seven days, depending on the size and number of lesions treated.

On the patient's return it will be possible to remove the lesion with a scalpel, leaving a clean ulcerated area which should be protected and an astringent antiseptic agent applied.

Other suitable review periods should follow. The ulcerated area heals rapidly. This method is suitable for deep single and multiple verrucae.

4. Electrocautery and electrosurgery—the introduction of 'hot wire' techniques coupled with improved apparatus has facilitated the cutting and coagulation of superficial skin lesions such as verrucae, fibrous plantar helomata or vascular and neurovascular lesions. The probe is either in the form of a fine wire terminal, which acts in the

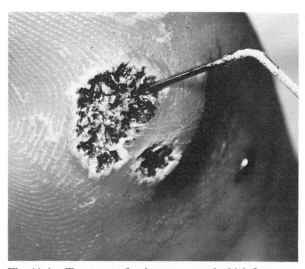

Fig. 11.4 Treatment of a plantar verruca by high frequency coagulation.

same manner as a scalpel and allows the accurate dissection of the lesion, or it can be of the ball type, which desiccates the tissue to which it is applied. The hot wire probe leaves a clean, sterile wound which can be protected with a sterile dressing with or without a broad spectrum antiseptic. It may be necessary to plug the wound with one of the sterile alginate styptic agents to control bleeding. The desiccated tissue which results from the use of the ball type probe can be removed immediately following application using blunt dissection techniques (see curettage) which allows accurate assessment of the result. If necessary, electrocautery can be reapplied immediately until the tissue to be removed seems clear. Any area of bleeding can be sealed using the probe. As with the hot wire techniques a sterile dressing should be applied. In addition, deflective padding may be required. A review period of between three and seven days should be given and the patient is discharged when the area is healed.

Electrosurgery is suitable for single treatments of large verrucae. In addition to burns, dangers exist in the use of electrosurgical equipment on patients fitted with pacemakers. Electric shock is usually associated with faulty equipment but patients should be protected from contact with exposed metal on other equipment.

Local anaesthesia and electrosurgery. The use of local anaesthetics to facilitate electrosurgery requires additional consideration as the electrical current used to cauterise can stimulate nerve impulses to surmount the local anaesthetic blockade. It is recommended that the level of block be made more profound by the use of agents such as bupivacaine.

Laser emission

This offers an alternative to electrosurgery. Laser emissions can be tailored to specific uses and have been employed with some success in dermatology and, more recently, in podiatry. The surgical laser is very versatile and allows more accurate localisation of tissue destruction than any previous technique. Surgery is conducted under local anaesthesia and the safety require-

ments for the use of class 4 surgical lasers must be observed: these include the use of protective goggles and a controlled environment with warning systems to indicate when the laser light is in use. The emission is directed onto the lesion and the tissue destruction is controlled by visual monitoring. A sterile dressing is applied postoperatively and the lesion seen in seven days. Healing is rapid.

Curettage

This technique tends to be regarded in an unfavourable light but without adequate reason. There is some risk of scarring, but handled skilfully, curettage can give satisfactory results in the treatment of stubborn verrucae. The technique requires the administration of a local anaesthetic and, depending on the site, it may be convenient to apply a pressure cuff to control bleeding.

The infiltration of local anaesthetics with vasoconstrictive additives may also be used if the site is suitable.

The edges of the verruca are located with a scalpel and, with a suitably sized Volkmann spoon, the wart can be scooped out of its location. Because this causes gross disruption of the papillae, it is necessary to apply a styptic, the most effective agent being 95% silver nitrate. It is wise to use a longer-lasting anaesthetic either at the outset or as a supplement. A sterile dressing and protective padding should be applied and the patient seen again in three to seven days and again after one month.

An alternative to the use of a Volkmann spoon is blunt dissection with a Macdonald's dissector. It is usually necessary to start the superficial separation with a scalpel but blunt dissection is more accurate than cutting techniques and produces little postoperative bleeding. This method tends to be preferable when using electrosurgery, although some practitioners use sharp dissection coupled with forceps to elevate the tissue.

Home treatments

In certain circumstances, where patients are

unable to attend on a regular basis, verrucae may require to be treated with chemicals which can be safely used by the patient at home with only a limited amount of monitoring by the practitioner. The patient must be sufficiently co-operative to follow instructions about the treatment precisely.

The best home treatment is the use of formaldehyde solution 10% applied twice a day with a moistened applicator stick. This desiccates the verruca and the desiccated tissue needs to be removed once a fortnight. 20% salicylic acid in collodion flex is another and slightly safer method as the rapid drying effect of the collodion prevents the spread of the acid on to adjacent skin.

Home treatments are suitable for mosaic verrucae and multiple verrucae. Preparations containing podophyllum resin can be successful but they may also cause severe irritation which can only be controlled by ceasing their application.

Home treatments are usually prolonged and it may be that natural regression intervenes. This may account for the wide range of self-treatments which are available and the success which is often ascribed to them. However, they are not always satisfactory and may result in more radical methods becoming necessary later.

INFLAMMATORY CONDITIONS

Perniosis (erythema pernio, chilblains)

Chilblains represent one of the conditions in which intervention to control the inflammatory process is necessary in order to prevent additional tissue damage. In the hyperaemic stage, the application of cold compresses is essential to control the volume of tissue fluid in the area and thus diminish the possibility of rupture. In the chronic stage, it is necessary to apply heat together with rubefacients, provided the state of the circulation permits. The use of the infra-red heat lamp is effective, coupled with the inunction of rubefacient creams containing methyl salicylate, particularly those with added menthol for its antipruritic value. In younger patients, contrast footbaths can be used, and also wax baths.

Usually the peripheral circulation is impaired and therefore the rubefacient should have a mild action. A weak solution of iodine painted on and followed by an application of tincture of benzoin compound is sufficient. Also useful is the application of ichthammol 12% in collodion flex. Compound tincture of benzoin and 12% ichthammol in collodion flex have the additional advantage of reinforcing the skin and minimising the risk of its rupturing. Warm foot baths (40°C) may also be used.

Broken chilblains usually occur on the dorsum or apex of digits and over the medial aspect of the joint in hallux abductovalgus and the lateral aspect of a prominent fifth metatarsal head. There is usually severe diminution of the arterial supply and the condition should be treated with great care to prevent the entry and spread of infection. Warm antiseptic footbaths using Savlon Hospital Concentrate 5 ml per litre should be followed by gentle dabbing to dry the foot. Tenderness of the condition restricts the choice of antiseptic agent to one with a cream base. Sterile dressings should be applied using a 'no touch' technique. This treatment should be repeated daily until signs of healing are seen. It is then possible to change to spirit-based antiseptics such as povidone-iodine. When healing is complete, applications of ichthammol in collodion flex will help to improve the condition.

Patients who are regularly subject to chilblains should be advised about preventative measures. If prolonged exposure to cold is unavoidable, the feet should be warmed only slowly. Warm lined footwear should be worn provided it is not tight fitting. Thermal insoles can be made from Plastazote or Evazote but insoles incorporating metal foil are better because they are less bulky. Thermal insoles and extra or thicker socks should be worn only if the footwear will accommodate the extra bulk. Feet which are subject to chilblains need to be carefully bathed in luke-warm water (not more than 40°C) and gently dried. Ointments and creams formulated for the treatment of chilblains, particularly those with an antipruritic effect, are often useful. Systemic treatments for chilblains have not proved effective in general. Proprietary remedies rely on vasodilatation and may produce unpleasant side-effects.

They should be used only if prescribed by a general medical practitioner.

Ulceration

Ulceration on the feet occurs in a number of forms and for various reasons. Its management following treatment for verrucae is referred to earlier, and its management in diabetic and other high risk patients, and in the elderly, is discussed in the relevant chapters.

An additional form is that resulting mainly from sustained trauma as a complication of heloma and callus formation. Typically, this is seen in pes cavus under the first and fifth metatarsal heads, and on the dorsum or apices of toes which are clawed, retracted or hammered. The condition is often aseptic in the early stages but may later become invaded by pathogenic bacteria and display signs of inflammation, including those of cellulitis and lymphangitis.

The overlying callus should be completely removed and the area drained for any pus, of which swabs should be taken for bacteriological examination. As with all such infected conditions, care should be taken to ensure that sterile blades are used and are kept separate from other instruments for sterilisation and disposal after use. Similarly, all dressings and materials used should be sterile, and after use should be discarded into a suitable disposable container. A 'no-touch' technique should be used in order to minimise the risk of cross-infection.

Following exposure, the ulcer should be irrigated with normal saline solution and then should be thoroughly dried. After being dried with sterile cotton wool, an astringent antiseptic agent such as povidone-iodine in spirit or chlorhexidine gluconate 0.1% in spirit could be used, but if the area is particularly sensitive, a cream-based agent may be better. Suitable protective padding should be applied and the patient seen again in twenty-four hours when the inflammation should have subsided. Astringent antiseptics should then be applied with suitable padding and the patient should be advised to rest and to return after seven days. Thereafter, the condition should be treated as described in Chapter 8, but if cellulitis is still present with pain, additional systemic antibacterial cover must be prescribed.

Similar symptoms may be evident if a lesion has become infected through self-treatment by the patient or through abrasion from footwear.

Subungual ulceration is commonly found in patients with arterial deficiency and may be present in cases of onychogryphosis. Careful removal of the overlying nail plate is necessary to expose the full extent of the ulceration. This should be treated as previously described but it may also be necessary to provide a protective orthotic device.

The management of ulceration must include consideration of the footwear and the provision of orthoses to redistribute weight and prevent excessive stress on vulnerable areas. Patients with ulcerative conditions which do not respond to treatment should be referred to their medical practitioners for more extensive investigation. (The management of ulceration is considered in detail in Ch. 8.)

Sinus formation

Cases of chronic bursal or corneous sacs often result in the tracking of fluid to the surface and the organisation of a sinus which prevents closure and permits the entry of bacteria. Such sinuses may become plugged with hardened fluid and they appear cornified. Enucleation uncovers these sinuses, exposing a straw-coloured and viscous discharge. They are found in the main on the dorsum of retracted toes, on triggered first toes, and on the medial aspect of the first metatarsophalangeal joint.

Closure of the sinus is the obvious objective but it is essential first to control the underlying deformity with orthoses and footwear modifications to prevent recurrence. The main agents used to close a sinus are liquefied phenol BP, iodi fortis, 95% silver nitrate or strong ferric chloride solution BPC. Of these, the most effective are phenol and liquor iodi fortis, with 95% silver nitrate used as a supplement.

Liquefied phenol BP should be applied for about four minutes, making sure it is confined to the sinus which is then washed out with alcohol and covered with a sterile dressing. Progress should be monitored at weekly intervals for three to four weeks, when healing should be complete.

HYPERHIDROSIS

In the management of hyperhidrosis, it is important to appraise all footwear worn by the patient and also the demands of his occupation. Instances exist where a patient's sensitivity to sweating has led to enclosing the feet in occlusive footwear when the reverse approach was indicated. Occupational factors are less easily controlled but a willing approach by the patient can often improve the condition.

Localised control of the most commonly affected areas consists of washing in tepid water and careful drying to avoid breaking the skin. The areas should be painted each day with 3% formalin. Once this has dried, an antiseptic powder such as Savlon dusting powder can be used to increase the surface drying area.

When the sweating and maceration have ceased, the application of formalin solution should be discontinued and replaced with spirit-based solutions with mild astringent agents, e.g. 3% salicylic acid in spirit, applied after washing. It may be necessary to continue with dusting powders, in which case antifungal agents are advisable. Interdigital fissures occurring with hyperhidrosis should be treated with astringent antiseptics.

A variety of commercial insoles are available, of which most tend to be absorbent and a few are impregnated with formalin, which vapourises when coming into contact with the warmth of the foot. Vapourising insoles are an effective local treatment which should be stopped on the cessation of the sweating and re-started on recurrence. Absorbent insoles only reduce the level of maceration of the epidermis. The patient should be advised to dispense with shoes and socks whenever possible, or to wear sandals, and to change hosiery frequently.

If the excessive sweating on the foot is not an isolated entity but is more general, help should be sought from a medical practitioner. It may be that the condition cannot be treated but underlying factors such as stress and diet may be controlled.

Bromidrosis can be dealt with in the same way, with the additional use of deodorants.

ANHIDROSIS

Many instances of this condition result from poor peripheral blood supply in the elderly. Where this is the cause, little more can be done than to apply emollients regularly, preferably daily after washing. The choice of emollient matters little since the purpose is to prevent moisture loss from the skin. Hydrous wool fat ointment BPC or proprietary preparations incorporating lanolin are suitable. If there is much thickening of the stratum corneum, this should be reduced to minimise the risk of fissuring.

The main complication of anhidrosis is the possibility of fissuring due to the reduction of epidermal elasticity and applied tensile stress. It can become a considerable problem, causing much pain and disability, as well as being a site for entry of infection. It is most commonly found on the borders of the heel.

Treatment consists of reducing the callus at the edges of the lesion with a scalpel or an abrasive bur and applying paraffin impregnated gauze and an occlusive covering for two to four days. Thereafter, the dressing should be removed and frequent and regular applications made of a suitable emollient. If the fissure is open and infected, antiseptic emollient dressings are indicated until the lesion heals, followed by the regular application of emollients.

FUNGAL INFECTIONS

Tinea pedis

Consideration of the epidemiological factors involved in dermatophyte infections is relevant when considering the treatment of tinea pedis. The incidence of fungal infections of the foot has been accelerated by rising affluence which allows feet to be kept warmer. The incidence rises in winter with the wearing of occlusive footwear. Greater control is possible if personal hygiene can be improved. This last point should always be considered when treatment is planned so that any regime can incorporate regular cleansing and careful drying of the feet. The type of footwear worn by the patient should also be considered and, if occlusive footwear cannot be entirely avoided because of the occupation, as with miners and servicemen, open sandals should be advised whenever possible to allow free circulation of air.

The use of communal washing facilities is a factor in the transmission of fungal infection. Advice should be given to minimise the amount of barefoot contact with all surfaces. The feet should be dried meticulously and the shared use of towels or clothing should be avoided since studies have shown that *Epidermophyton floccosum* can be transmitted thereby.

Tinea pedis is generally found in adults. The common causative organisms are *Trichophyton rubrum*, which is the most intransigent, *Trichophyton mentagraphytes* and *Epidermophyton floccosum*. Occasionally *Candida albicans* may be the causative organism but this may be accompanied by paronychia. *Microsporum canis* has also recently been identified as a causative organism, which is no doubt due to the increased numbers of cats and dogs kept as pets. Also incriminated is *Trichophyton tonsurans*. The only positive means by which the extent of a fungal infection can be established is by culture on dextrose agar, and this should be an integral part of assessment. Material for culture should be taken from the advancing edge of the condition, and if there are vesicles, the total roof of a number of them should be used for this purpose. It is necessary to avoid prior swabbing with the usual preoperative preparations, such as chlorhexidine gluconate. The area should be swabbed with alcohol instead.

If positive identification of hyphae does not result from microscopic examination or dextrose culture, it cannot be assumed that there is no fungal infection, but consideration should be given to the existence of other conditions such as erythrasma, pustular psoriasis or dyshidrotic eczema.

It is useful when considering the treatment of tinea pedis to recognise three forms, each of which requires a different approach.

Mild form

In its mildest form, it is frequently confused with erythrasma but if culture establishes the existence of fungal infection, the treatment should be followed assiduously. The medication should be of two types, the first of which is designed to remove the scaling material. Examples are Whitfield's ointment, phenyl mercuric acetate, phenyl mercuric nitrate, chlorophenesin, or compounds containing the undecenoates.

When the scaling skin has been removed, the use of these ointments should be stopped and general antifungal substances, in the form of a dusting powder, applied daily after careful washing. If the fissuring, which is sometimes found with this mild form, is deep, it is necessary to commence treatment with broad spectrum antiseptic agents until the fissures are healed. Then the scaling tissue can be removed. The application of antifungal dusting powders should continue for at least six months after the condition has apparently cleared, and they may be necessary indefinitely, particularly at times of high ambient temperature and where there may be constant exposure to re-infection, as in swimming baths and communal changing areas.

Moderately severe form

The condition may be more severe when the interdigital areas desquamate and the infection spreads on to the dorsal and plantar areas adjacent to the affected interspaces. At the periphery there may be vesicles and the whole area may be moist. It may be beneficial to initiate treatment with a lukewarm footbath containing potassium permanganate. After five minutes immersion, the foot should be thoroughly dried. Treatment with astringent antifungal agents such as paint of magenta produces good results. Salicylic acid 3% in spirit is also used but is better as a prophylactic measure.

Clotrimazole in spray form is a very effective antifungal agent and its action can be enhanced if used in conjunction with antifungal dusting powders. Socks should be changed daily and, if possible, have a high cotton content. Shoes should also be changed daily and disinfected with formaldehyde solution BP (formalin), care being taken to air the shoes before use to avoid irritation caused by the formalin. Disinfection of shoes is easily achieved by placing formalin in a wide shallow container such as a tin lid inside the shoe, covering the opening with paper and leaving for 24 hours. Provided the ambient temperature is about 15°C, the inside of the shoe will be exposed to a high concentration of formalin.

The moderately severe infection will usually respond well to treatment, leaving the skin with a completely clear appearance. Instances do occur when it may be necessary to use a desquamating preparation and, if so, it should be used as described for the mild form. The cream preparations of antifungal agents require strict attention to hygiene and must be accompanied by careful washing and drying of the feet. They are more difficult to apply in the digital interspaces than the liquid preparations but can be as effective if it is ensured that they are applied to all areas.

Severe form

The severe form of tinea pedis is rarely seen in the temperate zones of the world but it is common in tropical climates. The number of causative fungi increases outside the temperate climates and this should be remembered in attempts to identify by culture mechanisms.

The treatment does not differ greatly from that described. There are likely to be many more vesicles and the affected areas may reach towards the medial longitudinal arch. The vesicles should be drained and the exudate carefully removed. Thereafter, a fungicide which has antibacterial and anti-inflammatory properties, such as domiphen bromide and dibromo-propamide, is indicated. If there is marked bacterial infection also, it should be treated with antibacterial agents but not topical antibiotics as they may cause sensitisation. If the condition does not respond to treatment after a few days, the patient should be referred for specialist investigation and treatment.

Onychomycosis

The treatment of onychomycosis is seldom effective. This may be because of the difficulty in reaching the site of the infection and its low level of activity. The thickness of the nail should be reduced to ensure that the dorsal nail plate is breached. Topical agents should have a low surface tension to allow the agent to saturate the area. The required frequency of treatment coupled with slow rates of improvement often cause the treatment to be discontinued.

A commonly used medicament is paint of magenta BPC which requires renewal at weekly intervals. Borotannic acid complex may also be used and has a reputation for improving the condition.

The use of griseofulvin coupled with avulsion of the nail is also a possible cure. Griseofulvin, prescribed by a medical practitioner, should be taken for a month before avulsion and continued until the nail is fully developed. The side-effects of griseofulvin often cause the treatment to be stopped.

Consideration should be given to ablation of the nail plate with eradication of the matrix, thus ensuring no future growth of the nail. This may seem to be a radical move but the low success rate of other treatments often suggests that this course of action would be in the best interests of the patient. Some of the recently introduced topical antifungal agents, used in association with avulsion without phenolisation, seem promising, as do systemic doses of terbinafine (see Ch. 7).

Onychia and paronychia

These conditions may occur as a result of *Candida albicans* infection and are usually chronic in nature. They respond well to regular applications of the imidazoles.

Acute and chronic inflammatory conditions

Inflammatory states arising from trauma may require two methods of treatment complementing each other. The first aims to reduce and control inflammation and swelling, e.g. by the application of cold (cold compresses, ice packs) or by ultrasonic micro-massage (see Chs 10 & 14). The second method supports and rests the affected part by the use of paddings and strappings.

Some paddings can be utilised inside the patient's footwear as a transitional stage pending the supply of orthoses. Advances in orthotic therapy have reduced the need for techniques of padding and strapping, but the following have proved useful in providing relief of symptoms in certain painful conditions.

Tension strappings

'Figure-of-eight' strapping for foot and ankle (Fig. 11.5)

This strapping has various uses:

a. to support a sprained or weak ankle
b. to support a strained foot
c. to limit painful movement in the subtalar and midtarsal joints
d. to relieve tensile stress on the plantar fascia and its calcaneal attachment.

According to need, this strapping can be applied so as to invert the foot and to support the structures on the medial aspect of the foot and ankle; to evert the foot and to support the structures on the lateral side of the foot and ankle; and to hold the foot in a neutral position, neither inverted nor everted, but with movements in each direction restricted. Medial support is required, with or without valgus padding, in cases of sprain of the deltoid ligament, acute or chronic foot strain, and plantar fasciitis. Lateral support is required, with or without a tarsal platform ('filler pad') in cases of sprain of the external lateral ligaments of the ankle, and in some cases of pes cavus with associated postural instability. Neutral support is indicated in tarsal arthritis.

The material of choice is an elastic adhesive bandage of 5 cm, 6.25 cm or 7.5 cm width, depending on the size of foot. This is more readily tolerated by painful tissues than non-stretch strapping as it conforms more closely to the foot contours. The closest conformation is achieved by stretching one edge of the strapping more than the other as the need dictates. If it is necessary to protect the skin, as with hyperhidrosis or plaster allergy, the strapping may be applied over a soft cotton bandage. To prevent excessive stretch of the material in wear and consequent loss of support, two 3.75 cm or 5 cm wide straps of non-stretch strapping are used to reinforce and prolong the corrective effect of the dressing.

For medial support (Fig. 11.5)

(a) Anchor the first non-stretch strap antero-posteriorly to the lateral side of the foot, pass it around and behind the calcaneus and as low down on the heel as possible. Apply sufficient tension to invert the heel before securing the end of the strap along the medial and dorsal aspect of the first metatarsal, which must meanwhile be held in plantarflexion. This locks the calcaneus into inversion by supinating the subtalar joint (Fig. 11.5B).

(b) From immediately behind the base of the toes on the dorsum of the foot (to prevent swelling occurring here), apply the flexible strapping laterally and obliquely round the forefoot to complete one turn of the metatarsus, then continue round the tarsus

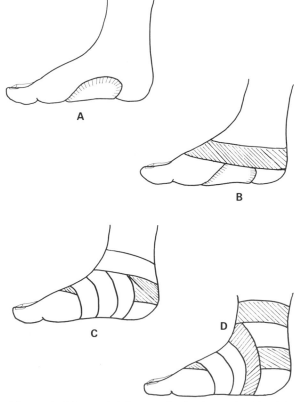

Fig. 11.5   Figure-of-eight strapping for foot and ankle with valgus pad: (A) Valgus pad in position; (B) First non-stretch tension strap to invert heel; (C) Figure-of-eight elastic strapping; (D) Second non-stretch reinforcing strap.

with upward tension on the medial border before encircling the ankle and heel as low down as before in order to maintain maximum inversion.

(c)   Continue across the front of the ankle and once more round the tarsus from lateral to medial before again encircling the ankle at a higher level. The second strap should overlap the first by half its width and should also well cover the malleoli so that it may be finally secured to the leg above the ankle (Fig. 11.5C).

(d)   Apply the final reinforcing strap of non-stretch strapping to form a 'figure-of-eight' around the tarsus and the malleoli, the lower loop proving a supporting cradle or 'stirrup' while the upper affords a firm attachment to the leg above the ankle (Fig. 11.5D).

The strapping should just avoid the anterior margin of the plantar fatty pad, leaving it free to change shape on weight-bearing, otherwise the edge of the strapping cutting across the fatty pad will cause discomfort. Alternatively, an additional 'figure-of-eight' strap may be applied so as to enclose the fatty pad completely.

Depending on the degree of support or correction required, valgus padding may be incorporated into this dressing, it being applied to the foot before the strapping is begun or inserted into the shoe. Firm supporting footwear must be worn at all times with this strapping, the unshod foot never being allowed to bear weight. This strapping will give support for up to ten days before requiring renewal.

For lateral support

The technique is similar to the foregoing but the strapping is applied in the reverse direction, the upward tension being exerted on the lateral side of the foot which is held in eversion. No preliminary reinforcing strap is necessary to evert the foot, but the final reinforcing strap should be applied as previously described but in the reverse direction. Additional lateral support can be provided if necessary by fitting a tarsal platform into the shoe.

For neutral support

The object of this strapping is to restrain painful movement in the tarsal joints. The most comfortable position of the foot should first be established by passive manipulation. No preliminary reinforcing strap is necessary. The flexible bandage is applied as for medial support but without the medial tension. The final reinforcing strap is applied with approximately equal tension on the medial and lateral borders of the foot before being secured to the leg above the ankle. Additional medio-lateral support can be provided, if required, by fitting a combined tarsal platform and valgus pad into the shoe—the 'tarsal cradle'.

Appliance techniques appropriate as follow-up to 'figure-of-eight' foot and ankle strappings may be any of the following: elastic anklets, corrective or palliative insoles incorporating valgus, tarsal platform or combined tarsal cradle support, buttressed heels and wedged heels. Unlike the strapping however, all such devices provide only passive support or correction.

Valgus padding

Valgus padding, so-called because it is used in cases of valgus foot, has two separate but related elements, a plantar cushion and a medial flange. The plantar cushion fills the concavity of the longitudinal arch with the object of affording support to the joints and the muscular and ligamentous attachments which become strained in abnormal pronation. It is essentially palliative in function.

The medial flange extends towards, and if necessary over, the prominences of the sustentaculum tali, the talar head and the tuberosity of the navicular. Its function is to endure some degree of inversion of the foot and thereby some correction of abnormal pronation. Where such correction is possible, it should be initiated primarily by means of medial heel wedging, but the medial flange is often necessary to supplement the correction.

It follows therefore that the design of valgus padding must be varied considerably to meet individual needs.

Applications

(a) As part of a 'figure-of-eight' strapping for footstrain, a thin felt pad having both elements is usually required (Fig. 11.5A).

(b) As a temporary palliative insole or shoe insert, the plantar element alone may be adequate to control symptoms.

(c) As a permanent feature of an accommodative insole for pes plano-valgus, both elements are usually required in combination with medial heel wedging. The shape, texture and density of the materials used must be varied to suit the needs of each case and will depend on whether the objective is correction or palliation.

(d) In metatarsalgia and in hallux rigidus, with the addition of metatarsal padding or a shaft pad respectively.

Valgus padding is contra-indicated in the presence of occlusive arterial disease as it may occlude the plantar arteries and excite symptoms in the foot akin to those of intermittent claudication. Nor should the plantar element be used alone and continuously as a form of so-called 'arch support'. The degree of compression of the plantar soft tissues entailed in the attempt to provide direct support to the skeletal arch in that way is likely to produce an unacceptable degree of wasting of the plantar soft tissues. Control of the calcaneal eversion by heel wedging and the medial flange is the preferred therapy in chronic abnormal pronation.

Tarsal platform ('filler pad') (Fig. 11.6)

The tarsal platform or 'filler pad' is never applied to the foot but is used only as a component of insoles or as an insert in footwear. Its main function is to bring the lateral border of a highly-arched foot into firm contact with the waist of the shoe. By raising the floor level to the foot, it enlarges the weight-bearing area and to that extent relieves the loading on the heel and the metatarsal heads. It also tends to evert the foot.

The basic design is that of a platform of firm material extending the full width of the insole from the anterior margin of the heel seat to just behind the tread (Fig. 11.6). It thus fills the

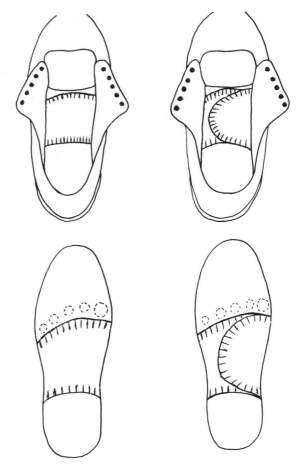

Fig. 11.6 Shoe padding: shapes and positions. Left: tarsal platform. Right: tarsal cradle, combining tarsal platform with valgus pad.

empty space between the lateral border of a highly-arched foot and the waist of the shoe. There is no contact between it and the plantar aspect of the medial longitudinal arch, the bulk of the padding on the medial side serving only to anchor it more firmly to the waist of the shoe. It is the limitation of contact to the lateral border only which tends to evert the foot, thus stabilising the ankle in cases of abnormal inversion. The medial portion of the padding also provides the base for additional valgus padding where this is needed to form a tarsal cradle.

When required, the anterior edge of the platform may be thickened to form a metatarsal bar, or may be extended under the three middle metatarsal heads to form a 'double-winged' metatarsal pad to protect the first and fifth

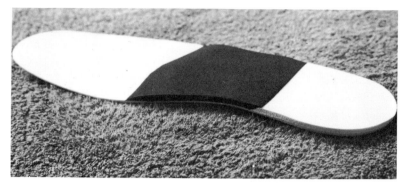

Fig. 11.7   Tarsal platform insole with heel cushion for painful heel (without cover).

metatarsal heads, or extended as shafts under the first and fifth to protect the middle three, or extended as a shaft under the first alone in hallux rigidus.

Applications

(a) In pes cavus, to redistribute weight from the heel and metatarsal heads.

(b) In persistent ankle sprain, to stabilise the foot by obviating forced inversion.

(c) In painful heel, in conjunction with a heel cushion. The combination is more effective than heel cushioning alone and is indicated in all such cases regardless of the height of the longitudinal arch (Fig. 11.7).

(d) In metatarsalgia and plantar lesions in conjunction with suitably shaped metatarsal padding.

(e) In tarsal arthritis in conjunction with valgus padding to form a tarsal cradle.

Tarsal cradle (Fig. 11.6)

This is a combination of a tarsal platform with a valgus support superimposed on it. This provides support for both medial and lateral borders of the foot and restrains the movement of inversion and eversion. Its main application is in tarsal arthritis when it may be used to augment the effect of a neutral 'figure-of-eight' strapping. Like the tarsal platform, it is not applied to the foot but is used as a component of an insole or as an insert in the footwear.

It also has an important application in restraining hypermobility and elongation of the foot in cases of abnormal pronation associated with calcanecuboid subluxation. The cuboid underlaps the front of the calcaneus by a process which extends from its medial, plantar and posterior aspect. Pressure on this process as the calcaneus everts causes some axial rotation of the cuboid and consequential hypermobility of the fourth and fifth metatarsal. In such cases, support to the lateral segment of the foot (calcaneus, cuboid, fourth and fifth metatarsals) is necessary in addition to that provided to the medial segment. The tarsal platform element under the cuboid stabilises the lateral segment much as the valgus element stabilises the medial segment, the entire foot thus being cradled and stabilised much more effectively than by valgus support alone.

Padding and strapping for hallux abductovalgus (Fig. 11.8.)

This is used as a temporary measure to lessen the deviation of the hallux and thereby to relieve strain in the periarticular tissue, and to protect the bony prominence. In moderate and still mobile cases, crescent-shaped pads posterior to the prominence are usually sufficient to relieve shoe pressure. With more severe and more fixed deformity, more all-round protection by oval cavity pads may be required. In each case, the padding must be shaped and bevelled on both interior and exterior surfaces to fit the bony contours very closely.

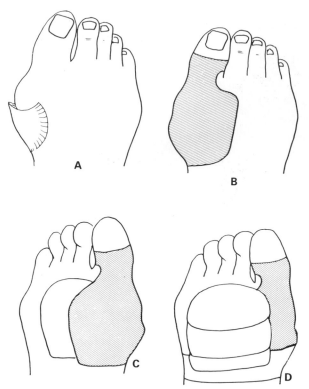

Fig. 11.8 Padding and strapping for hallux abductovalgus: (A) Crescent pad to protect prominence; (B and C) Stockinette butterfly strapping first adhered to hallux and then drawn back with sufficient tension to correct the line of the hallux to the extent required, before being stretched laterally to cover crescent and metatarsal pads; (D) Dressing completed with full metatarsal strapping.

The strapping of choice is adhesive stockinette which has one-way stretch only. This is cut into a flask or 'butterfly' shape and the anterior ends are first adhered to the hallux and secured there by a narrow strapping. The non-stretch dimension of this material must lie antero-posteriorly. The main part of the stockinette is then drawn back over the joint and padding with sufficient tension to correct the line of the hallux to the extent required. The 'wings' are then stretched laterally across the dorsal and plantar surfaces of the metatarsus and adhered, covering any necessary plantar padding also. The dressing is completed by a full metatarsal strapping together with covering straps for the plantar padding. An interdigital wedge for the first cleft may also be necessary for inclusion in the dressing, e.g. to relieve an interdigital corn.

A smaller version of this dressing is occasionally helpful in cases of digitus quintus varus with a painful 'tailor's bunion'.

Hallux valgus shields and metatarsal braces offer alternative means of long-term protection. Interdigital wedges for the first cleft, either singly or as part of an orthodigital splint, may also be indicated. If incorporated into an orthodigital splint embracing the middle three toes, this design eliminates any possibility of the lesser digits being abducted by the wedge since they are firmly fixed against the sole of the shoe by superimposed weight. For this reason, the interdigital wedge in this form also exerts better control on the hallux. Footwear modifications, such as stretching or the fitting of a balloon patch, may be necessary, failing surgical intervention.

Padding and strapping for hallux limitus/hallux rigidus

In acute and subacute cases, immobilization of the painful joint is required, together with relief of weight-bearing on the metatarsal head. A single-wing metatarsal pad is often the most readily tolerated dressing as it relieves the load on the painful joint, facilitates the inverted posture of the foot which is adopted in such cases, and thus helps to minimize dorsiflexion at the joint. The padding may be combined with a stockinette flask strapping as for hallux abductovalgus, except that the neck of the flask is cut extra wide so that it can extend on to both the dorsal and plantar aspects of the joint and help to splint it. The dressing is completed with a full metatarsal strapping.

In less acute cases, a shaft pad extending under the first metatarsal and proximal phalanx may be suitable, and this can be combined with any necessary plantar metatarsal padding. A similar form of strapping is used. The effect of all such dressings may be nullified, however, if a stiff-soled shoe is not worn.

In chronic cases the joint may be relatively painless but padding may be necessary to protect a dorsal exostosis or painful plantar lesions under the interphalangeal joint and the second metatarsal head. The former may require a modified oval cavity pad with a groove on its inner surface to accommodate the extensor tendon ('saddle pad'). The most effective type of appliance for chronic hallux rigidus is an accommodative insole of the pattern shown on page 82. This has applications both preoperatively and postoperatively as well as in cases where surgery is not indicated.

FURTHER READING

On hyperkeratosis

de Launey W E, Land W A 1984 Principles and practice of dermatology. Butterworth, Borough Green

Marks R, Christophers E 1981 The epidermis in disease, MTP Press, Lancaster

Thomson A D, Cotton R E 1983 Lecture notes on pathology, 3rd edn. Blackwell Scientific Publications, London

On fungal infection

Emmons C W, Binford C H, Utz J P, Kwong Chung K J 1977 Medical mycology, 3rd edn. Lea and Febiger, Philadelphia

Frey D, Oldfield R J, Bridger R C 1977 A colour atlas of pathogenic fungi. Wolfe Medical Publications, London

General

Benett R G 1988 Fundamentals of cutaneous surgery. Mosby, St Louis, chs 17, 22

Goodman-Gilman A, Goodman L S 1985 The pharmacological basis of therapeutics, 7th edn. Collier Macmillan, New York

Wade A (ed) 1977 Martindale's extra pharmacopeia, 27th edn. Pharmaceutical Press, London

12. Clinical pharmacology

Rae M. Morgan

INTRODUCTION

Pharmacology is the study of the effect of chemicals on the cells and tissues of the body. These chemicals may be endogenous substances, such as the neurotransmitter noradrenaline, or foreign molecules, such as drugs and poisons. In this chapter, some of the more commonly used groups of drugs which are administered to produce a therapeutic effect in the body will be considered. It is important to remember that not only does a drug molecule have an effect on the body, but the body also has an effect on the drug molecule. For example, a drug which is administered for its therapeutic effect may be metabolised by the body to inactive compounds which are then excreted. Thus, pharmacology may be divided into two major areas: *pharmacodynamics*, the study of the effect of the drug on the body; and *pharmacokinetics*, the study of the effects of the body on the drug. The drug may have effects other than the desired therapeutic effect, and so pharmacodynamics includes the study of the therapeutic effects of a drug, its side effects and its toxicity.

It is important for the podiatrist to be aware of the range of drugs commonly used in therapeutics, their effects and side effects, and the possible interactions between drugs (e.g. in the use of local anaesthetics) for two reasons. First, many patients of podiatrists, especially the elderly, receive drug therapy for a number of different conditions. This may well have a bearing on the management of the patient by the podiatrist. Secondly, the nature of the podiatrist-patient interaction is such that patients may well spend more time talking with their podiatrist than they do talking with their medical practitioner. Under such circumstances, patients may refer to problems which relate to their drug therapy. Therefore, the podiatrist is in a position not only to reassure patients about their problems, but also to identify potential areas of concern, which may then be brought to the attention of their general practitioner.

ACTION OF DRUGS

Drugs may bring about their therapeutic effects in one of three different ways:

1. interaction with receptors
2. interaction with enzymes
3. interaction with transport systems.

Interaction with receptors

Drugs which interact with receptors produce their effects by either augmenting, or inhibiting, the natural processes of nervous and hormonal control of the body. If a drug produces an effect similar to a naturally occurring compound which interacts with an endogenous receptor, it is called an *agonist*. An example of an agonist drug is salbutamol, which is an agonist at β_2 receptors in the airways of the lung. If a drug produces an effect whereby a naturally occurring agonist is prevented from acting at its receptor, it is called an *antagonist*. An example of an antagonist drug is propranolol, which prevents the action of noradrenaline on the heart, by blocking the β_1 receptors in cardiac muscle.

Interaction with enzymes

Drugs manifesting their therapeutic effect by an action on an enzyme usually act as antagonists, preventing the enzyme from performing its normal metabolic function. An example is enalapril, which blocks an enzyme called angiotensin converting enzyme (ACE), so preventing the production of vasopressin. The effect is a reduction of the blood pressure.

Interaction with transport systems

Many substances are transferred across biological membranes by transport systems which employ specific carriers to move the molecule from one side of the membrane to the other. Such a system may well be affected by drugs which resemble the natural substrate for the system. Drugs which interact with transport systems exert their effects by competing with a natural substrate for the transport system and inhibiting it. An example of this is the antidepressant imipramine which blocks the entry of noradrenaline into nerve endings.

ADMINISTRATION OF DRUGS

It should be clear at this point that the most important consideration concerning the effect of a drug in the body is its concentration available at the site of action (receptor, enzyme or transport system). If the concentration is too low, there will be little, or no, therapeutic effect; if the concentration is too high, an exaggerated therapeutic effect may result, or even an unacceptable toxic effect. It must also be remembered that, although pharmacologists attempt to target the drug at the required site of action, some drugs may well produce an effect at another site, thus producing a possible range of side effects. An example of this is seen with salbutamol, which is an agonist at β_2 receptors in the lung. Although, at normal therapeutic doses, the action of salbutamol is specific to the lung, it is possible for salbutamol to stimulate the β_1 receptors in the heart, causing tachycardia.

Critical factors

A number of factors are important in determining whether or not a drug reaches the desired site of action at a suitable concentration to produce the required therapeutic effect. These are:

- Dose and frequency of dose
- Route of administration
- Rate of absorption
- Protein binding and distribution
- Metabolism
- Excretion

Dose and frequency of dose

The dose of a drug and the frequency of its administration are of prime importance in determining whether a drug reaches the required concentration in the target tissue. If the dose is too small, or too infrequent, the drug will not reach the required concentration. Conversely, if the dose is too large, or administered too frequently, side effects or toxic effects may ensue. The actual therapeutic dose used will obviously depend upon the individual drug, as well as the other factors listed above, but the aim must always be to maintain the concentration of drug at the site of action as close as possible to the concentration required to produce the desired therapeutic effect.

Route of administration

There are a number of possible routes by which a drug may be administered. By far the most common, and the most convenient for the patient, is the oral route, as this allows the patient to administer their own medicine and continue their normal lives. However, the drug may produce problems of gastrointestinal upset, absorption may be slow and unpredictable or the level of drug metabolism may be too high for the drug to be given orally. Some drugs may be administered sublingually giving rapid absorption and little metabolism.

Administration of the drug by inhalation provides a means of delivering the drug directly into the lung. This is of special benefit if the lung is the site of action (as in the treatment of asthma), but also provides for rapid absorption into the blood from the lung mucosa.

Drugs which do not easily cross the wall of the gastrointestinal tract, or for which a rapid therapeutic effect is required, may be given by injection. Drugs administered directly into a vein (intravenous injection) produce an immediate effect; those administered into muscles (intramuscular injection) may produce either a rapid effect, or a slow prolonged effect, according to the type of formulation used. Other routes of injection are subcutaneous, just under the skin; and intrathecal, directly into the cerebrospinal fluid of the spinal cord.

Some drugs may also be administered by direct application to the skin. This is an obvious way of administering ointments and creams and it is now used for the administration of oestrogen in the treatment of post menopausal problems, and for the administration of glyceryl trinitrate in the long-term treatment of angina.

Rate of absorption

The rate at which a drug is absorbed into the body is also important in determining the concentration at its site of action. Lipophilic drugs are absorbed rapidly as they are able to cross cell membranes easily. Hydrophilic drugs are absorbed more slowly unless there is a specific carrier present to promote absorption. Absorption of drugs from the gastrointestinal tract is markedly affected by the presence, or absence, of foodstuffs in the gut at the time of the drug's administration. For this reason, patients may be instructed to take their medicine on an empty stomach, before meals or to avoid milk or iron preparations whilst taking the medicine.

Protein binding and distribution

The distribution of a drug after it has been absorbed into the bloodstream is also important in determining its action in the body. Many drugs are bound to plasma proteins (especially plasma albumin), and so are unavailable for therapeutic action. In some cases, more than 90% of a drug may be bound up in this way, leaving less than 10% of the administered dose available. It is only the drug which is available free in solution in the plasma which is important in determining the effective plasma concentration. The distribution of a drug between the various body compartments will depend primarily upon its physical properties. If the drug is highly ionised, or hydrophilic, it will not be able to cross the lipid membranes between the body water compartments, and so will tend to remain in the plasma and not reach its required site of action. Conversely, lipophilic (unionised) drugs can easily cross these membrane barriers and so will become distributed throughout the various body compartments.

A major barrier to the passage of drugs into the central nervous system is the blood-brain barrier. This barrier protects the brain and spinal cord, only allowing specific, lipophilic molecules access to the central nervous system. Thus, hydrophilic drugs do not gain access to the central nervous system, whereas lipophilic molecules pass this barrier easily, and can attain relatively high concentrations in the brain.

Metabolism

The metabolism of a drug plays an important role in determining not only whether a drug reaches the required concentration at its site of action, but also the length of time for which that concentration may be maintained. Most drugs are metabolised by the microsomal enzymes of the liver, and are converted to water-soluble metabolites which may be more easily excreted. However, the degree of metabolism varies from almost nothing to almost complete destruction of the drug as it passes through the liver. Drugs absorbed from the gastrointestinal tract pass directly to the liver via the hepatic portal vein. Therefore, if a drug is highly metabolised during this 'first pass' through the liver, very little of an administered dose may actually reach the systemic circulation at all. It should be borne in mind, however, that metabolic degradation of a drug does not always inactivate the drug, as some metabolites are as active, and possibly more active, than the parent compound.

Excretion

The excretion of drugs takes place mainly via the

kidney, although small amounts may be excreted in the faeces, sweat and exhaled air. Therefore the rate of excretion of a drug, or its metabolites, will depend upon the rate at which it can enter the nephron tubules of the kidney. Free drug in the plasma—i.e. that which is not bound to plasma protein—will enter the nephron by glomerular filtration, but some may be secreted into the proximal convoluted tubules by the acid or base secreting pathways. In some cases, these secretory pathways provide a too efficient excretion mechanism and result in only short durations of action.

For a comprehensive account of the subject of pharmacology, reference should be made to the text books listed at the end of this chapter. Included here is a selection of those groups of drugs which are commonly prescribed and whose effects need to be considered in relation to treatment of the feet, as well as monitoring and assessing the patient's health state.

GROUPS OF DRUGS

Drugs acting on the gastrointestinal system

Antacids

Antacids are a commonly used group of drugs, often bought over the counter, which can be of benefit for the symptomatic treatment of a number of gastric disorders, such as dyspepsia and reflux oesophagitis. They usually contain aluminum or magnesium salts, or sodium bicarbonate. They should not be taken at the same time as other medicines as they may impair absorption from the gastrointestinal tract. They should also be used with care, as some preparations, especially those containing magnesium salts, may well cause diarrhoea.

Antispasmodics

Antispasmodics are used to relieve the pain associated with spasm of the smooth muscle of the gastrointestinal tract in diseases such as irritable bowel syndrome and diverticular disease. Most drugs in this group are antimuscarinics which exert their action by blocking the action of acetylcholine at the muscarinic receptors on the smooth muscle of the gastrointestinal tract.

As a consequence, they show typically atropine-like side effects, such as dry mouth, blurred vision and possible difficulty with the passing of urine. Elderly patients are particularly at risk in developing side effects with this group of drugs, and in some patients glaucoma may be precipitated. Drugs used in this group are dicyclomine and mebevarine, as well as derivatives of atropine.

Ulcer-healing drugs

The most commonly used group of ulcer-healing drugs are the histamine-H_2 antagonists, cimetidine and ranitidine. These drugs act by inhibiting the secretion of hydrochloric acid by the parietal cells of the stomach, and thus allow the ulcer to heal. Both cimetidine and ranitidine are well tolerated, only rarely causing rashes, tiredness and mental confusion. However, cimetidine has been reported to produce gynaecomastia (breast development) in males. Other groups of drugs used for the treatment of ulcers in the gastrointestinal tract include pirenzipine, a selective antimuscarinic drug, and misoprostol, an analogue of prostaglandin E_1 which inhibits gastric acid secretion. Misoprostol has been reported to produce nausea and diarrhoea, as well as vaginal bleeding in females. Omeprazole, which inhibits the proton pump in the parietal cell, has been shown to be effective in the treatment of gastric ulcers resistant to other forms of therapy. However, headache, nausea and skin rashes have been reported following the use of this drug.

Laxatives

The use of laxatives is widespread, especially among the older population, often without medical advice or diagnosis of the need for their use. Bulk-forming laxatives, such as bran and methylcellulose, exert their effect by increasing the faecal mass and stimulating peristalsis in the lower gut. Stimulant laxatives, such as cascara preparations and bisacodyl, increase gastrointestinal motility, and hence cause evacuation of the bowel. However, they are prone to causing painful abdominal cramps, and their use can result in a period of apparent constipation, resulting in further unnecessary use. Faecal softeners, such as liquid paraffin, are not now recommended for use as laxatives. The prolonged use of liquid paraffin can result in anal seepage of the oil, lipoid pneumonia and interference with the absorption of fat soluble vitamins.

Osmotic laxatives act by retaining water in the bowel through an osmotic effect, and by changing the pattern of water distribution in the faeces. The most commonly used example is lactulose, a semi-synthetic disaccharide which retains water in the lower bowel and produces a mild laxative effect.

Antidiarrhoeal drugs

Antidiarrhoeal drugs act by either *adsorbing* water from the gastrointestinal tract, or by inhibiting gastrointestinal motility. Kaolin is a commonly used adsorbent antidiarrhoeal preparation which can be of some benefit in mild cases, but more severe cases require the use of antimotility drugs such as diphenoxylate or loperamide. Diphenoxylate is an analogue of morphine and loperamide acts by decreasing gastrointestinal motility, especially the propulsive movement. It has been reported to produce abdominal cramps and some skin rashes; excessive use may precipitate paralytic ileus.

Drugs acting on the cardiovascular system

Cardiac glycosides

Cardiac glycosides, such as digoxin, are used in the treatment of congestive heart failure and atrial fibrillation (see below). Digoxin increases the force of contraction of the failing heart and restores an adequate circulation of blood. Its action is primarily on the myocardium, restoring the pacemaker potential of the sino-atrial node and re-establishing sinus rhythm. Side effects of digoxin include nausea, vomiting and some visual disturbances. The therapeutic efficacy of digoxin is dependent upon the levels of potassium ions in the plasma and so care must be exercised in the use of digoxin in patients also receiving drugs which may cause hypokalaemia, such as the thiazides and loop diuretics.

Diuretics

Diuretics are drugs which bring about an increased urine output by a direct action on the kidneys. They are primarily used for the relief of oedema, but are often used in the treatment of mild to moderate hypertension, because of their ability to increase water loss from the body. There are three groups of commonly prescribed diuretics.

The most common group, *thiazide diuretics*, are essentially well tolerated and produce few side effects. The most common side effect, especially in the elderly, is hypokalaemia and occasional skin rashes. The hypokalaemia produced by the thiazides is of special significance if the patient is also being treated with digoxin, as a fall in plasma potassium levels may well precipitate digoxin-related side effects. Thiazides are often administered together with potassium chloride to offset the hypokalaemic effect.

The second group of diuretics are the so-called *loop diuretics*. These act by inhibiting the formation of the medullary osmotic pressure gradient in the kidney, by preventing the reabsorption of chloride ions from the ascending limb of the loop of Henle. Frusemide and bumetanide are the commonly used members of this group. The major side effect with these compounds is hypokalaemia, although gastrointestinal disturbances, tinnitis and deafness have been reported.

The third group of diuretics are the *potassium-sparing diuretics*, acting upon the sodium/potassium and sodium/hydrogen exchange mechanisms in the distal convoluted tubule. They may be used alone as mild diuretics, but are more commonly used in combination with a thiazide, or a loop diuretic, to offset the tendency of these drugs to produce hypokalaemia. The commonly used examples in this group are triamterene and amiloride which act to inhibit the sodium/hydrogen exchange mechanism. Both drugs have been reported to produce skin rashes and some mental confusion. The aldosterone antagonists, spironolactone and potassium canrenoate, inhibit the aldosterone-sensitive sodium/potassium exchange mechanism, but can cause nausea and vomiting. Spironolactone has been shown to be potentially carcinogenic in rodents. Consequently, its use in man is now restricted.

Anti-angina drugs

Angina pectoris may be treated either by the use of coronary vasodilators, or by reducing the oxygen demand of the cardiac muscle.

Coronary vasodilators include the nitrates, glyceryl trinitrate, isosorbide mononitrate and isosorbide dinitrate. Glyceryl trinitrate may be given sublingually or as an inhalation spray for the treatment of acute attacks of angina; the isosorbide compounds are more often used in the prophylaxis of the condition. All three compounds produce throbbing headache, flushing, dizziness and tachycardia as side effects.

The calcium channel antagonists, nifedipine, diltiazem and nicardipine are also used in the prophylactic treatment of angina pectoris as a result of their ability to dilate coronary arteries and increase the oxygen supply to the heart.

The use of beta blocker drugs in the prophylaxis of angina is dependent upon their ability to reduce the oxygen demand of the heart. Thus, the cardiac muscle is able to produce the required contractile effort, even though the oxygen supply is reduced.

Anti-arrhythmic drugs

Arrhythmias in the heart fall into one of a number of different categories, depending upon their site of origin and their frequency. In general, cardiac arrhythmias result in a decrease in the pumping efficiency of the heart, a fall in blood pressure and a decrease in the efficiency of blood circulation, and they may vary in severity.

Ectopic beats are occasional extra heart beats initiated usually within the atria. If they are infrequent, in an otherwise normal heart, they rarely require treatment. Atrial flutter and atrial fibrillation are more serious and result from multiple ectopic foci, producing atrial beating rates of 200–300 beats per minute. Ventricular arrhythmias, such as ventricular fibrillation, are extremely dangerous as they result in rapid cardiovascular collapse.

Anti-arrhythmic drugs may be classified into four groups, according to their mechanism of action:

Class I drugs are membrane stabilisers which increase the stability of the cardiac muscle membrane, thus decreasing the incidence of ectopic foci. Examples are quinidine, lignocaine, flecainide, disopyramide.

Class II drugs are those which inhibit the effect of the sympathetic nervous system on the heart, such as beta blockers.

Class III anti-arrhythmic drugs delay the repolarisation phase of the cardiac action potential, examples being amiodarone and oxyfedrine.

Class IV drugs, the calcium channel antagonists, inhibit the influx of calcium into the cardiac muscle cell, which is a prerequisite of muscle contraction.

All classes of anti-arrhythmic drugs cause a decrease in myocardial excitability, which is essential for their therapeutic action. However, the major side effect with these drugs is the extension of this myocardial depression into heart failure.

Beta blockers

Beta blocking drugs act upon the β_1 receptors in the heart and vascular circulation. They are of use in the treatment of mild hypertension, angina, myocardial infarction, cardiac arrhythmias and thyrotoxicosis. Unfortunately, although many beta blockers are relatively specific for the beta receptors in the heart, they may also exert an antagonistic effect on β_2 receptors in the smooth muscle of the airways in the lung, and thus precipitate bronchoconstriction. For this reason, their use in asthmatics is contraindicated.

Beta blockers are relatively well tolerated by most patients, however their mode of action on beta receptors in the sympathetic nervous system gives rise to a number of side effects, most of which are an extension of their therapeutic effects. Thus, they are prone to produce bradycardia (and possibly heart failure) in susceptible individuals, bronchospasm and peripheral vasoconstriction, leading to a feeling of coldness in the fingers and toes. Some beta blockers penetrate the blood brain barrier and enter the central nervous system. In these cases, side effects can include sleep disturbances, fatigue and hallucinations. Two beta blockers, practolol and metipranolol, have been withdrawn as a result of serious side effects in the eye. Whilst similar effects have not been reported with other beta blockers, it is prudent to assess any reports of eye problems from patients receiving long term therapy with beta blockers.

There are a large number of beta blockers available, the most common being propranolol, atenolol, oxprenolol and metoprolol.

Antihypertensives

Antihypertensive drugs are used to lower the elevated blood pressure of hypertension. Hypertension is a common disease state. Unfortunately, in the majority of hypertensives there is no clinical pointer as to the cause of the elevated blood pressure (*primary essential hypertension*), although hypertension may also result from identifiable causes such as renal dysfunction, drug therapy and pregnancy. Consequently, in the majority of cases, the treatment of hypertension is often symptomatic, bringing about a fall in blood pressure without treating the underlying cause of the problem. Only in the case of an identifiable cause for the hypertension can treatment attempt to cure the disease.

Hypertension may be treated in a number of ways:

- Inhibition of the sympathetic drive to the heart
- Reduction in the force of cardiac contraction
- Dilatation of the blood vessels
- Inhibition of the renin-angiotensin system.

Inhibition of the sympathetic drive to the heart. Drugs which inhibit the sympathetic drive to the heart may do so by either reducing the activity of the cardioaccelerator centre in the brain, preventing the activity of the neurohumoral transmitter in the sympathetic ganglia, or by reducing the activity of the neurohumoral transmitter at the junction between the sympathetic nerve and the heart tissue, i.e. the neuroeffector junction.

The most common drugs for the initial treatment of mild to moderate hypertension are the beta blocking drugs, such as atenolol and propranolol. These act by inhibiting the action of noradrenaline on the heart and so bring about a reduction in heart rate (bradycardia) and a fall in blood pressure. The side effects of beta blockers have already been discussed.

Another drug, methyldopa, reduces the sympathetic drive to the heart by substituting for dihydroxyphenylalanine (Dopa) in the synthesis of noradrenaline in nerve terminals, resulting in the synthesis of the 'false transmitter', methylnoradrenaline, which is less active than noradrenaline. This action of methyldopa occurs predominantly in the central nervous system, to inhibit the cardioaccelerator centre, rather than at the neuroeffector junction in the heart. Consequently, methyldopa shows some centrally mediated side effects, such as sedation and depression, as well as failure of ejaculation, skin rashes and fluid retention.

Clonidine produces an antihypertensive effect by an action on alpha adrenoceptors in the medulla oblongata, leading to a decrease in sympathetic drive to the heart as well as resetting arterial baroreceptors to increase vagal tone to the heart.

Ganglion blocking agents, such as trimetaphan, inhibit sympathetic nerve activity by preventing the action of acetylcholine at the sympathetic ganglia and so reducing the sympathetic drive to the heart. However, ganglion blocking drugs are not necessarily specific for sympathetic ganglia and also inhibit neurohumoral transmission at parasympathetic ganglia. Consequently, side effects include tachycardia, dry mouth and visual disturbances.

Adrenergic neurone blocking drugs, such as guanethidine and bethanidine, act by reducing the release of noradrenaline from the postganglionic sympathetic nerve endings. However, because they effectively reduce the amounts of noradrenaline present in the nerve endings, they are likely to produce postural hypotension, resulting in fainting on standing and mild exertion.

Reduction in the force of cardiac contraction. A reduction in the force of the heart beat may be brought about by inhibiting the influx of calcium ions, which is an essential prerequisite for the initiation of contraction in cardiac muscle.

Drugs in this group are called calcium channel antagonists, and they reduce myocardial contractility and alter the conduction of the cardiac action potential across the heart.

Dilatation of the blood vessels. Vasodilator drugs produce their therapeutic effect by causing a widening of the diameter of the blood vessels through which the blood is passing, and so reducing the pressure in the arteries. This group of antihypertensives includes hydralazine and minoxidil. The fall in blood pressure produced by these drugs, however, often causes a reflex tachycardia.

Inhibition of the renin-angiotensin system. Inhibition of the renin-angiotensin system prevents the formation of vasopressin, which is a powerful vasoconstrictor peptide. Vasopressin is produced from an inactive precursor, angiotensinogen, by the action of the enzymes renin and angiotensin converting enzyme (ACE). ACE inhibitors, such as captopril, enalapril and lisinopril, cause a marked fall in blood pressure by this mechanism. All three drugs cause a rapid fall in blood pressure and so treatment requires initial small doses, followed by a gradual increase in dosage until the desired effect is achieved. Side effects include a persistent dry cough, fatigue, weakness, nausea and diarrhoea.

Anticoagulants

Anticoagulants are used to reduce the incidence of unwanted blood clotting in conditions such as deep vein thrombosis. Heparin is a naturally occurring substance, found in basophils, which acts by inhibiting the blood clotting cascade at a number of sites. It may be administered by subcutaneous or intramuscular injection, especially in the management of postoperative thrombosis.

The oral anticoagulants antagonise the effects of vitamin K, and thus produce an inhibition of the blood clotting cascade. The most commonly used oral anticoagulant is warfarin, although phenindione may also be used. Great care must be exercised in the use of warfarin, as it is very strongly bound to plasma proteins. Consequently, the introduction of other drugs into a patient who is stabilised on a particular warfarin dose, may result in more warfarin being made available free

in the plasma, due to its displacement from protein binding sites. In this situation, the patient may experience internal haemorrhage.

Drugs acting on the respiratory system

Bronchodilators

The diameter of the airways in the lungs is controlled by β_2 receptors, and so the most effective method of increasing the diameter of airways is by the use of selective β_2 agonists, such as salbutamol, terbutaline, rimiterol and fenoterol. However, it must be remembered that these agonists may also cause some stimulation of β receptors in other parts of the body, especially the heart and skeletal muscle, so tremor and tachycardia may result from their use. Antimuscarinic drugs also increase the diameter of airway passages by inhibiting the action of the parasympathetic supply to the lung, so drugs such as ipratropium may also be used, although these will produce the atropine-like side effects of dry mouth and blurred vision.

Corticosteroids

Corticosteroids have been used in the treatment of asthma for many years, and nowadays there are a number of aerosol preparations of these drugs. Their mechanism of action is not clearly understood, but they probably reduce the hypersensitivity reactions associated with asthma and hence reduce mucus secretion in the airways. Beclomethasone is the most commonly used drug in this group.

Drugs acting on the central nervous system

Hypnotics and anxiolytics

Hypnotics and anxiolytics are used to sedate the patient. This may be to induce sleep, in the treatment of insomnia, or to provide relief from a variety of anxiety states. The prescribing of these drugs is widespread, and may well lead to problems of either physical or psychological dependence. The most commonly used group of hypnotics and anxiolytics is the benzodiazepines. Nitrazepam, temazepam, triazolam and lormetazepam are used as hypnotics, and diazepam, lorazepam and oxazepam are used as anxiolytics. The major side effects of these drugs are drowsiness and ataxia (particularly in the elderly). Other non-benzodiazepine drugs used for the treatment of anxiety include busiprone and chlormezanone. All hypnotics and anxiolytics have their actions potentiated by alcohol.

Antipsychotic drugs

Antipsychotic drugs (neuroleptics) are used for tranquillising patients without impairing their state of consciousness in severe anxiety states, schizophrenia and psychoses. They also may exert an antidepressant action. These drugs are likely to cause hypotension and a loss of temperature control in the elderly, and so should be used with care in patients over 70 years of age.

Antidepressants

Antidepressant drugs may be divided into the tricyclic (and related) antidepressants and the monoamine oxidase inhibitors. The tricyclic antidepressants are the drugs of choice in the treatment of the majority of depressive states because they do not show the potentially dangerous interactions seen with the monoamine oxidase inhibitors.

Tricyclic antidepressants, such as amitryptyline and clomipramine, are most useful in the treatment of endogenous depression associated with psychomotor disturbances. All tricyclic antidepressants produce a range of side effects: dry mouth, blurred vision and difficulty with micturition as a result of their antimuscarinic action; and tachycardia, cardiac arrhythmias, postural hypotension, sweating and tremor as a result of their central effects.

Monoamine oxidase inhibitors, such as phenelzine, may be used in the treatment of depressive illness which will not respond to the tricyclic group of antidepressants. They are of particular benefit in phobic states and hysteria. However, care must be exercised in their use because of the interaction with some foods. Monoamine oxidase inhibitors prevent the destruction of catecholamines in the body, and so produce a rise in the levels of noradrenaline in the body. Some foods, especially cheese, broad beans and meat extracts, contain tyramine which is a precursor for noradrenaline, and so patients eating these foods whilst undergoing treatment with a monoamine oxidase inhibitor will experience serious increases in blood pressure, possibly leading to haemorrhage. The administration of local anaesthetics is also contraindicated.

Analgesics

Analgesics are drugs used for the control of pain. They may be classified into two groups: non-opioid analgesics, used for the control of pain associated with skeletomuscular disorders, and opioid analgesics, used in the control of pain associated with the viscera.

Non opioid analgesics include aspirin, paracetamol and ibuprofen, all of which may be purchased over the counter in pharmacies, as well as being prescribed by medical practitioners. In many cases, non-opioid analgesics are prescribed in compound preparations, often with codeine or dextropropoxyphene. The availability of non-opioid analgesics, especially paracetamol, over the counter and by prescription can lead to serious problems of overdosage if patients take paracetamol containing analgesics from both sources. It is of paramount importance to ensure that patients receiving paracetamol based analgesics do *not* also take other paracetamol containing preparations, as this may lead to serious liver damage and death.

Opioid analgesics, such as morphine and diamorphine, are used in the control of severe pain of visceral origin. Most opioid analgesics cause marked respiratory depression and drowsiness, as well as nausea and vomiting in the initial stages of their administration. They may also markedly alter the response to other centrally acting drugs, such as anti-depressants.

Drugs acting on the endocrine system

Antidiabetic drugs

Two groups of drugs are used for the treatment of diabetes, dependent upon the type of diabetes from which the patient is suffering. In patients where there is no insulin-secreting capacity in the cells of the islets of Langerhans, insulin must be given, usually by intramuscular injection. There are a number of different types of insulin preparation available, varying in the rapidity of onset and duration of action.

In patients where there is still some insulin-secreting capacity, oral hypoglycaemic drugs may be used. There are two groups of oral hypoglycaemic drugs currently in use: the sulphonylureas, such as chlorpropamide and gliclazide, act by increasing insulin secretion from the islets of Langerhans and so return the insulin levels in plasma towards normal. The second group are called biguanides (metformin), and these act by decreasing gluconeogenesis and increasing peripheral glucose uptake into cells. These two groups of antidiabetic drugs are of value in non-insulin dependent patients who do not respond to dietary measures. The sulphonylureas tend to cause gastrointestinal upset, headache and some sensitivity reactions, and the biguanides cause nausea, vomiting and decreased absorption of vitamin B_{12}.

Thyroid drugs

Thyroxine is used in a number of clinical situations in which there is a deficiency in thyroid function, such as hypothyroidism. Consequently, it is used in long-term treatment regimes, and a number of side effects have been reported. These include arrhythmias, anginal pain, tachycardia, headache and skeletal muscle cramps.

Drugs acting on infections

Antibacterials

Antibacterial drugs, commonly called antibiotics, are widely used to treat a range of bacterial infections. They fall broadly into three groups: penicillins, cephalosporins and tetracyclines, plus erythromycin and trimethoprim. The actual drug used in any given situation is dependent upon the type and sensitivity of the infecting organism.

The penicillins are bactericidal and act by inhibiting the synthesis of bacterial cell walls, thus preventing replication of the invading organism. They have a broad spectrum of activity and there is a wide range of penicillin derivatives available, including phenoxymethylpenicillin, amoxycillin, flucloxacillin and ampicillin. All penicillin derivatives cause nausea and diarrhoea, and are liable to produce hypersensitivity reactions ranging from mild rashes to anaphylactic shock.

Cepahalosporins, such as cephalexin and cefuroxime, are broad spectrum antibiotics having a mechanism of action similar to that of the penicillins. Their side effects are similar to those of the penicillins and patients who show hypersensitivity reactions to penicillins often show similar responses to cephalosporins.

Tetracyclines are broad spectrum antibiotics, although their use has declined in recent years due to the development of bacterial resistance. However, they are of use in the treatment of some sensitive organisms, such as *Haemophilus influenzae* in chronic bronchitis. Tetracyclines are also used in the treatment of acne and periodontal disease. Tetracyclines are deposited in growing bone and should not be given to children under the age of 12 years or to pregnant women.

Erythromycin has a similar spectrum of antibacterial activity to that of penicillin, but does not cause hypersensitivity reactions. It may, therefore, be used as an alternative in cases of hypersensitivity to the penicillins.

Trimethoprim, used alone or in combination with sulphamethoxazole, is used in the treatment of urinary tract infections and respiratory tract infections which do not respond to antibiotics from other groups.

Antifungals

Antifungal drugs are used in the treatment of a wide range of infections such as intestinal candidiasis, dermatophyte infections of the skin and thrush. Miconazole is most commonly used for skin infections and thrush, and griseofulvin is used in the treatment of dermatophyte infections of the scalp and nails. Most antifungal drugs, when given systemically, cause nausea, vomiting, diarrhoea and occasional skin rashes.

Antivirals

The most commonly used antiviral drug for systemic infections is acyclovir. This is effective against *Herpes simplex* and *Herpes zoster* infections. Side effects include skin rashes, gastrointestinal disturbances, headache and fatigue, together with a rise in bilirubin and liver-related enzymes indicating possible hepatic damage in prolonged use.

Both acyclovir and idoxuridine are used topically in the treatment of viral infections such as cold sores and shingles.

Drugs used in rheumatic diseases and gout

Non-steroidal anti-inflammatory agents

Non-steroidal anti-inflammatory drugs are used frequently in the treatment of diseases such as rheumatoid arthritis, which produce inflammation and pain in the joints. They act by inhibition of the enzyme prostaglandin synthetase, which is responsible for the production of prostaglandins. Inhibition of prostaglandin production in a joint damaged by arthritis reduces the inflammation and so helps to reduce the pain associated with these diseases. Non-steroidal anti-inflammatory agents, such as aspirin and ibuprofen, are available over the counter in pharmacies, and many more are available on prescription. They commonly produce gastrointestinal upset as a side effect, and must only be used with great care in patients with a history of gastric ulcers, as their use can lead to severe gastric bleeding. Non-steroidal anti-inflammatory agents must also be used with care in asthmatic patients, as some people are particularly sensitive to these agents (especially aspirin) and may suffer an asthmatic attack.

Anti-gout drugs

Acute bouts of gout are often treated with high doses of a non-steroidal anti-inflammatory drug, such as azapropazone. However, for long term control of gout it is more common to use drugs which decrease the amount of uric acid in the plasma. Allopurinol decreases uric acid formation but can produce skin rashes, headache and gastrointestinal disorders. Probenecid and sulphinpyrazone increase uric acid excretion by the kidney, but may also produce gastrointestinal disturbances, dizziness and skin rashes.

SUMMARY

Therapeutically administered drugs exert their effects by actions on receptors, enzymes or transport systems and the most important criterion to be considered in determining the effect of a drug is its concentration at the site of action. However, no drug is absolutely specific in its effects in the body and all are capable of giving rise to side effects and toxic effects, ranging in severity from mild to life threatening. Whilst it has not been possible to cover every eventuality of side effect and interaction in the confines of this chapter, it cannot be overemphasised that it is important to listen to patients receiving drug therapy, in order to ascertain whether or not they are experiencing adverse effects from their treatment. In most cases, such information will lead to re-assurance of the patient that the problem is associated with their drug treatment and is recognised as a side effect; occasionally, information from the patient may lead to the identification of hitherto unrecorded side effects of drugs.

FURTHER READING

Foster R 1991 Basic pharmacology, 3rd edn. Butterworth Heinemann, London
Goodman L S, Gilman R 1985 The pharmacological basis of therapeutics, 8th edn. Macmillan, London
Jacob L S 1987 Pharmacology, 2nd edn. Wiley Medical, Chichester

Rang H P, Dale M M 1991 Pharmacology, 2nd edn. Edward Arnold, London
Wingard L B, Brody T M, Larner J, Schwartz A 1991 Human pharmacology: molecular to clinical. Wolfe Publications, London

13. Functional orthoses

James A. Black

It is widely recognised that most foot problems have some mechanical factors involved in their aetiology. Whether arising from some congenital variation in the structure of the foot and leg or acquired as a result of a disease process such as rheumatoid arthritis or one of the neuropathies, the basic philosophy of treatment remains the same. Mechanical foot defects can be controlled only by mechanical means.

This may be achieved by altering the structure by surgical intervention or by actively controlling the biomechanics of the foot and leg with an orthosis. It may be that, with increasing inter-professional awareness and cooperation in the management of patients, combined surgical and orthotic management provides the best treatment plan in many cases. The surgeon may decide that surgery is necessary in order to create an environment where orthotic therapy has a better chance of success in the long term. Similarly, an orthosis may be fitted postoperatively to control or rest the foot, thereby enhancing the healing process.

An appliance which controls or corrects structural abnormality is termed an 'orthosis', (Grk. *orthos*, straight). This term may be applied to all forms of appliances which have a corrective function. Appliances which primarily accommodate and protect deformities without correcting them, e.g. a hallux abductovalgus shield, are termed 'accommodative'. Many appliances combine both corrective and protective functions depending on the nature of the foot fault, its severity and duration. Appliances which replace missing parts whether as a result of trauma, disease or surgery are termed 'prostheses'.

Where correction is possible, even if only partially, the corrective element should always take precedence over the protective element and this consideration determines the choice of materials. Considerable force is often required to correct even a simple deformity, such as a hammer toe, or to prevent major deformation, such as abnormal pronation, from occurring under load. The more rigid the material, the better its splinting qualities but the lower its tolerance to wear by the patient. It is often necessary in these cases for the patient to become accustomed to the orthosis by gradually increasing the length of time it is worn.

Plastics used in functional orthoses can be simply classified by their ability to resist stress according to their thermo-forming temperature. The higher the temperature at which they become malleable, the stronger they are; the lower the temperature, the more likely they are to deform under load. However the thickness of the plastic is also of considerable importance and there is a direct correlation between rigidity and thickness.

Orthoses need to be designed so that they are both tolerable in wear and optimally effective in their therapeutic design. Accommodative appliances, e.g. latex shields, are utilized in established deformities to protect vulnerable tissues from trauma and to some extent to limit painful movement. They may not correct the underlying fault, but they make it tolerable by relieving painful symptoms and controlling secondary lesions. They are more flexible than rigid orthoses and usually can be well tolerated from the beginning. An accommodative device may be desirable for a time before the patient moves to a more corrective one.

Orthoses are worn either on the foot or within the footwear, and however well-designed and accurately fitted they may be, their beneficial effects will be largely nullified if the footwear is unsuitable. Orthoses and footwear must therefore be considered together when treatment is planned. The footwear must be of the correct size and shape, have adequate internal volume in the right places, and be correctly balanced both medio-laterally and antero-posteriorly. Modifications to footwear may be necessary to ensure these points and those most often required are listed later. It is a sound principle that patients purchase their shoes after the orthosis is fitted. Heel height is of critical importance when fitting a functional orthosis. If the heel height is such that the normal relationship between the forefoot and the rearfoot is disturbed, then the shoe is totally unsuited to wear with the orthosis.

Orthotic technology is constantly developing as new materials and techniques are introduced and a greater understanding of foot mechanics evolves. Only a brief summary of its main aspects is possible here and further reference is recommended to specialist literature on the subject.

MANAGEMENT

It is essential that practitioners develop a sound working knowledge of the materials and techniques available in order to offer their patients a complete service, even if this is to be provided by an orthotics laboratory. At the outset of treatment, a management plan should be explained to the patient, outlining the progress envisaged and explaining its rationale. Patients have a right to know what the practitioner has in mind for their treatment and they should have a clear indication of how long it might take, the extent of improvement in the condition and, in the private sector, how much it might cost.

If this is accepted as a reasonable principle of patient management, then it is incumbent on the practitioner to be able to offer the best possible treatment available. If the practitioner is unable to provide this, then the patient should be referred to a clinician with the necessary equipment and skills. Not every patient needs an orthosis, but where this is an integral part of the treatment, patient management and patient awareness of the treatment plan and any possible sequelae must

have a higher profile. This is particularly valid with the increasing use of functional orthoses aligned to biomechanical assessment, and the possible medico-legal implications which may arise if the treatment proves to be inappropriate and causes pathology elsewhere in the leg or trunk. If possible complications have not been explained to the patient, then the podiatrist is in a vulnerable position should the patient pursue a claim for negligence.

Before embarking on the treatment plan certain considerations are important. The physical characteristics of the patient must be assessed, i.e. height, weight and mobility; also the presence of any physical disability which might preclude the use of certain types of orthoses, e.g. the patient might be blind, rendering the positioning of a replaceable device difficult. In such circumstances, a 'locator' might be necessary to enable the patient to position the orthosis by touch. Should patients have any physical disabilities which prevent them from reaching their feet, orthoses which require careful positioning by them would also be unsuitable.

With such factors taken into account, the type of orthosis and the materials to be used in its manufacture can be considered. Important points are:

a. What effect will the material have on the patient's foot? Since the orthosis is going to be in contact with the foot for a long time, will the material be irritant, or likely to cause an allergic reaction? Is it likely to damage the foot? Is the material stable or will it, once placed in the shoe, deteriorate due to the increase in temperature and humidity and release products which may be irritant or even toxic? These factors are particularly relevant to patients with diminished sensation.

b. What effect will footwear have on the device? The quality or suitability of the patient's footwear may be a major factor in the effectiveness of the orthosis. Unsuitable footwear is probably the most frequent reason for not embarking on some form of appliance therapy and the practitioner frequently has to persuade the patient to invest in new footwear. This is most often experienced when treating adolescent or fashion-conscious women. Often the best compromise is for the patient to wear the orthosis at school or at work and to revert to fashion footwear only at other times. Such an arrangement is not totally satisfactory, as the effectiveness of the treatment may be diminished. This should be explained so that the patient understands clearly where the responsibility lies if the orthosis is not as successful as it might have been.

Replaceable pads

The simplest extensions of padding and strapping to more permanent orthoses are replaceable pads. These devices take many forms and are usually held in place with elasticated bands positioned around the toes or the foot (Fig. 13.1). Before embarking on use of a replaceable pad, the practitioner will usually try the design with clinical padding and assess its potential effectiveness. The role of clinical padding in this form is often undervalued and substantial biomechanical control can be achieved with the skilful use of clinical padding materials either attached to the foot or positioned in the shoe. Manufacture is straightforward and devices may be made in a variety of materials, depending upon the physical properties required. A device may be required simply to replace fatty padding atrophied by age. Such devices are protective in nature and a material is selected for its ability to resist compression over a long period. Newer visco-elastic forms are much more effective in resisting compressive stress than materials derived form rubber. Table 13.1 lists some materials and illustrates their compressibility and percentage relaxation under compressive stress.

All of the above samples were 7 mm thick.

Tests were carried out for 3 hours on an Instron, a device used to quantify the elasticity of materials. The percentage strain indicates the degree of deformation of the material under stress.

Forces entering the foot can be dissipated in one of two ways: (a) by absorbing the force in such a way that the material decelerates the rate at which forces enter the foot, i.e. shock absorption; (b) by increasing the surface area through which weight is taken. It must be remembered that the orthosis should be placed in a position such that during 'foot flat' and 'heel off', the maximum area is in contact with the ground during the gait cycle.

Technological advance in materials has produced a new range of visco-elastic products which provide effective cushioning or dampen

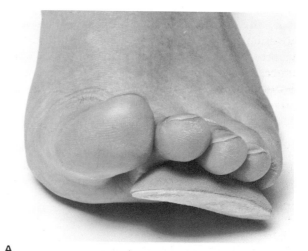

A

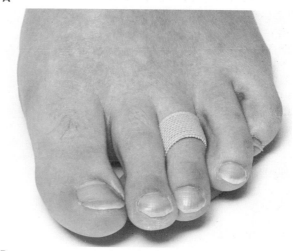

B

Fig. 13.1   (A and B) Replaceable long prop.

Table 13.1   Percentage strain of a variety of padding materials used in orthotics and prosthetics

Sample	Load (Kg)	% Strain	Load (Kg)	% Strain
PPT	20	87.10	40	98.39
Poron	20	75.61	40	87.80
Grey latex foam	20	61.29	40	80.65
NCCR	20	80.39	40	98.04
Clocell	20	70.00	40	78.33
Hindell	20	75.86	40	84.48

ground reaction force. These materials, such as Sorbothane and Viscolas, allow the podiatrist to provide the patient with high quality shock absorption without recourse to cutting, shaping and covering replaceable orthoses. The practitioner should be aware that viscoelastic materials are much heavier than traditional cushioning materials; this could be critical if supplying orthoses to sports persons or rheumatoid arthritics. Sheets of silicone rubber are now also available in varying thicknesses and have proved most effective in the treatment of plantar keratomas or lesions over pressure areas on the toes.

Replaceable digital orthoses may also be manufactured by the same processes as used for plantar devices. However, practitioners may find that the effectiveness of digital orthoses is governed by their ability to remain in place, and secure anchorage is essential. Figure 13.1 illustrates a long prop and it is important that an assessment of the amount of movement in the interphalangeal and metatarsophalangeal joints has been made before embarking on the manufacture of this type of orthosis. Digital devices may conform to virtually any shape provided the

principle has first been assessed with conventional padding.

Figure 13.2 illustrates a variety of replaceable pads.

Elastic anklets and braces

An elastic anklet is useful as an alternative to figure-of-eight strapping when continuing support is required. Commercial varieties are readily available and are usually satisfactory. They may be used with a tarsal platform or a tarsal cradle fitted either into the shoe or on to an insole. A buttressed heel may also be indicated for greater ankle stability.

A metatarsal brace is an elastic bandage encircling the metatarsus, and it usually includes a plantar metatarsal pad. Commercial varieties are usually unsatisfactory because the stereotyped pads attached to them are seldom if ever the right shape, size or density for a particular patient. The brace can be easily fabricated from elastic webbing or elastic net. Both materials are available in different widths, and it is advantageous to be able to design both brace and padding according to individual needs. The metatarsal

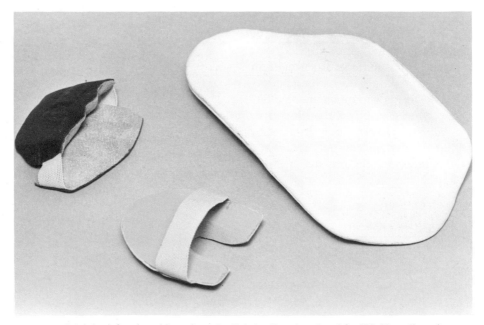

Fig. 13.2 Selection of replaceable pads: orthodigital splint; dorsal pad for IPJ; Hexcelite valgus support covered in latex foam.

brace may often be combined with a toe-loop or with orthodigital splints where correction and/or protection of the digits is also desired (Fig. 13.3).

There is now a plethora of elasticated supports specifically designed for use in sport. As people are intent on improving their fitness and using sports as a means to better health, sportswear manufacturers have met the demand by producing supports for all the joints which may be stressed during sporting activity. These are usually available from pharmacists or sports shops.

Insoles

Virtually any pathological condition affecting the plantar surfaces can be controlled by appropriate insoles provided that sufficient depth is made available in the footwear. It is essential that this requirement be specified whenever specially-made footwear is ordered. With normal footwear, every effort must be made to save bulk by the choice of material, and by stopping the insole just behind or just in front of the metatarsal heads, depending on the design required (unless the footwear will accommodate a full-length insole). There are basically two types:

a. a simple or non-casted insole which has as its principle the use of the prescribed padding.
b. casted insoles made to a cast or model of the foot.

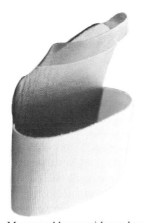

Fig. 13.3 Metatarsal brace with toe-loop.

Non-casted insoles

Non-casted insoles are manufactured in such a way that they form part of the shoe. The first prerequisite is the production of a template to the shape and size of the insole of the shoe. From the template, the base material of the insole is then shaped accordingly and placed in the shoe.

The pressure points on the foot may be coloured and the patient allowed to walk for a few minutes until the colour is transferred to the base material. This provides a static impression. Experience will show that if this method is used, the placement of the padding should be moved slightly anteriorly to allow for the elongation of the foot which occurs during locomotion. This adjustment varies from patient to patient, depending upon the elasticity of the foot. For this reason, this method of manufacture is not entirely accurate.

To eliminate error, dynamic impression marks are more valuable. To obtain these, the patient walks for anything up to two weeks with the template in the shoe before returning it. Other methods may be used, such as waxing the template. The template is rubbed over with dental wax until a light layer of wax is left on the surface. This gives an accurate impression when walked upon for a few minutes. Whichever method is used, the most important feature is to ensure that the base material fits exactly. Any movement of the insole within the shoe would render it less effective. From the wearmarks provided on the template, appropriate padding is shaped and bevelled to suitable thickness. This is then adhered to the base material, covered with a fine leather or synthetic covering such as Pampa, and, once trimmed, fitted into the shoe. Figure 13.4 shows the manufacture of a simple insole, without its top cover. It is also possible simply to remove the insole cover from the shoe, incorporate appropriate padding and replace the insole cover.

Casted insoles

Insoles made to a cast may be *accommodative orthoses*, which are designed to support and protect feet which have deformities incapable of

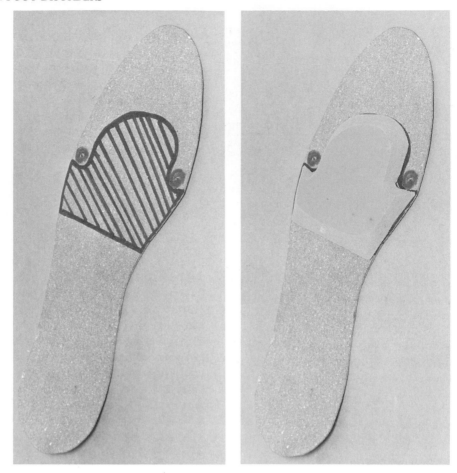

Fig. 13.4   Showing construction of non-casted insole (without top cover).

correction, or *functional orthoses*, which are designed to correct biomechanical imbalances between the hindfoot and the forefoot, such as forefoot varus or structural malalignment of the foot on the leg, as occurs in hindfoot valgus.

Accommodative orthoses are normally prescribed for conditions where joint pathology renders correction impossible. A large number of acquired and congenital deformities fall into this category. Figure 13.5 shows an accommodative orthosis manufactured for a patient injured in a motorcycle accident. His knee is fused and he presents with an ankle equinus and shortening of one leg by one and a half inches. The object of the insole is to load the maximum amount of foot surface contact area by filling in the exaggerated arch with a cork/latex compound. Birko cork, latex milk and the varieties of ethyl vinyl

acetate foams are excellent materials for this purpose. They provide a flexible support while incorporating forefoot padding to reduce pressure on the first and fifth metatarsal heads. The compound consists of cork, leather dust and fine woodflour to which latex is added until a consistency of porridge is achieved. The mixture is then spread on the covering of the orthosis, smoothed as evenly as possible and cured or vulcanised for 24 hours. The orthosis may then be finished by grinding, and fitted to the shape of the shoe. In the case illustrated, the orthosis was fitted into a running shoe. Such shoes are excellent for orthoses of this type because they have all the necessary features one would look for in a good shoe. The midsole has an extra piece added to it to reduce the leg length differential still further.

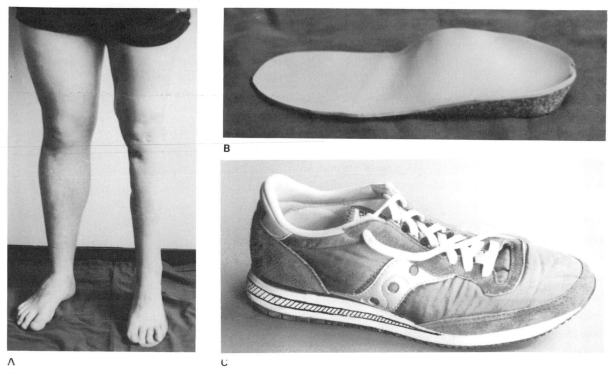

Fig. 13.5   Casted insole. (A) $1\frac{1}{2}$ inch shortening of left leg after accident. (B) Orthosis in cork/latex compound gives 1 inch heel raise. (C) Orthosis is worn in running shoe fitted with additional raise to the midsole (hatched).

Functional orthoses

Hindfoot/forefoot malalignments underlie many mechanical foot disorders and they are referred to as structural osseous deformities of the foot. The most common frontal plane structural problems which fall into this category are forefoot varus, forefoot valgus and plantar-flexed first ray, hindfoot varus and hindfoot valgus. The incidence of these structural deformities is difficult to identify since little random sampling of the population at large has been carried out; however one study (Black, 1986) identified 44% of those under investigation having a forefoot/hindfoot abnormality.

Sperryn (1983) highlighted the association between pain in other areas of the musculoskeletal system, such as knee, hip and back, and biomechanically abnormal feet. Foot pathology is recognised as a major contributory factor in compartment syndromes of the lower limb.

As a general rule, the more severe the structural abnormality, the more rigid the material required

to achieve correction, provided the requisite joint motion is available in the foot to allow for realignment. In severe deformities, however, it may be necessary to compromise between what is possible and what is tolerable. It may also be impossible to post the orthosis to the degree required to achieve full correction and still get it into a shoe.

The choice of materials is also subject to other factors outwith the range of joint motion previously mentioned. Factors which have to be taken into account are age, weight, occupation, chronicity of the condition, preferred style of footwear; also, in the case of the sports person, the nature of the event: if it involves running, jumping or contact sport, the ground/shoe interface has to be considered. Materials range from rigid to flexible. Acrylic resins, such as Rohadur, are rigid plastics and splinting materials; Hexcelite, Aquaplast and the new range of fibreglass fracture splinting materials can provide orthoses which last for many months. It is possible to manufacture temporary orthoses in situ on the foot using these splinting materials since their thermo-forming temperature can be tolerated by the skin on the sole of the foot. Children normally tolerate semi-rigid or flexible orthoses rather than those of a rigid variety.

Functional orthoses are constructed on plaster models of the patient's foot. The mould or cast is taken with the subtalar joint in its neutral position. The neutral position of the subtalar joint may be determined by one of four methods: palpation, observation, measurement and evaluation. No one method is entirely reliable and the practitioner should always seek to support observation by measurement in determining the position of the subtalar joint neutral position. The neutral position of the subtalar joint occurs twice in the gait cycle, shortly after heel strike and later at the mid-point of mid-stance, when the foot moves from being a pronating mobile adapter to a supinating rigid lever. This ensures that the contours of the foot accurately reflect the relationship between the forefoot and hindfoot. One procedure is as follows:

1. The patient is placed supine with the feet extending beyond the edge of the leg or plinth in order to secure full muscular relaxation. The patient may lie prone if this is preferred. A pillow or towel is placed under the hip on the same side as the foot to be casted. This brings the foot to a vertical position ideal for neutral casting.

2. The neutral position of the subtalar joint having been previously determined, the foot is held in this position while a slipper cast is taken. Low plaster loss bandage is applied in broad strips two layers thick. The first layer is moulded round the back of the heel and both sides of the foot to just behind the first and fifth metatarsal heads. The upper edge of the bandage is positioned three-quarters of an inch below the malleoli and the lower edge is folded inward to cover the plantar surface. The second layer is placed in similar fashion around the front of the toes and both sides of the forefoot and moulded towards the heel so as to overlap the first layer. The lower edge is turned in to meet and overlap the first layer so that the whole plantar aspect of the foot is encased. To facilitate removal, only the tips of the toes are covered. Before the plaster sets, pressure is applied beneath the fourth and fifth metatarsal heads to force the foot into slight dorsiflexion until resistance is met. This ensures that the midtarsal joint is maximally pronated whilst the subtalar joint is held in neutral. All excess water is squeezed from the bandage and the position of the foot is held until the plaster sets and the cast is ready for removal.

3. On removal, it is checked to ensure that it represents exactly the foot which has been casted. Any flaws are made good at this stage while the patient is still present. It is good practice to write an accurate and full description of all the features which are to be incorporated in the orthosis. When fully set, the cast is filled with plaster to make the model on which the orthosis is made.

The cast is best filled with a mixture of dental plaster and stone plaster (Kaffir D), which produces a model of the foot capable of modification and of withstanding heat and the forces created by the vacuum press. Additional plaster should be added to compensate for flattening of soft tissue during weight-bearing, particularly on the lateral plantar aspect of the heel. Similarly, additions must be made to the medial longitudinal arch to accommodate flattening. Failure to make these modifications will result in an orthosis which is not comfortable and fails to perform its functions. Philps (1990) describes in detail methods of manufacture, uses of materials and means of correction.

Subtalar neutral casts may also be taken with the patient in a supine position and certain authorities describe the technique with the patient seated. However, irrespective of which method is used, the practitioner must always ensure that the principles are the same. The knee must be fully extended and the foot dorsiflexed to resistance.

Children present particular difficulties when casting. This is especially true of the hypermobile child and having the child prone makes it less likely for the child to move or to interfere with the casting technique. However, establishing where resistance occurs when dorsiflexing the foot can present problems and it is best to dorsiflex the foot to 90°. Children frequently wriggle their toes and their feet if they tend to be tickly when the plaster is being moulded and every effort should be made to distract the child during the procedure.

Many companies now produce plastics in precut template sizes ready for heating. Once malleable, the plastic is trimmed to its rough shape and moulded either by vacuum forming or pressure from a rubber sheet until the plastic cools and conforms exactly to the shape and contours of the plantar surface of the foot. Different plastics require heating at different temperatures and for differing lengths of time (Table 13.2). Prior to manufacture, it should be decided whether intrinsic or extrinsic posting is to be used, based on the presenting condition, range of joint movement and the degree of correction required. Posts are best described as platforms added to the plastic shell to provide the correction measured during examination. There is debate as to whether extrinsic or intrinsic posting is more effective. However, it is generally accepted that intrinsic posting is more comfortable while extrinsic posting provides more correction.

Irrespective of which technique is used the principle is the same. Rigid or high density materials, such as dental acrylic, tensol (liquid plastic), high density polyethylene foam, or birko may be used for posting. These posts or wedges hold the foot in its optimal functioning position under load, restrain it from deforming as it would otherwise do, given the nature of the intrinsic fault, and reconstitute the normal time sequence of events occurring in the foot during the gait cycle. If some accommodation is required, posts

Table 13.2 Working temperatures and thermoforming times for plastics in common use.

	Temp	Time (mins)
Hexcelite	72°C	3
Aquaplast	100°C	3
Pacton	110°C	5
Evazote	130°C	6
Plastazote	140°C	8
Polythene	140°C	10
Ortholene	165°C	14
Polyprophylene	165°C	15
Rohadur	170°C	18
TL61 (Carbon fibre composite)	180°C	20

Times are based on the oven being at working temperature. All materials were 3 mm thick. Thicker materials take longer to become malleable.

may be made of a material which will 'give', such as high density rubber.

A hindfoot post consists of a shaped heel pad placed under the heel of the shell and tapered off on the lateral side to the required angle, varus posting only being used for the hindfoot. This prevents abnormal or excessive subtalar pronation but permits normal pronation to take place. Forefoot posting may be either varus or valgus as required for inversion or eversion deviations of the forefoot respectively. A bar of material is placed 0.5 cm to 1 cm behind the metatarsal heads, tapering off to the medial or lateral sides to the required angle (Fig. 13.6).

Rigid orthoses thus incorporate all the required correction yet allow for ease of fitting as they require little room in the footwear. However, complete functional control may not always be tolerated by the patient at first, and the orthosis should be worn for short periods only, increasing daily until the patient becomes accustomed to wearing it all day. Alternative methods of controlling the imbalance in a more tolerable manner are available by the use of laminations of leather or compounds of granulated cork and latex, or by the use of semi-rigid plastics. Forefoot padding may also be added to functional orthoses, if necessary, to make them more comfortable to wear.

A corrected negative mould in modelling clay or Plasticine may also be used to fabricate a rigid orthosis. Moist clay is placed in a tray the size of a shoe box about 25 cm deep. The foot is first wrapped in thin plastic film and then placed on the softened clay and subjected to weight-bearing while the subtalar joint is held in neutral. A block of about 10 cm is placed under the other foot to even up the stance. As the foot sinks into the clay, the sides of the foot are buttressed by extra clay being pushed around them to form strong walls about 20 mm high. The foot is withdrawn leaving an accurate negative impression. The plastic film is unwrapped from the foot and left in the impression. This method avoids any contamination of the clay and possible cross-infection between patients.

Aquaplast is heated until malleable and placed into the negative cast, followed by insertion of the foot. The clay is pushed into the sides of the foot

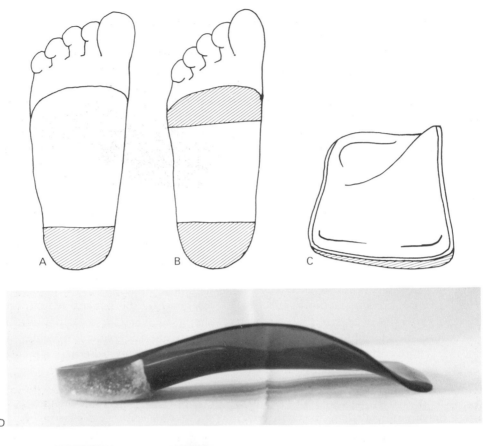

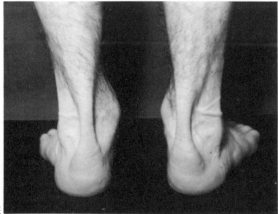

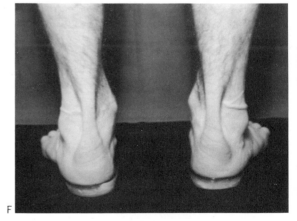

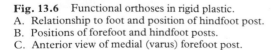

Fig. 13.6 Functional orthoses in rigid plastic.
A. Relationship to foot and position of hindfoot post.
B. Positions of forefoot and hindfoot posts.
C. Anterior view of medial (varus) forefoot post.

D. Medial view of medial (varus) hindfoot post.
E. Pronation associated with hindfoot and forefoot varus.
F. Correction of pronation by means of rigid plastic orthoses with medial (varus) hindfoot and forefoot posts.

to gain a close contour. The sheet of aquaplast may need stretching and this can be done to specific areas before placing the foot on top. It is

not, however, mandatory that the foot be placed on top as the aquaplast can be adequately moulded to the negative. Good accurate results can be achieved by smoothing the aquaplast into place whilst hot and soft. The device may be trimmed and finished when the patient returns.

It is also possible to manufacture such an orthosis directly onto the patient's foot, should time or circumstances not allow the patient to return later. Low temperature thermoplastics which become malleable in hot water are ideal for moulding straight onto the foot. The only drawback of this method is that two pairs of hands are needed, one to hold the patient's foot in subtalar neutral and the other to place the heated plastic onto the foot. This method may be of particular value in domiciliary visits or where the patient may be unable to attend for a fitting appointment.

Heel orthoses

There are a number of orthoses which may be made specifically for conditions affecting the heel. A heel cup may be fabricated on a cast of the heel using plastics already described, or fibre glass. Such devices are well tolerated since they take up little room and can be worn in a wide variety of shoes. Wedges or posts may be incorporated into such devices at the time of manufacture or at a later stage. These devices are corrective in nature. However, palliative heel orthoses may be required for lesions on the plantar aspect of the heel, such as calcaneal bursitis, and for the area around the insertion of the tendo Achilles where the bursae are often subject to irritation from footwear. Skaters are particularly vulnerable to retrocalcaneal bursitis because of the rigidity of the counter surrounding the heel of skating boots. These heel orthoses can be manufactured on casts or made directly onto the heel using silicone. The silicone technique is discussed later.

Painful intractable hyperkeratotic lesions frequently occur on the area of the heel following trauma, or in some cases resulting from harmful X-ray therapy for verrucae. The formation of scar tissue in such cases leaves the practitioner no other course than to rely on palliative orthoses. Most often, these devices are best fabricated in latex for wear on the foot. However, simple heel pads can also be made to fit into the shoe and be removed for use in other shoes as required.

Latex technique

Deformities of the toes such as hallux abductovalgus and hammer toes are often chronic and require protection more or less permanently. In such cases, devices made in latex are often the most effective type of orthosis. Irrespective of the area involved, the principle of manufacture is the same. For the purposes of illustration, the fabrication of a hallux abductovalgus shield is described, but the technique is suitable for digital orthoses as well.

The most important feature is the accuracy of the negative cast. This may be taken in a variety of materials but the most effective are the elastic impression compounds. Dental impression materials are ideal for this purpose and the most cost-effective of these is dental alginate.

Sufficient alginate having been mixed, the gel is spread on to the area to be cast with a sufficiently wide margin all round. The amount of movement available in the joint dictates whether or not this cast should be taken weight-bearing. If the joint is fixed, a non weight-bearing cast will suffice, but if it is mobile, the cast is best taken in a weight-bearing position. Before removal of the negative, it is essential to encase the alginate in a light covering of plaster of Paris bandage. This guarantees that there will be no deformation upon removal of the negative. This technique can be adopted for all large alginate casts.

The negative is then filled with plaster and when this has set the alginate is stripped bit by bit to ensure that the positive remains intact. Any blemishes on the positive are removed with fine sandpaper, and, if necessary, porosities may be filled in with a thin mixture of plaster. The positive is then allowed to dry. Care must be taken not to overheat the cast as this might reverse the chemical process, causing the cast to become crumbly.

The positive is then dipped in latex, each layer being allowed to dry, until several layers have been built up on the cast. At this stage, the correct type of pad is applied according to the therapeutic function required. If an open-cell foam is used, the pad is first covered with adhesive. This seals the pad and prevents latex from permeating into the foam, and it also traps air within the open-cell structure thereby improving the physical properties of the material. The cast is then dipped twice more to complete the process before being removed from the cast and trimmed. In some cases, it is preferable to cover the cast in a layer of soft leather such as chamois to provide a soft lining for the appliance. If this method is employed, the edges of the leather must be sealed and the appropriate adhesive used, otherwise degradation of the leather may result due to interaction with the solvents used to stabilize the adhesives.

It is sometimes necessary or convenient to speed up the process for latex orthoses. This may be done by either heating the cast before dipping or by using a hot air blower such as a hair dryer to dry each dip. In this way it is possible to manufacture a latex orthosis from start to finish in fifteen minutes. A variety of latex digital shields is shown in Figure 13.7.

Digital appliances for the lesser toes

All necessary designs of digital appliances for the lesser toes can be produced by any of the methods previously outlined for hallux abductovalgus shields. The necessity for negative and positive casting when the latex technique is used, coupled with the smaller size of digital appliances, lends great advantages to the direct moulding techniques utilising silicone rubbers or thermoplastic materials. Silicone rubbers are well proven as the most suitable materials for digital orthoses. They can also be fabricated from orthotic plastic, but it is then usually necessary to line them with softer material for good tissue tolerance. Plastics used for this purpose are designed for finger splinting as they are soft and malleable. This combination increases the corrective effect of an appliance whilst maintaining patient tolerance.

The principle of reciprocal dorsoplantar padding is the most effective basis for digital appliances, and this has been previously described (p.203). When moulded in silicones or thermoplastics, orthodigital splints are infinitely adjustable to individual needs. They may be either full or partial. When full, they fully cover the dorsum of the proximal phalanges and the plantar surfaces of the intermediate and distal phalanges of the middle three toes. When partial, they are reduced in size to fit one or two toes only, or to form a long prop. Maximum effect is thus obtained with minimum bulk. Deformities and lesions of the fifth toe are particularly amenable to well designed partial splints in silicones or thermoplastics.

SILICONES

The use of silicone elastomers in orthotics and

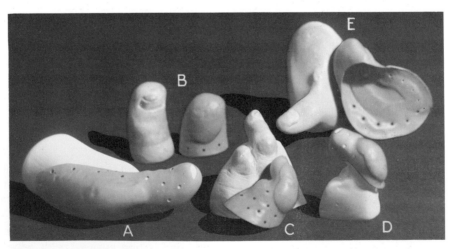

Fig. 13.7   Latex sigital shields for various sites. (A) Hallux valgus. (B) Subungual exostosis, when surgery was refused. (C) Fourth and fifth dorsal protection. (D) Hammer toes. (E) Saddle pad for extensor longus hallucis tendon.

prosthetics is probably the most significant advance in this field for many years. In the short time since their introduction, rapid progress has resulted in new opportunities of treatment for digital deformity in both the old and the young. Silicones used in podiatry are derivatives of elastomers used in dentistry, although in recent years specific materials designed for podiatry have become available.

Silicones are presented as a paste or putty to which a catalyst is added. This promotes cross-linking and end-to-end butt-joining of the polysiloxane chains in the paste. After a period, the viscous paste or putty is transformed into a flexible solid. The material, whilst undergoing its change of state, achieves a putty-like consistency which remains for a period ranging from two to eight minutes, depending on the paste/catalyst ratio and the room temperature. This space of time allows the practitioner to fabricate the device. After final setting, the material must be able to withstand repeated functional loading without dimensional change or fracture. There is a wide variety of formulae possible, but the practitioner must be aware of any alterations which he may make as they will directly affect the properties of tension and compression, and setting time, and therefore the subsequent usage of the material. Other external factors also affect the ultimate vulcanisation of the silicone, such as the type of paste, the quantity of catalyst, and room temperature. Silicones set more quickly in high temperatures whilst cold dramatically delays the onset of chemical change.

Basically, there are two approaches in the use of silicone elastomers. The practitioner may use the material before the phase transition begins. At this stage, the paste is still in a 'flow state' and is best applied by spatula. This technique is best used for manufacturing heel cups, plantar pads and protective forms of digital devices. The practitioner applies the paste and thereafter the silicone will flow to cover the proposed dimensions of the orthosis. Initially, this method may be difficult to master because, if the paste is applied too soon after the catalyst is added, it may run out of control. However, it is by far the most effective method of covering large areas evenly and mastery can be assured after a few attempts.

The other technique involves utilisation of the chemical changes occurring in the paste as the silicone converts from paste to elastic solid. During this phase transition, the material becomes malleable and provided that the practitioner has included sufficient plasticiser in the formulation and uses liquid paraffin or some similar oil, the silicone can be handled and manipulated like Plasticine.

By far the most rewarding application of this material lies in the correction of congenital digital deformities in children. The same techniques may be used to correct toe deformities in older patients if sufficient motion is present in the affected joints, and the same methods have been applied to the maintenance of correction following corrective digital surgery. Basically, the splint is fashioned around the toes, and, as the silicone sets, the toes are held in their corrected position until the elastic properties of the material are strong enough to withstand the deforming forces. Figures 13.8 and 13.9 illustrate a variety of basic techniques for correcting the common congenital toe deformities.

When using these materials in the field of postoperative maintenance, one must work in close harmony with the surgeon who has performed the operation. It is essential that the podiatrist has a good knowledge of the surgical techniques which have been employed so that any splint manufactured for the patient acts as an integral part of the patient's therapy. In Figure 13.10 (p.252), a silicone orthosis has been fitted two weeks after the patient has undergone a Keller's arthroplasty and capsulotomy of the 2nd and 3rd toes. Assessment of the inherent strength of the lesser digits is important if attempting to manufacture a splint to maintain the position of the hallux in order to avoid moving the lesser digits laterally.

In order to assist the handling properties of the elastomer, 'plasticiser' may be added. The function of a plasticiser is to soften the silicone and make it more flexible. A light grade oil such as baby oil or liquid paraffin may be used, or additives such as 'Atrixo' or 'Siopel'. Plasticisers are able to penetrate between the randomly-orientated chains of the polymer and, as a result, the molecules become further apart and the forces

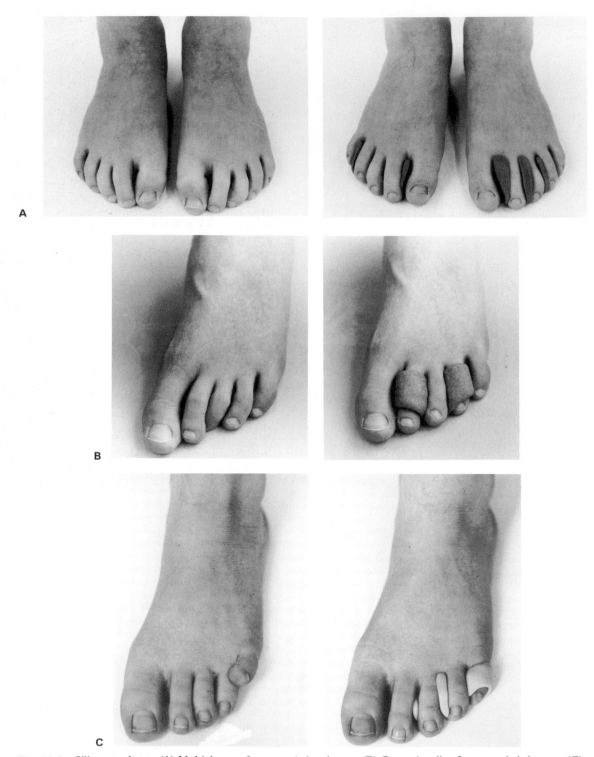

Fig. 13.8 Silicone orthoses. (A) Multiple prop for congenital curly toes. (B) Corrective sling for congenital claw toe. (C) Corrective sling for digitus quintus varus.

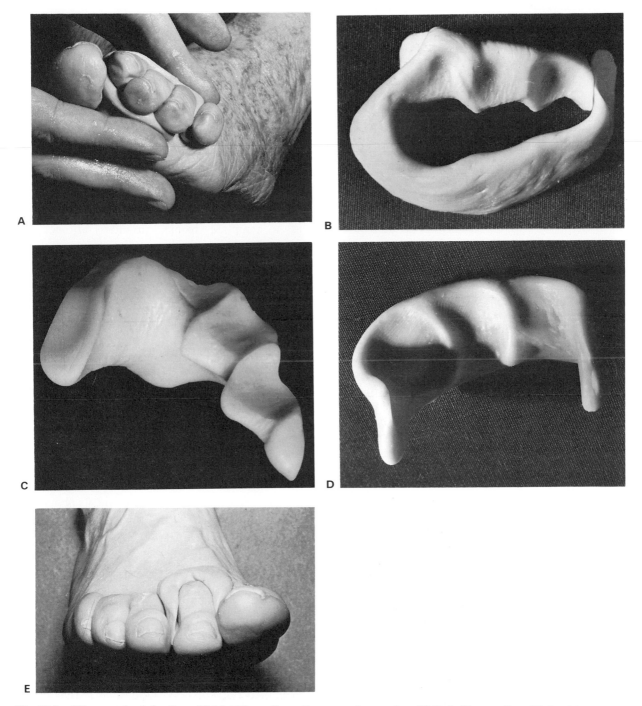

Fig. 13.9 Silicone orthogital splints. (A) Moulding splint at first stage of correction. (B) Full silicone splint. (C) Partial splint with interdigital wedge for first cleft. (D) Silicone long prop. (E) Single dorsoplantar splint for hammer toe.

between them are lessened. Plasticisers also allow the silicone material to be handled more easily by preventing the silicone elastomer from sticking to the operator's fingers. The amounts of plasticiser added should not exceed 30% of the bulk used. The more plasticiser added, the softer the device

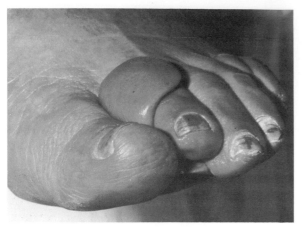

Fig. 13.10 Silicone prop and interdigital wedge to maintain position of hallux after Keller's arthoplasty.

and the more liable to plastic deformation under load.

Recent innovations on the market are silicone putties. Some have been specially designed for the podiatrist and they achieve their properties by the addition of inert fillers, such as liquid paraffin and zinc oxide, to demethyl polysiloxane until the material takes on a putty-like consistency. These materials are best catalysed with a cream catalyst. However, their applications are strictly limited to the manufacture of simple corrective devices where load imposition is minimal. The reason for this is implicit in their chemical composition, since much of their bulk is taken up with fillers which take no part in the chemistry of the reaction. Thus some podiatrists have found when using putty-type silicone elastomers that the physical properties do not match the therapeutic objectives of the device. The material chosen must be able to withstand the forces applied during use.

THERMOPLASTICS

Thermoplastic materials are usually products of addition polymerisation. They will soften on heating and harden once cooled without any chemical change taking place. Polymers which are thermoplastic can be moulded to a desired shape when heat and pressure are applied. The most common thermoplastic materials used in podiatry are derivatives of polyethylene, although polypropylene materials are also used.

This range of synthetic materials has four main areas of application: (1) firm splinting, (2) impression medium, (3) moulded lining, (4) modelling and construction.

The firm splinting material is polyethylene sheet which is not expanded in manufacture and consequently contains no pockets of gas. It is used for direct moulding to positive casts in the production of orthotic shells.

The impression material is the expanded polyethylene which, when inserted into the shoe as a template insole, provides an accurate dynamic impression of pressure areas. The template can then be built up with appropriate padding to produce a permanent insole.

As a lining material, the thermoplastic may be expanded polyethylene or expanded vinyl acetate. After it is heated, moulding is carried out directly on the foot and additional padding and outer layers are added in sequence. This method can be used for hallux abductovalgus shields and similar appliances, e.g. heel cups for bedridden patients to prevent bed sores.

These materials may also be used for taking negative casts. However, if they are to be used for this purpose, care has to be taken to ensure there is no deformation after removal from the foot and it is sometimes of help to mould a rigid material around the thermoplastic to retain its shape and dimension.

The softer of the two materials is the expanded vinyl acetate (Evazote) which looks identical to expanded polyethylene (Plastozote) but feels much smoother and softer and has lower tensile strength. Quite complex curvatures can be achieved by moulding these materials and one of the benefits is that a seamless lining is obtained.

Footwear which conforms accurately to the shape of the foot can be simply constructed by using the various densities and thicknesses of expanded polyethylene. One style is that of the clog with an enclosed front and no heel counter. The sole block is first cut out with a leather knife or on a bandsaw and the foot is placed on top. The upper is then shaped and covered in some appropriate material, e.g. Yampi. This is then moulded round the foot with the foot in place on the sole block and the upper is adhered around the edge of the base. An outer sole can then be added and trimmed. The pair of clogs may weigh no more than 200 g, an important consideration in many cases.

An even lighter style is that of the sandal with a block sole and two or three straps to hold it on to the foot. More complicated styles can also be produced which, when compared with traditional surgical footwear, are extremely attractive in terms of weight, fitting, style and price.

Almost any shape can be produced by cutting, heating, moulding and buffing thermoplastic materials (Fig. 13.11). To produce a moulded article, the material is heated in an oven at about 130°C until it is soft enough to mould. It cools in a minute or two and retains its moulded shape, at which stage adhesive can be applied. In some cases, the adhesive may be applied before heating so that the moulding and fixing is done in one stage. Synthetic contact adhesives are suitable for fixing these thermoplastics. Good surface finishing is achieved easily, particularly when this is done on a grinding machine. When heating thermoplastics, it should be remembered that they are all inflammable, giving off strong toxic fumes if allowed to get too hot. An oven with thermostatic controls is advised and a fire extinguisher should always be at hand.

'Hot-water plastics' (Polyform) (Aquaplast) (Hexcelite)

These orthotic splinting plastics are of particular

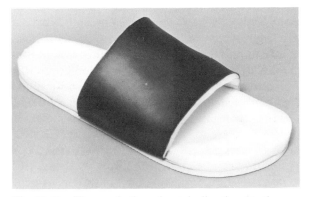

Fig. 13.11 Thermoplastic mule made directly on to the foot.

use when an immediate appliance is required and this technique is of great value in saving practitioner time. Its essential features are: low temperature moulding; chairside technique; production time of a few minutes; rapid remoulding of part or the whole device; no waste material, small offcuts being re-usable; readily adjustable thickness as the material can be built up or thinned out as required.

Low temperature moulding. In standard thickness (3 mm), the material can be softened in boiling water for between 1 and 3 minutes to become completely workable and to thin out to an extremely thin layer. At 65 to 70°C, it becomes workable in about 54 to 60 seconds but the moulding characteristics are not as precise as with the 100°C temperature. The plastic will not soften below 60°C.

The material should be dried on a towel before being moulded and it will remain workable for about 3 to 5 minutes. Fingers should be moistened to maintain a good 'slip' feeling on surface moulding. When moulding, any excess can be trimmed away easily with scissors. Most patients have good tolerance to the hot material directly on the skin but an intermediate layer of expanded thermoplastic can be included if thought advisable. Cooling can be speeded up by immersing in cold water. If the material is thinned out when moulding and cooled with ice-water, the hardened state can be expected in about 10 to 15 seconds.

Chairside technique. The whole device can be produced in as little as 2 minutes but should not normally take more than 10 minutes, allowing for modifications and adjustments.

Rapid remoulding. The advantage of this plastic over silicone rubber is that it can always be remoulded and reshaped by heating part or all of the device. As conditions respond to the orthotic, so the device can be adjusted to correspond to such correction.

No waste. Any small pieces can be reheated and moulded into one new piece. The new material can be flattened into a new sheet of any thickness on a smooth worktop. It will retain its cohesive properties after being heated and dried. Cold material is easily bonded to warm material by using a nonflammable Polyform adhesive. A finished device can be completely remade by placing it back into hot water. If the material has been thinned out while moulding, then in order to obtain the original or greater thickness it will be necessary to fold over and double the material or to add other sheets.

Complex construction. Where more complex structures are required, and trial and error may be necessary to achieve optimum results, small balls of the plastic may be added such as under the longitudinal axis of a three quarter length valgus insole, to gain the desired degree of spring. A valgus insole is very quickly made and can be altered at any time with ease. Heel cups are also easily made and by careful stretching of the material can be quickly and accurately produced. Double curvatures are not difficult to make as long as the material is well heated. Combinations of Polyform with silicone rubbers or expanded thermoplastics give good results.

Where a soft appliance lacks strength, Polyform can be added to the original device as a reinforcement or cradle. An analogy is the gum shield worn by boxers which consists of a strong plastic shell lined with soft material which has been moulded directly to the interior of the mouth. Expanded thermoplastics can be stuck to the Polyform sheet prior to heating and moulding to give an excellent fit when finished. Individual areas of the material can be heated using a hot-air gun and additional moulding or alterations can be performed.

Hexcelite. This is a remouldable plastic impregnated over soft cotton. The material forms a mesh and, as such, combines features of excellent moulding with ventilation. It is self-bonding, light and has considerable strength. It is a relatively inexpensive material and can be heated in water at 72°C. It sets 3 minutes and, when malleable, it will bond itself whether wet or dry. It has many uses and the podiatrist need only use imagination to provide a wide array of semi-rigid orthoses. It can be used to manufacture night splints for hallux abductovalgus and can be used to splint lesser toes following surgery. By bonding several layers together functional orthoses can be made in a matter of minutes. These insoles may be made directly on the patient's foot or manufactured on a cast. Posts may be added in the same material. The Hexcelite should be moulded together by rolling with a rolling pin. Any synthetic contact adhesive is suitable for use with Hexcelite.

Orthotic laboratories

The provision and manufacture of orthoses by commercial outlets is steadily increasing. It is now possible to provide patients with traditional types of orthoses, including latex appliances and functional orthoses, for sport and everyday wear. Many outlets produce orthoses on receipt of casts taken by the practitioner. Three or four weeks is about average of this type of service.

Two features are vitally important when using such services. The negative casts have to be accurate and well packed so that there is no damage during transit. The instructions on the prescription form provided must be explicit and detailed. No manufacturer can provide accurate, well fitting orthoses from badly produced negative casts. It is ultimately the practitioner's responsibility if the orthoses prove to be unsuitable. This method of providing a service is more expensive and, if the practitioner does not have the necessary equipment or expertise, alternations are time consuming. The practitioner should master the techniques of adjustment as this not only provides a more effective service, but enhances the practitioner's professionalism.

PROSTHESES

It is now within the podiatrist's capability to provide patients with life-like prostheses. Digital replacements, whether single or multiple, can be manufactured with silicone elastomers. KE 20 is a white elastomer which can be tinted to a flesh colour by adding a specific colorant provided by the manufacturer or by adding a little Verone RS. The technique is relatively simple and, for a single digit replacement, can be done with the patient present. A negative cast is taken of the digit or digits which are to be used as donor toes. If a fifth toe is to be replaced, a fourth toe may be used. A second toe can be substituted by a third toe, and so on. However, if all toes need to be substituted, then recourse is needed to an individual with similar foot size and configuration.

Figure 13.12 illustrates the technique for replacing the fourth and fifth toes. Using dental alginate or one of the dental elastomers other than silicone, a negative cast of the remaining two lesser digits is produced. This is then filled with an appropriately shaded amount of silicone. Exhaust holes must be pierced in the negative cast before commencement of the procedure. After the negative cast has been filled, the operator must wait until the paste has become a flexible rubber before removing the negative cast. The resultant mould is trimmed or drilled to the appropriate size and then bonded to a small silicone prop which runs under the remaining toes to provide

anchorage for the prosthesis. These are particularly successful devices and patients find the cosmetic improvement exceedingly satisfactory.

For total replacement of all toes, a positive cast of the remaining stump is necessary to provide a base to which the donor toes are bonded with silicone. When using this technique, an adequate amount of shaded elastomer with the correct proportions of added plasticiser must be pre-mixed so as to ensure that there will be no possibility of producing a two-tone prosthesis.

Where larger portions of the foot are lost, traditional methods of incorporating open-cell foams in latex are still considered effective. Attempts to provide lifelike prostheses for these feet with silicone prove to be both too costly and too heavy to be effective because of the large amount of silicone required. Until flesh-like foaming elastomers are produced which can withstand the destructive forces of weight-bearing, traditional methods prove more satisfactory.

SHOE MODIFICATIONS

Heels

Thomas heel

The heel is built out anteriorly under the instep to give solid support to the waist of the shoe to prevent it giving way under excessive pressure. Normally an extension half the width of the heel is sufficient for this purpose, and this saves additional weight. It ends either as it meets the sole or shorter than this as may be required. It is usually applied to the medial side in some forms of pes plano-valgus to provide medial support, but can equally well be of value when applied laterally ('reverse Thomas heel') to give lateral support where required in pes cavus or talipes varus. The extension may be combined with wedging if necessary ('crooked and elongate heel').

Buttressed heel (flared heel, floated heel)

The heel is built out laterally or medially as required to provide additional lateral or medial support and also, if necessary, to restrict abnormal inversion or eversion respectively. The

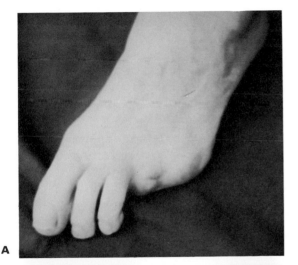

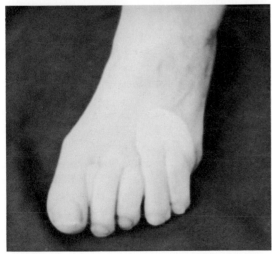

Fig. 13.12 (A and B) Silicone prothesis for fourth and fifth toes.

lower the heel, the more effective is the additional support.

Heel wedges

Heel wedges may be applied internally to the heel seat or externally to the shoe heel. Internally, they are used to correct or stabilise excessive eversion of the calcaneus within the shoe and hence of abnormal pronation of the foot. Externally applied, they tilt the heel seat into an inverted position. Either form may therefore be of value in the management of different forms of pes plano-valgus.

Internally, cork sections tapering from medial to lateral are shaped to conform to the size and shape of the heel seat, tapered off anteriorly and inserted under the heel sock. The degree of corrective wedging must be individually assessed. The cork sections are slightly cupped in the centre to ensure a close fit to the heel of the foot.

Externally, a leather or rubber wedge is inserted between the lifts of a leather heel or added to a solid heel as close as possible to the heel seat. If necessary, both forms may have to be applied, the internal wedging often constituting a main feature of a permanent insole. Additional measures such as a Thomas heel or valgus support may also be necessary. Wedging on the lateral side of the heel may occasionally be required with a reverse Thomas heel to control talipes equino-varus.

Excavated heel

The heel seat is hollowed out and filled with shock absorbent material in cases of painful heel, but this is possible only in well-built or specially made surgical footwear. It is indicated particularly where it is desired to lower the heel of the foot in relation to the heel quarters and counter of the shoe, as in posterior calcaneal lesions (posterior tuberosity, retrocalcaneal bursitis). For painful plantar lesions of the heel and for normal footwear, a tarsal platform with a heel cushion is simpler and may well suffice.

Shank stiffener

Firm, splinting material (stiff leather, glass fibre) is inserted in the shoe between the heel seat and the tread of the shoe to prevent the waist buckling. It may be combined with a Thomas heel.

Heel height adjustments

The height of the shoe heel is designed to accord with the 'pitch' (forward slope) of the shoe and the 'toe spring' (upward tilt of sole) to ensure that the shoe is properly balanced antero-posteriorly. With any given shoe, the heel height should not therefore be greatly varied, except as a temporary measure pending the provision of new shoes with the correct heel height. Heels may be raised temporarily to compensate for a short tendo Achilles, or to relieve pain in a strained calf muscle.

Soles

Sole wedges

Soles wedges are used to tilt the plane of the sole medially or laterally. They are only of value if worn over long periods and they should therefore not be fixed to the underside of the sole where they would quickly wear away and require frequent replacement. Instead, they should be placed between the insole and the outer sole. Although this is possible with specially made shoes and the superior kind of mass-produced shoes designed with separate insole and outer sole, it is not possible with many modern styles of shoe. Sole wedges therefore have a very limited application and the desired effect is usually better achieved by an appropriate design of orthotic insole.

A medial sole wedge may be indicated in conjunction with a medial heel wedge to stabilise a hindfoot varus. A lateral sole wedge is sometimes used in conjunction with a medial heel wedge (contralateral wedging). The intention is to invert the hindfoot and evert the forefoot in cases of supinated forefoot in children. The effective-ness of the lateral sole wedge depends both upon the degree of corrective pronation which can be obtained at the midtarsal joint and upon this being maintained throughout the mid-stance and propulsive phases of the walking cycle. These effects are difficult to ensure, and for this reason, together with the impracticability of sole wedges in many modern types of children's shoes, it is usually preferable to rely on over-correction of the calcaneus by medial heel wedging, leaving the pronation of the forefoot to be maintained by the shift of body weight to the lateral border of the forefoot as it bears weight. An appropriate orthotic insole is indicated, eliminating the need for sole wedges.

Metatarsal bar

As with sole wedges, this transverse bar should also be placed between the insole and outer sole of the shoe to avoid excessive wearing and the danger of tripping. It is similarly unsuitable for many modern footwear styles and so has a limited application, the desired effects being more readily and precisely achieved by the design of individual insoles.

Rocker sole. This is an effective means of providing a relatively painfree first metatarsophalangeal joint in cases of hallux rigidus. The shoe is built up with an additional outer sole which has its greatest thickness under the metatarsophalangeal joints and tapers away at its distal and proximal edges. The heel is also raised to a similar maximum thickness to maintain the balance of the shoe but it is tapered off at the back. The effect when in use, as the name suggests, is to enable the foot to rock forward instead of bending at the metatarsophalangeal joints. The same principle applies to some designs of platform soles. Some, but by no means all, provide for toe-spring and are quite easy to walk in and many so-called health sandals employ the same geometry in their solid wooden footwear.

The fitting of a rocker sole is best carried out by a reliable shoe repairer although test additions can be made from cork sheets of 8–10 mm thickness as a temporary trial before committing the shoe to a permanent alteration. Both shoes need the same modification regardless of whether the condition is unilateral or bilateral.

Uppers

Simple stretching. This can be achieved with a swan-neck shoe stretcher or by using a mechanical stretching machine with a variety of expandable lasts. The aim is to provide a pocket in the upper or an overall increase in accommodation. The shoe is worn by the patient and the area of protuberance is carefully delineated by applying an accurately-sized piece of adhesive tape over the area. The bulge of the instrument used to stretch the upper must coincide exactly with the area of tape. A softening solution can be applied to the upper, particularly if it is leather, to allow easier stretching. In many cases this is all that is required to alleviate a hammer toe or enlarged joint.

Slit release. This involves cutting through the layers of material of the upper to allow more accommodation for the forefoot. The cuts are made longitudinally and there should be several, spaced closely together, to achieve the best effect. If placed low down on the sides of the upper adjacent to the sole, they are more discreet. While appearing a drastic method, it is sometimes the only expedient pending the provision of more suitable footwear, and it is very suitable for footwear worn only indoors and for housebound patients.

Balloon patching. This is a method of providing an even greater pocket in the upper. A piece of soft leather is inserted into an over-sized hole that has been cut in the upper. When stitched or stuck into place, it effectively provides extra space. It is a skilled job for the shoe repairer.

Extra eyelets. This is a simple technique to provide an extension of the lacing section towards the front of the shoe so that it can be opened up more widely to allow a deformed foot to enter more easily. If the extra eyelets are provided at the proximal end of the laced section, the girth of the shoe will be increased to provide extra space for a swollen foot or ankle.

Vamp replacement. In certain cases of severe digital deformity, and also in the case of misfits in surgical footwear, it may be necessary to remove the entire vamp and replace it with another to give more depth.

FURTHER READING

Black J A 1986 The influence of the subtalar joint on running injuries of the lower limb. Sport and Medicine

Cavanagh P R 1980 Symposium on the foot and leg in running sports. Mosby, St Louis

Coates T T 1983 Practical orthotics for chiropodists. Actinic Press, London

D'Ambrosia R D, Drez D 1988 Prevention and treatment of running injuries. Slack, New York

Philps J W 1990 The functional foot orthosis. Churchill Livingstone, Edinburgh

Sperryn P N 1983 Sport and medicine. Butterworths, London

Sperryn P N, Restan L 1983 Podiatry and the sports physican—an evaluation of orthoses. British Journal of Sports Medicine 17(4)

Vixie D E 1980 Symposium on the foot and leg in running sports. Mosby, St Louis

14. Physical therapy

A. G. J. Saunders

Physical therapy, which was previously defined as treatment by physical and mechanical means, such as massage, has now developed to include treatments by heat, cold, manipulative techniques and exercise. Treatment objectives range from the relief of pain by palliative methods, such as heat and cold, to rehabilitation by means of functional exercises.

HEAT

Responses to heat

The body always attempts to retain a constant core temperature of 37°C. To achieve this in response to a changing environment, the peripheral vessels adapt either to lose or conserve heat.

Loss of heat involves a reflex vasodilatation of the superficial arterioles, which increases the amount of blood flowing to the body surface. Heat is then lost from the blood to the surrounding area by evaporation. Due to the increased blood flow through the periphery, more oxygen and nutrients are carried to the area and the corresponding increase in venous return enhances the removal of pain-stimulating metabolites.

Mild heating can produce a sedative effect on the nerve endings, whereas if the temperature is increased it can produce pain and may be used as a counter-irritant.

Dangers of applying heat

The main danger of applying heat is a burn. To avoid this, certain precautions must be carried out before any application. If in any doubt, do not give heat treatment.

1. The clinician must ensure that the patient can appreciate the sensation of heat. To check this, a thermal sensitivity test must be carried out. This is performed by touching hot and cold test tubes randomly on the patients' skin over the area to be treated and getting them to identify these with their eyes shut. If the patient cannot do this, no heat should be applied.

2. Heat should not be applied directly to the area of a patient with a deficient arterial blood supply as the heat will not be dissipated, therefore the part may overheat and burn.

Therapeutic aims

1. Relief of pain

This may be brought about by the sedative effects on the nerve endings, the reduction of any spasm or spasticity and the increase in blood flow, removing pain-stimulating metabolites.

2. Increased blood supply

A good blood supply is essential if healing is to take place by means of an increase in the amount of oxygen and the number of white blood cells being transported to the affected area. The resultant increase in venous and lymphatic return will enhance the removal of waste products and inflammatory exudate.

Methods of heating

There are two main ways of raising the temperature of the body: transferring heat to the body from an outside source, and getting the body to produce heat locally.

Transferring heat to the body

1. Wax foot baths. These are baths filled with paraffin wax which is heated to a temperature of 50°C. The patient's foot is immersed in the bath for a few seconds only and then removed to allow the wax to set. This process is repeated eight or ten times to allow a good coating of wax. The foot should then be wrapped in a towel to conserve heat and left for about 20 minutes. This efficient method is useful for most chronic inflammatory states, arthritis, chilblains and foot strain.

2. Hot water foot baths. As hot water is usually readily available, these baths are particularly suitable for home use. They should be given at a temperature of 45°C, should fully cover the foot and ankle and last for 15 to 20 minutes. A hypertonic saline foot bath is extremely soothing for tired aching feet, and for alleviating pain caused by verruca breakdowns. For septic conditions, medicated footbaths may be used; the following strengths should be used per gallon of water:

Sodium chloride: 125g
Potassium permanganate: enough to make a pale pink solution—usually only 4 or 5 crystals
Iodophores: according to the directions on the sachet.

3. Contrast baths. Although they incorporate cold, these baths are also suitable for home use, and are particularly good for stimulating the circulation and thus relieving muscle fatigue and reducing oedema. Two baths are used, one containing hot water at about 45°C and one containing cold water or ice slush. The feet are placed alternately in each bath for about one minute, starting and ending with the cold. These baths should not be used in cases of circulatory impairment, cardiac disease, hypertension, nor for the aged.

4. Infra-red irradiation. Infra-red rays are electromagnetic rays which are converted to heat energy when absorbed into the body. Those used in physical therapy are classified into two types.

Non-luminous rays (long infra-red rays). These rays are produced by lamps which have a heat source enclosed in fire clay. These lamps emit invisible rays with a wavelength of between 750 and 15 000 nm with a peak at about 4000 nm. The depth of penetration of non-luminous rays is into the superficial epidermis.

Luminous rays (short infra-red rays) are sometimes called radiant heat, as the lamps contain bulbs which also emit visible rays. These lamps emit rays with a wavelength of between 350 and 4000 nm with a peak at about 1000 nm, and have a penetration into the dermis as far as the superficial fascia. They are therefore effective in heating the peripheral vascular tissue.

The method of application and the uses of this form of treatment are generally the same for both types of lamp. Infra-red irradiation should be given to the bare skin and the lamp placed so the rays reach the skin at a right angle to ensure the maximum absorption of the rays into the body (Fig. 14.1). If the part being irradiated gets too hot, the lamp should be turned down or prefer-

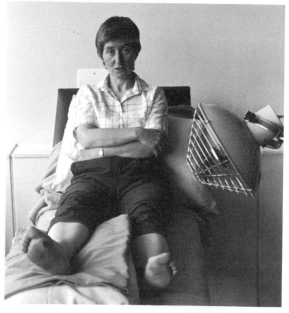

Fig. 14.1 Infra-red irradiation to the medial site of the right ankle. Note that the lamp is not placed directly over the patient for reasons of safety.

ably moved further away from the patient.

Both forms of infra-red irradiation are used in case such as osteoarthrosis, rheumatoid arthritis, plantar faciitis, painful heel conditions and sprains once the acute stage has passed. However, the non-luminous rays have a greater sedative effect and are more effective in relieving pain. The shorter and more irritant rays of the luminous lamps are of greater value for their counter-irritant effect.

Production of heat within the body

Ultrasound. Ultrasonic energy is a mechanical form of energy which is transmitted through a medium in the form of acoustic vibrations or waves at a frequency above that of human hearing; the frequencies used in therapy are between 1 MHz and 3 MHz. Ultrasound is emitted from a treatment head as a parallel beam of energy, the radius of the beam being the same as that of the treatment head. Particles within this beam will tend to move or vibrate as a result of the wave propagation and this produces friction between these particles, which generates heat. Because the heat is produced within the tissues, the amount of heat obtained in the tissues may be greater than that received by the previous methods.

The amount of heat generated depends on the intensity of power used, whilst the depth of penetration depends on the frequency. The effective depth of penetration is the depth at which the surface intensity is reduced to half; this is known as the *half value thickness*. The half value thickness for soft tissue is 4.5 cm at 1 Mz and 2.5 cm at 3 MHz.

Ultrasound waves are subject to reflection. Unlike audible sound, which is transmitted easily through air, ultrasound is totally reflected by air, so to avoid the beam being reflected before entering the body, the treatment head must be applied at a right angle to the skin and in contact with it (Fig. 14.2). To remove the possibility of an air pocket being trapped between the treatment head and the skin and to ensure maximum contact, a coupling medium, usually in the form of a proprietory gel (Fig. 14.3), must be placed between the treatment head and the skin. Water can be used as the coupling medium and is often used when giving ultrasound in a foot bath, when the treatment head need not be in contact with the skin; this is a particularly good method for treating sharp irregular surfaces like the ankle. Reflection also occurs at the interfaces between different tissues, particularly bony interfaces, therefore the tissues immediately surrounding bone may be subject to overheating due to presence of the reflected waves.

Ultrasound in podiatry is useful wherever a localised form of heat is required and has been found to be effective in the treatment of localised

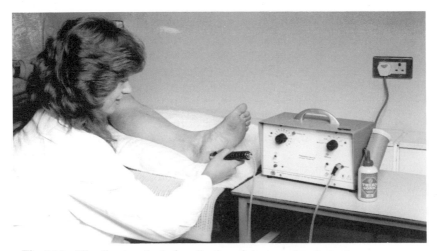

Fig. 14.2 The direct method of application of ultrasound to the heel.

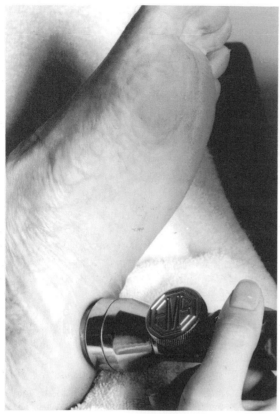

Fig. 14.3 Ultrasound application to heel showing the direct contact between the skin and the treatment head and the presence of the coupling gel.

heel pain, following injury with contusions, periarticular damage, Morton's metatarsalgia and in the incipient phase of hallux rigidus.

As ultrasound produces a vibration of particles within the body, it is often given in a pulsed (on-off) form which uses the vibrations as a form of micromassage without heating the part. The heat produced is removed by the blood flow during the off phase. This method of application is becoming more and more common as a method of loosening fibrosed structures in the treatment of chronic inflammation and plantar fasciitis.

Therapeutic doses of ultrasound are:

Acute conditions: low intensity approximately 0.25 W/cm^2 for between 2–5 minutes

Chronic conditions: 0.8 W/cm^2 for up to 8 minutes.

COLD

Responses to cold

The initial response to the application of cold to the skin is a vasoconstriction of the superficial blood vessels in order to reduce the heat loss. This is followed by a vasodilatation and then repeated alternations of vasodilatation and vasoconstriction; this process is known as the Hunting reaction of Lewis.

There is a reduction in spasticity and spasm, and although the mechanism of this response is not fully understood, it is thought that the reduction in the rate of conduction of nerve fibres is a contributory factor.

The reduction in spasticity is purely temporary, therefore cold should not be applied in isolation but must be used with other treatments aimed at a more permanent control of spasticity. Pain-induced spasm may be reduced permanently if the pain/spasm/pain cycle is broken.

Dangers and contra-indications of applying cold

1. *Ice burns.* These may occur when the skin is super-cooled and may be produced when ice or cold material, such as metal, freeze onto the patient's skin. Where there is a danger of an ice burn, it may be prevented by covering the skin with a thin layer of vegetable oil.
2. *Shock*, particularly in the treatment of the aged, or those with heart conditions.
3. *Circulatory impairment.*
4. *Bacterial infection.*

Therapeutic objectives

1. *Relief of pain.* Cold application is a very effective method of pain relief, although the relief obtained is only temporary.
2. *Reduction of spasticity and spasm.*
3. *Reduction of oedema* The stimulating effect on the circulation of cold application results in a reduction in the amount of oedema produced and aids the removal of any already formed. It is of particular benefit in the treatment of trauma immediately following injury.

Methods of applying cold

1. Cold compresses

These are an easy way of applying cold to an affected part. There are a number of application techniques. Whichever method is chosen there is little danger of producing an ice burn.

The towels are soaked in a bucket with two parts ice and one of cold water. A towel is then wrung dry and applied to the affected part for no more than 2 minutes when it is removed and another towel is applied; this process is continued for about 15 minutes.

Another method is to soak layers of lint or gauze in evaporating cooling lotions such as witch hazel, alcohol or Burow's solution and apply them directly to the skin over the affected part.

2. Immersion

Immersion is usually in the form of foot baths, which can be of cold water or ice slush, and are particularly suitable for home use. The method of use is to immerse the foot for one to five minutes twice or three times daily.

3. Ice packs

Crushed ice is placed in a container and applied to the part. The containers may be specially made waterproof bags, bags made from terry towelling or hand made, by wrapping the crushed ice in a terry towel which is folded into shape. Care must be taken that the ice does not leak and come into contact with the skin or it may produce a burn. To prevent this the skin at and surrounding the treatment area should be coated with a thin layer of oil before application.

4. Cold packs

It is now possible to buy proprietary flexible cold packs which contain a gel which crystallises at −15°C, but does not freeze solid. These packs can be kept refrigerated until necessary. To apply, follow the instruction which are usually printed on the pack.

5. Cold sprays

Various aerosols are manufactured which cool the skin through evaporation. These are sprayed directly onto the affected area for five seconds and this process can be repeated four or five times at half-minutes intervals. They are effective in reducing pain and swelling in acute traumatic inflammation and muscle spasm, but must not be used where the skin is broken.

REHABILITATION

Electrical stimulation

Electrical stimulation is often used to initiate a muscle contraction when the ability to contract has been lost due to pain inhibition, or when the movement pathway has been lost, perhaps due to disuse. Electrical stimulation is also effective in the early stages of rehabilitation of muscle action following surgery involving joint remodelling or muscle realignment.

Electrical stimulations should not be given as purely passive nor long-term treatment. The patient must be instructed to join in and to try to contract their muscles with the machines. When they can perform the action voluntarily, electrical stimulation is no longer required and the patient can continue with a fully active rehabilitation programme.

Electrical stimulation is given in the form of Faradic type current, which produces tetanic muscle contraction; this is then surged to produce a rhythmic contraction which is similar to a normal muscle action. Most Faradic stimulating machines produce the currents and surge automatically; many are small battery-powered units which are fully portable.

The common method for treating the foot is to use a foot bath with enough water to cover the sole of the foot, but not enough for the foot to be immersed. To stimulate intrinsic muscles, for conditions such as pes planus and metatarsalgia, an electrode is placed under the heel and another under the metatarsal heads (Fig. 14.4). The intensity is then increased and the patient is instructed to join in with the machine. As the patient begins to control the action, the intensity of the machine is gradually reduced to zero. To

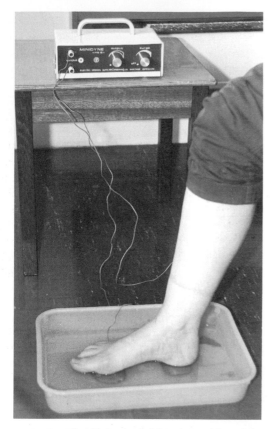

Fig. 14.4   A Faradic footbath. Note the position of the electrodes for stimulation of the plantar intrinsic muscles.

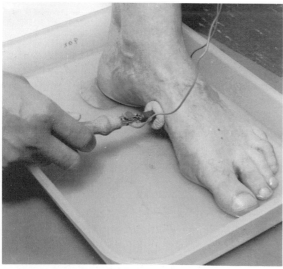

Fig. 14.5   Faradic footbath showing use of a button electrode to stimulate the abductor hallucis via its motor point. The plate electrode under the heel serves to complete the electrical circuit.

stimulate the abductor hallucis, the same procedure is used with the electrodes placed towards the medial side of the foot, or one electrode under the heel and another on the motor point of the abductor hallucis (Fig. 14.5).

PASSIVE STRETCHING AND EXERCISES

Movement can be brought about in two ways: passively, when an operator moves the part with no involvement of the patient, or actively, when the patients move the part for themselves by their own muscle action. Passive movements are used to maintain movement and, when used to increase movement by stretching tightened structures, are known as passive stretching. Active exercises are used to increase strength, improve coordination, balance and gait, and to retain movement pathways between the brain and the muscles.

Passive stretching

This is an effective method of stretching soft tissue, and is used in the reduction of some deformities. Before undertaking any passive stretching, it is essential that the clinician forms an accurate picture of the deformity. This requires careful examination, including X-ray study, observations of the position of the foot, its movements and the patient's gait, and a detailed physical examination of the part.

Correction by manual stretching is carried out with the proximal part being firmly held in one hand and the other hand giving a stretch to the distal party in the required direction. The corrected position is held for a few seconds with a slight overstretch. This should be repeated at least 10 times per day.

For deformities with more than one joint affected, each joint must be stretched in turn, starting proximally. For example, when treating talipes equino-varus, the deformities of the ankle, talonavicular and calcaneocuboid joints must be corrected in that order, each corrected position being held whilst the next is corrected.

Often it is necessary to teach a relative to carry out passive stretching. Careful explanation and demonstrations must be given and it is essential that the relative not only understands the procedure but that the clinician is satisfied that it is carried out correctly. Regular checks on progress and evaluation must be carried out by the clinician.

Active exercises

Active exercises are given with three main objectives of mobilising the joints, strengthening muscles, and ultimately restoring the function of the foot. In addition to these primary objectives are the associated objectives of improving posture and gait.

It is often necessary to start a rehabilitation programme with Faradic footbaths in order to retrain the movement pathways, before progressing to active exercises.

Mobility

Not only must the joints of the foot be considered individually, the foot should also be considered as a single functioning unit which must be mobile enough to adapt to varying surfaces, from level even ground to cobbled streets and grassy slopes.

To achieve or maintain mobility, passive stretching may be performed first to stretch tight soft tissues and reduce any deformity, but this must be followed by active exercises. Exercises should be performed slowly to enable the full range of any movement to be achieved. These may be perfomed as free exercises, in which the foot moves freely itself, or exercises using the body weight to increase the range of movement.

Examples of free exercises are:

1. Sitting with a leg crossed over the other leg, and with the lower leg remaining still, draw a large circle in the air with the big toe. Attention must be given to obtaining the full range of the movement.
2. Sitting and trying to place the soles of both feet together.
3. Fun-like exercises, which are good for children and adults alike, like tying knots in cord and picking up balls with both feet.

Examples of weight-bearing exercises are:

1. Standing with one foot in front of the other,

lean forwards by bending the front knee while keeping both feet flat on the ground.
2. Standing with one foot in front of the other, lean forwards, and rise up onto the toes of both feet.

Strengthening

Care must be taken when strengthening to ensure that the correct muscles are strengthened. Strengthening the wrong muscle group can lead to muscle imbalance and an increase in a deformity. If the intrinsic muscles of the foot need to be strengthened, exercises must be given to the intrinsics which will not include the long flexors, as imbalance between these two groups may result in an unmodified action of the long flexors, which can lead to claw toes and metatarsalgia.

Examples of strengthening exercises are:

1. Sitting with the feet flat on the floor and with the toes kept straight, raise the ball of the foot and draw the flat toes towards the heel. The toes must not be allowed to curl as this would bring into use the long flexors of the toes.
2. Sitting with toes relaxed, spread the toes.
3. Fun activities, e.g. tearing a newspaper into small pieces; or, if treating more than one person, tug-of-war games with clothbands, blankets, etc.

Functional exercises

When devising functional exercises, it is important to consider the age, occupation and social aims of the patient in addition to the accepted function of balance and gait. Are the needs of an athlete with a sedentary occupation different from those of a window cleaner, and to what extent is foot and ankle mobility important to a lorry or bus driver? Questions like these must be answered for functional exercises to be relevant.

The main function which concerns most people is that of gait. For a person to walk with an acceptable gait there must be:

1. Sufficient muscle strength to enable a good push off and control of the heel strike during the swing phase, and to maintain the balance of the body during the support phase.

2. Sufficient mobility to enable the foot to clear the ground during the swing phase.
3. Evenness in length and timing of each stride.
4. An identical sequence of events for both limbs

Examples of functional exercises to help re-educate gait are:

1. Standing with both feet together, with support if required, raise alternate feet off the ground. This will encourage balance, and should be done rhythmically to begin to train the timing required for normal gait. If a support is used, it should be progressively lessened and finally removed in order to progress to full unsupported standing and walking.

2. Standing with one foot in front of the other as in walking, rock forwards and backwards with a heel and toe action.
3. Walk forwards and backwards. It is often helpful to walk in front of a mirror so that abnormalities in a gait pattern can be seen, noted and rectified.

When giving any physical therapy regime as part of a rehabilitation programme, it must be remembered that although the treatment is under the control of the clinician, full and satisfactory progress can only be achieved with the cooperation of the patient, and preferably with added support and encouragement from friends and relatives.

FURTHER READING

Forster A, Palastagna N 1985 Clayton's electrotherapy: theory and practice, 9th edn. Baillière Tindall, London

Gardiner D M 1981 The principle of exercise therapy, 4th edn. Bell and Hyman, London

15. Principles of infection control

John C. McDermott

The prevention of all treatment-associated infection, both in their patients and in staff themselves, is an integral part of the professional responsibilities of podiatrists. An increasing awareness of hepatitis B and AIDS has heightened the concern of health care personnel over risks of infection. While concern over infections caused by hepatitis B virus (HBV) and human immunodeficiency viruses (HIV) has focused attention on danger in clinical practice, they must be viewed in the context of infection control in general.

The basic principles and terminology of infection and its control are considered here but, because initial training, professional experience and working circumstances vary greatly, it is impossible to dictate a single infection control regime suitable for all practitioners. However, equipped with a sound knowledge of the principles involved, individuals can select and implement measures most appropriate to their own practice.

INFECTION

Terminology

The fields of infection and infection control have evolved specialised terminology but, unfortunately, universally agreed definitions of all terms are not available, some variation in usage being demonstrated in published literature. However, there *is* agreement on the essential concepts and these are the basis of the following summary of terminology and associated information.

Pathogen

Pathogenicity is the ability of a microorganism to invade a host and cause disease, hence organisms which do so are termed pathogens. However, it is important to realise that the original concept of there being pathogens and non-pathogens must be modified in the light of modern knowledge. While only true (virulent) pathogens may cause infection in a completely healthy host, there are many other which can cause infection if the body is weakened in some way. These *opportunistic pathogens* demonstrate that infection is but one outcome of a complex relationship between the body and microorganisms, infection occuring when the balance of circumstances favours a potential pathogen. Given appropriate circumstances, virtually all microorganisms are potential pathogens.

Infection

Infection is the multiplication of microorganisms in or on the tissues of the body. Note that this differs from '*contamination*', which merely implies the presence of microorganisms which may or may not become established. Infection triggers a response by the body's specific immune system and products of this response, e.g. antibodies against the organism, can be used to detect infection or to monitor progress of an infection.

Importantly, not all infections result in clinical infection, i.e. visible disease symptoms. Lower level infections occur in which microorganisms become established and there is immune response but no clinical symptoms become apparent, i.e. subclinical infection is present. Even infections which eventually become overt will not show clinical symptoms in the early stages.

Infective dose

The number of cells/particles of a microorganism which are required to establish infection is referred to as the infective dose. Pathogens differ in infective dose, some requiring smaller numbers for successful invasion than others. More importantly, for any infectious agent, the greater the number contacting the body the more probable is establishment of infection. It follows that practical measures taken to reduce the number of microorganisms reaching the patient's tissue will reduce the likelihood of infection.

It is not possible to achieve the complete absence of microorganisms in the proximity of a patient. However, for minor non-invasive procedures, appropriate cleaning or disinfection will reduce the probability of microorganisms reaching the body in sufficient numbers to cause infection. When the body is more susceptible to invasion, e.g. due to surgery or other tissue damage, more stringent efforts must be made by the use of sterile instruments and aseptic techniques to minimise the numbers of microorganisms entering tissue.

Colonisation

This differs from infection; in colonisation an organism becomes established in or on the body but neither symptoms nor an immune response occur. However, colonisation may progress to infection should circumstances subsequently favour the microorganism.

Carriers

Carriers are people colonised or subclinically infected with a pathogen who show no clear symptoms but who are nevertheless infectious. The carrier state may be preceded by clinical infection but not necessarily. Carrier states may be temporary or long term, even permanent. Relevant pathogens include *Staphylococcus aureus*, HBV and HIV.

Sources of infection

A source is a site where potential pathogens can grow and multiply. A similar but more variable term is *reservoir of infection*, which has been used for sites where survival rather than growth occurs, as an alternative to *source*, or to describe a particular category of source. It will be used here for sites where survival rather than growth is to be expected.

Vehicles of infection

Many movable objects can become contaminated and transfer microorganisms to a susceptible person or body site. Some are naturally mobile because of their lightness, e.g. minute skin scales or respiratory droplets; while others are deliberately moved, e.g. instruments. Such objects are vehicles of infection, capable of transmitting an infective dose but not usually supporting microbial growth. Viruses, in particular, cannot multiply outside host cells but transmission can occur via contaminated instruments, e.g. wart viruses, HBV and HIV.

The preceding points have important implications for infection control. While it is relatively straightfoward to identify high-risk vehicles (e.g. instruments) and to render them safe by appropriate techniques, individual sources of infection are less easily identified. In particular, staff or patients colonised or in a symptomless stage of infection are sources but will not exhibit convenient symptoms warning of a possible infection risk. Continual awareness of the potential threat from sources, even unidentified ones, is required and safe working practices which minimise the risk of infection from such sources must be implemented.

Cross infection

The term cross infection is used specifically in clinical contexts to describe the spread of infections to patients from staff or other patients. It often involves staff-patient contact or transfer of organisms via clinical equipment. Cross infection is a significant risk to patients and many control procedures are aimed at its prevention.

Portals of entry

These are sites by which microorganisms gain access to the body, most pathogens having one usual portal although some are more versatile.

Once established, organisms may remain near the entry site, causing localised infection, or spread internally to involve other areas of the body. The respiratory, gastrointestinal and genitourinary tracts are common portals of entry but microorganisms rarely penetrate intact healthy skin.

Entry through skin is usually via damaged areas including minute abrasions, sites damaged by pressure, venous ulcers, and areas weakened by excessive exposure to moisture. Deliberate penetration occurs in surgery but damage may also result from other procedures, e.g. nail reduction or treatment of keratoses and verrucae. As the skin is an important defence of the body, every effort should be made to avoid unnecessary damage and accidental penetration during procedures. Furthermore, any article penetrating skin or contacting damaged tissue is a potential vehicle of infection and must be free of microorganisms which it could transport across the integument barrier.

Portals of exit

These are sites from which pathogens exit the body and from where they are spread to other people, or other sites on the same body. Portals of entry and exit are often one and the same, e.g. infected wounds exuding pus, but pathogens causing systemic infections may exit from different sites. HBV and HIV may exit from any site where bleeding is caused by deliberate or accidental penetration of skin. Pathogens infecting superficial tissues (e.g. dermatophyte fungi, warts viruses, *Streptococcus pyogenes*) will be shed in skin particles or lesion exudates, while other pathogens whose primary target is not skin may, particularly in advanced cases, cause skin lesions containing the infectious agent, e.g. tuberculosis.

The spread of infectious material from exit sites must be minimised by, for example, use of adequate dressings on infected lesions, safe disposal of contaminated dressings and decontamination of instruments.

Normal flora of the body

Every human body is colonised by a large number of commensal microorganisms — the 'normal flora' of the body. Many species, mainly but not exclusively bacterial, occur amongst the flora and different body sites support mixed populations of organisms suited to the particular conditions. The skin, mouth, upper respiratory tract and the large intestine are important sites of body flora.

The skin has not only a resident flora which is permanently present (e.g. *Staph. epidermidis*) but it is also frequently contaminated with flora from other body sites. These do not usually become established permanently on skin but are so often present that they may be considered as transient normal flora. Above the waist, organisms from the respiratory tract often occur, e.g. *Staph. aureus*, while below the waist intestinal species may be present, e.g. *Pseudomonas* spp. At any time, additional transient contaminants acquired from the environment and other people may occur on the skin.

In health, the normal body flora is harmless or even beneficial, it presents competition to the establishment of incoming pathogens. However, it includes species which, while usually harmless in their normal sites, can be serious pathogens in wounds or damaged skin, e.g. *Staph. aureus* and *Strep. pyogenes*. In circumstances when local conditions allow excessive growth of a commensal species (e.g. erythrasma), or contamination of wounds occurs, or the body is weakened by systemic disease (e.g. venous ulcers in diabetics), many other commensal species act as opportunistic pathogens of skin tissue.

Chief sources and reservoirs of infection

The chief sources of infection may be categorised as:

Endogenous: sites of flora or infection on a person's own body

Exogenous: infected or colonised people; infected or colonised animals; environmental sources.

Endogenous sources

Infections of wounds and damaged skin are most commonly caused by organisms from the patient's own body which gain access to vulnerable areas on the foot. Examples include:

Staph. aureus from nasal flora or, in some people, from colonised skin sites. This organism is commonly involved in external wound infections.
Strep. pyogenes from the throat or mouth.
Corynebacterium minutissimum from skin flora.
Candida albicans, a fungal opportunist, e.g. from skin or mouth.

Various intestinal bacteria such as:
Escherichia coli
Pseudomonas aeruginosa
Klebsiella spp.
Proteus spp.
Clostridium perfringens (previously C. welchii).

In addition to sites of body flora, any existing infected area (e.g. boils, ulcers) is a dangerous potential source from which pathogens can be transferred to damaged tissue.

The importance of endogenous sources in potential wound infections means that local flora must be reduced before invasive procedures, and transmission of organisms from other body sites must be prevented.

Exogenous sources

Infected or colonised people. In clinical situations, important and obvious sources of cross infection are staff or patients with clinical infections of the skin or other accessible sites, e.g. the respiratory tract. However, it is worth reiterating that human sources of various pathogens, including HBV or HIV, are often in symptomless states.

Commoner sources of cross infection are sites of flora on staff or other patients which, while harmlessly colonising those people, can cause infection if transferred to vulnerable foot tissue, e.g. approximately 30% of patients and staff will be nasal and/or skin carriers of Staph. aureus.

Infected or colonised animals. Animals can be colonised or infected by microorganisms which can cause human infections. Patients attending for treatment may have been infected from domestic animals, e.g. by zoophilic dermato-

phytes such as *Microsporum canis*. Infestation of premises by mice, cockroaches or Pharoah's ants may occur (Pharoah's ants are a minute, inconspicuous species sometimes encountered in warm hospital environments). Such vermin and pests can harbour pathogens, including species acquired from clinical and human waste.

Environmental sources and reservoirs. Survival or growth of microorganisms outside the body is determined by their requirements and the environmental conditions. Many microorganisms associated with the human body are unlikely to grow in the environment as they have specific requirements which would be absent, e.g. for complex nutrients or living host cells. All organisms need moisture for growth, therefore even less demanding species are prevented from multiplying by the dryness of most clinical areas. However, wet sites in clinical areas are potential sources or reservoirs, allowing growth of some organisms and aiding survival of others. Any body of standing water supports growth of bacteria, particularly Gram negative bacilli which need minimal nutrients. Wet sites such as soap receptacles, leaks or spillages from pipes or equipment, and residual water in stored utensils, are potential risks. Even aqueous solutions of chemicals, including disinfectants, especially if diluted or ageing, will allow survival and even growth of microorganisms.

Dry sites are reservoirs of viable microorganisms surviving in dirt and dust. In general, Gram negative bacteria survive poorly in dry conditions whereas Gram positive bacteria and fungi survive rather better. The resistance of bacterial spores to desiccation and even disinfection is well established. Protection by materials of bodily origin aids survival, e.g. dried blood, exudate and skin particles. Reduction in numbers due to cleaning procedures is counterbalanced by day to day contamination shed from staff and patients, by clinical waste (e.g. skin and nail debris), and by dirt or dust from clothing and footwear. Therefore, continual effort is required to restrict contamination to acceptable levels.

Transmission of infection

For infection to occur, microorganisms from an

exogenous or endogenous source must be transmitted by some means to a new host or host site. Details of transmission routes vary widely in individual instances but may be generally categorised as follows.

Direct contact transmission

This involves direct physical contact with, or close proximity to, a human source or reservoir. It includes close-range transmission of pathogens in droplets or skin particles shed from the body which fall immediately onto surfaces within 1–2 m, i.e. they do not become truly airborne. Those most likely to transmit exogenous infection to patients are staff who are themselves infected or colonised or whose hands and clothing are contaminated from other patients. Staff involvement in direct contact transmission, especially via hands, is of *major importance* in clinically acquired infections.

Also in this category could be included endogenous infection involving transmission from own-body sites, e.g. wound infections caused by organisms from skin or other sites via hands or clothing. Some pathogens usually spread by direct sexual contact, e.g. HBV and HIV, may also be transmitted by clinical contact if blood contaminates skin or mucous membranes. Measures to prevent contact transmission include hand/skin disinfection, protective clothing and 'no-touch' techniques.

Indirect transmission routes

These usually involve intermediate vehicles which transfer microorganisms from an animate or inanimate source or reservoir to a vulnerable host site. If the pathogens originate from a human source this is often termed indirect contact.

Transmission by clinical items. Any contaminated article coming into proximity or contact with vulnerable tissue is capable of transmitting infection. Background items, e.g. furniture, are relatively low risk while articles in direct patient contact are high risk. Potential vehicles include scalpels, burrs, handpieces and other instruments, swabs, dressings and drapes, antiseptics, syringes and injected solutions. Reusable instruments and multiuse containers of pharmaceuticals are more likely to become contaminated than single-use items. Surfaces including trolley tops may contaminate items placed on them. Adjustable lamps used during procedures may transfer contaminants to and from hands. Surfaces allowed direct contact with patient's skin, e.g. foot rests if not protected by a sheet, can transfer organisms between patients.

Airborne transmission. True airbone transmission, commonly associated with respiratory infections, should have little significance in chiropody procedures. Apart from close range contamination near the body, previously noted, airborne contamination appears to be significant only when tissue is exposed for prolonged periods, e.g. during extensive surgery (Ayliffe & Lowbury 1982; Meers 1983).

However, clinic dust is a reservoir of infection and may contain remnants of skin, nail, blood, pus and lesion exudates. Various activities may render it airborne, to settle afterwards on exposed surfaces. Dry sweeping of skin and nail debris, vigorous movement of curtain screens, overcrowding and unnecessary human activity all increase airborne contamination. While this risk is difficult to quantify, these activities are undesirable near clinical procedures or unprotected sterile items.

Transmission by animals. Vermin and insects may shed contaminants when feeding or defaecating. They may also act simply as vehicles, transferring contamination on their body surfaces from dirty areas, such as drains and disposed wastes. Either way, contamination of the clinical environment, surfaces and unprotected materials may occur.

Faecal transmission. Faecal-oral transmission is of major importance in food and waterborne infections. While this has no direct relevance to podiatry, note that hands and skin are often contaminated with faecal organisms, including potential wound pathogens, after toilet use, and dispersion of such contamination is more likely if diarrhoea is present.

HBV and HIV infections

In view of current concern over HBV and HIV

infections, a brief overview of these infections is given here, drawing on the concepts established above.

Hepatitis B virus

HBV is one of several viruses which can cause hepatitis, i.e. inflammation and necrosis of liver tissue. The combination of HBV infection and the body's immunological response follows a complicated course which may result in a range of consequences. For example:

Subclinical infection: this is the commonest form of infection in adults and is usually undiagnosed.

Acute infection: after a long incubation period (1–6 months) the clinical phase lasts usually for up to a month, after which most patients slowly but fully recover. In rare cases infection leads rapidly to liver failure and death.

Chronic hepatitis (carrier state): develops from the above forms of infection in a minority of cases. These carriers may be symptomless or may undergo progressive liver damage which is eventually fatal. Either carrier state may result ultimately in primary liver cancer.

As with other viruses, the components of HBV are antigenic and some of these antigens, together with the antibodies formed against them, may be present in blood and are used to monitor the infection and to indicate the carrier state. HBsAg is the viral surface antigen which, though not infectious itself, indicates that the person is infected and infectious. This disappears as recovery progresses but its persistence longer than six months after infection indicates a chronic carrier state. Components of the virus inner core are also antigenic, e.g. HBeAg, the presence of which in the blood of carriers indicates that the person is highly infectious.

Human immunodeficiency viruses

Previous names for this group of viruses were lymphadenopathy associated virus (LAV) and human T cell lymphotrophic virus 3 (HTLV3). The main cellular target of HIV infection is a type of T lymphocyte known as T_4 (helper) cells. These cells play a vital part in the body's response to infection by stimulating the activity of other T lymphocytes, B lymphocytes and phagocytic cells. Any reduction in number or function of T_4 cells leads to impaired humoral and cell mediated immunity, with a consequent vulnerability to infection.

HIV infection usually results in HIV antibodies being produced, but these are not protective. Appearance of these antibodies may take several months and some people do not produce them. Thus presence of these antibodies indicates HIV infection (not AIDS), but their absence does not necessarily mean that a person is not infected and infectious.

Individuals positive for anti-HIV antibody present differing states of health, reflecting progressive stages (of very variable duration) of the infection:

- Many remain symptomless carriers for prolonged periods, e.g. several years. Others, though essentially symptomless, have persistent generalised lymphadenopathy (PGL)
- AIDS related complex (ARC): a variable state of ill health short of fully expressed AIDS which may involve PGL, weight loss, diarrhoea and other symptoms, such as minor opportunistic infections (including tinea infections)
- Acquired immune deficiency syndrome (AIDS): drastic reduction in immune defense results in severe opportunistic infections, even by weak opportunists, and unusual tumours
- Nervous system involvement may also occur which can result, e.g. in presenile dementia and peripheral neuropathy.

The proportion of HIV infections which will result in symptoms is unknown; to date, many anti HIV antibody positives have developed some form of ill health up to and including AIDS, and it may be that all will develop some degree of illness eventually.

Implications for podiatrists

Both viruses are blood borne but are also present in other body fluids including semen and vaginal secretions, hence their association with entry of blood through mucous membranes or damaged skin, and with sexual transmission. Both infections have an increased incidence in certain groups, e.g. illegal drug injectors, homosexual/bisexual males and heterosexuals with multiple sexual partners; but in this context it is much more relevant that these infections are *not* confined to such high risk groups. Both HBV and HIV infections are currently on the increase, both have potentially serious consequences and there is no cure for either, therefore prevention of infection is the only effective strategy.

A podiatrist is unlikely to know whether or not a patient belongs to a high risk group and anyway, other patients not in these categories could still be infected. Therefore practitioners must treat *all* invasive procedures, contacts with blood/tissue fluids, and blood/tissue fluid contamination of instruments as dangerous, however unlikely it seems that the patient constitutes a risk. All sharps used in procedures *must* be sterile. HBV is more infectious and rather hardier than HIV, but this distinction is irrelevant in most circumstances as effective prevention must take into account the possible presence of either virus.

No vaccine is currently available against HIV infection and, although an effective HBV vaccine is now available, only a small minority of the population will be protected by this in the foreseeable future. As health care workers with direct patient contact, podiatrists are an at-risk group and should seek HBV vaccination. In no way does staff vaccination reduce the necessity for other infection control measures which are essential to protect patients from both these, and other, infections.

INFECTION CONTROL

The modern term, infection control, reflects the realistic objective of reducing infection to the practicable minimum rather than claiming the ideal of total prevention. Infection has always been of major concern to professionals involved in surgery and treatment of wounds. Much is now known about prevention of infection generally and wound infections in particular. If the established principles and practices of infection control are implemented, infection following podiatric procedures should be uncommon, especially as many procedures are relatively minor in terms of tissue invasion. Infection control in clinics must encompass measures to prevent patient infections from both endogenous and exogenous sources, and also to protect staff from becoming infected from patients.

Knowledge of infection control in clinical situations stems largely from efforts to prevent infections in hospitals and comprehensive texts on these aspects have been produced (e.g. Lowbury et al 1981; Bennett & Brachman 1986; Aycliffe et al 1990). In addition, The Society of Chiropodists (Anon, 1987) has indicated to its members recommended procedures for particular aspects of routine practice. The following section will summarise the underlying principles of infection control in the context of podiatry and indicate how they provide a rational basis for safe procedures.

Terminology

Sterilisation

This is a process which renders an item free from all living microorganisms, i.e. it becomes sterile (British Standard 5283: 1986). There are no degrees of sterilisation; all microorganisms, including bacterial spores, must be killed or removed. Any process which does not achieve this is a disinfection and not a sterilisation process. Sterilants are chemical agents capable of sterilising, but few can achieve this in routine podiatric circumstances.

Disinfection

Disinfection is a process by which microorganisms are reduced to a level harmless to health. In contrast to sterilisation, there are degrees of disinfection, the level of microbial reduction considered necessary being dependent on the item to be disinfected and the infection risk it presents. Bacterial spores are often little affected. Disinfection, unlike sterilisation, can be applied to living tissue, e.g. skin, as well as to inanimate articles.

Disinfection methods, particularly chemical

disinfectants, often demonstrate a particular spectrum of antimicrobial activity, varying in effectiveness against different types of micro-organisms. The terms *bactericidal* and *fungicidal* indicate capability of killing bacteria and fungi respectively. Similarly, *sporicidal* and *virucidal* indicate ability to kill spores or to inactive viruses. These properties are determined under laboratory test conditions and such terms should *not* be taken to mean that disinfection so described or labelled will kill all of the specified type of microorganism under conditions of ordinary use. A term such as *germicide*, while implying anti-microbial activity, is too vague and should not be used.

Antisepsis

Antisepsis is the destruction or inhibition of microorganisms on living tissues, having the effect of limiting or preventing the harmful results of infection (British Standard 5283: 1986). Anti-septics are chemical agents used to achieve antisepsis; they are usually unsuitable for general use on inanimate articles either for reasons of lower antimicrobial action or cost effectiveness. Some antiseptics inhibit rather than kill micro-organisms, this capability being described by terms such as *bacteriostatic* or *fungistatic*.

Asepsis

The term asepsis means an absence of contamina-tion or, perhaps more realistically, absence of infection (sepsis) resulting from contamination. This should be the objective underlying all clinical procedures. Aseptic techniques are safe methods of working on patients by which contamination is minimised and thus infection prevented—in this context largely by the prevention of cross infec-tion and the protection from contamination of damaged foot tissue. As appropriate, both sterili-sation and disinfection are employed to achieve asepsis.

Strategies and methods of control

As microorganisms may be transmitted by so many routes, a similarly wide range of measures must be employed in infection control. All individual control measures stem from the three basic strategies of infection control (Ayton 1981; Lowbury et al 1981):

a. elimination of sources and reservoirs of infection
b. disruption of transmission routes
c. increasing or restoring host resistance to infection.

In any particular circumstances, which will vary for individual practitioners, these strategies provide a framework for a sensible choice of suitable control measures. Strategies a. and b. above are especially relevant to practical podiatry and are discussed in the following sections.

Elimination of sources and reservoirs

Important sources of infection are patients with existing clinical infections, e.g. septic lesions, fungal infections, verrucae. Successful treatment not only benefits that patient but also eliminates them as a source of cross infection. During a course of treatment, dressings minimise exit of pathogens from such sources. Endogenous infected sites must be covered by dressings before invasive techniques or exposing nearby tissue.

Less commonly, podiatrists providing hospital ward services may encounter *source isolation*. Some patients with serious infections are isolated by a variety of measures to prevent cross infection from them to others. Essentially, both the patient and his immediate environment are considered to be contaminated and measures are enforced to prevent transfer of pathogens from these by either personnel or equipment. Appropriate protective clothing must be donned and, after patient care, must be discarded within the isolation area. Instruments may require special arrangements for decontamination before re-use and thorough hand cleansing after patient contact is most important. Practitioners treating such patients should familiarise themselves with, and adhere to, the isolation procedures in force at that time.

Podiatrists with clinical infections are clearly a risk to patients. Particularly relevant are infections on the hands or other exposed areas of skin, e.g.

furuncles, infected cuts or paronychia. The risk to patients is not necessarily eliminated by wearing gloves and direct contact with patients should be avoided until the infection is resolved. Infections of other parts of the body also constitute a significant risk, e.g. streptococcal sore throat. Skin affected by chronic skin conditions such as eczema or psoriasis may become colonised with *Staph. aureus* and lead to profuse shedding of the organism. Practitioners who become carriers of HBV and HIV are very unlikely to transmit such infection to patients. As infection and circumstances vary greatly, practitioners should seek medical advice if in any doubt of the advisability of contact with patients. Other possible sources amongst staff include symptomless carriers of wound pathogens such as *Staph. aureus* and *Strep. pyogenes*. Routine screening of staff for such carriage is not justified but may be necessary in certain circumstances, e.g. to investigate an outbreak of wound infections.

Accumulations of dirt anywhere in the clinical environment are reservoirs of infection which should be eliminated by cleaning, with additional disinfection if necessary. Clinical waste must not be allowed to contaminate the area and should be disposed of hygienically. Collection of patient debris at source using a disposal bag, partially inserted underneath the sheet protecting the footrest and anchored by the foot (Paterson 1985) is a sensible measure. Wet sites caused by faulty equipment or plumbing can be eliminated by repair or replacement. Other wet sites need a commonsense approach to alteration of working procedures or choice of materials. Examples include disinfecting and drying cleaning utensils before storage, and replacing bar soap lying in a wet dish by cleaner draining storage or, better still, by a suitable detergent/disinfectant dispenser.

Prevention of animal pest infestations is aided by maintenance of building structure (to inhibit access) and high standards of general cleanliness throughout the premises to deny them food, water and breeding sites. Should infestation occur, eradication can be difficult and professional pest control operatives should be contacted. If the source of a patient's infection is found to be a family pet (e.g. *M. canis*) then successful treatment of the person may require veterinary treatment of the animal to prevent reinfection.

Disruption of transmission routes

Essentially, this is achieved by effective decontamination of inanimate vehicles and by procedures designed to exclude contamination at the point of patient contact, the latter including hand/skin disinfection and other aspects of aseptic technique.

Decontamination of inanimate articles is based on cleaning, disinfection and sterilisation. These techniques represent increasing degrees of decontamination and are employed according to the infection hazard posed by particular articles or circumstances. As a general rule, the closer an article approaches susceptible tissue or vulnerable items such as sterile instruments, the more thorough the decontamination required. Cleaning is usually adequate for most general items such as furniture, utensils and laundry. Disinfection is necessary when a specific infection risk is known to exist, e.g. articles in the vicinity of treatment procedures, blood spillages, and for articles which are unsuited to sterilisation but require more thorough decontamination than cleaning. Sterilisation is necessary for all items penetrating the body or contacting exposed tissues.

Cleaning

The clinical environment should present a high standard of general cleanliness. Inadequately cleaned clinics will not only contain unnecessary reservoirs of microorganisms but also reduce patients' confidence and staff morale. Cleaning should not be dismissed as a background chore that has little to do with the professional staff but should be part of an integrated programme of clinical decontamination. In this context, it implies thorough cleaning at sufficiently frequent intervals using effective agents and appropriate, well maintained equipment. Such cleaning is a surprisingly efficient method of decontamination and is all that is usually necessary for routine surfaces and equipment such as floors, furniture, sinks, toilet facilities and similar items.

Disinfection of these is unnecessary because first, such items normally present an insignificant infection risk, and secondly, recontamination is inevitable and reaches a similar equilibrium level whether or not disinfectants are used (Ayliffe et al 1966, 1967). However, disinfection is justified for such items on specific occasions of known risk, e.g. blood spillage.

In addition to preventing excessive accumulations of contaminated dirt, cleaning should not itself increase any risk of infection. Both the methods and materials employed must themselves be hygienic. There are two main dangers here: the distribution of dust-borne contamination and the growth of bacteria on wet cleaning utensils. Dry dusting or sweeping, including the sweeping up of debris after patient treatment, is not acceptable in clinical areas and suitable vacuum cleaners or dust-attracting mops should be used instead. Vacuum cleaners should incorporate efficient filters, regularly checked and replaced as necessary, and inner disposable paper bags which retain debris and microorganisms. Dust-attracting mops must themselves be cleaned as soon as they are visibly dirty or at least every 1–2 days.

Wet cleaning should be done with clean water and a detergent, changed frequently to maintain effectiveness. Cloths, preferably disposable for damp dusting surfaces and 'string mops' for cleaning floors, are more suitable than sponge utensils which are less easy to decontaminate after use. Utensils for wet cleaning are known to support the growth of bacteria, particularly Gram negatives, if they are not effectively decontaminated after use. Ideally, such items as reusable cloths, mopheads, buckets and wet parts of cleaning machines should be cleaned after use, heat disinfected if possible, and then stored dry. Unless serviced by a centralised hospital cleaning service, practitioners may consider this an unattainable standard but serious efforts should be made to avoid heavy contamination of wet utensils which in turn would contaminate the very items they are supposed to clean. Utensils should at least be cleaned in fresh hot water and detergent then rinsed and dried. Storage of all ancillary equipment including cleaning materials should, of course, be separate from the area used for patient treatment. Routine cleaning activities, even if well

done, carry a risk of dust disturbance or splashing and should be completed as long as possible (ideally at least an hour) before treatment of patients, to allow airbone contamination to finish settling.

Floors, toilet facilities and furniture should be washed or damp dusted daily as appropriate. Sinks also require thorough cleaning daily, and additional cleaning if soiled during use, with either detergent or mild abrasive cleaning products. Sites which could harbour stagnant water, e.g. soap ledges, must be dried. Walls in good repair are of little significance in infection and unless soiled require infrequent cleaning; every few months should suffice. In contrast, adjustable lamps positioned immediately above the patient and which are frequently handled should be cleaned daily and disinfection between patients could be recommended.

Some exceptions to daily cleaning of floors and furniture may be necessary. If floor areas on which patients walk barefoot exist, there is the risk of cross infection and careful organisation of patient movements or use of overshoes could eradicate this. As some foot conditions will render patients vulnerable to infections, while other patients may have existing infections, it is difficult to justify contact with a floor that is not at least cleaned between patients. Similarly, furniture or surfaces in the immediate vicinity of treatment procedures justify extra cleaning and even disinfection between patients, especially before invasive procedures.

Used instruments should be cleaned before further decontamination and reuse. After a rinse in cold water they may be cleaned manually using a brush and mild detergent. Rubber gloves should be worn, as thick as is consistent with dexterity, and every care taken to avoid accidental injury while cleaning, rinsing and drying sharps because of the risk of HBV and HIV infections. Used instrument brushes should be cleaned and disinfected, preferably sterilised, and not simply left by the sink. Instruments and other utensils should not be cleaned in the same sink used for clinical handwashing but, if this is completely unavoidable, the sink should be cleaned and disinfected after use for instruments. Alternatively, ultrasonic cleaning in detergent solution can be employed for instruments, in which case manufacturer's instructions on method and suitable agents should be followed. Note that ultrasonic baths are a cleaning aid only and do not kill microorganisms —they may even disperse aerosols of microorganisms if lids are not tightly fitted. Furthermore, they should not be allowed to retain water or stagnant cleaning solution, which could support the accumulation of bacteria. For further details of cleaning methods and agents the reader is referred to comprehensive texts on clinical hygiene (e.g. Maurer 1985).

Disinfection

Many agents have been employed for disinfection in clinical situations, including steam, hot water, chemical vapours, chemical solutions and ultraviolet radiation. The agents most relevant to podiatric clinics generally are hot water and chemical disinfectants. Hot water has the advantage of being effective against all types of microorganisms except bacterial spores; it needs little expertise, leaves no residues and is inexpensive. However, it is unsuitable for very heat labile items, cannot be used on living tissue, and is not practicable for larger items. Chemical disinfectants can be used on surfaces and furniture, and some are suitable for skin disinfection. Unfortunately, as a group they have many disadvantages including possible toxicity, corrosiveness, variable antimicrobial effectiveness, inactivation by many materials, undesirable odours or residues, limited in-use life, and a general requirement for skilled use to be effective.

Despite the widespread use of chemical disinfectants in the past, it is now accepted that they should be used only when there is a clear need for disinfection additional to thorough cleaning, and when no practical alternative is available. If possible, hot water should be used instead, particularly as items too sensitive for heat sterilisation often withstand the lower temperatures used for disinfection.

In summary, heat disinfection is the preferred method for inanimate items of suitable size for immersion whereas chemicals are employed for larger items and surfaces, for skin disinfection, and when heat is not practicable.

Disinfection by hot water. Articles should be cleaned first then fully immersed in hot water, ensuring parts are not protected by trapped air. Temperatures of at least 65°C are necessary; higher temperatures decrease the time required for effective disinfection. For routine use:

Temperature(°C)	Minimum time
65	10 min
70	2 min
90	1 sec

Such treatments are recommended to kill vegetative bacteria on items such as heat labile instruments (Central Sterilising Club 1986). Thermostatically controlled washer/disinfectors with timed cycles, and washing machines incorporating a disinfecting hot water rinse, are available. Heat resistant instruments should be immersed in boiling water for at least 5 minutes (BMA 1989). 'Instrument boilers' need careful use as they usually lack time controlled cycles and also can pose problems of operator safety. It must be emphasised that disinfection, even at high temperatures, is not sterilisation and it should not be used when sterility is required.

Disinfection by chemicals. Despite their disadvantages, chemical disinfectants are required for certain tasks and are effective when used correctly. However, users should be aware of various factors which influence the efficiency of disinfectants.

Concentration of disinfectant solutions is important in determining efficiency and recommendations of manufacturers or suppliers must be followed. For this reason solutions should never be 'topped up' by the addition of more water, with or without additional disinfectant. Once prepared, in-use solutions deteriorate, resulting eventually in a lower actual concentration which is ineffective. If possible make up fresh solutions daily; this need not be wasteful if appropriate quantities are prepared. Otherwise, it is essential to note shelf life information and to prepare fresh solutions when required, marking the date prepared and use-by date as appropriate. Remember that disinfectant solutions can act as sources or reservoirs of pathogens.

All disinfectants can be inactivated to some extent by various natural or synthetic materials such as hard water, detergents, soaps, tissue or other body material, cork, cellulose (e.g. cotton wool) and plastics. This is potentially serious as many articles used to contain or apply the disinfectants, and items for disinfection themselves, may reduce the effectiveness of the process.

Dirt, especially dried organic materials, may inhibit disinfectants by inactivation and by presenting a physical barrier to penetration of the solution. The level of initial microbial contamination also influences the number of microorganisms surviving after a given treatment. Therefore, if possible, articles should be cleaned to remove dirt and reduce contamination before disinfection.

Disinfection is not instantaneous and adequate contact time must be allowed. This varies from seconds to prolonged soaking, depending on the agent and the item involved. Disinfection is accelerated at higher temperatures and solutions in warm/hot water should be used when practicable.

An important and very variable factor in chemical disinfection is the user, and many studies have shown human ignorance or error to be responsible for ineffective clinical disinfection. The number of different chemical agents should be kept to a minimum and clear instructions must be available on preparation, circumstances for use, method of use and acceptable in-use life.

Types of chemical disinfectants. Many categories of chemicals have been used in disinfection but relatively few are suitable for clinical use. Others, while effective, have been superseded by more modern agents. Properties of the chief types in current use are summarised here.

Phenolic compounds: these are widely effective against bacteria and fungi but are poorer against viruses. Organic matter has little inactivating effect, therefore they are suitable for use in dirty conditions or on soiled items, but not when there is contamination by blood. In-use concentration is usually 1 or 2% v/v for clean and dirty conditions respectively. Combination with a suitable detergent (anionic or non-ionic) aids penetration of dirt but they are inactivated by cationic detergents. Clear soluble phenolics (e.g. Stericol, Clearsol and similar products) are preferable to cruder coal tar derivatives and are used for environmental disinfection in hospitals, e.g. for contaminated areas and floors, and for operating rooms. 'Pine' type products, though chemically related are often poor disinfectants and are too easily inactivated to be generally accepted for clinical use.

Chlorine compounds: these are very effective against most microorganisms including viruses. They are usually the agent of choice when there is risk of viral infection, including blood spillages. However, they are more easily inactivated by organic matter than phenolics therefore items must be cleaned first, or sufficiently high concentration used to compensate for the loss. It is important to ensure adequate activity of the in-use solution, usually expressed in terms of % or ppm (parts per million) of available chlorine. Solutions for routine clinical use should contain 1000 ppm (0.1%) and strong solutions (e.g. for blood spillage) 10 000 ppm (1%) available chlorine. Products may be purchased as liquid concentrates, powders or tablets which are diluted or dissolved in water. Typical chlorine-releasing agents employed as ingredients include hypochlorites and dichloroisocyanurates (NaDCC). Product information must enable accurate calculation of available chlorine concentration.

Sample calculation:

Thickened liquid concentrates (e.g. Domestos) typically contain 10% (100 000 ppm) available chlorine. If diluted in water, a 1% v/v solution (1 volume disinfectant to 99 volumes water) would contain 100 000/100 = 1000 ppm (0.1%) available chlorine. A cautionary note on liquid concentrates: concentration varies between brands and degeneration can occur in storage (Coates 1988).

Dichloroisocyanurate tablets are available, which have the advantages of long storage stability and simplicity of preparing in-use dilutions (Coates 1985).

Iodine compounds: alcoholic solutions of iodine are effective disinfectants but cause tissue irritation and staining. Improved alternatives are available. Iodophors, which are organic complexes containing iodine (e.g. povidone-iodine), are less irritant and less likely to stain. Iodophors have a wide spectrum of activity against bacteria, fungi, viruses and, unusually, bacterial spores on prolonged contact. Iodophor preparations are used for skin and hand disinfection, and wound antisepsis.

Alcohols: ethyl and isopropyl alcohols have a wide and rapid antibacterial action, but a poorer action against some viruses. They are most effective in aqueous solution, typical concentrations being ethanol at 70% and isopropanol at 60 – 70%, though higher concentrations are sometimes used. They may be used for rapid disinfection of skin and hands, clean surfaces, and for combination with other antimicrobial agents. Ready to use disposable wipes containing isopropanol are available.

Biguanide compounds: the most widely used is chlorhexidine (Hibitane) which is effective against Gram positive and Gram negative bacteria but poor against viruses. Combination with alcohol increases its effectiveness and accelerates disinfection. It is inactivated by many materials, including soaps and anionic detergents, and cannot be recommended for general environmental use. However, it is widely used for skin and hand disinfection, showing very little toxicity and having both immediate and residual action.

Triclosan (2,4,4'-trichlor-2'-hydroxydiphenylether): effective against Gram positive and Gram negative bacteria with little reported toxicity. Available both as aqueous and alcoholic preparations (e.g. Aquasept, Manusept). Several have been reported to be effective in hand disinfection and show cumulative action (Bartzokas et al 1983).

Quaternary ammonium compounds: a group of chemicals which have both surfactive and disinfectant properties, to varying degrees. Although active against Gram positive bacteria, they are poor against other microorganisms and are too easily inactivated for clinical use. However, cetrimide is one which, in combination with chlorhexidine, provides effective wound cleansing agents (Savlon-type products).

Glutaraldehyde: this has been used widely for cold 'sterilisation' in podiatry, although probably only disinfection was achieved in normal practice. It is a widely effective disinfectant, with good antiviral action, and is sporicidal in certain conditions. Thorough disinfection requires 20 – 30 minutes immersion (sterilisation requires 3 – 10 hours). As it is irritant, disinfected items should be rinsed in sterile water. Glutaraldehyde (e.g. Cidex) still has restricted specialised use in hospitals but its routine use in podiatry cannot be recomended. Alternative disinfection, or sterilisation by heat, should be used for items previously treated by glutaraldehyde.

Hexachlorophane: this once popular compound is effective against Gram positive bacteria but poor against other microorganisms. Chlorhexidine and povidone-iodine products are more generally effective after single or repeated applications, therefore are to be preferred.

Disinfection of specific items. Items suitable for heat disinfection include cleaning utensils (especially if used in operating rooms or on contaminated areas), routine laundry, instrument brushes, reagent bottles before refilling, containers for antiseptics, general purpose bowls, and containers for non-sterile cotton balls, etc. Sterilisation of some of these may preferable, e.g. instrument brushes. In the absence of sophisticated disinfection facilities, cloths and mops may be cleaned then placed in a container to which boiling water is added and kept immersed for at least ten minutes before drying and storing dry. Alternatively, after cleaning they can be immersed in a 1% phenolic or chlorine based disinfectant for thirty minutes then rinsed and stored dry. Note that some materials, e.g. plastics, may inactivate disinfectants and that utensils should be stored dry, not in disinfectant. Clinical laundry can be cleaned in an ordinary automatic using a prewash followed by a wash at the highest temperature setting, unless known contamination by HBV is present.

Floor areas contaminated with tissue other than blood should be cleaned and disinfected with 1% phenolic. Blood spillages require disinfection targeted at possible contamination by HBV or HIV; rubber gloves should be donned and the spillage covered with paper towels or similar disposable material. Strong hypochlorite solution (10000 ppm available chlorine) is then poured on and left for at least 10, preferably 30 minutes. The towels are discarded as contaminated waste for incineration and the area is then cleaned. The gloves may be thoroughly washed and reused. Alternatively, purpose made packs of granular Na DCC are available for spillage treatment, in which case the manufacturer's instructions should be followed.

Small areas of clean impervious surfaces, e.g. trolley tops, footrests, adjustable lamps, and other hand-contact surfaces in the chair's vicinity, can be disinfected with agents that are unsuitable or uneconomic for wider environmental use. Although 1% phenolics could be used, alcohols or alcoholic chlorhexidine, as wipes or sprays, are faster acting/drying and likely to be more convenient for use between patients (e.g. Azowipes, Hibispray and Dispray type products). Cartridges of local anaesthetic should be wiped with alcohol before use. Handpieces are potential vehicles of infection between patients via the operator's hands, and ideally should be sterilsed. If disinfection is used, manufacturers may advise on appropriate methods; alternatively, clean thoroughly then disinfect with alcoholic chlorhexidine .

Skin disinfection. Hands of staff and skin of patients both require adequate decontamination, the degree necessary being dictated by the circumstances. Whatever method is used, effectiveness depends largely on the care and thoroughness of the operator. Handwashing facilities vary but taps operated without hand contact (e.g. foot operated) are best, and if ordinary taps are fitted they should be turned off using a paper towel.

Hands: the main purpose of routine handwashing is to remove transients acquired from previous contacts, particularly patients. Although loosely adhering transients can be removed by washing with ordinary soaps, detergent/disinfectant preparations containing chlorhexidine, povidone-iodine or Triclosan are more effective and on repeated use they also progressively reduce the more accessible flora. Intervening washes with ordinary products eliminate this residual benefit and therefore, as daily case loads may include treatments which require hand disinfection, it is sensible to use disinfectant preparations for all clinic handwashing. However, choice of agent is less important than thoroughness of application (Ayliffe et al 1990). If hands are visibly clean, rapid and highly effective disinfection between patients or during procedures can be achieved with alcoholic disinfectant preparations. Handwashing with non-disinfectant products is not adequate for surgery, invasive techniques, treatment of damaged tissue or dressing changes.

Further reduction of skin contamination is required for some procedures, e.g. nail surgery. The aim is to reduce flora as much as possible on hands and on forearms from where organisms may also be shed. Initially, the hands and forearms are subjected to prolonged double washing with detergent/disinfectant preparations (as above), attention also being paid to cleaning nails and nail folds. If brushing is employed to remove loose skin squames, it should only be done at the start of a clinical session. Use of an alcoholic disinfectant preparation after washing will increase the degree of this initial disinfection. For subsequent cases, these alcoholic preparations alone, well rubbed in, are very effective although washing is necessary if hands are soiled. Note that hand disinfection is not an alternative but an addition to wearing gloves for aseptic procedures.

Hand cream may be employed to offset the drying effects of disinfectant products but it should be one which is compatible as commercial products often inhibit disinfection (Walsh et al 1987); pharmacists can advise on suitable products.

Patients' skin: intact skin should be cleaned before disinfection if possible. As immediate, effective disinfection is required, alcoholic skin disinfectants are the agents of choice. Chlorhexidine is less likely to cause any reaction although povidone-iodine has wider antimicrobial action; normally either is suitable. Friction is an important factor in skin disinfection, rubbing the site thoroughly with the agent (subject to patient comfort) is more effective than merely wiping or spraying. Combined detergent/disinfectants (e.g. Savlon) may be used for damaged skin which requires cleaning. Injections (e.g. local anaesthetic) present little danger of infection but skin is usually prepared by swabbing with alcohol.

Sterilisation. Of the many methods of sterilisation available, only steam at increased pressure or dry heat are likely to be used directly by the podiatrist.

Steam at increased pressure: this is generally recommended for use on clinical materials whenever possible (British Pharmacopoeia 1983).

Steam hot enough to sterilise necessitates pressure vessels, termed sterilisers or *autoclaves*. Saturated steam sterilises articles it contacts, the time required depending on the temperature. Minimum treatments required are:

15 mins at 121°C
10 mins at 126°C
3 mins at 134°C.

Additional time must allowed for heating to sterilisation temperature and for cooling after sterilisation. Saturated steam can be obtained only in the absence of air. In sophisticated equipment, air is evacuated enabling penetration of steam even into wrapped/porous materials (e.g. dressings), and evacuation after sterilisation facilitates drying of such items. The basic models affordable by practitioners rely on simple displacement of air by steam generated within the steriliser. Removal of air, steam penetration and subsequent drying are therefore not as efficient in these models. Although wrapped/porous items may be sterilised, they are usually too wet for clinical use. However, these small sterilisers are very suitable for rapid sterilisation of unwrapped instruments. When removed, instruments must be covered immediately to prevent contamination. A sterile cloth may be used but alternatively, a lid sterilised separately in the same cycle could be clipped onto the instrument tray.

Dry heat: an electrical, fan-assisted hot air oven should be used. Microorganisms are more resistant to dry heat than to steam, therefore higher temperatures, usually 160–180°C, are required for sterilisation within a practicable time, e.g. 20–30 mins at 180°C, (DHSS 1980, British Pharmacopoeia 1983). All items must reach sterilisation temperature before holding time commences. As heating time varies with the load, it is often underestimated, especially for items wrapped or in containers, e.g. individually wrapped small instruments require about 15 minutes initial heat penetration time. Dry heat has the advantage that instruments can be packaged and is suitable for non-stainless steel, but the longer cycle time is a disadvantage.

Whichever method is chosen sterilisers must be of a suitable design (BMA 1989) and should be regularly serviced and tested (DHSS 1980). On a more frequent basis, chemical indicators which change colour when exposed to specific temperatures for sufficient time (e.g. Browne products) are useful to detect failure to achieve sterilising conditions, although they are not an absolute guarantee of sterility. Types are available for steam and dry heat and these are to be recommended, particularly for hot-air sterilisers where it is very difficult to predict the time required for packaged items.

Items which should be sterilised include scalpels, files, burrs, forceps, probes, nail clippers, tissue nippers, drill handpieces (if suitable), scissors, cryosurgical probes and instrument brushes. For other materials obtained pre-sterilised, e.g. dressing packs, it is important to check the integrity of packaging and sterility indicator if present, discarding any that are suspect.

Glass bead sterilisers: these units reach very high temperatures (e.g. 235–250°C) and very short process times are suggested by manufacturers. A recent report on such a unit stated that such temperatures, given adequate time and with certain precautions, 'should be sufficient for the purpose of sterilizing chiropody instruments' (Corner 1987). Further to this provisional acceptance, note that only part of an instrument is treated, use must be immediate and sterilising conditions cannot be checked directly by indicators. For some practitioners such units may represent an improvement on previous instrument treatment but, overall, their use cannot be recommended in a modern fully effective sterilisation programme.

Further microbiological aspects of clinical work

Protective clothing

Any serious attempt at aseptic technique precludes contact of the practitioner's bare hands with damaged skin or exposed tissue, i.e. 'no-touch' techniques should be used. The wearing of sterile gloves for such procedures should be more widely adopted and any claimed reduction in tactile sensitivity can be solved by careful choice of glove size and material. Apart from patient protection, there is the risk of contamination of podiatrists' skin by HBV or HIV and gloves should always be worn for giving injections, changing dressings, cleaning wounds and any invasive procedure. Cuts or abrasions on the hands should be covered by waterproof plasters even when gloves are worn. Hands require washing after a gloved procedure, as not all gloves are structurally perfect.

The wearing of masks is unnecessary for minor procedures including routine dressing changes. Situations requiring masks for the podiatrist's protection include nail drilling and nail surgery, where effective masks to filter/deflect organisms from the mouth away from the operation site are necessary. Masks must be discarded after each use and not worn around the neck to be donned at intervals. Note that drilling of mycotic nails is unwise; not all debris is removed by the drill vacuum and significant amounts escape to contaminate the clinical environment and the practitioner.

The usual clinical coat is satisfactory for many procedures but needs protection when significant debris is expected, particularly from any infected patient, to prevent cross infection occurring via the coat. A gown, plastic apron or adequately sized impermeable paper sheet or drape would serve the purpose. Purpose-made gowns or suits of appropriate material should be used for surgical procedures and hair should be completely covered by a surgical cap. If surgical footwear is fitted, avoid contamination of previously disinfected hands.

Aseptic technique

Initial disinfection of the patient's skin should be followed by the use of sterile instruments whenever skin is penetrated, accidental breach is likely or previously wounded tissue is being treated. Other materials used on or near such vulnerable areas, e.g. dressings, must also be sterile. Single use sachets of antiseptics, etc. are preferable but, if communal ones are used, individual quantities should be dispensed without contaminating the remainder. For example, small quantities can be poured from bottles into sterile pots taking care not to touch the pot with the outside of the bottle, or solutions can be transferred by bulb pipettes which should be disposable or cleaned and disinfected before reuse.

Sterile fields. A sterile field is an area in which contamination is kept to an absolute minimum, although unlikely to be sterile in the full microbiological sense. Such a field may be established by starting with a sterile surface and thereafter taking every care to avoid contamination of that area. The surface must not be touched by bare hands and any necessary items are transferred aseptically onto it. The initial surface may be formed by a sterile drape/towel, or the unfolded inner (sterile) wrapping of a dressing pack, placed on a disinfected trolley top. If pack wrapping is used it must be unfolded by the corners, taking care not to reach over the contents as they are uncovered because contaminants are shed from skin and clothing. Additional items may be slid gently from their sterile wrapping onto the sterile field, or transferred by sterile forceps. Outer wrappings are always contaminated and should not be opened near the sterile field.

Sterile instruments should be arranged in the field conveniently within reach. After use (i.e. contaminated) they should be placed elsewhere for disposal, or on a separate secondary field (e.g. clearly to one side) for possible reuse but not back amongst sterile items. (Note that reuse on a patient may be contra-indicated, e.g. if an infected or dirty lesion is being treated an instrument used earlier may reintroduce contamination into cleaned tissue). It may prove convenient to use a sterile, empty steriliser tray as a secondary field which can be used later to transport used instruments. Contaminated disposable items, e.g. swabs, should be disposed of immediately and should not re-enter the sterile field. Overall there should be a one way movement from sterility to patient to disposal or secondary field.

Dressing changes. Hand disinfection is necessary before commencing, after removal of the old dressing, after completion of the treatment, and at any time during the procedure should hands become contaminated. The old dressing is removed using disposable gloves (or forceps) which, with the dressing, are immediately disposed of carefully. After hand disinfection, sterile gloves are donned for the remainder of the treatment.

Microbiologically clean wounds should need no further cleaning but practice varies. Sterile saline may be used, or antiseptic preparations for contaminated areas as considered necessary. After treatment, all used *and* unused materials from dressing packs should be disposed of as they are no longer sterile.

Waste disposal

Clinical waste should be placed carefully in bags and sealed before removal to prevent contamination of the area. Bags should be colour coded to distinguish ordinary from contaminated waste (e.g. used dressings). There is no universal code, though yellow is used in the United Kingdom to denote contaminated waste for incineration, and practitioners should check local policy. Bags should not be overfilled and must be removed from the clinical area frequently, at least daily. They should be stored safely, and protected from damage, until removed by disposal personnel.

Reusable instruments should be bagged or containerised for return to a central sterile supplies unit, or cleaned before return, or cleaned and resterilised in-house, depending on individual arrangements. Disposal of sharps requires great care to protect the practitioner and others from the risk of HBV and HIV infection; they must be discarded into an approved rigid container (e.g. meeting DHSS specification TSS/S/330.015.) and sent for incineration.

Operating rooms

The design of operating facilities has evolved essentially for the needs of hospital surgery. Such facilities with positive pressure, high efficiency-filtered ventilation systems (DHSS 1983) and various ancillary support areas may sometimes be available to hospital practitioners, and indeed access to these may be necessary for treatment of high risk patients. However, infection rates associated with minor surgery and ambulatory care services are low and such complex facilities should not always be necessary.

In general surgery, airborne contamination appears to have little responsibility for postoperative sepsis (Ayliffe & Lowbury 1982) and during minor operations of short duration, true air borne contamination is unlikely. The greatest risk will be from staff and the standards of their aseptic techniques but nevertheless, adequate ventilation is important to reduce contamination dispersed from personnel while minimising entry of airborne contamination from outside. If extraction alone is used, there is a risk that extracted air is replaced by contaminated air from surrounding areas, i.e. there is an inflow of 'dirty' air towards the operation area. A compromise would be extraction to the outside in combination with sufficient filtered air inlets at selected sites to replace the extracted air. Practitioners intending to expand significantly into surgery should seek expert advice on their particular facilities to ensure that adequate safe ventilation is provided.

Operating rooms should be clearly separated from the general clinic and access restricted to essential personnel. They must be large enough to allow unimpeded movement without contact contamination from other people, furniture and surfaces. Only essential equipment and surgical supplies should be stored in the room and its use should be restricted to surgery and associated procedures such as immediate instrument sterilisation. Initial interview and preparation of the patient should take place elsewhere and adequate facilities for scrubbing up and dressing of surgical staff must be provided.

Thorough cleaning of general surfaces should be done daily and the floor cleaned after each session; routine disinfection of floors should not be necessary. Known occurrences of contamination, especially by tissue or blood, do require disinfection. Overcrowding and vigorous movements should be avoided in operating rooms as they increase airborne contamination. Clinical waste must be removed carefully to avoid contamination of the room or associated clean facilities.

Laboratory specimens

Podiatrists could make more use of the expertise of microbiology laboratories. Laboratory investigation of samples from skin, nails or infected wounds can confirm infection and/or identify the pathogen, thus aiding choice of the most effective patient management. In fungal infections, where symptoms are often insufficiently specific, definitive diagnosis can only be achieved by microscopy and culture techniques.

If possible, samples should be taken before commencing antimicrobial treatment as this may inhibit the isolation of pathogens. The receiving laboratory will advise on containers and packaging for samples. Usually, swabs from wounds are collected into capped containers while skin scrapings and nail clippings may be collected in paper sachets which maintain dry conditions and prevent overgrowth by saprophytes. As much material as possible should be collected to increase the probability of isolating the pathogen. Specimens must be taken carefully, avoiding contamination of self, the clinical surroundings and the outside of the container. As much clinical information as possible should be provided to aid investigation.

Infection control policies

Any practice, large or small, should have a written control policy. This should include instructions on sterilisation of various items, use and concentrations of disinfectants or antiseptics, waste disposal, treatment of spillages, etc. For the individual practitioner this will serve as a useful *aide memoire* while in larger units all staff should be able to consult it for information on agreed procedures. Health service and hospital podiatrists should ensure compliance with the local health authority or hospital policy on infection control. In units with several staff, there should be a designated person with responsibility for implementation and monitoring of control measures. Cleaning staff must be given clear instructions on methods required, adequate facilities, and time to discharge their duties effectively.

Elaborate infection surveillance systems are not necessary in view of the low risk associated with well run ambulatory care facilities. Full note should be taken of any infections which apparently result from podiatric treatment, and overall incidence of these should be reviewed periodically. Undue incidence should alert staff to review control measures, seeking expert advice if necessary.

Infection control personnel are employed by health authorities and hospitals and these local sources are the best initial points of contact for any practitioner. Much published information is also available, including material from public health laboratories and government departments, and is continually being augmented.

FURTHER READING

Anon 1987 Control of cross infection. Journal of the Society of Chiropodists 42: 115
Axnick K J, Yarbrough M (eds) 1984 Infection control—an integrated approach. Mosby, St. Louis
Ayliffe G A J, Collins B J, Lowbury E J L 1966 Cleaning and disinfection of hospital floors. British Medical Journal 2: 442
Ayliffe G A J, Collins B J, Lowbury E J L 1967 Ward floors and other surfaces as reservoirs of hospital infection. Journal of Hygiene 65: 515
Ayliffe G A J, Lowbury E J L 1982 Airborne infection in hospital. Journal of Hospital Infection 3: 217
Ayliffe G A J, Collins B J, Taylor L J 1990 Hospital-acquired infection: principles and prevention, 2nd edn. Butterworth, Sevenoaks
Ayton M 1981 National surveillance of communicable diseases. Nursing 1: 1248
Bartzokas C A, Gibson M F, Graham R, Pinder D C 1983 A comparison of triclosan and chlorhexidine preparations with 60% isopropyl alcohol for hygienic hand disinfection. Journal of Hospital Infection 4: 245
Bartzokas C A, Corkill J E, Makin T 1987 Evaluation of the skin disinfecting activity and cumulative effect of chlorhexidine and triclosan handwash preparations on hands artificially contaminated with Serratia marcescens. Infection Control 8: 163
Bennett J V, Brachman P S (eds) 1986 Hospital infections, 2dn edn. Little Brown, Boston
British Medical Association 1989 A code of practice for sterilisation of instruments and control of cross infection. BMA, London
British Pharmacopoeia 1980 Addendum 1983 Sterilisation. A56 Appendix XVIIIA. HMSO, London
British Standard 5283: 1986 British standards glossary of terms relating to disinfectants. British Standards Institute, London
Central Sterilising Club 1986 Sterilisation and disinfection of heat-labile equipment. CSC, Birmingham
Coates D 1985 A comparison of sodium hypochlorite and sodium dichloroisocyanurate products. Journal of Hospital Infection 6: 31
Coates D 1988 Household Bleaches and HIV. Journal of Hospital Infection 11: 95
Corner G A 1987 An assessment of the performance of a glass bead steriliser. Journal of Hospital Infection 10: 308

Department of Health and Social Security 1980 Sterilisers—health technical memorandum 10. HMSO, London

Department of Health and Social Security 1983 Ventilation of operating departments (currently under revision). DHSS, London

Gardner J F, Peel M M 1986 Introduction to sterilisation and disinfection. Churchill Livingstone, Melbourne

Lowbury E J L, Ayliffe G A J, Geddes A M, Williams J D, (eds) 1981 Control of hospital infection— a practical handbook, 2nd edn. Chapman and Hall, London

Maurer I M 1985 Hospital hygiene, 3rd edn. Edward Arnold, London

Meers P D 1983 Ventilation in operating rooms. British Medical Journal 286: 244

Paterson R S 1985 In: Neale D, Adams I (eds) Common foot disorders, 2nd edn. Churchill Livingstone, Edinburgh

Pratt R J 1988 AIDS a strategy for nursing care, 2nd edn. Edward Arnold , London

Royal College of Nursing 1986 Nursing guidelines on the management of patients in hospital and the community suffering from AIDS. RCN, London

Royal College of Nursing 1987 Introduction to hepatitis B and nursing guidelines for infection control. RCN, London

Russell A D, Hugo W B, Ayliffe G A J (eds) 1982 Principles and practice of disinfection, preservation and sterilisation. Blackwell Scientific, Oxford

Walsh B, Blakemore P H, Drabu Y J 1987 The effect of handcream on the antibacterial activity of chlorhexidine gluconate. Journal of Hospital Infection 9: 30

16. Local analgesia

Donald L. Lorimer

The ability to perform procedures which are in themselves painful makes it essential for podiatrists to be able to anaesthetise selected areas of the foot. The methods employed range from local infiltration of the anaesthetic agent at the site to nerve block techniques, which will remove sensory stimulus to a predictable area of the foot. The choice of method and site of injection must be based on factors which are in patients' best interests, and which use the lowest possible dosage of anaesthetic.

A single site on the weight-bearing plantar surface will generally involve blocking the tibial nerve, whereas a single site on the dorsum can be anaesthetised by local infiltration. Multiple sites on the dorsum may be better anaesthetised by a block of the nerve which supplies the area, which could be the sural, saphenous, deep or superficial peroneal.

If both of the latter are to be blocked, it is better practice to block the common peroneal. The most frequently used sites for the administration of anaesthetics in the foot are the digital nerves and, of these, the commonest is the hallux. The nerve supply to the digits is by four nerve trunks, two of which are on the dorsum and two on the plantar aspect. Textbooks of anatomy identify these as having a predictable location, but in many instances the nerve trunk can be shown to have sub-divided before entry to the toes (Bruce Scott 1989). This is usually accompanied by a similar sub-division of the small blood vessels, which will increase the vascularity of the area into which the injection is to be made.

As a general consideration, before giving an injection to produce analgesia, the operator should have a clear understanding of the anatom-ical structures in that site, together with the normal variations possible (Wildsmith & Armitage 1987). In addition, the following objectives should be observed:

1. The anaesthetic agent to be injected should be deposited accurately to ensure effective contact with the nerve trunk. If there are any suspected anomalies, such as early bifurcation of the nerve, the deposition of the fluid should be wider.
2. Care should be taken to avoid systemic toxicity due to inadvertent intravascular injection or the administration of the fluid in highly vascularised sites. The essence of good practice is in the use of minimum dosage, therefore excessive quantities should be avoided.

Local anaesthetic agents in current use are very safe, but this safety is dependent upon an accurate assessment of patients' physical and clinical states and the site of the injection as well as the type and the composition of the anaesthetic solution (Covino & Vassallo 1976). Before administering a local anaesthetic, the patient's medical history should be elicited and if there are doubts, the opinion of the patient's physician sought. However, it should be stressed that allergy or adverse reactions to amide anaesthetics are extremely rare and if they do occur, are usually the result of systemic toxicity, overdosage or patient anxiety. The procedures which should be followed are discussed in Chapter 3 but particular attention should be paid to the following points:

1. Interaction with systemic drug therapy relates mainly to the mono-amine oxidase inhibitors (MAOI) and procarbazine drugs.

MAOI are used to control acute anxiety states in patients and the procarbazines are anti-tumour drugs used mainly in the control of Hodgkin's disease. These drugs inhibit the action of the hepatic microsomes, in particular the microsomal cytochrome P450 enzymes responsible for biotransformation to simpler chemical structures (Vickers et al 1984).

An additional factor, which is not a drug interaction but merits similar consideration, is the application of local anaesthetics to those patients being treated with the benzodiazepines. As anticonvulsant drugs, these may mask the early signs of toxicity so that if a reaction to the local anaesthetic does occur, the patient may become suddenly and deeply unconscious (Wildsmith & Armitage 1987). Other drugs which can cause problems in association with local anaesthetics are the antihypertensive drugs, such as diuretics. In this case it is not a drug interaction, but postural hypotension may be experienced with risks of fainting when the patient resumes an upright position after treatment.

2. Patients on steroid therapy are more easily put under stress and have a lower resistance to infection. Such patients will have a card identifying the details of treatment. Patients who are receiving anticoagulant therapy will also have a card identifying the treatment and need special consideration in the control of bleeding. This precaution also applies to those who are haemophiliacs or have other haemorrhagic diseases and to patients with leukaemia who also have a lowered resistance to infection.

3. The administration of local anaesthetics to pregnant women is not seen as a risk, provided the pregnancy is proceeding normally. However, in the interests of good practice, local anaesthetics should only be employed at this time in emergency situations. It is considered inadvisable to use anaesthetics during the first three months of pregnancy. Of greater importance is the choice of anaesthetic agents and the dosage levels applied to the patient because of the effects on the fetus via transplacental transfer. The longer-lasting anaesthetics, particularly, may not be metabolised so easily due to lack of development of the enzyme systems in the fetal liver. The agent which crosses the placenta most readily is prilocaine (de Jong 1977) and its use should be avoided if possible in such patients.

4. Patients who suffer from impaired liver function from such causes as infective hepatitis or cirrhosis will have a reduced or negative ability to metabolise amide type anaesthetic agents. Care should be taken in the initial patient assessment to establish the possibility of liver disease or alcohol drinking patterns which have potentially harmful effects. Systemic reactions have been notified in patients with severe hepatic disease (Seldon & Sashara 1967).

A consideration associated with liver function occurs in the metabolism of prilocaine. One of its main metabolites is a substance called o-toluidine which can induce methaemoglobinaemia in humans (Covino & Vassallo 1976). For this reason, it is advisable to avoid high levels of dosage of this agent.

5. Of similar importance is a consideration of renal function. The kidneys excrete up to 10% of lignocaine and mepivacaine, and up to 16% of bupivacaine, in unaltered form; therefore impaired renal function could be a contraindication to the use of local anaesthetics (Wildsmith & Armitage 1987).

6. Patients with hypertensive cardiovascular disease should not have anaesthetic agents containing adrenaline administered to them. Similarly, patients with peripheral vasospastic conditions such as Raynaud's phenomenon should not receive anaesthetics with added vasoconstrictors and fluid tourniquet effect with plain solution should be avoided.

7. Local sepsis at the proposed site of injection precludes the administration of the anaesthetic agent as it facilitates the spread of sepsis. Around the site of sepsis the tissue pH is usually more acidic and this will inhibit the action of the anaesthetic agent. Where an anaesthetic agent has to be used to treat a septic condition, the site for the nerve block should be well away from the sepsis.

8. A number of patients may have a lowered resistance to secondary infections caused by the injection. The general conditions which may cause this would be nephritis, the anaemias and uncontrolled diabetes. Controlled diabetics should not be in danger from the use of plain solutions of anaesthetic.

9. Epileptics not well stabilised by drug therapy could be influenced by the central nervous system stimulation which results from local anaesthetics.

10. The administration of local anaesthetics requires good patient compliance and they may not be suitable for use in the very old or young, in nervous, mentally impaired and insane or hysterical patients.

Toxicity

The toxicity of an anaesthetic agent of the amide type is dependent upon its chemical structure and the ability of the liver enzymes to metabolise it. Prilocaine, which is metabolised at a much faster rate than lignocaine, is considerably less toxic. As a result, the choice of agent and the subsequent dosage requires careful consideration.

The ability of local anaesthetic agents to affect the central nervous system (CNS) produces a range of progressive symptoms. At normal dosage levels, accurately administered, the patient may display the early signs of CNS stimulation becoming excited and talkative and euphoric. Another symptom is numbness of the tongue and also the tissues around the mouth, but this is also ascribed to the highly vascular nature of these tissues which provide a focus for a purely local reaction.

The first real sign of CNS toxicity is light-headedness and dizziness, soon to be followed by difficulty in focusing the eyes, and tinnitus. There may be slurred speech, shivering and light muscle twitch in the face and sometimes the extremities. The patient may appear drowsy, disorientated or even become fleetingly unconscious. Should the toxic reaction continue, the patient will become convulsive with a generalised tonic-clonic state. Following this, depression of CNS activity ensues with respiratory depression and arrest (Stricharz et al 1987).

The effects on the cardiovascular system at toxic levels result in decreased myocardial activity and cardiac output which, combined with peripheral vasodilation, produces circulatory collapse.

Toxic reactions resulting from the maladministration of local anaesthetics are usually due to intravascular injection, excessive dosage or careless administration on vascular sites. The treatment of such reactions consists of adequate ventilation of the lungs, and anticonvulsant agents such as diazepam. Vasopressor drugs, such as adrenaline, may be used to support circulation or physical methods may be used if necessary. Physical methods of life support are discussed in Appendix 3.

CHOOSING AN ANAESTHETIC AGENT

The first factor in the chain is determined by the procedure, its length and possible postoperative pain. Procedures of short duration and little postoperative pain can be adequately covered using lignocaine or, if a higher dosage is required, prilocaine, which has lower toxicity levels. Longer procedures, or those which are perceived to be more painful postoperatively, may require bupivacaine or etidocaine. With both of these, careful postoperative management is necessary as there is prolonged loss of proprioception.

Procedures where bleeding needs to be controlled, or where prolonged action is necessary without the toxic dangers of bupivacaine, may require the use of an added vasoconstrictor. Where a vasoconstrictor is required but its effects are contraindicated in the presence of end arteries, then the non-vasodilatory action of mepivacaine may be used. A more detailed consideration of the commonly used agents follows.

Procaine

This was the first of the synthesised local anaesthetic agents which was used extensively until lignocaine and the other amide compounds were introduced. It is an ester type substance which is metabolised predominantly by the plasma pseudo cholinesterases to paraminobenzoic acid. It has about a quarter of the systemic toxicity of cocaine, which it largely supplanted, but duration of action was short and its chemical structure was less stable to heat sterilization than the amide substances which supplanted it.

It is little used clinically but reference is made to its toxicity relative to other substances.

Lignocaine

This drug is normally prepared as a hydrochloride salt and is one and a half times more toxic than procaine. Its rate of onset is rapid and its effect is more intense and lasts longer than procaine, with effective anaesthesia of up to three hours, but more normally $1\frac{1}{2}$ hours. The maximum safe dose in the United Kingdom is 200 mg in plain solution and 500 mg in solution with added vasoconstrictors (See Table 16.1).

Vasoconstrictor additives are used to prolong its action unless contraindicated by the site of injection or the patients' state of health. Lignocaine is an amino-acyl-amide and as such is detoxified in the liver with small amounts being excreted unchanged by the kidneys (less than 10%) and in the bile (less than 7%) (Dripps, Eckenhoff & Vandam 1988).

Its use in podiatry is as a surface analgesic, (EMLA) for local infiltration or nerve trunk block. It is mainly used in 2% plain solutions.

Bupivacaine

Bupivacaine is also prepared as a solution of its hydrochloride salt. It is four times as potent and toxic as lignocaine but when used for specific nerve blocks it has a duration of action up to six hours. The maximum safe dose in the United Kingdom is 150 mg and it is generally used in 0.25% or 0.5% concentration in plain solution (see Table 16.1).

It is used when a longer lasting analgesic effect is required after techniques which produce some postoperative pain. Its rate of onset is very slow and allowance should be made for this when using it. As with lignocaine, it is detoxified in the liver.

Etidocaine

This substance (which is not available currently in the United Kingdom) is also a longer lasting anaesthetic agent with effective analgesia of up to

Table 16.1

	Maximum safe dose, plain solution	Maximum safe dose, vasoconstrictor	Dose per kg body weight
Lignocaine	200 mg	500mg	3 mg per kg
Bupivacaine	150 mg	150 mg	2 mg per kg
Etidocaine	200 mg	—	3 mg per kg
Mepivacaine	400 mg	—	6 mg per kg
Prilocaine	400 mg	600 mg	6 mg per kg

Maximum safe dosage (after Martindale)
The information in this table is in milligrams per 24 hours and is calculated on an average body weight of 70 kg, based on information applicable to usage in the United Kingdom. Variations may be found in other national formularies. The maximum safe dosage with added vasoconstrictors is also shown, where appropriate. A more accurate method is to apply the formula of milligrams of anaesthetic agent to kilograms of body weight. This takes account of variations in size of patients and should be a principal consideration in assessing patients of small physique.

four hours duration. Although its duration of action is shorter than bupivacaine, its rate of onset is faster than that of lignocaine, which increases patient confidence in the effectiveness of local analgesia. It is capable of producing intense motor blockade, and because of its high plasma binding property has the lowest transplacental transfer. It is detoxified in the liver.

It is prepared as a hydrochloride salt and is normally used in 1% concentrations. The maximum safe dose is 300 mg.

Mepivacaine

This drug has properties similar to lignocaine and is prepared and detoxified in the same way. Its duration of action is similar to lignocaine but it has a slight vasoconstrictor action and is often employed when vasoconstrictor additives are contraindicated. The maximum safe dose is 400 mg. In ankle block techniques, the higher maximum safe dosage level of mepivacaine is particularly useful in allowing higher volumes.

Prilocaine

Prilocaine has properties similar to lignocaine but

is only half as toxic. Its effect on the central nervous system and the cardiovascular system is less pronounced than lignocaine, but one of the main metabolites of prilocaine is o-toluidine, which is considered to be responsible for the production of methaemoglobin in humans. This may limit its use in podiatry where pregnancy may not be admitted by patients at the earlier stages. It is detoxified in the liver. The maximum safe dose is 400 mg.

TECHNIQUES OF ADMINISTRATION

In podiatric practice, two techniques of administration are used. Local infiltration is used to produce an intradermal wheal to facilitate nerve blocks, or to deposit anaesthetic agent around a superficial lesion on a non weight-bearing surface. Nerve block techniques are the most commonly used, either to single nerve trunks or to produce a digital block.

The correct preparation of the patient greatly facilitates the procedures and it is important to have the patient supine or semi-recumbent. This reduces the risk of fainting, but equally importantly, allows the patient to relax and direct their gaze away from the area. Skin preparation of the area is important to reduce the risks of bacterial entry through the site of injection. The point of entry and adjacent skin should be prepared with a suitable antiseptic skin cleanser and should be preceded with a soap and water wash if necessary. The operator's hands should be thoroughly scrubbed and barrier gloves worn. The injection site should be swabbed with an alcohol swab immediately prior to administration of the anaesthetic agent and allowed to dry (Wildsmith & Armitage 1987).

The selection of hypodermic needles is important as the finest needles, 25 or 27 gauge, produce the least pain, but when it is necessary to advance to a deeply placed nerve trunk, it may be better to use a more rigid needle. The use of plain solutions avoids unnecessary impairment of tissue nutrition due to local vasoconstriction. Accurate location of the site and minimising dosage, coupled with aspiration, ensure minimal risk of toxic reaction (Bruce Scott 1989).

Local infiltration

This technique of administration starts with the raising of an intra-dermal wheal at a suitably selected site. This is done by inserting the needle at an angle of 45° to the skin with bevel uppermost. When the bevel is covered, plunger pressure should be applied to raise a small bleb or pool of fluid under the skin, which will show white against the surrounding skin. The needle should then be passed through the skin and directed under the lesion, depositing fluid. The needle may have to be withdrawn to the point of entry and directed in other directions under the lesion, in a fan-shaped pattern. This technique is seldom possible on weight-bearing areas of the foot when the subdermal structures will resist the easy passage of fluid and the needle.

NERVE TRUNK BLOCKS

Digital nerve block

The most commonly used form is the digital block which, because of the special nature of nerve supply, requires separate consideration. As discussed earlier, the nerve supply to a digit is by way of four small nerves, two on the dorsum and two on the plantar which may have sub-divided before entering the septal planes of the digit. The techniques discussed assume that the anatomical norm applies; premature sub-division would be dealt with by small compensatory deposits, the site of which could be identified by the areas remaining unaffected by the anaesthetic agent.

The digit should be examined to select two sites on the dorsum so that the medial dorsal and plantar nerves can be reached from one site and the lateral dorsal and plantar nerves can be reached from the other (Fig. 16.1). At the same time, it is useful to mentally sub-divide the proximal phalanx into thirds so that the site of injection will be over the proximal end of the medial one third. At this point, the 'waisted' effect of the phalanx will allow the easiest access to the plantar nerve trunk with the least possibility of striking the phalanx with the needle and causing damage to the periosteum (Fig. 16.1).

The intra-dermal wheal should be raised in the manner previously described. The amount of fluid

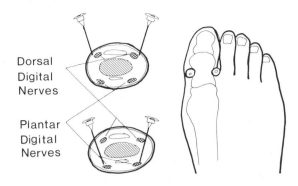

Dorsal
Digital
Nerves

Plantar
Digital
Nerves

Fig. 16.1 Location of dorsal and plantar digital nerves and sites for intradermal wheals.

required for this stage will be unlikely to exceed 0.25 ml on each site. The needle should then be directed towards the point of entry for the wheal at a steeper angle (closer to 90°) and towards the dorsal nerve trunk. Approximately 0.5 ml of fluid should be deposited slowly and steadily after having aspirated the syringe to ensure it is not inserted into a blood vessel. Upon completion of this, the needle should be withdrawn. Aspiration should be carried out before each deposition of anaesthetic agent. If, on aspiration, blood is seen to enter the barrel of the syringe, no further use of that fluid and syringe should be made. This precaution is to protect against the remote possibility of re-entry into another blood vessel and the consequent deposition of damaged blood cells into the circulation.

One finger of the operator's hand holding the digit should be laid over the plantar nerve to be anaesthetised and the needle inserted through the original point of entry and advanced towards the plantar (Fig. 16.1). It is possible to detect the pressure from the advancing needle with the locating finger and the progress of the needle should be stopped as soon as this is felt. The needle should be withdrawn until this pressure is no longer felt (about 1 to 2 mm) and deposition of the fluid commenced. It will be possible to detect this deposition with the finger which is monitoring, and up to 0.5 ml should be deposited on each plantar nerve trunk.

Satisfactory anaesthesia should be possible with up to 2.5 ml of a 2% anaesthetic agent. It is important in digital anaesthesia to avoid depositing excessive amounts of fluid or encircling

the digit with a subdermal ring of fluid and producing a tourniquet effect, with consequent risks. This two-point entry technique is a modification of the Stockholm technique. The lesser digits seem to allow further modification of this technique to a single entry on the dorsum, but unless the toe is very narrow it is a modification capable of producing internal damage and it would be better to retain two points of entry.

Upon completion of the injection procedures, it is better to avoid testing for loss of sensation until a digital hyperaemia appears which indicates the blockade of the sympathetic fibres and the onset of sensory loss. The patient may describe the toe as numb or tingling. Delaying testing for sensation until the outcome is more predictable will ensure greater patient confidence in the whole process.

Specific nerve block

Anaesthesia of all or part of the foot may be obtained by selective nerve blocks. The sensory supply from the larger nerve trunks, although more predictable, is not absolute and areas on the margin may be served by more than one trunk, making careful testing of the anaesthetic effect necessary. Alternatively, their larger size allows them to be accurately located by palpation and careful digital pressure will produce distal paraesthesia.

This precision in locating the nerve reduces the need to use large quantities of solution by enabling it to be deposited accurately. It also reduces the incidence of blockade failure. The increased size of the blood vessels which often accompany the nerve trunks necessitates careful location of the hypodermic needle to avoid intravascular injection (Fig. 16.2).

The raising of an intra-dermal wheal is not always seen as essential but it allows pain-free relocation of the needle if this should be necessary. Deposition of the fluid at the site should be slow to minimise discomfort from the disruption of the fascial planes. The volume employed can be reduced to about 0.5 ml but it is advisable to use higher concentrations to ensure an adequate length of blockade. Where suitable, the use of an added vasoconstrictor will allow a lower concen-

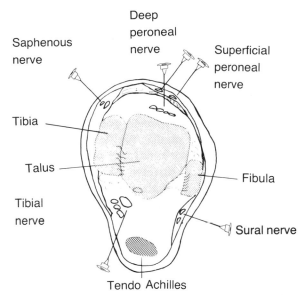

Fig. 16.2 Location of the nerve trunks at a transverse plane through the ankle joint.

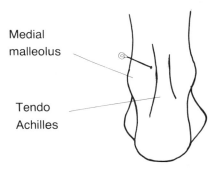

Fig. 16.3 Site of injection for the tibial nerve.

tration of local anaesthetic. The nerves which can be blocked are:

1. tibial
2. sural
3. saphenous
4. deep peroneal
5. superficial peroneal (before or after subdivision)
6. common peroneal

The tibial nerve (Fig. 16.3)

At the ankle, the tibial nerve passes behind the medial malleolus, lying lateral to the posterior tibial artery. As it passes behind the flexor retinaculum, division starts to take place into its three terminal branches (calcaneal, medial and lateral plantar nerves). Examination of cadaveric specimens and clinical practice suggest that this bifurcation can take place proximal to the flexor retinaculum in a significant number of cases, indicating that the best clinical practice is to locate the nerve slightly proximal to the medial malleolus (approximately 2.5 cm from the central point of the medial malleolus towards the shaft of the tibia). On most patients, it is possible to elicit paraesthesia using careful digital pressure.

The best sites to block the nerve are just as it passes behind the malleolus or a little proximal to it. The raising of an intradermal wheal greatly assists the operator in advancing the needle slowly and steadily towards the nerve and, depending on site, it may be necessary to penetrate the retinaculum. With either site, accuracy is greatly enhanced by keeping the locating finger on the site. Before depositing the anaesthetic solution it is necessary to aspirate (Zenz et al 1988). Blockade of this nerve can be obtained using 2 ml of a 2% solution but only accuracy allows this lower dose to be attained.

The sural nerve (Fig. 16.4)

This nerve is located on a line between the lateral aspect of the tendo Achilles and the lateral malleolus. It is closely associated with the course of the short saphenous vein. Its sensory supply is to the lateral aspect of the foot, the fifth toe and, in a significant number of instances, a small portion of the lateral plantar aspects of the calcaneal area. It may have sub-divided into a number of its terminal branches, and this, combined with its

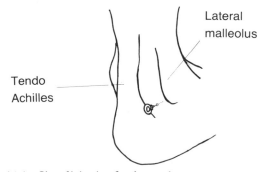

Fig. 16.4 Site of injection for the sural nerve.

passage over relatively well covered areas, makes palpation difficult but not impossible.

In most instances, it can be located and blocked using small amounts of anaesthetic but occasionally, due to early bifurcation, it is necessary to lay a 'track' of fluid between the posterior aspect of the lateral malleolus and the lateral aspect of the tendo Achilles (Fig. 16.4). Even this latter can be accomplished using 0.5 ml 2% solution. It is generally better to initiate the process with an intradermal wheal.

The saphenous nerve (Fig. 16.5)

This terminal branch of the femoral nerve supplies the medial aspect of the dorsum of the foot, occasionally extending to include the surface over the medial side of the metatarsophalangeal joint. It is found entering the foot on the anterior aspect of the medial malleolus closely associated with the great saphenous vein (Bruce Scott 1989). It is not easily located but careful palpation will produce paraesthesia by pressure at a site close to the vein.

The raising of a wheal on the surface between the tendon of the tibialis anterior and the great saphenous vein (Fig. 16.5) allows the needle to be advanced towards the medial malleolus where, after aspirating, the fluid should be deposited close to the vein. Satisfactory blockade is usually obtained by using 0.5 ml of 2% solution.

The deep peroneal nerve (Fig. 16.6)

This nerve is found closely associated with the anterior tibial artery, deeply placed between the tendons of the tibialis anterior and the extensor hallucis longus. Its sensory supply is limited to opposing sides of the hallux and the second toe.

The artery is usually easily located by palpation, although the nerve is not normally palpable. An intradermal wheal should be raised at a site which will allow the needle to be advanced lateral to the artery until paraesthesia is elicited, or until contact is made with the periosteum.

The syringe should be aspirated, and if this is clear, a small amount of fluid is deposited. It is usually necessary to deposit about 1 ml of 2% solution because of the interface of septal planes.

The superficial peroneal nerve (Fig. 16.7)

This nerve becomes subdermal at the proximal end of the lower one third of the leg, on the anterolateral surface. At this site, it is palpable and it is possible to produce paraesthesia. It very quickly divides into a medial and lateral branch and is responsible for the sensory supply to the

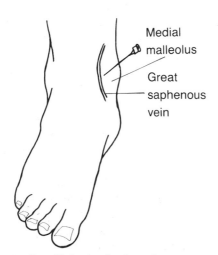

Fig. 16.5 Site of injection for the saphenous nerve.

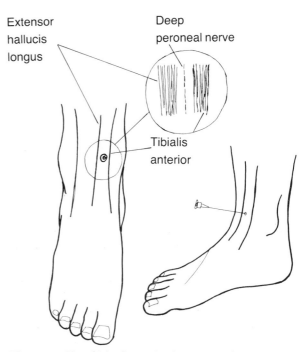

Fig. 16.6 Site of injection to the deep peroneal nerve.

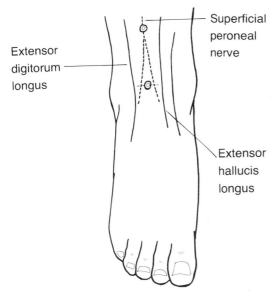

Fig. 16.7   Site of injection to the superficial peroneal nerve.

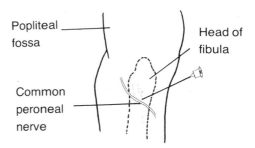

Fig. 16.8   Site of injection to the common peroneal nerve.

lower anterior surface of the leg, as well as most of the dorsal aspect of the foot.

As the nerves pass into the foot, the medial branch lies immediately lateral to the tendon of the extensor hallucis longus and may be palpated there. The lateral branch lies lateral to these structures at the same level and may also be palpated.

The branches may be anaesthetised using small quantities of fluid (about 1 ml of 2% solution) at either of the sites described or where the nerve becomes superficial in the lower part of the leg.

The common peroneal nerve (Fig. 16.8)

This nerve, arising from the popliteal fossa, passes over the neck of the fibula before dividing to become the deep and superficial peroneal nerves. Where the nerve curves around the neck of the fibula, it can be easily palpated and access to it is simple as it is in a situation not complicated by the presence of major blood vessels. Raising an intradermal wheal allows the needle to be advanced slowly towards the nerve, the site of which can be indicated by a finger palpating the nerve (Fig. 16.8). Satisfactory anaesthesia can be obtained with 1 or 2 ml of 2 % solution.Using the common peroneal nerve reduces the number of injections if both the deep and superficial nerves have to be

blocked and significantly reduces the total dosage required.

Field block anaesthesia

This is also known as Mayo block or ray block and involves the blocking of nerve conduction to a whole segment of the forefoot from the level of the base of the metatarsals. The location of the nerves at this site is more predictable but is complicated by the close association of the nerves with the blood vessels and the need to pass through the dorsal and plantar interosseous muscles as well as the plantar intrinsic muscles. Variations in location may make it necessary to lay a 'track' of anaesthetic fluid so it is essential that the needle is withdrawn along the same line as it was advanced, with due consideration being given to the vascularity of the site. Variation of the location of the plantar nerve may make it necessary to supplement with a block to the tibial nerve.

The most commonly used field block in the foot is that to the 1st metatarsal segment and it is this that is referred to as a Mayo block. Blockade of the 5th metatarsal segment is less common, as is that to the lesser metatarsals, but both of these are described as they have minor variations in technique.

The dosage of anaesthetic substance may be quite high, with 6 to 8 ml of 2% lignocaine being normal for a profound blockade of a metatarsal segment. It may be necessary to use an added vascoconstrictor or to employ mepivacaine, as the increased vascularity of the area reduces the effective time for anaesthesia. Patients who have a lower body weight may require the application of lower percentage concentrations to avoid approaching maximum safe dosage.

Anaesthetic block of the metatarsal segments requires the passage of hypodermic needles between the metatarsal shafts and it is convenient to establish clinical guide lines to determine the optimum passage between the bones. A simple guide is to locate a point on the medial aspect of the 1st metatarsal about 1 cm distal to the base, and a point on the lateral aspect of the 5th metatarsal, 2.5 cm distal to its base. A line drawn between these two points will ensure easy passage between the shafts (Fig. 16.9)

First ray or Mayo block

The nerve supply to the 1st metatarsal segment is from one of the terminal branches of the deep peroneal nerve (dorsolateral) with the other terminal branch supplying the dorsomedial aspect of the 2nd segment. The dorsomedial aspect of the 1st segment is supplied by the medial terminal branches of the superficial peroneal and in some cases terminal branches of the saphenous nerve. The plantar aspects of the 1st segment are supplied by the terminal branches of the tibial nerve.

The nerve supply to the medial plantar aspect of the 1st segment is superficial at the base of the 1st metatarsal and medial to the line of the plantar aponeurosis. The nerve supply to the lateral plantar aspect of the segment lies deep to the plantar aponeurosis at the level of the base of the 1st metatarsal and is the 2nd terminal branch of the medial plantar nerve.

The venous arch over the dorsum of the foot provides the best clinical guide to locate the various nerve trunks, when used in conjunction with osseous landmarks of the base of the 1st metatarsal. Using these two features, it is possible to identify easily the optimum sites of entry which should not exceed two in number: one on the dorsum between the 1st and 2nd metatarsals (A), and the other on the medial aspect of the 1st metatarsal shaft (B) (Fig.16.10). The dotted line (C) represents the line of the venous arch.

To anaesthetise the dorsomedial branches of the 1st metatarsal segment, the hypodermic needle should be passed through the intradermal wheal (B) and directed towards the point where the venous arch crosses over the tendon of the extensor digitorum longus, where the major trunk will be located. After aspirating, up to 1 ml of anaesthetic should be deposited and the needle withdrawn, leaving a 'track' of fluid all the way up to the point of entry (Fig. 16.11). This will ensure that all small irregular branches are anaesthetised.

Using the same point of entry, the needle

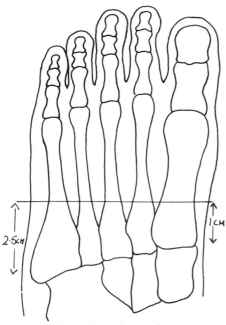

Fig. 16.9   Guideline to intermetatarsal route.

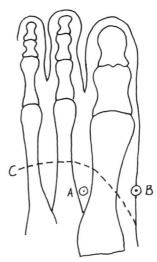

Fig. 16.10   Site of injection for 1st ray block: A and B, intradermal wheals; C. line of venous arch.

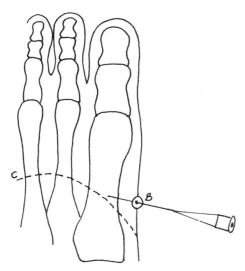

Fig. 16.11 Anaesthetising mediodorsal nerve trunks.

should be advanced laterally over the plantar surface of the metatarsal to a point in line with the lateral aspect of its base. This should also be close to the medial edge of the plantar aponeurosis (Fig. 16.12). Aspiration should not be necessary at this site and about 1 to 1.5 ml of anaesthetic fluid should be deposited. As the needle is withdrawn, the fluid should continue to be deposited, thus leaving a 'track' to deal with any irregular branches of either the medial plantar nerve or the saphenous nerve which may be found at that level. This process will complete the

blockade of the plantar medial aspect of the segment.

Small terminal branches of the superficial peroneal nerve often supply the dorsolateral aspect of the 1st metatarsal segment and it is necessary to ensure that these are also blocked. To accomplish this, the needle is passed through the intradermal wheal (A) and directed medially over the surface of the metatarsal shaft towards the point where the venous arch crosses the tendon of extensor hallucis longus. At this point, a small amount of fluid (0.5 ml) is deposited after aspirating and the needle is then withdrawn leaving a small 'track' of fluid in case there are irregular nerve trunks (Fig. 16.13).

To complete the dorsal block, it is now necessary to pass the needle through the intradermal wheal (A) and direct it towards the base of the 1st metatarsal (Fig. 16.14). It is necessary to monitor the progress of the needle with careful palpation to avoid vascular penetration or intraneural injection. Before depositing anaesthetic fluid, it is essential to aspirate, as this is a highly vascularised area. 1 ml of fluid should be adequate and care must be taken not to deposit a fluid 'track' on the withdrawal of the needle, because of the vascularity.

The remaining nerve trunk serving the 1st metatarsal segment is the 2nd terminal branch of the medial plantar nerve, which also serves the

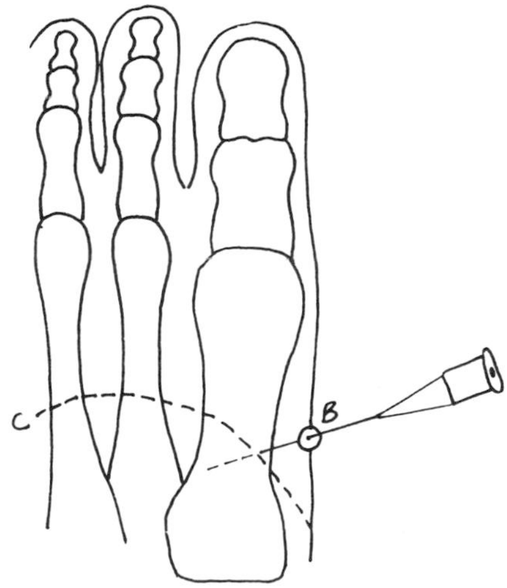

Fig. 16.12 Injection site for medioplantar nerve supply to 1st ray.

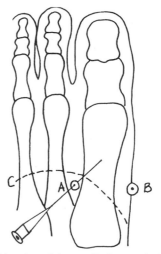

Fig. 16.13 Direction of the needle for terminal branches of the superficial peroneal nerve (dorsolateral nerve supply).

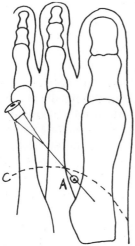

Fig. 16.14   Injection to anaesthetise the deep peroneal nerve (dorsolateral nerve supply).

medial aspect of the 2nd segment. The best palpable indicator of its position is the tendon of the flexor hallucis longus, to which it runs parallel at a distance of about 8 to 10 mm.

Entry should be made through the intradermal wheal (A) and the needle directed in an antero-medial direction towards the plantar surface. The target area is the lateral aspect of the distal one-third of the metatarsal shaft (Fig. 16.15). It is necessary to pass through the muscle of the flexor digitorum brevis.

The operator's finger should have been placed over the site of the nerve and this will locate the pressure caused by the advancing needle. Once this is felt, the needle should be stopped and the syringe aspirated. It will be necessary to deposit at least 1 ml of fluid, but it is usually prudent to double that amount. It should be deposited slowly and all pressure on the plunger must cease on withdrawal to avoid any inadvertent intravascular injection.

Fifth ray block

This segment is supplied by nerves from three sources. The lateral branch of the superficial peroneal nerve supplies the medial dorsal aspect. The terminal branches of the sural nerve supply the lateral, the dorsal and, in some cases, the lateral plantar aspect. The plantar and, in most cases, the lateral plantar aspect of the segments are supplied by the lateral branch of the lateral plantar nerve, which lies superficial to the plantar aponeurosis, parallel to the line of the flexor digitorum brevis. The medial plantar aspect of the segment is supplied by the medial terminal branch of the lateral plantar nerve, which also supplies the lateral aspect of the 4th segment.

To achieve anaesthesia of the 5th ray segment, it is necessary to raise intradermal wheals on

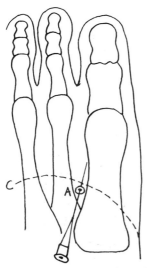

Fig. 16.15   Injection to anaesthetise the 2nd terminal branch of the medial plantar nerve.

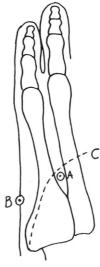

Fig. 16.16   Sites for intradermal wheals in 5th ray block.

two sites (Fig. 16.16). The first, at site (A), is proximal to the course of the venous arch (C) and this gives access to the terminal branch of the superficial peroneal as it lies superficial and medially to the tendon of the extensor digitorum longus (Fig. 16.17). It also allows access to the medial branch of the lateral plantar nerve by passing between the 4th and 5th metatarsals and through the dorsal and plantar interossei muscles

(Fig. 16.18). It is essential to aspirate the syringe because of the vascularity of this site. Approximately 1 ml of fluid should be deposited slowly. On withdrawal of the needle, fluid should not be expelled.

The terminal branches of the sural nerve are blocked by inserting the needle through the intra-dermal wheal (B) and advancing it postero-dorsally towards the lateral side of the venous arch, taking care not to penetrate the vessel. About 1 ml should be deposited and the needle should be slowly withdrawn, depositing a large 'track' of fluid which should block any irregular branches (Fig. 16.19).

The lateral branch of the lateral plantar nerve is also reached through the intradermal wheal (B), with the needle being advanced anteromedi-ally towards the line of the flexor digitorum longus. This should be palpated and its position identified by the operator's finger so that the advance of the needle to the site can be identi-fied.

Once this is located, the fluid can be deposited without aspiration. It should be sufficient to deposit 1 ml on the site and to withdraw the needle slowly, leaving a substantial track as before to the point of entry. This should ensure that any other irregular nerve trunks are blocked (Fig. 16.20).

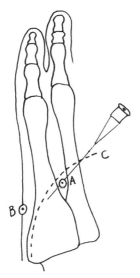

Fig. 16.17   Injection site for terminal branch of superficial peroneal nerve.

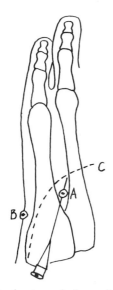

Fig. 16.18   Injection towards the medial branch of the lateral plantar nerve.

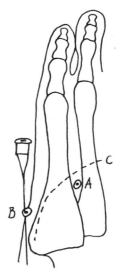

Fig. 16.19   Injection towards the terminal branches of the sural nerve.

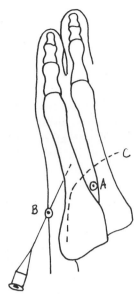

Fig. 16.20   Injection site for the lateral plantar nerve.

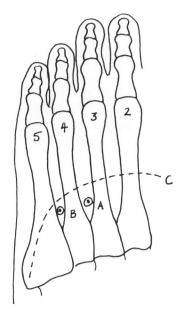

Fig. 16.21   Site for intradermal wheals for 4th ray block.

Middle ray blocks

The anaesthetic block of the 2nd, 3rd and 4th metatarsal segments requires only minor modification to the techniques already described. The 3rd/4th segments are supplied on the medial and lateral borders respectively by the medial terminating branch of the lateral branch of the superficial peroneal nerve, which normally passes superficial to the venous arch. The plantar supply is from the lateral branch of the medial plantar nerve but may have an irregular supply from the medial terminating branch of the lateral plantar nerve.

Both plantar and dorsal nerve trunks may be reached from intradermal wheals at sites (A) and (B). The line indicated by (C) is that of the venous arch (Fig. 16.21). On the plantar sites, the nerves are accompanied by a number of blood vessels, therefore aspiration is essential and the fluid should not be expelled during the advance or withdrawal of the needle.

Location of the needle can be identified by placing a finger over the area between the tendons of the flexor digitorum longus. The plantar nerves are deep to the plantar aponeurosis and the dosage of about 1 ml should be delivered slowly to each nerve trunk.

Anaesthesia of the 3rd metatarsal segment can

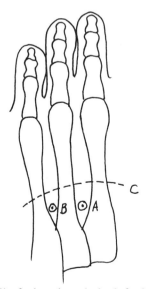

Fig. 16.22   Site for intradermal wheals for 3rd ray block.

be attained by raising intradermal wheals at sites (A) and (B) (Fig. 16.22) and following the same general directions.

The 2nd metatarsal segment can be anaesthetised by raising wheals at points (A) and (B) (Fig. 16.23). In addition, the technique described for the 1st ray procedure, so far as the deep peroneal nerve is concerned, needs to be applied.

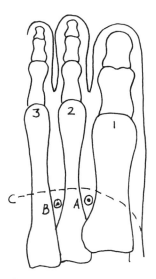

Fig. 16.23 Site for intradermal wheals for 2nd ray block.

A general consideration which applies to all the procedures concerning the location of the nerve supply deriving from the medial and lateral plantar nerves is the proximity of the site of injection to a very vascular area. In addition, there is the need to pass through muscle tissue. One way of minimising this risk is to block the innervation from these nerves at the common trunk of the tibial nerve, at the posterior aspect of the medial malleolus. This has the advantage of being a more accessible site, generally requiring lower dosage, and is usually the site of choice. Ultimately, the method chosen must reflect the clinical needs of the procedure and the patient.

POSTOPERATIVE SUPERVISION

The duration of postoperative supervision following the use of local anaesthetics is determined primarily by the nature of the condition and its postoperative state. However, it is prudent that precautions should also be taken against the possibility of any ill-effects arising from injection, even though these are rare. A suggested form of advice information is given below.

Advice to patients

The local anaesthetic injection you have been given is not expected to have any unwanted side effects.
You are advised to keep the area dry for . . . . . When the effects of the anaesthetic have worn off, you may feel some discomfort. If so, you are advised to take mild painkillers such as you would for a headache. Should you experience:
  (i)   persistent *coldness* of the affected area;
  (ii) undue *pain* in the affected area;
  (iii) *discolouration* of the affected area;
then telephone or return to the Clinic, quoting this number . . . . In the event of emergency, or outside clinical hours, contact your family doctor and show him this paper.

Procedure carried out:
. . . . ml of . . . .% . . . . (drug)
. . . . in order to carry out . . . .
Date . . . .
Signed . . . .

FURTHER READING

Bruce S D 1989 Techniques of regional anaesthesia. Appleton & Lange/Mediglobe, Warwalk, Connecticut
Covino B G, Vassallo H G 1976 Local anaesthetics. Grune & Stratton, New York
de Jong R H 1977 Local anesthetics. Charles C Thomas, Springfield, Illinois
Dripps R D, Eckenhoff J E, Vandam L D 1988 Introduction to anesthesia, 7th edn. W B Saunders, Philadelphia
Seldon R, Sashara A A 1967 Journal of the American Medical Association

Stricharz G R (ed) 1987 Local anesthetics. Springer Verlag, Berlin
Vickers M D, Schnieden H, Wood-Smith F G 1984 Drugs in anaesthetic practice, 6th edn. Butterworths, London
Wildsmith J A W, Armitage E N 1987 Principles and practice of regional anaesthesia. Churchill Livingstone, Edinburgh
Zenz M, Panhans C, Niesel H C Kreuscher H, 1988 Regional anesthesia. Wolfe Medical Publications, London

17. Principles of surgical practice

Alistair J. Clark

Before elective surgery is undertaken, it is essential to establish a clear picture of the patient's condition, life-style and expectations from the prospective surgery. The most important question is whether surgery is necessary. The practitioner must discuss with the patient the advantages and disadvantages of surgery compared with those of conservative treatment. This is necessary in order to establish 'informed consent'. It is a legal requirement that the patient fully understands what is causing the condition and what can be done about it, including all possible outcomes and complications. This must be achieved using terms the patient understands.

Major factors in this process are the duration and severity of the symptoms. It is necessary to ascertain what previous treatment has been given and what the prognosis is. Also relevant are the patient's expectations and the level of patient compliance that may be forthcoming. In establishing a comprehensive assessment, the patient's attitude towards the condition is a crucial factor. Patient compliance may be indicated from the record of previous treatments and the number of cancelled or missed appointments. Occupational demands may affect availability for treatment, as may domestic circumstances. If the patient is living alone, it is important to establish the level of support available from friends and family. Poor patient compliance complicates the pre- and postoperative stages of a surgical procedure, and may affect the healing time as well as its quality.

The patient should have a realistic expectation of the surgery during the operative and postoperative stages. The procedure could be traumatic if the patient were unprepared for surgery and it is important to discuss the procedure with the patient and evaluate their response. The use of premedication to relieve anxiety of the patient may be of benefit to both parties and the oral administration of diazepam 5–10 mg, two hours before surgery, is often employed. The age of the patient must also be considered, as elderly patients carry a greater surgical risk due to the ageing process, and so they must be viewed in conjunction with a detailed medical history. The very young patient also presents special problems; the level of anxiety and a lack of compliance during the procedure are factors to be considered, and here again the use of premedication may be advisable. During this process, it must be remembered that the podiatrist is part of the the overall health care team and discussion with the general practitioner, the hospital consultant or any other member of the team involved with the patient, can only strengthen the practitioner's understanding of the patient's health and circumstances. Co-operation is important in improving the quality of information received during the history taking and the examination of the patient. The podiatrist can then call on other professionals for support in premedication or in the postoperative care of the patient. Communication with other health care professionals is to the benefit of both the patient and the practitioner.

Healing by second intention, as after nail surgery, is dependent on a number of variable factors. In trying to predict the healing time, the important factors are: the depth of the wound; its surface area; the degree of stress exerted on the site; the degree of operative trauma; and the amount of tissue loss. The clinical implications of any systemic disease must also be considered in assessing patient suitability for surgery.

THE SURGICAL WOUND

The sutured wound offers many advantages to the practitioner, as the apposed surfaces limit the introduction of bacteria into the wound and reduce its surface area. Any tissue loss which would normally be replaced over a period of weeks is replaced in a much shorter time scale. In the initial stages of wound healing, when the wound is becoming organised, the sutures act to support and maintain the integrity of the clot and the healing tissues, improving healing time. Over areas of high stress, the sutures also act to limit distortion of the tissues.

There are a number of methods of wound closure, the simplest being Steristrips (3-M), which give good closure and give support to the tissues. These adhesive strips are made in a variety of sizes to accommodate most wounds;

they are simple to apply and can be used to reinforce sutures where necessary.

Equipment

There is a large range of surgical instruments available to the practitioner, but the basic kit should include sufficient instrumentation for a variety of techniques (Fig. 17.1).

3 No. 3 scalpel handles
2 double prong 6 inch retractors
2 Kilner 6 inch retractors
1 pair of bone cutters
1 pair of bone rongeurs
1 pair of 5 inch Kilner needle holders
1 pair of 5 inch toothed dissecting forceps
2 Gillies skin hooks
6 pairs of Backhaus or Mayo towel clamps
2 pairs of scissors
2 pairs of Rampley sponge holders
1 blunt elevator
2 MacDonald's dissectors
4 pairs of 5 inch straight artery forceps

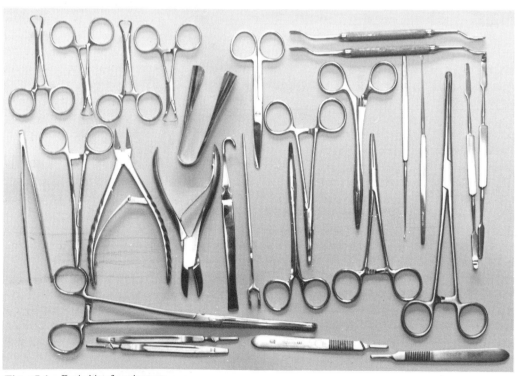

Fig. 17.1 Basic kit of equipment.

2 pairs of 5 inch curved artery forceps
2 pairs of 4 3/4 inch Adsons toothed dissecting
   forceps
17 inch double ended bone rasp
   Suturing material (absorbable and non-
   absorbable)
18 inch kidney dish
13 inch bowl

The number of each type of instrument will depend upon the range of surgery to be undertaken. The kit does not include consumable items or any power equipment. Each instrument can be used in a number of ways, and the variety of different types available provides a range of choice. Several scalpel handles will be included in a pack as they may be used at various points in a procedure. One is used for the first skin incision and is then discarded. Further scalpels will be needed to enlarge the wound or remove tissue.

There are many types of retractor available and it is best to include retractors of different sizes, both small and wide-headed. The choice is related to the size and position of the wound as the retractors allow much greater visualisation of the wound and can protect soft tissue structures from damage. The practitioner can also use a self-retaining retractor which allows the assistant much greater freedom, but this increases the possibility of tissue damage, because of the constant pressure it exerts. It is the role of the assistant to retract the tissues and protect the surrounding structures, thus increasing the size of the window through which the operator can work.

The dissecting forceps allow small amounts of tissue to be handled firmly and accurately with the minimum of trauma. There are a number of types; the Adsons forceps, with their wide arms and small jaws, give secure and accurate tissue handling, and the straight dissecting forceps are used to hold the wound margins during suturing. The MacDonald's dissector can be used to elevate or protect structures and can separate tissue by blunt dissection. Backhaus towel clamps can also be used during procedures, to aid in the removal of sections of bone. Their jaws can pierce the section, giving the operator greater control during the process of excision.

There are two distinct groups of instruments used for cutting bone. Rongeurs have 'spoon-like' jaws for 'nibbling' bone, and are used to remove osteophytes or to reshape bone. The second group includes bone cutters of various types which are used to cut through the phalanges or any bone. They have a variety of jaw shapes and can be single or double action. The double action type gives greater accuracy and greater mechanical advantage, reducing the strain necessary to cut through bone.

The oscillating bone saw is another alternative and is used most effectively on larger bones. e.g. the first metatarsal. It offers the advantage of minimal bone fragmentation, giving smoother edges which need less rasping. This reduces the possibility of any bone fragments being included in the wound. (When using power equipment, care must be taken to protect the surrounding tissues.) The bone can be damaged if the saw blade is blunt; this can be due to the tearing action of the blade and the excessive heat produced, resulting in further damage to the bone. The surgical drill is another power tool which is often used to reduce irregular bony surfaces and an alternative is the power rasp, used in osteotripsy. Most pneumatic equipment allows the interchanging of hand pieces which facilitates the use of all three types of equipment. The use of the drill or rasp is common in minimal incision surgery, but it is important that the resulting debris is removed from the area, by flushing the wound with sterile saline. Power equipment offers greater accuracy and is essential if more complex surgery is undertaken.

Skin hooks allow tissue to be handled with minimal trauma and they aid in wound closure. They are used to hold the subcutaneous tissues and epidermis during closure, producing minimal tissue damage. Artery forceps are another multipurpose tool which can be used to separate tissue, to clamp tissue and to secure a tourniquet. It is important to have sufficient instruments to deal with any problem that may occur. Contamination of a set of instruments must not interfere with a procedure and a second set of instruments should be prepared and held readily available.

To cover all contingencies, three sets of instruments should be sterilized to give the maximum cover. It is best to use a standard pack of instruments, as this offers the operator the maximum range of instruments during surgery.

Tissue viability

In planning the most suitable approach for any procedure, it is essential to visualise the position and identify of all the structures in the operative field. This review must include the position of any sensory nerves emerging through the deep fascia, the position of the neurovascular bundles, the tendons passing over or inserting into the area, and the underlying bones and joints. It is also necessary when choosing the site of an incision, and hence subsequent suturing and scar formation, to consider the direction of the cleavage lines of the skin. These were first described by Langer, but more recent authors advocate the use of the skin creases as a more accurate definition of the lines of stress and therefore a more accurate guide to the most suitable direction of incision.

This minimises any tension on the wound and allows the scar to blend with the existing skin creases. After reduction of a deformity is completed, the operator may have to reduce the overlying tissue to accommodate the change in position. Any excessive force used during the procedure will be reflected in the amount of tissue loss occurring postoperatively. This is most relevant when osseous deformity has displaced structures. Elliptical incisions allow the removal of excess tissue and, in the case of digital surgery, often result in the removal of all or part of the associated corn or callus.

It is important that sufficient tissue is removed to produce good cosmesis; however, removal of too much tissue will produce excessive wound tension. If insufficient tissue is removed, the remaining excess may result in the development of a dead space lesion and fluid aggregation, which will retard healing. Dissection uses the line between the tissue planes to develop tissue cleavage. This minimises tissue disruption, reduces the amount of cell damage and limits the inflammatory response. This technique also

allows for orderly closure of each layer where necessary. The tissue planes can be divided at specific histological barriers. It is important to remember that the dermis and epidermis gain blood supply from vessels passing up through the superficial fascia and separation of the junction can adversely affect the superficial tissues.

Surgery can be restricted by poor haemostatic control obliterating the field, deformity displacing structures, or trying to work through a very small incision, making recognition difficult. If excision of a particular area of tissue is to be undertaken, it will not be possible to choose the site of the incision. The size of the incision should be sufficient to remove adequately all the tissue necessary. The tissue should be sent for histological examination and pathological report to identify the cell types and to ascertain whether the excised tissue is benign or not.

It is important to irrigate the wound regularly with sterile saline during the procedure. This will allow greater visualisation and if the saline is mixed with Betadine solution, it will act as an antiseptic to reduce any possibility of infection. Irrigation prevents the tissues from drying out due to excessive exposure, and sterile saline can also be used to flush debris from the wound after osteotripsy or rasping. Irrigation is carried out using a syringe to create sufficient pressure to clear the debris from the area without damaging the tissues or lodging debris in the wound margins.

Scalpel techniques

The scalpel has a variety of uses and this is reflected in the range of associated techniques. The type of grip on the scalpel will vary depending on which of the particular features the practitioner considers most important at any particular stage of the procedure. The fingertip grip is often used for making the initial incision as it allows for greater control with the maximum cutting edge in contact with the skin, particularly in longer incisions.

The palm grip can be used where greater pressure is required as it offers great stability while pressure is being exerted.

A pencil grip can be used throughout the procedure, the angle of the blade being varied. This ensures great precision and control of the scalpel, allowing the accurate initial incision, with only a minimum of the blade in contact with the patient. A vertical placement of the blade will give a small incision which can be enlarged using the same grip. With this 'press cutting' technique, the incision is highly controlled in length and direction. Sliding the blade over the tissues under pressure produces an accurate continuous incision which will vary in depth depending on the degree of pressure used. It is important that the area is stabilised to avoid excessive skin movement during the incision, as this can result in a jagged wound or an alteration in the direction of the incision. The operator must apply sufficient tension to the wound to allow an accurate incision of the area (Fig. 17.2), and it is important that the scalpel is kept vertical to the skin to avoid an oblique incision of the tissues. The scalpel should be changed after the first incision to reduce the possibility of wound infection. It is best to incise the superficial fascia with short strokes as this will allow more haemostatic control and a greater visualisation of the tissues. The superficial fascia has a limited cosmetic importance and has a different structure from the underlying tissues.

The initial incision should completely cut the skin, leaving vertical wound edges for apposition on completion of the procedure. Repeated incisions increase the probability of irregular wound edges which increase tissue damage and may retard wound healing. Skin tension on the area will give greater separation and greater control to the operator, hence greater accuracy (Fig. 17.2).

Once the wound is established, it is important to identify the structures and this is aided by the use of retractors. The tissues should be displaced with the minimum of damage and the procedure can continue using either sharp dissection or blunt dissection. Sharp dissection using scalpel or scissors is necessary to deepen a wound or to release structures, blunt dissection using forceps or dissector can be used to increase the size of a wound. At all stages the tissues should be handled with the greatest care to minimise trauma to the area.

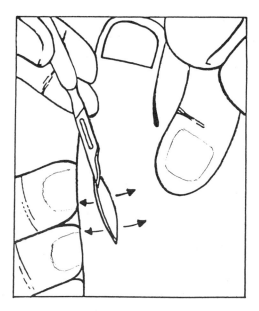

Fig. 17.2 Initial incision using a press cutting technique with the assistant creating suitable skin tension.

Haemostatic control

This has to be considered throughout the three phases of surgical practice: preoperatively, during operation and postoperatively.

Preoperatively, it is important to investigate thoroughly any history of bleeding, e.g. prolonged bleeding after tooth extraction or any earlier surgery, any history of anaemia or of recurrent infection, and of medication which may prolong clotting time. For patients who describe periods of excessive bleeding after minor injury, it is prudent to establish formally the patients' clotting time and bleeding time.

A history of back or lower limb problems may exclude the elevation of the lower limb. These factors do not preclude patients from undergoing surgery but they should be considered as part of the decision making process as to the patient's suitability.

Elevation of the limb preoperatively for approximately 3 minutes reduces the vascularity of the area, and exsanguination, using a pressure bandage, further reduces the blood in the limb. For some procedures, surgery may be carried out with the limb in an elevated position without the use of a tourniquet and although there may be some bleeding, it will not interfere with the operation.

If the procedure involves only the nail or distal interphalangeal joint, then a digital tourniquet can be used and this must be released after 20 minutes to avoid any tissue damage due to anoxia.

The use of a pneumatic cuff placed at the lower third of the calf and inflated to approximately 250 mmHg gives constant haemostasis. The use of a mid-thigh tourniquet inflated to 400 mmHg has the advantage of increasing the tourniquet time to two hours, whereas an ankle tourniquet can be used for one hour only.

A thigh tourniquet is preferable because there is less danger of compressing the neurovascular structures against the underlying bone. The tourniquet site should be wrapped with gauze to protect the area and underlying structures. The cuff is normally inflated only after the limb has been elevated for 3 minutes to reduce its vascularity, but it can produce discomfort.

Preoperative measures also include the choice of a local anaesthetic which does not cause vasodilatation, e.g. mepivicaine 3% plain solution. Lignocaine produces local vasodilatation, increasing the vascularity of the area, but this does not preclude its use.

The use of 1:200 000 adrenaline offers a much longer period of anaesthesia, but the resultant vasoconstriction precludes its use on the lesser toes, although several studies have concluded that it produces a negligible effect on the vascular flow when used with lignocaine, due to the vasodilatory action of the latter. The use of adrenaline in ankle block anaesthesia is well documented and offers a great reduction in the blood supply to the plantar surface of the foot, as well as prolonged anaesthesia with lower doses.

During the procedure, any vessel which is bleeding can be seen and can be ligated using an absorbable suture material, e.g. Dexon, thus facilitating better visualisation in the field.

Another method of haemostatic control is electrocautery which is available in a number of forms, including disposable units (Aaron Medical Industries USA; Cardiokinetics Ltd UK). It is important that the cauterising tip is at the correct temperature; if it is not hot enough it will adhere to the tissues and if too hot, it will burn through the vessel instead of sealing it. The use of chemical haemostatics is to be avoided as they produce increased tissue necrosis and produce a higher level of postoperative infection.

Postoperatively, a variety of agents are available to control bleeding. Absorbable sponges, such as the gelatin or calcium alginate sponges, help to control bleeding by increasing the surface area in the clot and absorbing several times their own weight of blood. These substances are absorbed over a 4–6 week period, are non-irritant and do not elicit a tissue reaction. Oxygen regenerated cellulose is an agent which acts by absorbing blood; it is bactericidal against a wide range of organisms. Bone wax can also be applied to control haemorrhage from cut sections of bone, although both bone wax and oxygen regenerated cellulose may affect bone healing.

SUTURING

Sutures hold the wound edges in apposition, encouraging the healing process. This depends upon accurate coaption and the minimum of tissue trauma. It is important that the wound edges are either slightly everted or level, not inverted as this retards healing and can lead to the development of elevated and unsightly scars. It is also important that the stitches are not too tight as this may lead to avascularity of the wound edges and, in conjunction with postoperative oedema, may produce a localised tissue necrosis. The tension of the suture is also important; it must allow for postoperative oedema and excessive tension which may lead to rupture of the suture. Sutures should achieve coaption throughout the full depth of the wound, not only the superficial tissue, thus avoiding the development of a 'dead space' which will retard healing and act as a possible focus of infection (Fig. 17.3).

There are several different forms of sutures, each with a particular function. The most common form is the single interrupted suture; it holds the wound edges in apposition and, using a surgeon's knot of three throws followed by two throws, it prevents slippage and is therefore very

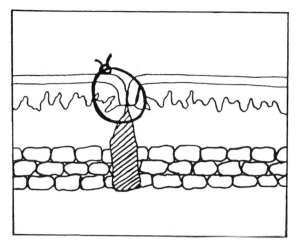

Fig. 17.3   Poor suturing technique showing inversion of the wound edges and dead space in the tissues.

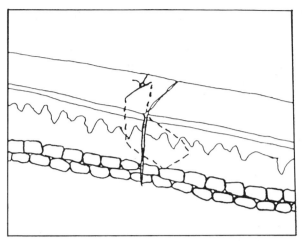

Fig. 17.5   Half buried horizontal mattress suture, used to give deep and superficial closure and greater wound stability.

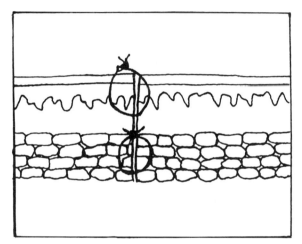

Fig. 17.4   Interrupted suture (non-absorbable) and buried subcutaneous suture (absorbable).

secure (Fig. 17.4). The stitches may be placed in close proximity or used in conjunction with horizontal mattress sutures, which will coapt a larger section of the wound.

An alternative type of suture is the vertical mattress suture which gives both a deep and superficial level of wound coaptation, passing through the tissues at two depths. Another method is the half buried mattress suture, which is excellent for holding wound margins together after tissue excision. This type of suture passes from the surface of one wound margin into the deeper tissues in the opposite wound margin and then superficially back to the initial wound margin, leaving the suture visible only at the first wound margin (Fig. 17.5).

Continuous sutures, such as the simple running suture, can be advantageous to the practitioner as they avoid repetitive knot tying and offer continuous wound coaption. They are also used in closing subcutaneous tissues. On completion of a suture, the practitioner should check the position of the knot which should lie to one side of the incision. It should not lie over the incision, as it may there act as an irritant to the wound and become trapped in the clot formed by postoperative bleeding.

Drains serve to reduce the accumulation of fluid at the site of the wound. This reduces the possibility of seroma or haematoma formation and reduces pain and the possibility of tissue necrosis, thereby increasing the rate of healing. The drain is normally kept in place for 48–72 hours but it can act as an irritant and a route of infection, and can also produce discomfort or pressure ischaemia on the tissues. The simplest type of drain is a sterile rubber tube inserted into the wound with a small section protruding from the wound. This is often known as a 'Penrose drain' and it depends upon the position of the limb to maximise drainage. To reduce the possibility of infection, a closed suction drain can be used. This has a sealed container which can collect only a fixed amount of fluid. It is often used to reduce any accumulation of fluid after wound infection.

Equipment

The following list is sufficient for most minor procedures:

2 pairs of Kilner needle holders
2 pairs of 5" toothed dissecting forceps
2 pairs of suture removal scissors
dressing scissors and forceps.

There are two groups of suturing material: non-absorbable and absorbable sutures. In each group there is variety of different structures, monofilament or multifilament, and a number of different materials, natural and synthetic, with a range of needle shapes and suture lengths. The practitioner must consider the particular qualities required from any suture material, including its tensile strength, its elasticity and plasticity, and the strength of the knot. Braided or multifilament sutures allow greater tracking of body fluids along the material. Natural fibres elicit a greater tissue reaction than synthetic materials. All suture materials elicit some tissue reaction which lasts for between 5–10 days. After this period, most non-absorbable sutures will be removed. Monofilament nylon and polypropylene produce the least tissue reaction. In ascending order of their tensile strengths, braided nylon, braided polyester or stainless steel may be used, although polyester and stainless steel both produce more tissue reaction. The stainless steel suture can also produce some discomfort but it gives good skin closure and a very stable wound scar. Stainless steel wire is even stronger and is used commonly as skin closure clips, but their use is not favoured for minor surgery.

Non-absorbable sutures

The most common suture material used is braided silk. It is dyed black to make the suture clearly visible in the wound. Silk is not a particularly strong material and as a natural fibre, elicits a slightly stronger tissue reaction. Its advantages are that it moulds well onto the surface of the wound and is an easy material to tie, offering small secure knots with minimal distance between sutures if necessary. Silk is described as non-absorbable but if left in the tissues over a long period of time, it first loses its tensile strength and then continues to degenerate. This is unlikely to occur in the types of procedures carried out initially by podiatrists, and any subcutaneous sutures can be of the absorbable type. Synthetic materials which can be used as an alternative to silk include Dermalon and Novafil (Davis and Geck). Dermalon is a monofilament nylon material which is non-capillary and elicits a minimal tissue response due to its structure. This is also true for Novafil, a monofilament polybutester which has similar properties. If necessary, braided nylon, braided polyester and stainless steel may be used in ascending order of their tensile strength.

Absorbable sutures

As mentioned in the previous section, there is a range of natural and synthetic suture materials. The natural materials are commonly labelled as either chromic or plain catgut, which consists of processed sheep intestine. As a 'foreign' protein, this type of suture elicits a high tissue response and is not recommended for wound closure as it attracts a higher level of bacterial infection than many other materials, especially when compared to the alternative synthetic materials such as Dexon. Dexon is a coated polyglycolic acid, having similar properties to catgut, and producing minimal tissue reaction. It can be used for wound closure, as well as subcutaneously, since it does not lead to scarring.

Removal of sutures

The time scale for the removal of sutures depends on the site of the sutures, the wound strength, the healing rate and the type and number of sutures involved. Generally, sutures are removed after approximately 5–10 days and, if over a joint, after 6–12 days. It is important to ensure that all sutures are removed in order to avoid the possibilities of infection tracking along the course of the suture, or of any tissue reaction caused by the suture in the wound. Removal of the sutures should be carried out with the minimum of tissue trauma by cutting the suture so as to avoid pulling the knot through the tissues. After removal of the sutures it is important to protect the wound from any trauma which would disrupt the healing process.

Osseous surgery

As part of the evaluation of osseous surgery, the practitioner must consider how the corrected position can be maintained postoperatively. The use of an external dressing or bandage may be sufficient to control the position of the joint, but in many cases a more stable fixation is required and the fixation technique will depend on the procedure undertaken. Stainless steel wire is commonly used for internal fixation to close an osteotomy, giving stability and strength, but it can produce severe compression at the site of insertion with a risk of necrosis of the bone. Kirschner wires are used to give some compression and stability in digital arthrodesis, the gauge of the wire determining its strength. Often a number of Kirschner wires may be used to give maximum control of the corrected postoperative position. The Kirschner wire should normally be removed after three weeks, although this has the disadvantage that it can create a tract for infection. Staples and clips offer permanent internal fixation but are more difficult to use because of the equipment needed and the variability in the amount of compression they produce, which may be due to the positioning of the clip and irregularity of the bone surfaces.

Screws produce stability and can be used to aid fusion, but the positioning of the screw can also act to distort the alignment and care should be taken to consider its positioning relative to the direction of the two sections. The screw can act to displace the two sections of bone and its application is a skilled exercise involving a large amount of specialised equipment.

The use of an external, supporting or controlling cast will also maintain the correct position. This can be constructed from plaster of Paris bandage or a more lightweight synthetic material, and the elderly patient will benefit from the easier ambulation that a lightweight cast provides. An advantage of synthetic casts is that they achieve their maximum strength in a much shorter period of time but they cost considerably more than the equivalent plaster of Paris cast and the material also has a limited shelf life.

POSTOPERATIVE CARE

It is essential to establish the highest level of asepsis possible while undertaking postoperative care after surgery. The wound must be protected from contamination and trauma, particularly from any mechanical irritation between wound and dressing. Ambulatory surgery, as its name suggests, encourages patient mobilisation and, with this, comes the increased possibility of trauma. To combat this, there are a range of options open to the practitioner.

Choice of dressing

This must relate to its function and to what properties are considered essential. The ideal wound dressing must be impermeable to microorganisms and be able to meet the following criteria:

(i) to absorb any wound discharge
(ii) to maintain a suitable environment for wound healing
(iii) to minimise the shedding of fibres which could interfere with the healing process
(iv) to be removable without causing trauma to the wound.

Medication

There are many types of wound dressings available, e.g. semipermeable films such as Opsite (Smith & Nephew) which can be sprayed over the wound; also hydrocolloids, e.g. Granuflex wafers or granules (Squibb Surgicare). Another wound dressing is Debrisan (Pharmacia), a dextranomer which absorbs wound exudate. It is produced as a paste and as a powder.

Dressing

The dressing must be able to absorb any discharge from the wound, without compromising its function. It should not act as a mechanical irritant by being too large or too loose. If the dressing absorbs any blood, it may become rigid and adhere to the wound, acting as an irritant, promoting entry of microorganisms and thus failing to maintain a suitable environment for healing. Some dressings are applied with the knowledge that they will harden, e.g. povidone-iodine soaked dressing will harden to act as a splint and can be used to aid in the maintenance of the corrected position.

If this rigid dressing is used, it is first necessary to apply a non-adherent layer, and this is followed by a covering of sterile gauze to protect the wound and maintain correction. This will also act as an absorbent for discharge. The dressing is completed securely and neatly by using a Kling bandage applied with some tension to prevent displacement. Where the dressing encircles the toe, it should not compress the tissues excessively, or it may cause pressure necrosis of the wound.

Aftercare

The postoperative care of the patient can influence the cosmesis and healing time. Prior to surgery, the patient must have been advised that, to maximise postoperative care, they must be available to attend the surgery should the need arise. It is equally important that the practitioner is also available and that there is sufficient time in the schedule for such a contingency.

After surgery, the practitioner should give the patient clear instructions to follow and should reinforce the important of postoperative care (see Advice to patients, p. 317). The use of written instructions is advised and they should be discussed with the patient before leaving the surgery. It is important that the patient has a realistic expectation of the postoperative outcomes and has suitable instructions. The most immediate of these outcomes is postoperative bleeding, followed by postoperative pain. The patient should remain in the surgery for approximately 45 minutes after the procedure to allow the practitioner to monitor any bleeding which may occur. Should there be any marked haemorrhage later, they should return to the surgery for investigation.

The degree of postoperative pain is individual to each patient and each procedure. Prior advice should minimise this and recourse to medication,

e.g. aspirin, is also helpful. Aspirin has the advantage of reducing inflammation and pain; however it is a gastric irritant and can be replaced by buffered aspirin or by any of the alternatives, e.g. paracetamol. If thought necessary, a mild sedative may be prescribed but this would be for a 48–72 hour period only.

The foot should be protected from trauma and rested during this period, and the elevation of the limb will reduce some of the postoperative oedema and reduce the associated throbbing sensation. Ice packs wrapped in a sealable polythene bag will also aid the reduction of postoperative swelling. The patient must keep the dressing dry; if it becomes moist the number of bacteria present will increase. It is impossible to stop the spread of skin flora into the area of the dressing, but with suitable changes of dressings the possibility of infection is minimised.

Mobilisation of the patient as soon as possible is important to avoid postoperative complications, notably deep vein thrombosis. Mobilisation will aid the reduction of postoperative oedema and encourage patient morale.

The use of a trauma shoe to minimise compression of the wound during the postoperative period will benefit the patient (Fig. 17.6). There are a variety of types which all protect the foot and allow mobility with little restriction of the foot. It is important to give advice on footwear which may prevent a recurrence of the deformity. The practitioner must advise the patient to wear a shoe which will allow the insertion of an orthosis if that is necessary.

The use of exercises as part of the postoperative process can improve the range of mobility and prevent muscle wastage. This is an important factor in maintaining correction and avoiding any delay in osseous development.

In most cases of conservative surgery the procedure will not correct any underlying bio-mechanical deformity, and while the surgery may improve the cosmesis of the foot the condition may recur unless the range of motion is controlled by the orthosis. This is another area which must be discussed as part of the patient evaluation for surgery. Once the wound has healed and a suitable orthosis is in place, the patient should be monitored as part of the follow-up process. This

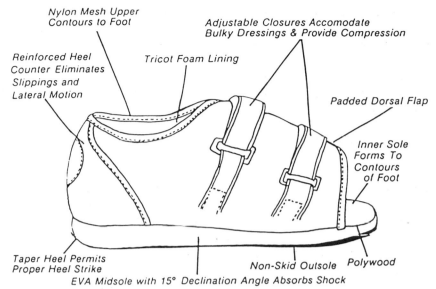

Nylon Mesh Upper Contours to Foot

Reinforced Heel Counter Eliminates Slippings and Lateral Motion

Tricot Foam Lining

Adjustable Closures Accomodate Bulky Dressings & Provide Compression

Padded Dorsal Flap

Inner Sole Forms To Contours of Foot

Taper Heel Permits Proper Heel Strike

Non-Skid Outsole   *Polywood*

EVA Midsole with 15° Declination Angle Absorbs Shock

Fig. 17.6   A postoperative trauma shoe. (With kind permission of Nova Instruments Ltd.)

will give maximum benefit from surgery and will give the practitioner invaluable information about the long-term outcome of procedures. This cannot be over-stressed as it gives the practitioner accurate and objective information about the technique.

POSTOPERATIVE COMPLICATIONS

Wound dehiscence

Wound dehiscence, or the splitting open of a wound, is a possible outcome during the postoperative period. It is important to consider the sequelae to wound closure that can lead to post operative infection or poor wound healing. The suture should produce wound apposition without producing tension on the wound and restricting the postoperative oedema which occurs as part of the healing process.

Haematoma

Haematoma formation within the wound can be caused by poor haemostasis, i.e. the failure to coagulate or ligate a vessel. In some cases, a haematoma can occur despite good haemostatic control and, if untreated, it can cause distension

which may lead to marked postoperative swelling. This may lead to rupture of the wound or to the development of superficial gangrene of the overlying tissues. Should this occur, the wound should be opened, the coagulum removed and the edge resutured.

Seroma

Distension may also occur as a result of seroma formation. A seroma is an accumulation of lymph and tissue fluid produced when the skin and subcutaneous fascia have been separated from the underlying fascia, allowing the fluids to collect. The fluid can be drawn off using a syringe with the puncture site distant from the wound.

This distended area can act as a focus for infection and produce a dead space within the wound. If this area becomes infected, the bacterial toxins can produce cellular necrosis and microvascular thrombosis which will delay tissue replacement and epidermal migration, resulting in tissue necrosis of the wound edges. The infection will impair the function of the fibroblasts which produce wound collagen and this will further weaken the wound. The availability of oxygen in the tissues is essential for wound healing and any reduction in that level due to infection or any other factor will also impair the healing process.

Oedema

Marked postoperative oedema may also lead to deformation of the tissues which may distort wound apposition and affect the healing process. Weight-bearing sites or joints can produce greater wound tension and this extra stress may lead to wound dehiscence.

Drains

The use of drains in small surgical wounds is often undesirable as they may act as routes for infection. There should be sufficient drainage through the apposed wound. Loss of apposition by the use of drains leads to healing by second intention, increasing healing time and leading to an irregular and pronounced scar. The wound may heal but produce a hypertrophic scar which is elevated and it may appear red and itching. It is commonly very sensitive to touch and pressure. The scar can be treated with anti-histamine creams or infiltrated with hydrocortisone, or by ultrasonic therapy. If the scar fails to resolve, its excision should be considered, although early excision carries a high incidence of recurrence.

Keloid

Another type of hypertrophic scar is a keloid, in which the hypertrophy extends beyond the wound margins into the surrounding normal skin. There is a higher incidence of keloid formation in children, adolescents and the Afro-Caribbean population. This hypertrophy can lead to recurrent ulceration, corn and callus formation and thus higher levels of discomfort. If the scar becomes fixed to the underlying tissues, such as deep fascia or tendon, this may restrict mobility and negate the purpose of the operation.

Any displacement of the underlying superficial fascia can lead to irregular continuity of the tissues. Should the superficial fascia become involved with the wound closure, this can retard healing and lead to the development of a cyst or fibroma.

Epidermoid cyst

If a portion of the epidermis becomes inverted and becomes buried within the subcutaneous tissues during closure, this may lead to the development of an epidermoid cyst. This normally appears as a circumscribed fluctuant swelling lying on or close to the scar. It will cause little discomfort unless over an area subject to stress, but it is often cosmetically unacceptable. It can be excised and the wound closed.

Fibroma

Fibroma development may result from the inclusion of starch from the practitioner's gloves into the wound, which will act as an irritant producing a foreign body reaction. After wound closure the irritant will be trapped in the tissues gradually becoming established. It appears as a fairly rigid swelling which has symptoms and treatment similar to the epidermoid cyst.

Neurological complications

Neuropraxia, causalgia and hyperaesthesia

These can take a number of different forms. Neuropraxia, or transient sensory loss, can be the result of compression of the sensory nerves by the tourniquet, or the result of trauma due to poor tissue handling. There is no actual damage to the nerve and the recovery of the tissue can take place over a period of a few hours to about seven days. More serious nerve damage could result in a considerably longer period of recovery and may produce causalgia. This is most commonly seen in the lower limb involving the tibial nerve. It may produce a burning or itchy sensation which can give great discomfort or even longstanding acute disabling pain. Hyperaesthesia of the sensory nerves is another sequel and in this, the patient cannot tolerate any contact with the area involved. The discomfort can be particularly severe at night and there appears to be some link with impaired vasomotor tone, anaemia and vitamin B_{12} deficiency.

Pressure neuritis and nerve entrapment

Pressure neuritis, due to contraction of deep fascia, can produce paraesthesia in the area. This may also be associated with the amount of postoperative oedema present and only after a 5–14 day postoperative period is this identifiable. If the fascia or retinaculae become thickened, this can produce a nerve entrapment. Any lesion can compress the nerve to cause entrapment, producing motor and sensory impairment leading to paralysis and tingling or itching. Ultimately, tropic changes will occur in the skin. The position and distribution of the symptoms will indicate the nerve involved and palpation at the site of the entrapment will produce pain both proximal and distal to the site (*Valleix phenomenon*).

In a small number of cases, there may be residual chronic intractable pain due to nerve damage. The use of corticosteroid injections, with or without local anaesthetic, can help to alleviate the symptoms. If medication fails to alleviate the problem, exploratory surgery may be necessary to identify the cause of the condition.

In a few cases a sensory nerve may be severed giving permanent sensory loss. This *neurotmesis* may cause the patient concern and it is important that the practitioner is supportive and clearly explains this outcome. *Vasomotor disturbance* can lead to trophic changes, producing great pain and tenderness. This affects bone and soft tissues presenting symptoms of swelling , discolouration, hyperhidrosis and temperature change and hyperaesthesia. Should these symptoms present, early treatment is essential as the longer the condition exists, the poorer the prognosis.

Vascular complications

The history taking and examination of the patient should have established any conditions present which may impair the vascular response. However, any surgery carries the risk of some local or systemic reaction which can compromise or impair the success of the procedure. The causes may be pre-existing systemic disease, the surgery, or the postoperative care. Any abnormality in clotting time can affect the postoperative management and the excessive use of ice packs can produce vasodilatation, complicating postoperative care.

Poor placement of a tourniquet can also lead to vascular complications by compressing the vessels against underlying bone, leading to inflammation and damage. This can lead to phlebitis and thrombophlebitis which can also occur as a result of venous stasis induced during surgery. The patient will then have the added risk of possible pulmonary embolism. Local thrombosis formation is another sequel which may be caused by poor tissue handling; here the area will be cold, pale and tender. This is often a precursor to gangrene when there is limited collateral circulation, but the involved vessels may recanalise.

Excessive tourniquet time can lead to an increase in clotting time and the metabolites which are normally controlled by the body's buffering system alter the pH of the affected tissues, giving tissue acidosis. The ischaemia also leads to tissue destruction and muscle fatigue, which increases healing time and may lead to the formation of splinter haemorrhages appearing in the affected area. Tissues with the highest metabolic rates are the first to become damaged. Nervous tissue will progressively lose its conductive ability and muscle tissue will gradually swell, increasing the tension in the area. Skin and superficial tissues can survive 6–8 hours before irreparable damage occurs.

Atrophy complications

Immobilisation of the foot may lead to atrophy of the tissues which can affect the postoperative recovery of the patient. Part of the foot can be compressed within a cast, thereby restricting tissue nutrition. In the early stages of wound healing compression may lead to ischaemia of part of the wound and surrounding tissues, leading to ulceration of the overlying skin and underlying tissues. If untreated, this ulceration may progress to involve bone, leading to osteomyelitis.

The immobilisation of any part of the limb will affect muscle bulk and strength due to lack of muscular activity and, over several weeks, it may produce fibrosis of some of the fibres, leading to extended healing times and osteoporosis, which may extend the period of external support, thereby creating a vicious circle. The muscle atrophy will restrict ambulation and in the elderly patient may be a permanent feature. It is therefore important to establish a programme of physical therapy to exercise the musculature to avoid any loss of motion. This will also stimulate blood supply to the area, encouraging healing and muscle strength, which in turn will encourage healing of the bone. If the area is immobilised, a gradual disuse atrophy can ensue, producing osteoporosis, retarding the callus development and delaying fusion. Normally in younger patients, the removal of the cast and subsequent ambulation will lead to the rehabilitation of the muscle. However, in some patients a generalised osteoporosis of the foot can lead to stress fractures after the cast is removed which would interfere with mobilisation of the patient.

These changes are often most evident around the calcaneus where scarring may be evident with a marked reduction in the quantity of superficial fascia and in the quality of the tissues in general.

Infection

The tissue planes discussed earlier normally restrict the spread of infection by acting as anatomical barriers. Deep fascia is the most important of these, sealing the deeper structures and compartmentalising them. However, in most surgery this barrier is breached, allowing the entry of bacteria into the deeper structures.

Infection may occur as a result of defective surgical technique or inadequate postoperative care. The area may be red, hot, swollen and tender as a natural sequel to surgery, and there may be some postoperative bleeding. This should subside during the first 72 hours postoperatively, but if the area becomes more inflamed and painful it is essential that the practitioner examines the wound.

Any serious discharge from the wound is a cause for concern and a swab should be taken and sent for examination. The tension of the wound should be examined for any abscess formation and, if there is any doubt, it is wise to commence antibiotic therapy. This can be adjusted after the results of the swab become available. Infection may occur as a result of a dead space lesion, allowing either haematoma or seroma formation, and the infection may form an abscess in the tissue space.

It is important to drain the abscess to avoid encouraging bacterial growth, which would lead to increased tension and possible necrosis of the overlying tissues. In order to avoid disturbing the wound unnecessarily, particularly during the first 72 hours, it is important to establish whether any clinical signs which may present are of systemic origin or are due to local infection.

Postoperative advice to patients

A suitable format in which to present postoperative advice to patients follows.

POSTOPERATIVE ADVICE TO PATIENTS

The following instructions are for your benefit and will help to reduce any swelling or pain and encourage healing. Please follow them.

1. Please go directly home. Do not drive yourself if you are so advised. If your journey will take more than 15 minutes, elevate your feet.
2. To encourage a quick and uneventful recovery, do *not* sit with your feet down or with your legs crossed for any length of time as this may cause swelling and pain.
3. Some bruising and swelling is to be expected but that is no cause for alarm.
4. Whenever possible, sit with your feet elevated at least as high as your hips.
5. Keep the bandages dry and clean. Do not remove them to inspect the wound. A small amount of bleeding is normal and it may mark the bandage.
6. Ice packs will reduce any discomfort and swelling but make sure the pack is sealed to avoid wetting the dressing. (A simple dressing can be made by soaking a kitchen towel in cold water, squeezing out excess water then putting the towel inside two plastic bags and placing in the freezer for 30 minutes. It can then be draped over the foot.)
7. Do not get the dressing wet. Cover the foot with a plastic bad and place on the side of the bath. Do not use the shower as the water will penetrate the bag and dressing.
8. Exercise your legs frequently by bending your knees and ankles to stimulate the circulation and healing.
9. Protect your foot at night to avoid any pressure from the bed clothes.
10. Reduce your smoking and consumption of alcohol.
11. Drink plenty of fluids.
12. CALL YOUR DOCTOR IF:
    (i) your dressing becomes soaked with blood or if it becomes tight and your toes tingle or feel numb
    (ii) discomfort is not reduced by your medication
    (iii) you knock or injure the foot
    (iv) you develop a high temperature.

FURTHER READING

Anderson R, Romfh R 1980 Techniques in the use of surgical tools. Appleton Century Crofts, New York
Brown J 1986 Minor surgery. Chapman and Hall, London
Epstein E, Epstein E Jr 1979 Techniques in skin surgery. Lea & Febiger, Philadelphia
Gerbert J , Sokoloff T 1981 Textbook of bunion surgery. Futura Publishing, New York
Hara B, Locke R, Lowe W 1976 Complications in foot surgery. Williams & Wilkins, Baltimore
Hymes L 1977 Forefoot minimum incision surgery & podiatric medicine. Futura Publishing, New York
Irvin T 1981 Wound healing: principles and practice. Chapman and Hall, London
McGlamry E D 1987 Fundamentals of foot surgery. Williams & Wilkins, Baltimore

Mercado O A 1979 An atlas of foot surgery, Vol. 1. Carolando Press, Illinois
Passmore R, Robson J 1976 Companion to medical studies, Vol. 1, 2nd edn. Blackwell Scientific Publications, Oxford
Saleh M, Sodera V 1988 Illustrated handbook of minor surgery & operative technique. Heinemann Medical, London
Smith C, Aitkenhead A R 1985 Textbook of anaesthesia. Churchill Livingstone, Edinburgh
Yale J F 1987 Podiatric medicine, 3rd edn. Williams & Wilkins, Baltimore
Yu G, Cavaliere R 1983 Suture materials. Journal of the American Podiatric Medical Association 73 (2): 57–64
Zederfelt B, Jacobson S, Ahonon J 1986 Wound and wound healing. Wolfe Medical Press, London

18. Digital surgery

Alan S. Banks   E. Dalton McGlamry

Surgery on the digits can be seen as falling into two distinct areas: that which involves the nail and soft structures only and that which involves the subdermal structures of bone and related tissues. These two areas of ambulatory surgery, developed by podiatrists in the interests of patient care, share the need for very accurate assessment of patients and thorough postoperative care.

NAIL SURGERY

If conservative treatment of onychocryptosis or severe involution fails to provide long term relief, or is considered inappropriate in cases of onychauxis or onychogryphosis, then recourse to nail surgery will invariably achieve that objective. In cases of onychocryptosis or involution, two procedures are available: total or partial ablation of the nail with destruction of the matrix. In cases of onychauxis or onychogryphosis, the only procedure possible is usually total avulsion with destruction of the matrix.

In the case of onychomycosis, it is possible to consider total avulsion with or without destruction of the matrix. The decision depends on the ability of nail to regrow; the administration of systemic or tropical antifungal agents is indicated when the matrix is not destroyed and nail regrowth is aimed for (Ch.11).

Partial nail avulsion

The foot must be prepared using the measures described in Chapter 17 and a local analgesic administered (see digital nerve block, Ch. 16). It is essential to operate without causing pain, and also to ensure a low risk of infection. To allow the procedure to be carried out in a bloodless field, an Esmarch bandage (tourniquet) should be applied.

The Esmarch bandage is applied from distal to proximal so that the toe is gradually exsanguinated. Once the bandage is applied, it should be secured at the base of the digit in as broad a form as possible to ensure that the underlying structures are not injured. The toe should be swabbed again and the foot draped.

The instruments used for this procedure will be chosen from those described in Chapter 17. They should include MacDonald dissectors in two sizes, small, medium and large artery forceps, Thwaite's nippers, a range of instruments for dressings and, if required, nail chisels and Volkmann spoons.

Using the finest MacDonald dissectors, the nail plate is freed from the sulcus and the eponychium (Fig. 18.1A). Any debris should be removed at this stage. The object of a partial avulsion is to remove a section of nail sufficiently large to leave the remaining surface of the nail plate flat. This is done by using the Thwaites nippers to make a clean straight cut along the nail plate to the level of the eponychium.

At this stage opinions vary, with some operators easing the Thwaites nippers below the eponychium and completing the separation to the level of the matrix (Fig. 18.1B). Alternatively, the cut can be completed using a nail chisel. Either method is acceptable but it should be remembered that when using a chisel, the instrument should be held steady and the movement continued in the same direction as the first part of the cut.

The cut section of nail is then removed using a suitably sized pair of artery forceps locked onto it

(Fig.18.1C). The section is then carefully rotated so that the lateral margin rolls upwards and inwards. Part of the nail matrix may become detached with removal of the section of nail, but the nail should be examined to check for the *frond* effect at the base. Presence of the frond indicates the satisfactory separation of the nail from the matrix.

The sulcus must be cleared of all debris and hyperplasic tissue (Fig. 18.1D). At this stage, as at all other stages, the area should be thoroughly cleansed. It is now necessary to destroy the section of matrix from which the section has been taken. Several methods may be used: chemical (phenolisation, trichloracetic acid, sodium hydroxide) or using specialised apparatus (cryotherapy or electrosurgery).

Phenolisation

This is the method most commonly used. Liquefied phenol BP is applied to the area to be treated and worked thoroughly using a metal instrument or a fine sterile cotton wool bud. The phenol should be applied for a minimum of two minutes, but often three minutes may be needed. Care should be taken to apply it only on the area to be destroyed, and the field of application should be dry. If cotton wool buds are used, they should be changed every 30 seconds (Fig. 18.1E).

Alternatively, the phenol can be applied for up to two minutes, the area dried out with a fine sterile cotton wool bud and the process repeated for the same time. Whichever method is used, the most important factor is to apply the phenol so that it is well worked in to the tissue to be destroyed. After this application, the area should be irrigated with alcohol to wash out the phenol and terminate its action. It is now useful to dry out the area with a fine cotton wool bud.

Finally, the Esmarch bandage is removed and the digit observed for the return of arterial blood. This is usually rapid but its return must be observed. The entire area should be covered with a sterile dressing which may include a broad spectrum antiseptic. After treatment, it is good practice for the patient to sit for a short time before returning home.

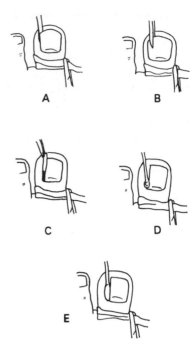

Fig. 18.1 (A) Separation of the nail plate from the nail bed using a MacDonald dissector. (B) Cutting a section of the nail using Thwaites nippers. (C) Removal of the section of nail using artery forceps. (D) Removal of debris and hyperplastic tissue with a Volkmann spoon. (E) Phenolisation using a cotton wool bud.

Trichloroacetic acid

This may be used in the same way as liquefied phenol BP but the time application usually needs to be extended slightly (by about 1 minute).

Sodium hydroxide

This may be used as a 10% solution instead of liquefied phenol; its effect is more rapid. It is usually applied until the tissue blanches thoroughly. The area is then dried with a sterile cotton wool bud and carefully washed out with 5% acetic acid to neutralise the sodium hydroxide. Normally, one application in the manner described for liquefied phenol will be found adequate provided that it is applied to a completely dry field. Appropriate sterile dressings should be used with follow-up care as described previously.

Total nail avulsion

The foot should be cleansed thoroughly and a suitable skin preparation antiseptic applied. A local anaesthetic should be administered and an Esmarch bandage applied, completing the process by draping in the manner described before.

The nail sulci and eponychium are freed carefully from the nail plate and all debris removed. A MacDonald elevator is then inserted under the free edge of the nail and the plate separated gently until loosened. When this stage has been reached, locking forceps are attached to an edge of the nail so that the lateral margin of the nail rolls upwards and inwards. This procedure is then repeated on the other border and the nail then eased away from any remaining attachments. Finally, all epidermal material should be removed and the area thoroughly cleansed using sterile cotton wool buds.

The matrix should be destroyed by one of the methods described for partial nail avulsion, but since the area to be treated is larger it may be necessary to extend the time of application a little to ensure complete destruction. It is essential, also, to ensure that the agent being used is introduced to all areas of the matrix.

Postoperative care

Following nail surgery, it is essential to give the patient clear and concise advice concerning any immediate postoperative problem which might arise. An excellent practice is to give the patient an advice sheet similar to that described in Chapter 16.

The return date will vary depending on the particular circumstances of each case but should be within three to seven days following the procedure. At this visit, the original dressing should be removed, the condition reviewed and another dressing applied. Strict antiseptic precautions should be observed using sterile dressings and a 'no touch' technique.

After removal of the original dressing, the area should be irrigated and swabbed with a sterile solution which may or may not contain an antiseptic agent. The area should be clean and show some granulation tissue; there may be some serous exudate. Any pain which may still be experienced by the patient may be a result of the trauma to the area, but this usually disappears after the first redressing. On rare occasions the patient may experience *phenol flare* — an acute inflammatory response to the application of liquefied phenol. It is a rare phenomenon, and largely unexplained, but will settle in four to five days and will call for extra reassurance and support from the podiatrist.

If the area appears healthy and free from infection, a sterile dressing with or without an antiseptic agent should be applied and held in place with tubular gauze dressing. It is advisable to give explicit instructions regarding the avoidance of trauma and keeping the area dry in the early stages. Later, provided progress to resolution is uneventful, the patient may be allowed to bathe and redress the area, always assuming the patient's compliability. These procedures should be carried out weekly until healing is complete. At this stage, advice on prophylactic care should be given.

Alternative techniques

There are several alternative surgical methods which are now increasingly practised to give long term relief to persistent onychocryptosis and involution:

Winograd's operation

This procedure is carried out by means of a double incision. The first begins at the distal edge of the nail plate on the affected side and extends longitudinally down to bone under the eponychium and through the matrix. The second incision starts in the same place and is carried in a slight curve through the paronychial soft tissue to meet the proximal end of the first. The entire elliptical wedge of nail plate, matrix and granulation tissue present is then underscored and removed down to bone in one piece. The sides of the incision are brought together and then sutured (Fig. 18.2).

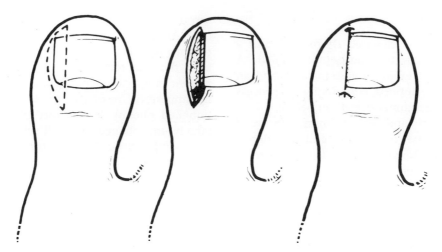

Fig. 18.2   Winograd partial matrixectomy procedure for relief of ingrown toenail. (From Comprehensive Textbook of Foot Surgery, McGlamry E D (ed), by permission of Williams and Wilkins.)

Frost's root resection

In this procedure, an L-shaped incision is made from the distal tip of the nail plate into the epony-chium on the dorsum and then laterally. The flap of tissue is reflected, the entire section of nail plate, bed and matrix is excised in one piece and the flap is replaced. Sutures are not normally required but may sometimes be indicated. (Fig.18.3).

Zadok's operation

The nail plate (or a section of nail plate if only one side requires treatment) is removed, longitu-dinal incision is made on each side of the base of the nail and the resulting flap of eponychium is turned back. The nail matrix is then excised and the flap realigned and then sutured (Fig. 18.4).

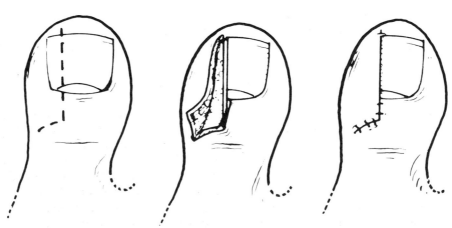

Fig. 18.3   Frost partial matrixectomy procedure (modified with suture closure). (From Comprehensive Textbook of Foot Surgery, McGlamry E D (ed), by permission of Williams and Wilkins.)

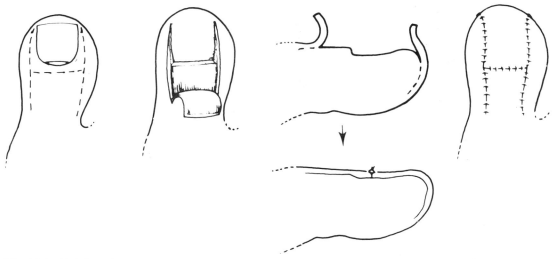

Fig. 18.4 Zadok total matrixectomy procedure (From Comprehensive Textbook of Foot Surgery, McGlamry E D (ed), by permission of Williams and Wilkins.)

It cannot be stressed too strongly that skilled aftercare is as essential a part of nail surgery as the operation itself. Unskilled treatment and lack of competent postoperative supervision could well give rise to questions as to the efficacy of nail surgery; but when properly performed, adequately followed up and when careful attention is paid to the elimination of the causative factors, the surgical techniques outlined certainly give excellent results and favourable prognoses.

SUBUNGUAL EXOSTOSIS

A subungual exostosis (Fig. 18.5) is a small outgrowth of bone under the nail plate near its free edge or immediately distal to it. Most frequently, it occurs on the great toe and is a source of considerable pain. As the outgrowth increases, the toe nail adheres closely to it and undergoes some displacement from the nail bed. The epidermis covering the exostosis becomes stretched and thinned and takes on a bright red colour. This will blanch on the application of pressure. The protuberance offers a hard resistance to pressure and there is usually a clear line of demarcation around the area. This, combined with the bright colour, readily distinguishes the exostosis from a corn. When the exostosis occurs distal to the nail plate, the bright red gives way to a yellowish-grey colour. Accurate diagnosis of this condition requires X-ray examination.

Aetiology

It may occur, though rarely, from a single sudden trauma such as stubbing, or may be due to repeated trauma such as continual, though perhaps slight, trauma from shoes which are either too short or excessively high-heeled.

Pathology

Following an injury to the periosteum of the distal phalanx, a periostitis occurs. Initially there is an outgrowth of cartilage which later ossifies.

Treatment

Temporary relief may be given by means of protective padding and supervision of footwear, but surgical excision is always the most satisfactory treatment. After the nail plate has been avulsed, a horizontal linear incision is made around the medial and lateral aspect of the phalanx. The nail bed is then carefully elevated and reflected. The exostosis can now be resected. The area is then smoothed flush with the phalanx and the nail bed is replaced and sutured.

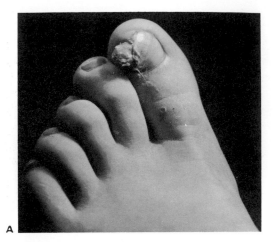

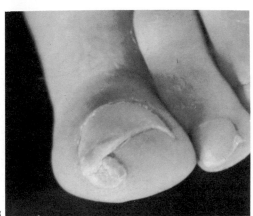

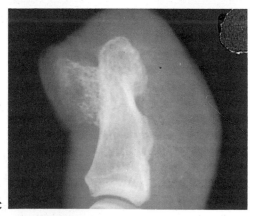

Fig. 18.5 (A and B) Subungual exostoses. (C) X-ray shows elevation of nail plate by exostosis.

DIGITAL BONE SURGERY

Digital deformities provide a source of complaint for many patients. Fortunately, most of these can be corrected surgically. Selection of the appropriate procedure rests upon an understanding of the type of deformity and its aetiology (Jimenez et al 1987).

Applied anatomy

Normal digital function and stability is achieved by smooth coordinated muscle function. The primary muscles involved in maintaining digital stability are the dorsal and plantar interossei and the lumbricales. They act to stabilise the proximal phalanges firmly against the metatarsal heads, thereby ensuring a rectus digital alignment and

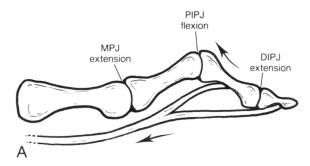

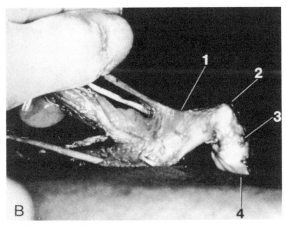

Fig. 18.6 Flexor stabilisation: in weight-bearing, the phalanges cannot be plantarflexed through the ground. In such instances, plantarflexory force is retrograded proximally creating dorsiflexion at the metatarsophalangeal joint. (A) When flexor digitorum brevis is primary force, proximal interphalangeal joint is plantarflexed. (B) When flexor digitorum longus is primary plantarflexory force, distal and proximal interphalangeal joints are both plantarflexed. (1) MPJ extension; (2) PIP flexion; (3) DIP flexion; (4) Ground reactive force. (From Comprehensive Textbook of Foot Surgery, McGlamry E D (ed), by permission of Williams and Wilkins.)

Plate 1 Arthroplasty: (A) Midline dorsal longitudinal skin incision affords excellent exposure of toe while avoiding neurovascular structures. (From Comprehensive Textbook of Foot Surgery, McGlamry E D (ed), by permission of Williams and Wilkins.) (B, C, D) Alternative technique to transecting tendon is demonstrated with undermining and retraction. Collateral ligaments are then cut to deliver the phalangeal head. (E) Bone is resected either with power saw or bone forceps.

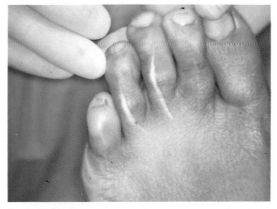

A

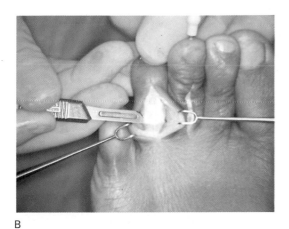

B

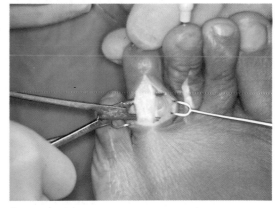

C

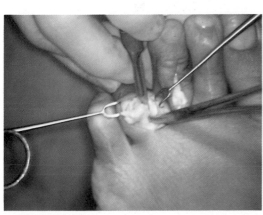

D

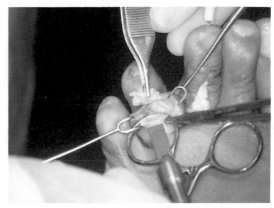

E

Plate 2a–e Peg-in-hole arthrodesis. (A) The medial, lateral and plantar condyles are resected as well as the distal articular cartilage. The dorsal cortex is carefully preserved. (B) A ball burr is then used to contour the phalanx into a suitable peg. (C) Starting with a very small ball burr or a side cutting burr, the initial hole is made in the base of the middle phalanx. Progressively larger ball burrs are used to ream the middle phalanx into a satisfactory receptacle. (D) A hand held Kirschner wire is used to identify the medullary canal of the proximal phalanx. Note the fully developed hole in the middle phalanx. (E) The Kirschner wire is then introduced into the middle phalanx and directed distally through the tip of the toe. The surgeon holds the distal aspect of the toe rectus or in slight hyperextension. The wire driver is then moved to the end of the toe and the wire is retrograded across the arthrodesis site into proximal phalanx. Fixation of the peg-in-hole arthrodesis is not mandatory, but enhances the overall stability.

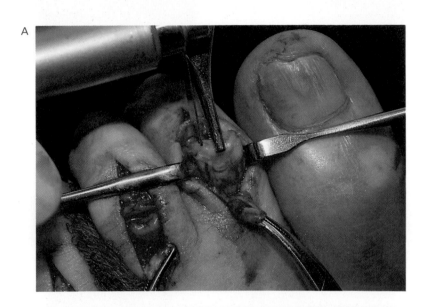

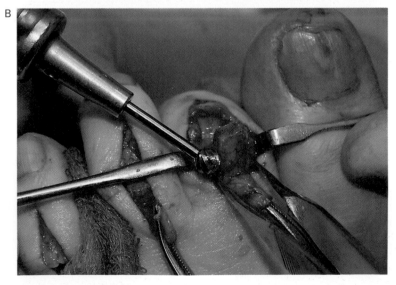

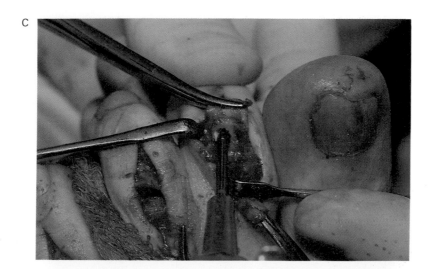

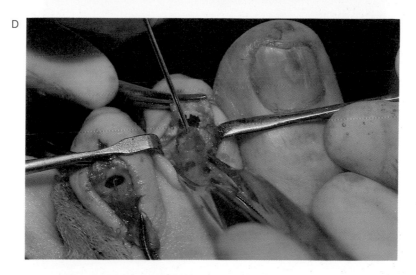

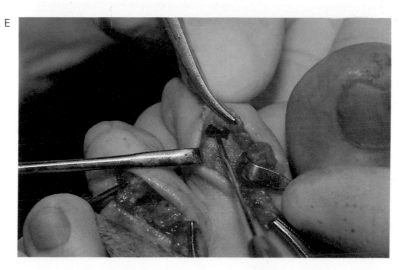

Plate 3 (A) Skin incision for access to medial and plantar aspects of hallux interphalangeal joint. Note lesion plantar to location of interphalangeal joint. (B) Capsule opened and flexor tendon retracted plantarly, exposing sesamoid. (C) Note thickness of sesamoid.

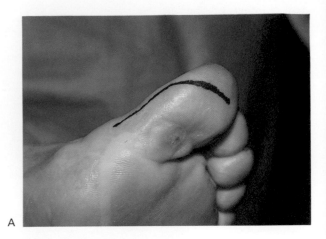

A

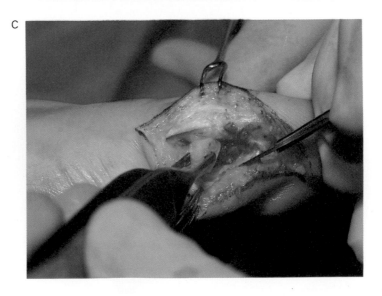

B

C

firm contact of the distal phalanges with the supporting surface. With this function effectively executed the subsequent contraction of the leg muscles will not alter the rectus digital alignment. If a stable proximal phalanx is not present upon contraction of the more powerful longus muscles then the toe will buckle. Such functional imbalance will lead to the development of hammer toe deformity (Jarret et al 1980).

Flexor stabilisation

In the normal foot, sufficient stability exists within the osseous structures to adequately support the body comfortably. However, when the foot pronates excessively much of this normal intrinsic stability is lost (Fig. 18.6). In such instances, other structures will be required to render the necessary support for adequate function. Most often the flexor digitorum longus, tibialis posterior and flexor hallucis longus muscles will need to begin function earlier, and maintain contraction longer than is normal. This results in the flexor digitorum longus contracting before the intrinsic muscles have been able to stabilise the proximal phalanges. The digits buckle, the proximal phalanges are dorsiflexed and hammer toe deformities are thus initiated (Jarret et al 1980). When such instability is present in gait, the lesser digits will be seen to grasp the weight-bearing surface during midstance and the propulsion phase.

Extensor substitution

As previously discussed, the lumbricales function in concert with the interosseous muscles to stabilise the proximal phalanges of the lesser digits during the stance phase of gait (Fig. 18.7). However, the lumbricales have a dual action. These muscles are also active during the swing phase of gait, stabilising the proximal phalanx of the digit against the metatarsal head. When subsequent contraction of the extensor digitorum longus occurs, the digit is maintained in a rectus alignment. In such proper circumstances the extensor digitorum longus will exert most of its power in assisting dorsiflexion of the ankle joint during the swing phase of gait.

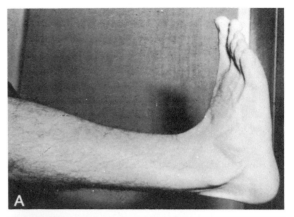

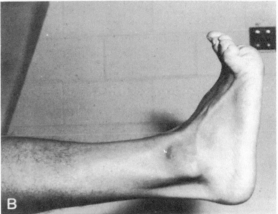

Fig. 18.7 Extensor substitution: (A) Clinical demonstration of normal digital extension with foot dorsiflexed. (B) Extensor substitution with excessive dorsiflexion of digits. Notice retrograde force of toes is transmitted to Metatarsal head, accentuating plantar protrusion of metatarsals. (From Comprehensive Textbook of Foot Surgery, McGlamry E D (ed), by permission of Williams and Wilkins.)

However, if the extensor digitorum longus has to contract prior to the lumbricales, or if intrinsic muscle function is impaired, the lesser digits will be seen to assume a hyperextended position during the swing phase of gait. This is referred to as extensor substitution, and it results in retraction of the toes. One will also note that toe purchase of the ground is delayed (Jimenez et al 1987).

Some of the causes of extensor substitution are neuromuscular diseases, other forms of weakness of the tibialis anterior, and ankle joint equinus. In certain neuromuscular diseases (i.e. Charcot-Marie-Tooth) intrinsic muscle function is lost and allows the long extensors to pull the digits into a dorsiflexed position. Any condition which leads to weakness of the tibialis anterior will result in prolonged contraction of the long extensor muscles—a true extensor substitution (Green et al 1976). Patients with limited dorsiflexory motion at the ankle will also over-exert the long extensors in an attempt to achieve more dorsiflexion.

This type of digital contraction may also be noted in the cavus foot which is not afflicted with neuromuscular disease (Whitney & Green 1982) (Fig. 18.8). When the cavus foot drops to a plantarflexed position at rest, increased tension is placed upon the long extensor tendons. This tension is in turn transmitted to the extensor hood apparatus surrounding the metatarsophalangeal joint, pulling the digit into a more dorsiflexed position. Eventually, adaptive contracture occurs dorsally at the metatarsophalangeal joint and is followed by loss of efficient intrinsic muscle function. The flexor digitorum longus resists this dorsal pull and thus contributes to the buckling of the digits at the interphalangeal joints and hence the clawing of the toes.

Flexor substitution

Flexor substitution is the least common cause of hammer toe deformity (Jimenez et al 1987). It is seen where there is extensive weakness of the triceps surae and the reminder of the posterior leg muscles must supply the necessary force for propulsion. This overactivity includes the flexor digitorum longus and will result in a rather abrupt accentuation of the hammer toe as the patient propels forward. A marked supinatory twist of the foot may be seen to occur concomitantly.

SURGICAL CORRECTION

Surgery should be aimed at relieving the immediate symptoms of the patient as well as providing a long-lasting correction of deformity. Procedures may consist of soft tissue releases and/or osseous approaches. Generally speaking, soft tissue procedures alone fail to maintain adequate correction of deformity over the long term (Jimenez et al 1987). However, several of these same techniques may mean the difference

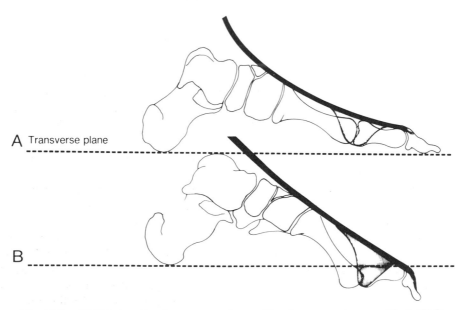

Fig. 18.8 (A) Relationship of extensor tendons and hood apparatus in normal foot. (B) In foot with anterior cavus deformity, the forefoot at rest drops into plantarflexed attitude. This places tendons under increased tension resulting in buckling of toes at metatarsophalangeal joints. (From Comprehensive Textbook of Foot Surgery, McGlamry E D (ed), by permission of Williams and Wilkins.)

between a successful or less than adequate result when combined with more definitive osseous procedures. Ultimately, the choice depends upon the severity of deformity, which digits are affected, the ambulatory status of the patient, and the aetiology of the contracture.

One concern with osseous surgery is which procedure is indicated: either arthroplasty or arthrodesis. Arthrodesis is rarely performed upon the fifth digit as this creates a very rigid toe which is not readily accommodated by shoes. In more severe contractures arthrodesis may be preferred as the correction tends to be better maintained. Patients suffering from extensor substitution generally require arthrodesing techniques as the function of the lumbricales may be irretrievably lost (especially in the presence of neuromuscular diseases). Patients with mild or moderate hammer toe deformities due to flexor stabilisation may undergo either type of surgery and do equally well. However, if an arthroplasty is performed then the excessive pronation must be adequately controlled postoperatively so as to discourage return of the hammer toe deformity (Jimenez et al 1987).

Arthroplasty (Plate 1 A-E)

A 2.5 to 3 cm longitudinal skin incision is made over the dorsal aspect of the digit with care taken to avoid completely penetrating through the skin. With medial and lateral tension being applied to the margins of the incision, dissection is deepened to the level of the superficial fascia. One may distinguish this layer as the skin margins are retracted and the vascular structures become visible. The superficial fascia is then incised parallel to the skin incision and vessels are identified and coagulated. Once the extensor tendon is visualised the surgeon has reached the deep fascia (Post 1882; Jimenez et al 1987).

By using a brushing stroke with the scalpel, the superficial fascia is separated from the underlying deep fascia, extensor hood and the joint apparatus. All major vessels will be contained within the superficial fascia and the surgeon may proceed with the proposed procedure without fear of inflicting neurovascular compromise.

The digit is now flexed and a medial and lateral vertical incision made at the joint level to sever the collateral ligaments. A transverse incision is then completed to transect the extensor tendon at the level of the proximal interphalangeal joint. The joint surfaces should be readily apparent upon flexion of the toe. Further dissection is usually required to sever the collateral ligaments totally and to free the head of the proximal phalanx. The same medial and lateral vertical incisions are repeated at the joint level, this time with the blade entering the joint itself. If ligamentous attachment is still present then the blade is introduced into the joint from within and advanced medially and laterally around each of the condyles of the phalangeal head. The head of the proximal phalanx should be totally freed at this point.

A power instrument or bone cutting forceps may then be used to remove the head of the proximal phalanx. The remaining bony stump should be rasped smooth to discourage future irritation.

The extensor tendon is then reapproximated using a 3–0 or 4–0 absorbable suture. The subcutaneous tissue is closed using a 4 0 or a 5–0 absorbable suture. The skin may be closed as the surgeon prefers.

Postoperative care

The toe (s) is typically maintained in some type of a surgical dressing for at least 10–14 days. Nonabsorbable sutures may be removed at this point. Afterwards, dressings may be removed and bathing allowed, although the toe(s) may require further dressings or some type of splintage to maintain alignment and discourage tenderness or excessive swelling.

During the initial postoperative period a surgical shoe is probably best suited for ambulation. Once dressings have been removed, the patient may still prefer to use the surgical shoe as it is common for the digits to remain tender if placed in a closed shoe at this point. After several weeks the patient will probably tolerate a tennis shoe or a depth oxford. Ladies may have difficulty wearing a dress shoe comfortably for several months following surgery as it is not unusual for some induration to remain within the toe until most of the scar tissue has remodelled.

Arthrodesis

The dissection sequence for arthrodesis of the proximal interphalangeal joint is the same as that for an arthroplasty. Surgery takes on a different approach once the head of the proximal phalanx is freed.

End-to-end arthrodesis (Fig. 18.9A, B)

The cartilaginous surfaces of the proximal phalangeal head and the base of the middle phalanx are removed. This may be performed with either power or hand instrumentation. However, hand instruments tend to provide a better 'raw' bone surface which theoretically encourages earlier osseous fusion. If power instrumentation is used then further dissection may be required to free the attachments of the extensor tendon from the dorsal aspect of the base of the middle phalanx to allow access for the saw (Soule 1910).

A 0.045 inch Kirschner wire (K-wire) is then introduced into the central portion of the proximal phalanx to identify the medullary canal. This will allow for smooth passage of the wire later in the procedure. The K-wire is then loaded into the wire driver. The distal aspect of the toe is then grasped medially and laterally with two fingers, with a third finger being placed plantarly to effect hyperextension of the distal interphalangeal joint. The K-wire is then introduced into the base of the middle phalanx centrally and advanced distalward through the tip of the toe. If the position is not satisfactory then the wire should be completely retrograded and the procedure repeated. One may find that the second attempt is somewhat more difficult as the wire tends to follow the path of least resistance, that is, the initial canal created by the wire. By increasing the speed of the wire driver one may help to overcome this problem.

Once a suitable position is attained, the K-wire is guided distally until only a small portion is visible at the base of the middle phalanx. At this point an assistant will stabilise the proximal phalanx with a forceps while the surgeon drives the wire from distal to proximal into the previously opened medullary canal of the proximal phalanx. If the wire is driven slowly one may feel the faint resistance of the subchondral bone plate at the base of the proximal phalanx and stop the wire driver. Another uncut wire lined up with the tip of this wire may be used to gauge depth position to ensure that one has not crossed into the metatarsophalangeal joint. Next, the arthrodesis site is examined to ensure that adequate apposition has been attained. The wound is then closed in the standard manner.

Peg-in-hole arthrodesis (Plate 2 A-E)

Once the head of the proximal phalanx has been exposed, the medial, lateral and plantar condyles of the head are resected. The remaining cartilaginous distal cap is also resected with care taken to preserve the integrity of the dorsal cortex. The 'peg' is smoothed with a burr on its corners and a hole is fashioned in the base of the middle phalanx. One should start the drill hole with a fairly small drill and gradually increase its diameter using progressively larger ball burrs until the hole approximates the size of the proximal peg. A trial seating of the arthrodesis is performed with a forceps being used to guide the proximal peg while the other hand firmly stabilises the middle phalanx (Young 1938).

Once seating has been accomplished, the forceps should be used to grasp the proximal phalanx at its juncture with the middle. With the forceps held in this position and the joint thence unseated, the surgeon will have an estimate as to how much of the peg was actually seated.

If the fit is secure then wire stabilisation is not necessarily required, though the security of such fixation is generally preferred. Where deemed appropriate, a 0.045 inch Kirschner wire may be used for stabilisation as previously described.

Follow-up care

As mentioned previously, K-wires are not essential for peg-in-hole arthrodeses provided a good snug fit has been achieved. If wires are used they should optimally remain in place for 4–6 weeks before removal. For end-to-end arthrodeses the wire should preferably remain in place for at least 6 weeks. Some type of splintage of the digits (i.e.

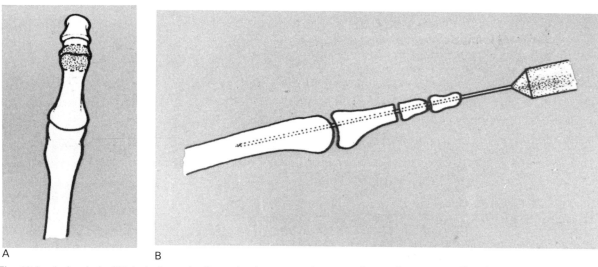

A   B

Fig. 18.9 Arthrodesis: (A) Articular ends of apposing bones must be resected, exposing raw cancellous bone, to ensure rapid arthrodesis. (B) Internal fixation with Kirschner wire eliminates motion at joint and assists in early union. Where metatarsophalangeal joint release has been effected, the wire may be extended across the joint to maintain alignment during early healing.

toe crests) may still be helpful for a few additional weeks. A closed shoe may be used once the wires have been retracted, although ladies may not be able to wear dress shoes comfortably for 1 to 2 months after this point (Jimenez et al 1987).

THE SEQUENTIAL APPROACH TO DIGITAL SURGERY (Fig. 18.12 A-F)

One quandary the surgeon may encounter when repairing hammer toe deformities is how far to go before adequate correction is obtained and can be reasonably maintained. A sequential approach to digital surgery has been devised which provides the surgeon with a reliable means to assess intra-operatively the efficacy of the procedure. After each manoeuvre, if adequate correction has not been obtained then the surgeon proceeds in a logical fashion to the next step. The sequence is described below (Jimenez et al 1987).

Preoperative evaluation

The first step is to evaluate the degree of deformity prior to surgery in order to ascertain which, if any, osseous procedures are indicated. One may also sense the steps which may be required to release the contracture completely by examining the digit while a loading force has been applied to the forefoot. Loading the forefoot simulates the weight-bearing attitude and allows one to note the relationship of the proximal phalanx to the metatarsal. If the proximal phalanx returns to a rectus alignment, then more elaborate intervention may not be needed. However, if the phalanx remains dorsiflexed relative to the metatarsal, or if there is a transverse plane deviation, then several steps will most likely be required.

In performing an arthroplasty the head of the proximal phalanx is initially removed. The amount of bone removed is that which is required to relieve soft tissue tension while maintaining the length of the toe in relation to its neighbouring digits. This will eliminate the osseous prominence and in a milder deformity may provide enough relaxation of the soft tissue structures to provide good correction.

If an arthrodesis is to be done, then the head of the phalanx is free. Dorsiflexory pressure should once again be applied to the forefoot. If the proximal phalanx returns to a rectus alignment without resistance then this may be all the release that is necessary. However, if resistance is met then one needs to proceed to the next step.

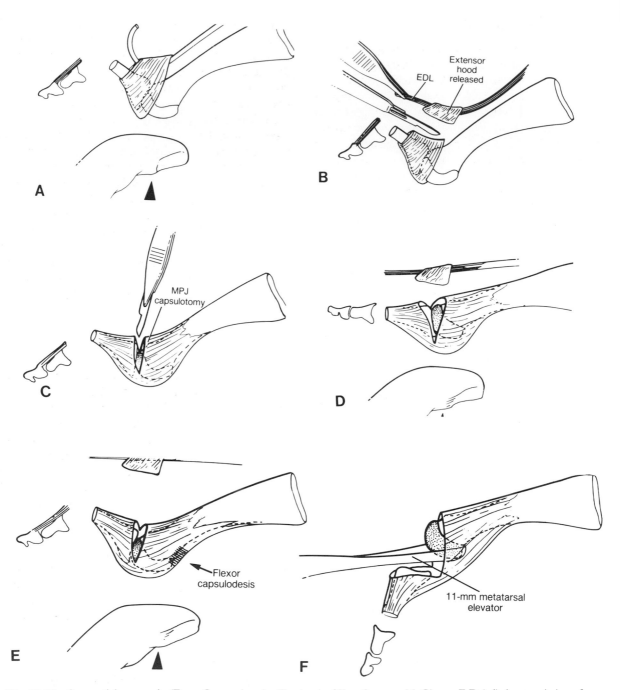

Fig. 18.10 Sequential approach. (From Comprehensive Textbook of Foot Surgery, McGlamry E D (ed), by permission of Williams and Wilkins.) (A) Following phalangeal head resection, push-up test is repeated. Note continued dorsiflexed position of proximal phalanx. Next sequential step is indicated. (B) Extensor hood release is performed and push-up test repeated. Unless metatarsophalangeal joint realigns easily, next step is performed. (C) Capsulotomy of dorsal, medial, and lateral aspects is effected. (D) Push-up test shows realignment of joint indicating adequate correction of digit. (E) Failure to realign indicates capsulodesis of flexor apparatus to metatarsal neck. (F) Metatarsal elevator is used to release flexor capsule from metatarsal neck.

Extensor hood recession

Although the extensor digitorum longus tendon has its terminal insertion at the distal phalanx of each digit, the tendon slips richly invest the metatarsophalangeal joint area by fibrous expansions forming what is known as the extensor hood. The primary force of the extensor tendons at the digital level is applied not within the toe itself, but more proximally at the hood apparatus. After digital deformity has been present for a sufficient time, the extensor hood adapts and assists in maintaining the deformity. At times these hood fibres will need to be released to allow adequate repositioning of the toe (Jiminez et al 1987).

To accomplish this one lifts the extensor tendon distally and slightly dorsally to place tension on the hood fibres. The scalpel is then placed parallel to the tendon at its medial edge. The blade is rotated ninety degrees and the medial expansions are severed. The same manoeuvre is performed laterally. The tendon should then be lifted free of its underlying attachments to the phalanx. The butt end of the scalpel handle should be able to pass beneath the tendon to the level of the metatarsal neck and beyond. If resistance is met then the above procedure is repeated. Once the hood has been thoroughly released the push-up test is again effected.

Metatarsophalangeal joint capsulotomy

If the extensor hood recession failed to relieve the contracture adequately, then one will need to incise the dorsal, medial and lateral capsule of the metatarsophalangeal joint. Using a forceps to grasp the proximal phalanx, distal distraction is applied. This causes a dimple to form dorsally in the joint capsule. The blade is introduced dorsally at that point and passed medially and laterally. Should contracture remain following the push-up test then further surgery will be necessary (from 16 mm film, *Approaches to Digital Surgery*, Podiatry Institute, Tucker, Ga. 1973).

Plantar capsular release

With long standing deformities, the flexor plate, which is normally supported beneath the central plantar aspect of the metatarsal head and neck, may be displaced medially or laterally or may be fibrosed to the metatarsal neck just proximal to the plantar cartilage. Such capsulodesis will prevent plantarflexion of the toe when the forefoot is loaded. If the flexor cap is displaced medially or laterally it will draw the toe medially or laterally as the forefoot is loaded. Such displacement is almost always the cause of digits exhibiting medial or lateral deviation at the metatarsophalangeal joint. Plantar capsular release will be required in such instances and this is greatly facilitated by the use of the McGlamry metatarsal elevator. Having completed release of the flexor plate the toe should easily return to a rectus position when the foot is loaded (from 16 mm film, *Approaches to Digital Surgery*, Podiatry Institute, Tucker, Ga. 1973).

Extensor tendon lengthening

When a moderate to severe contracture is present, one should anticipate the need for an extensor tendon lengthening. This is performed just prior to and in conjunction with the extensor hood recession. A longitudinal incision is made along the medial or lateral margin of the tendon and a haemostat is introduced beneath the extensor tendon and opened. The tendon is then incised longitudinally at its midpoint so that it is split into two equal parts. At the proximal aspect of the incision the lateral one-half of the tendon is severed. This is then retracted distally and the more medial half of the tendon incised distally at the proximal interphalangeal joint level (Jimenez et al 1987) (Fig. 18.11). At closure, the tendon is repaired in an appropriately lengthened position.

Additional notes

If the metatarsophalangeal joint capsule requires release, the surgeon may elect to use a Kirschner wire to maintain the digit in the corrected position while the capsular structures heal. This is highly recommended if the plantar capsule has been released. Once the wire has been retrograded through the digit to the base of the proximal phalanx, the metatarsophalangeal joint is

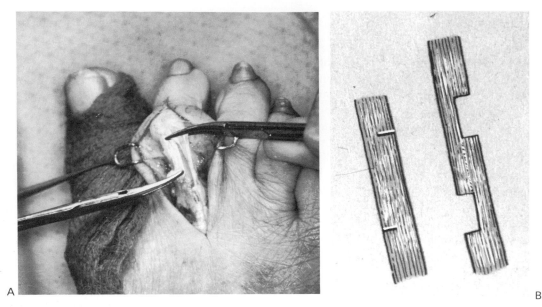

Fig. 18.11   Z-plasty lengthening of extensor tendon: (A) Tendon split longitudinally into two equal parts; (B) Showing how lateral and medial incisions enable retraction distally to new length required.

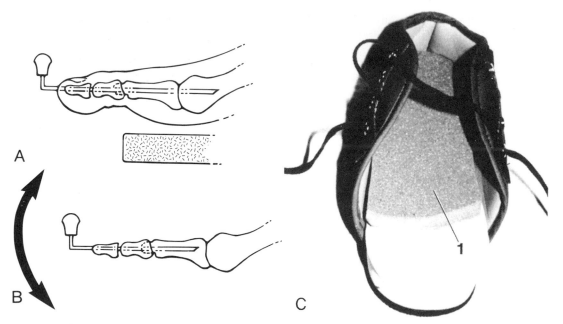

Fig. 18.12   Kirschner wires are protected from bending forces to avoid metal fatigue and breakage and to prevent tissue irritation resulting in pin tract infection. (A) Built-up insole removes pressure from under side of toe. (B) Pin which does not cross metatarsophalangeal joint allows bending of toe without strain to the wire. (C) Darco trauma shoe is built up with cork or with heavy felt forward to sulcus under toes. Toes are allowed to float over the end of the insole. (From Comprehensive Textbook of Foot Surgery, McGlamry E D (ed), by permission of Williams and Wilkins.)

repositioned and the wire driven into the metatarsal several centimetres.

Postoperatively one will need to protect the wire from bending forces to prevent breakage or a pin tract infection (Fig. 18.12 A–C). This protection is best achieved by using a Darco type trauma shoe with a built-up insole of $\frac{1}{4}$ inch cork or $\frac{1}{2}$ inch felt all the way forward to the area beneath the sulcus (1, on Fig. 18.12C). This allows the toes to be relieved of any weight-bearing stresses.

If the flexor plate has been released, then the wire should remain across the metatarso-phalangeal joint for only 3 to $3\frac{1}{2}$ weeks. At this point the wire should be retracted across the joint into the proximal phalanx so that motion at the metatarsophalangeal joint limitus may be created if the wire is left in position for a longer period of time. By retracting the wire into the toe at $3\frac{1}{2}$ weeks, the joint may still require splinting to help maintain alignment for several more weeks, but a passive range of motion exercises must be initiated.

Primary contractures of the distal inter-phalangeal joint may result in mallet toe deformities which require surgical intervention (Fig. 18.13). The procedure of choice in most cases is arthroplasty of the distal interphalangeal joint (Jimenez et al 1987). The preferred approach is usually two transverse semi-elliptical incisions at the level of the joint. The corresponding skin wedge is excised and the head of the middle phalanx exposed in a manner similar to a hammer toe correction. The head of the middle phalanx is then resected and the wound closed as previously mentioned. Subcutaneous sutures are not usually necessary. The excised wedge of skin removes redundant tissue and effectively tightens the skin

to retain the straightened alignment once the phalangeal head has been removed.

Follow-up care

Post operative care is essentially the same as that outlined previously for hammer toe repair.

THE FIFTH DIGIT

The fifth digit is often considered separately because it presents special requirements for accommodation in shoes (Korn 1980) (from 16 mm film, *Approaches to Digital Surgery*, Podiatry Institute, Tucker, Ga. 1973). The fifth digit is rarely arthrodesed as this creates a rigid member which is easily irritated by most shoes. However, arthroplasty alone is often insufficient to provide an asymptomatic toe.

Synostosis of the middle and distal phalanges (Fig. 18.14A–C)

This hereditary condition results in loss of much of the flexibility of the toe and following the removal of the head of the proximal phalanx the hyperkeratotic skin lesion may at times shift distally over the middle phalanx. This transfer may be prevented in most instances by performing a hemi-phalangectomy of the middle and distal phalanges in conjunction with the original arthroplasty (Jimenez et al 1987).

The surgery is approached through a lazy-S

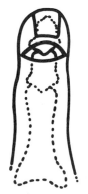
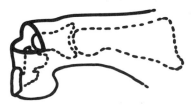

Fig. 18.13   Incisional approach for correction of mallet toe.

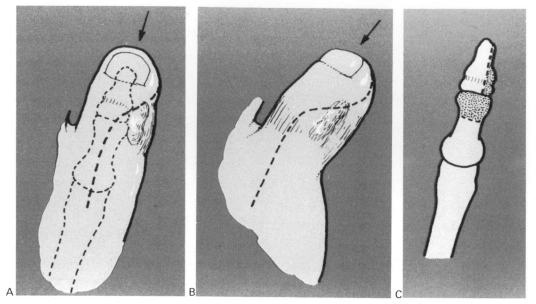

Fig. 18.14   Correction of fifth toe. (A, B) Incisional approach in exposing proximal interphalangeal joint and lateral aspect of middle and distal synostosis. (C) Represents typical bony resection in which appropriate bone is resected from proximal phalangeal head and lateral aspect of middle-distal synostosis is resected and smoothed.

incision over the fifth digit. Arthroplasty is performed at the proximal interphalangeal joint. Further distally, the soft tissues are dissected free from the lateral aspect of the synostosis comprising the middle and distal phalanges. Dissection is carried slightly dorsally and plantarly onto the phalanx with careful preservation of the tendinous attachments. This should expose the osseous structures and the lateral one-fourth of the phalanges should be removed with a bone cutting forceps. The remainder of the surface is then smoothed with a rotary burr.

Adductovarus deformity (Fig. 18.15 A,B)

In some patients the fifth toe may be seen to underlap the fourth digit assuming an adducto-varus attitude. This position may lead to the presence of a heloma at the lateral nail groove. The excessive pressure against the nail may also lead to onychauxis.

Adductovarus deformity may be corrected concomitantly by incorporating an elliptical skin wedge excision to aid in derotating the toe (Mahan 1987).

Heloma molle

A common condition seen by any foot specialist is the heloma molle which forms in the fourth web space. This is the result of shearing forces between the head of the proximal phalanx of the fifth toe and the base of the proximal phalanx of the fourth toe. Satisfactory resolution of the lesion may be provided by arthroplasty of the fifth toe. Generally speaking, additional procedures are not required on the adjacent fourth digit for this problem.

THE HALLUX

Occasionally the hallux itself may require surgery apart from hallux abductovalgus repair. One common condition which may manifest is the interphalangeal sesamoid (Plate 3 A–C). This accessory bone will lie intra-articularly within the more dorsal aspect of the flexor hallucis longus tendon. Often the ossicle will serve as the genesis of a hyperkeratotic plantar lesion. Surgical excision is most often performed through a medial incision at the level of the interphalangeal joint,

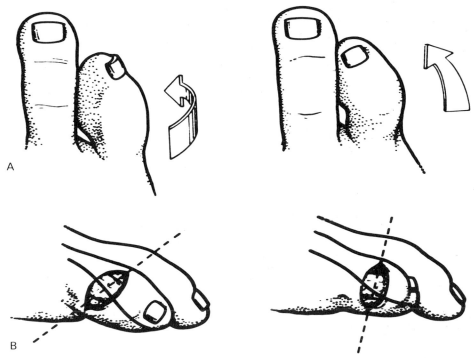

Fig. 18.15 Adductovarus and adductus deformity. (B) Shows appropriate placement of axes to effect correction of adductovarus and adductus deformities of fifth toe.

slightly more dorsal than plantar. The capsule of the joint is incised in a longitudinal fashion along with the periosteum as a single layer. The sesamoid may then be palpated with an instrument and excised. The dissection may be facilitated by maintaining the interphalangeal joint in a flexed position.

Alternatively, a transverse incision on the plantar aspect of the hallux or an 'S' incision may be used for exposure.

One may also see hyperkeratotic lesions on the plantar medial aspect of the hallux. Typically these 'pinch calluses' will be due to biomechanical imbalances. However, there may also be hypertrophy of the condyles of the head of the proximal or base of the distal phalanx. Surgical reduction of these osseous prominences may be accomplished through the medial incision described above.

Follow-up care

Postoperative care for the hallux is essentially the same as that for the lesser digits. Ambulation may

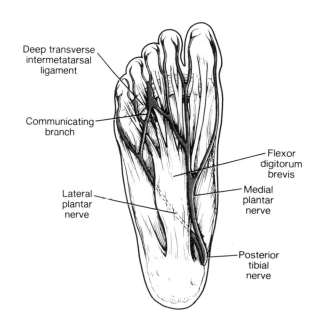

Fig. 18.16 Neuroma. Illustration of involved anatomy from plantar approach. (From Comprehensive Textbook of Foot Surgery, McGlamry E D (ed), by permission of Williams and Wilkins.)

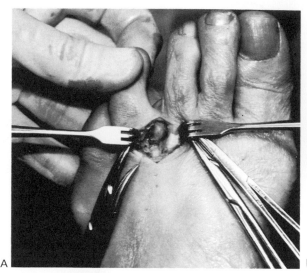

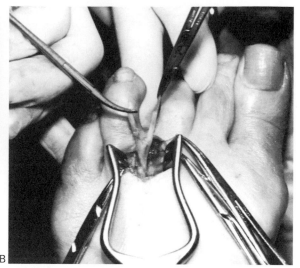

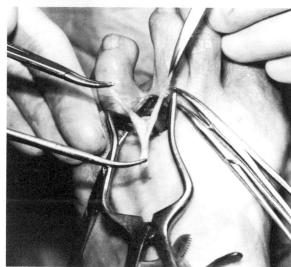

Fig. 18.17   (A) Neuroma shown exposed in floor of interspace. (B) Distal branches of neuroma have been resected and nerve traced proximally. (C) Nerve resected proximal to transverse metatarsal ligament.

1987). The surgical technique involves making a small puncture incision at a level where the tendon is readily accessible. Using a number 11 blade, the tendon may be placed on tension and 'snapped'. Closure usually requires only one suture.

It is very important to initiate early splintage or a digital traction device to prevent the tendon from fibrosing with the toe in a contracted position. One must also be aware of the risk involved with isolated tenotomies, specially the accentuation of deformity in the other digits. Once the tendon has been cut, the load from that tendon will be dispersed to the remaining intact slips and may increase any deforming influence to the other toes.

be allowed immediately and dressings maintained until sufficient healing has occurred, but very restricted activity should be anticipated for the first week or 10 days. A return to shoes is allowed as symptoms permit, usually 3 weeks post-operatively.

Tenotomy

Occasionally one may encounter an older patient with a reasonably flexible contracture of the toe and an associated heloma. If the patient is fairly appropulsive then an isolated tenotomy may be used to help alleviate the condition (Jimenez et al

NEUROMA (Figs 18.16, 18.17 A-C)

Surgical excision of Morton's neuroma may be required in patients who have failed to obtain relief from conservative measures. Excision may be accomplished through either a dorsal or plantar incision (Miller 1981; Miller 1987). The authors' preference is a dorsal incision, beginning at the base of the third web space and extending proximally over the third intermetatarsal space for 2 or 3 cm. Dissection is carried through the fascia and loose connective tissue to the floor of the intermetatarsal space. Attention is directed distally where the digital branches of the nerve are identified, isolated from the surrounding tissues and transected .

Using Metzenbaum scissors the neuroma is dissected proximally from its soft tissue attachments and cut at the most proximal to the transverse metatarsal ligament. Closure is accomplished with either 3−0 or 4−0 suture for the subcutaneous tissue. The skin is closed according to the surgeon's preference.

Postoperatively, a compression bandage is maintained for two weeks followed by some type of elastic compression for several additional weeks.

A transverse plantar incision may be made just proximal to the interphalangeal sulcus to effect flexor tenotomy and capsulotomy where needed. A linear plantar incision is sometimes used, though the authors prefer the transverse approach as a finer scar usually results.

REFERENCES

Green D R, Ruch J A, McGlamry E D 1976 Correction of equinus related forefoot deformities. Journal of the American Podiatric Medical Association 66: 768−779

Jarret B A, Manzi J A, Green D R 1980 Interossei and lumbricales muscles of the foot   an anatomical and function study. Journal of the American Podiatric Medical Association 70: 1−13

Jimenez A L, McGlamry E D, Green D R 1987 Lesser ray deformities. In: McGlamry E D (ed) Comprehensive Textbook of Foot Surgery. Williams & Wilkins, Baltimore, pp 57−113

Korn S H 1980 The lazy S approach for correction of painful underlapping fifth digit. Journal of the American Podiatric Medical Association 70: 30−33

Mahan K T 1987 Plastic surgery and skin grafting. In: McGlamry E D (ed) Comprehensive Textbook of Foot Surgery. Williams & Wilkins, Baltimore, pp 685−713

Miller S J 1981 Surgical technique for resection of Morton's neuroma. Journal of the American Podiatric Medical Association 77: 181−188

Miller S J 1987 Morton's neuroma syndrome. In: McGlamry E D (ed) Comprehensive Textbook of Foot Surgery. Williams & Wilkins, Baltimore, pp 38−56

Post A C 1882 Hallux valgus with displacement of the smaller toes. Medical Record 11: 120−121

Soule R E 1910 Operation for the correction of hammer toe. New York Medical Journal 649−650

Whitney A K, Green D R 1982 Pseudoequinus. Journal of the American Podiatric Medical Association 72: 365−371

Young C S 1938 An operation for the correction of hammer-toe and claw-toe. Journal of Bone & Joint Surgery 20: 715−719

19. Genetic factors in disorders of the foot

J. A. Raeburn

A number of foot disorders are inherited and may therefore occur in several members of a family. Consequently a basic knowledge of genetic principles can help the podiatrist, first in making a complete diagnosis and secondly by awareness that a condition may recur in other family members. Genetic counselling can be arranged by a patient's family doctor to ensure that relevant aspects of inheritance are understood and that the available therapeutic measures are discussed.

The foot deformity may be only one aspect of a more general abnormality, e.g. pes cavus with Charcot-Marie-Tooth disease. An important feature of this condition is muscle weakness and atrophy, particularly in the peroneal muscles. This causes a characteristic abnormality of gait. Thus the podiatrist might suspect that lesions of the feet were part of a more general condition and, after discussion with the family doctor, further investigation or a specialist referral might be advised in some cases. Not all congenital deformities are inherited, some being attributable to adverse factors operating in utero, such as drug therapy or infections. In addition, pressure on the lower limb or 'amniotic bands' may cause peripheral limb defects.

Genetic anomalies fall into three categories:

1. Single gene disorders, in which only one gene site is affected (Mendelian disorders).
2. Multifactorial disorders, in which both genetic and environmental factors are involved.
3. Chromosomal defects, e.g. trisomies and monosomies or structural defects such as translocations.

MENDELIAN GENETICS

The normal individual has 46 chromosomes consisting of 22 pairs of autosomes plus 2 sex chromosomes (two X chromosomes in females and an X and a Y chromosome in males). Except for the sex chromosomes in males and in certain cells of the gonads, all chromosomes occur in pairs so that at the same location on each of the chromosomes in a pair a gene exists which directs the development of a particular physical attribute. If both of a gene pair are normal the individual is normal for that attribute. If there is an abnormality of one of the pair, the abnormal characteristic may be expressed, depending on whether the abnormal gene is dominant or recessive. If an abnormal gene is dominant, the defect is expressed in single dose and the action of the normal gene is suppressed. If an abnormal gene is recessive, the defect is expressed only if *both* the genes are abnormal. The four types of Mendelian inheritance are:

1. autosomal dominant
2. autosomal recessive
3. X-linked recessive
4. X-linked dominant.

Autosomal dominant disorders

Since each parent donates one of the two autosomes in a pair, the child has a 1 in 2 chance of inheriting an autosomal dominant (AD) defect from an affected parent. Conditions caused by autosomal dominant genes therefore commonly occur in each generation of an affected family. In autosomal dominant inheritance, both sexes are equally at risk of involvement. Figure

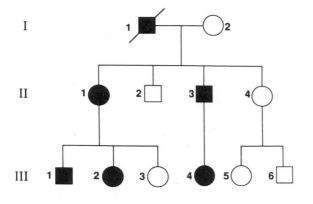

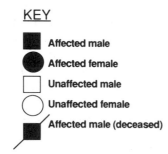

KEY

■ Affected male

● Affected female

□ Unaffected male

○ Unaffected female

◪ Affected male (deceased)

Fig. 19.1   An autosomal dominant pedigree. This pedigree shows three generations of a family in which an autosomal dominant disorder occurs. Several orthopaedic disorders which require chiropody treatment are inherited in this way.

19.1 shows a typical family tree where autosomal dominance occurs.

List I. Examples of conditions which are usually autosomal dominant

Lobster claw deformity (ectrodactyly)
Tarsal fusion syndromes, e.g. calcaneonavicular bar or talocalcaneal coalition
Some forms of postaxial polydactyly and of syndactyly or brachydactyly.

Since the diagnosis of one of the above syndromes does not always imply autosomal dominant inheritance, it is clear that advice from a genetic specialist will often be needed. A difficulty in estimating the risk of others in a family being affected by an AD disorder is that not all individ-

uals who have the abnormal gene will show any abnormalities. All of the examples in List I can occur in such slight forms that the presence of the gene in one subject may be missed. Nevertheless, the risk of that person's offspring inheriting the gene is 50%; consequently, the risk of a child having severe manifestations of the condition may be very high. The percentage of individuals with an abnormal AD gene who manifest the disorder is referred to as the *penetrance* of the abnormal gene. The genetic approach can be complicated by variable penetrance. In many conditions, this phenomenon will be more fully understood if the location of a gene on a specific part of one chromosome, or even the exact structure of the abnormal gene is identified. Non-manifesting gene carriers could then be recognised by the associated genetic marker patterns or by direct gene probing.

Autosomal recessive disorders

To be affected by an autosomal recessive disorder, an individual must have an abnormal gene at the relevant location on both chromosomes of the pair. Autosomal recessive (AR) defects can be expressed in either sex but tend to be seen in one particular sibship and not in several generations of a family. Offspring of a person with an autosomal recessive disorder have a low risk of inheriting the condition unless the affected person marries a carrier. However, the offspring of that affected person will be 'obligate' carriers of the condition. Both parents of a person with an autosomal recessive disorder are obligate carriers. The risks to the offspring of two such carries are: 1 in 4 for the child inheriting the condition, 1 in 4 for being clinically and genetically normal and 1 in 2 for being carriers.

It will be appreciated that if recessive genes occur in a family there may be several healthy carriers in that family. Therefore if cousins in such families were to marry, their children could inherit one copy of the abnormal gene from each parent. Thus AR diseases occur more often in offspring of consanguineous relationships. Figure 19.2 illustrates such a pedigree.

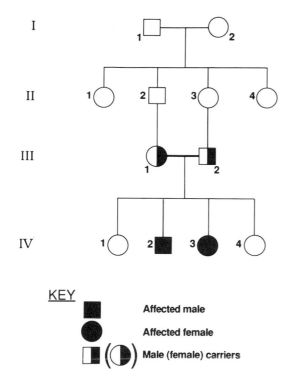

KEY

■ Affected male

● Affected female

◧ (◖) Male (female) carriers

N.B. II 2 and II 3 are probable carriers

Fig. 19.2 An autosomal recessive pedigree in which the parents of the affected children are consanguineous. As can be seen III: 1 and III: 2 are first cousins, their father and mother respectively being brother and sister. This consanguinity almost certainly led to the presence of the AR disorder in generation IV which has affected IV: 2 and IV: 3.

List II. Examples of autosomal recessive disorders

Polysyndactyly plus craniostenosis (Carpenter's syndrome)

Microcephaly, mental retardation, hypotonia plus syndactyly of the 2nd and 3rd toes (Smith-Lemli Opitz syndrome)

Congenital indifference to pain (Charcot's joints may occur)

Club foot with dwarfism.

X-linked disorders

Single gene disorders of the X chromosome account for a large number of conditions of which the best known are haemophilia and Duchenne muscular dystrophy. These two disorders are X-linked *recessive* in nature and this type of inheritance will be considered first.

A. X-linked recessive disorders

Males are almost exclusively affected with these disorders; females have relative protection from the abnormalities caused by an abnormal gene on one X chromosome because of the normal gene on their other X chromosome. In X-linked recessive families, females may be healthy carriers of the disorder. On average half of the sons of a carrier female will be affected whilst half of the daughters will be carriers.

Detection of carriers of X-linked disorders is difficult but for many of these conditions there are new techniques based on genetic markers which are identifiable by variations in individual specific segments of DNA or on direct identification of the genetic mutation. Since knowledge has changed very rapidly it is wise to ensure that patients and their families check up on the developments in their own condition, in case new approaches might be suitable.

List III. Examples of X-linked recessive disorders

Haemophilia

Duchenne muscular dystrophy (pseudohypertrophic)

Fragile X syndrome (an X-linked recessive form of mental retardation).

B. X-linked dominant disorders

Either sex may be affected with these disorders but the affected mother may transmit the gene to both sons and daughters, half of whom will be affected. Affected fathers can only transmit the abnormal gene (on the X chromosome) to daughters, all of whom will be affected. With some X-linked dominant disorders the hemizygous males are thought to have a more severe form of the condition.

Examples of X-linked dominant disorders

Hypophosphataemic type of Vitamin D resistant rickets

Pseudo-hypoparathyroidism (type 1).

MULTIFACTORIAL INHERITANCE

These types of disorder are caused by the combined effects of several genes and environmental factors. The chances of a particular individual inheriting a multifactorial condition depends on the heritability (i.e. the proportion of the disorder which is due to genetic factors) and on the closeness of relationship to the affected member of the family.

Examples of multifactorial inheritance

Congenital dislocation of the hip
Arthrogryposis
Spina bifida and related neural tube defects (e.g. myelomeningocele)
Talipes deformities.

Recognition of multifactorial inheritance is important because in relevant families, the knowledge of genetic factors operating could help in the identification of increased risk to individuals and families. Then, by modifying environmental aspects, e.g. diet, the condition may be prevented. For example, genetic factors contribute significantly to the cause of neural tube defects. It has recently been shown conclusively that in pregnancies at high risk, the incidence of neural tube defects can be reduced by treatment of the mother before conception and up to the 12-week stage of gestation.

CHROMOSOME DEFECTS

Chromosome abnormalities can be due to numerical changes or to structural defects. With numerical changes, there is either an extra or a missing chromosome, although in general those fetuses with an absent chromosome would not survive beyond the early stages of pregnancy. Of live-born chromosome abnormalities, Down's syndrome (Trisomy 21) is by far the commonest disorder and in this condition certain foot defects, including pes planus, can occur. Translocations are examples of structural defects of chromosomes and foot defects can occur as part of the resultant general chromosome imbalance syndrome.

Chromosome defects are very common in early fetuses but most major abnormalities will miscarry before pregnancy is far advanced. Chromosome defects also illustrate another feature of genetic disorders, i.e. that these disorders affect many body systems—brain, cardiovascular system, skeletal system, etc.

GENETIC HETEROGENEITY

With many clinical abnormalities it has been found that the same apparent syndrome can be due to different genetic causes. For example, in some families polydactyly can be due to an autosomal dominant gene or it may occur as part of an autosomal recessive syndrome. Polydactyly can also occur in chromosome disorders and certain forms have a multifactorial basis for inheritance. There is also evidence of polydactyly due to an entirely sporadic event which does not recur in a family. Genetic heterogeneity is one reason why caution should be taken in giving genetic advice and information to an isolated patient. To get the correct information, it may often be necessary to take a very careful family history and examine several other members of the family.

GENERAL ASPECTS OF GENETICS

Genetic disorders of the foot are quite common and can be due to a variety of different mechanisms. It is important to realise that the same genetic abnormality might vary in its expression in different members of the family and in the time of onset of complications. It will often be advisable for a podiatrist to ask for advice from an orthopaedic surgeon and a clinical geneticist if clients ask about the genetic recurrence risk. In general, referral to such specialists is essential for dealing with this type of problem. However, the clinical podiatrist will find a lot of interest in understanding the genetic mechanisms underlying some of the abnormalities he or she treats.

If the treatment is carried out in the patient's home, then family pictures or discussions with others in the family might suggest a genetic element which has not been previously appreciated. The enthusiast is referred to the following monographs for background detail.

FURTHER READING

Beighton P 1978 Inherited disorders of the skeleton. Churchill Livingstone, Edinburgh

Wynne-Davis 1973 Heritable disorders in orthopaedic practice. Blackwell Scientific Publications, Oxford

20. Circulatory disorders

Michael Davies

Circulatory disorders of the lower limb and foot arise from arterial disease, resulting in a diminished supply of oxygenated blood to the tissues. Impairment of drainage of blood and tissue fluid from the foot because of defective lymphatic and venous flow also produces changes in the feet.

DISEASES OF ARTERIES

Whilst there are many pathological states which affect arteries, the simple classification into degenerative, inflammatory and vasospastic will be used.

Degenerative arterial disease

Arteriosclerosis

This term should be applied strictly to those changes in the arterial tree which are part of the normal ageing process and which in themselves are of no significance. Medial sclerosis (Monckeberg's sclerosis) is an example of the changes which occur in the larger arteries with advancing years. In this condition, the media loses its muscular and elastic tissue and becomes calcified. The vessels become elongated and tortuous, but since the calibre of the lumen remains unaltered, there is little or no reduction in blood flow and clinical symptoms do not usually result.

Atherosclerosis or atheroma

This is a degenerative condition affecting the aorta as well as large and medium sized arteries and whilst commoner in the elderly, it is not an inevitable accompaniment of ageing. Because the pathological changes result in a reduction in the calibre of vessels, hypoxia of the tissues supplied by the diseased arteries occurs. This may result in angina and myocardial infarction from involvement of the coronary arteries, strokes due to involvement of the cerebral vessels, and intermittent claudication and peripheral gangrene as a consequence of the disease in the lower limb arteries.

Atheroma (*athere*, meaning gruel) begins with the development of small fatty streaks of lipid-containing material on the arterial intima and is followed by intimal thickening with the formation of an atheromatous plaque. This slowly increases in size and may ulcerate, producing an atheromatous ulcer upon which a secondary thrombosis may occur. Occasionally, haemorrhage may occur into an atheromatous plaque. Various stages of progression of atheroma may be found in different vessels in the same individual. Calcification of atheromatous ulcers may occur. When an atheromatous plaque ruptures, the yellow, porridge-like material, from which the disease takes its name, is discharged into the lumen and occasionally may occlude a peripheral vessel if sufficient 'gruel' is discharged. Ischaemia may therefore arise from (a) atheromatous plaques, (b) rupture and embolisation of the plaque and (c) haemorrhage into or thrombosis upon an existing plaque.

The precise aetiology of atherosclerosis is unknown but the incidence of ischaemic heart disease and other cardiovascular diseases related to atheroma vary throughout the world. Whilst there are genetic factors which predispose to the development of atheroma, there is a crude correlation between the level of serum cholesterol and

345

the incidence of atheroma. In Western societies, other factors known to predispose to atheroma are cigarette smoking, hypertension, diabetes mellitus, obesity and a sedentary existence. Female sex hormones also have a protective role, atheroma being commoner in men than women with the incidence increasing in post-menopausal women.

Those nations where the average serum cholesterol is low, e.g. Japan, have a low incidence of cardiovascular disease in young and middle-aged people. Characteristically, the diet contains a low amount of fat, particularly *saturated* fat which is found in mammalian meat. There is extremely good evidence to show that the incidence of cardiovascular diseases (which has reached epidemic proportions in the United Kingdom) can be reduced by adopting measures which lead to a lowering of the serum cholesterol. The simplest way of achieving a reduction in morbidity and mortality from cardiovascular diseases would be to reduce the consumption of saturated fats and to increase the ratio of polyunsaturated fats (such as linoleic acid) to saturated fats in the diet. Whenever this policy has been adopted, there has been a reduction in the incidence of ischaemic heart disease.

The true incidence of atherosclerotic disease is unknown but it is a major factor in all deaths from myocardial infarction, heart failure, hypertension, strokes and peripheral vascular disease. In this country, with an ageing population and a high incidence of atheromatous arterial disease, peripheral vascular disease represents an increasing cause of morbidity and mortality. In England during 1989, 2500 patients received amputations as treatment associated with the consequences of vascular disease or diabetes mellitus (in which vascular disease plays a significant role). In a survey of nearly 1500 patients with arterial occlusion, over 25% died within five years.

Clinical features. The most common symptom of atherosclerotic peripheral vascular disease is pain in the leg, which is brought on by exercise and is relieved by rest. This condition is known as *intermittent claudication* or *intermittent limping*, first described by Sir Benjamin Brodie in 1846. Whilst both legs may be affected by arterial disease, symptoms are usually present in only one. The patient complains of a cramping pain or tightness and numbness in the affected muscle groups on exercise. The symptoms increase in severity, eventually forcing the patient to cease walking. After a few minutes the pain subsides and they are able to continue exercising, only to be forced to stop again by a recrudescence of symptoms. The amount of exercise producing the pain is relatively constant in a given patient although the march tolerance (distance they can walk without symptoms) may be less on walking uphill, compared with the flat, because of the greater effort and therefore oxygen demand of the muscles. A few patients are able to walk through the claudication probably by unconsciously slowing down without actually stopping. Intermittent claudication occurs most frequently in the calf because femoropopliteal occlusions account for over 60% of patients with lower limb ischaemia and they are especially common in patients over 60 years of age.

When the arterial occlusion is more proximal, whilst calf claudication occurs, similar symptoms may be experienced in the thigh, buttocks and lower back. Leriche described a syndrome in men, due to aortic occlusion, of impotence and claudication in the thigh and gluteal regions. Aorto-iliac occlusion tends to occur in somewhat younger individuals in whom there is little femoropopliteal disease and it is more amenable to corrective surgery.

Rest pain is the other important symptom of ischaemic disease in the leg. This signifies a more precarious blood supply to the limb, indicating that even the small nutritional requirements of the skin have become compromised. The pain is usually felt in the toes and across the metatarsal heads, initially at night when the patient rests in bed. Relief from pain occurs on hanging the leg out of bed or by getting out of bed and sleeping in a chair. These methods allow gravity to aid the blood supply to the foot. The pain often has a burning character to it and may be associated with numbness or tingling in the foot and ankle. These symptoms may also occur on exercise and are due to ischaemic neuritis. Later, rest pain may be continuous despite efforts to relieve it by cooling and dependency.

Other complaints by the patient may be of coldness of the affected limb and of changes in the colour of the foot, i.e. pallor due to diminished blood flow, cyanosis when the blood flow is sufficient to prevent blanching or a persistent red or red-blue discolouration produced by anoxic damage to capillaries and venules, resulting in continued vasodilatation. In this situation, the skin becomes dry and atrophic. There is a loss of hair and a shiny tight appearance to the skin. The nails become hard, ridged and brittle. Any crack in the skin is likely to result in infection and the development of gangrene. This usually begins in the toes and slowly extends into the foot. The heel may be the first area to become gangrenous if the patient has been kept in bed and has not received the skilled nursing care needed to prevent the pressure areas (heels, elbows, buttocks) from breaking down and ulcerating.

Examination of the patient with claudication reveals diminished or absent pulses below the site of obstruction. Very occasionally, the pulses are only absent after exercising the patient. It must be remembered that about 10% of people have a congenital absence of the dorsalis pedis pulse in the usual site and 2% of patients may have an absent posterior tibial pulse. Both pulses are absent in only of $\frac{1}{2}$% of the population. Signs of ischaemia may also be present as mentioned above. Buerger's postural test can also be performed. The patient lies on their back and lifts both legs high, keeping the knees straight whilst the examiner supports the legs. The patient then extends their ankle and toes to the point of mild fatigue. When there is defective arterial supply to the limb, the sole of the foot becomes pale and the veins on the dorsum of the foot become empty and guttered. The feet are lowered and the patient sits with the legs hanging down. A ruddy cyanotic hue spreads over the ischaemic foot within three minutes.

Differential diagnosis. Other diseases which can produce pain in the leg need to be considered. Anaemia may produce intermittent claudication in the patients with a degree of atherosclerosis, but correction of the anaemia renders them symptom free. It is important, therefore, that all patients with ischaemic limb pain are examined for anaemia and, if found, that the anaemia is properly assessed, investigated and treated. Other painful syndromes which may be mistaken for arterial insufficiency include peripheral neuropathy, lumbar disc protrusion, osteoarthritis of hip and knee, and lumbar canal stenosis (claudication of the spinal cord). This last rare condition produces exercise-induced pain and paraesthesia in the limbs but the limb pulses are normal even after exercise. The condition can be cured by lumbar laminectomy. Occasionally, a glomus tumour of the toe may produce claudication and rest pain.

Prognosis. The outlook for patients with atherosclerotic peripheral vascular disease is extremely variable. Because it is a generalised disease, these patients may succumb from myocardial infarction, strokes and other complications of arterial disease, before requiring any specific treatment for limb symptoms.

Approximately one third of patients with intermittent claudication can be expected to improve spontaneously, presumably due to the development of collateral circulation. Of the remaining two thirds, approximately half remain static with no alteration in march tolerance, whilst the remainder gradually deteriorate with increasing claudication. In a series of nearly 4000 patients with claudication over a five year period, 10% required amputation. Factors which adversely affect the outcome are a failure to stop smoking and diabetes mellitus.

Treatment. There are several measures which may assist patients with peripheral vascular disease. Once a diagnosis is made, it is essential that a detailed examination of the patient is made to document any other manifestations of vascular disease (heart disease, hypertension) and the presence of obesity or diabetes.

Adequate control of diabetes mellitus, the maintenance of an ideal body weight and avoidance of smoking are essential. Regular exercise to the point of pain is believed to encourage the development of collateral circulation and is to be recommended. Treatment of hypertension can be expected to reduce the pace of the atheromatous process but in some patients it exacerbates intermittent claudication.

If it is considered that the patient's symptoms are incapacitating, and if they have managed to stop smoking and maintain a normal body weight, reconstructive arterial surgery may be possible. If successful, it may relieve the symptoms completely. Detailed radiological investigations are necessary before surgery can be contemplated. Some patients with localised arterial disease, particularly in the femoro-popliteal regions, can be managed by angioplasty. This procedure is done under a local anaesthetic, often by a radiologist and under X-ray control. Atheromatous plaques are crushed by passing a catheter along the vessel through the narrowed segment and inflating the catheter tip. Often the disease is found to be too extensive for surgical intervention, but when the circulation to the leg is severely compromised reconstructive surgery is often attempted as a last resort.

Where rest pain and incipient gangrene are present, division of the sympathetic nerve roots to the arteries in the leg occasionally produces improvement in skin circulation but is not of benefit for claudication.

When all other measures have failed, amputation becomes necessary to relieve the constant pain of the ischaemic gangrenous limb. The level of amputation is determined by the most distal level at which sound healing of a well-functioning stump can be obtained. When the level of amputation is immediately below the most distal arterial pulsation, healing usually occurs. The medical management of the ischaemic limb is singularly disappointing. Apart from the general measures already outlined, vasodilator drugs and anticoagulants have sometimes been used but with no benefit.

Alcohol is probably the best agent for ischaemic rest pain and the patient should sleep with the head of the bed elevated and the leg exposed to keep it cool. The limb must never be warmed directly as this will increase the metabolism of the tissues without improving the blood supply and may itself precipitate gangrene. These measures are usually holding operations prior to reconstructive surgery, sympathectomy or amputation.

The most important medical treatment for the care of ischaemic feet involves the cooperation of a podiatrist experienced in these problems and this is discussed later.

Acute ischaemia

Acute ischaemia of the lower limb may arise as a result of thrombosis upon an atheromatous plaque, or by embolisation from the heart in patients with (a) atrial fibrillation, or (b) myocardial infarction with mural thrombosis (the formation of a blood clot in the left ventricle overlying an area of infarcted muscle). Occasionally, rupture of an aortic atheromatous plaque may result in discharge of atheromatous material into the lower limb vessels, producing acute ischaemia of the leg and foot.

In contrast to chronic limb ischaemia, the onset is abrupt, with pain, coldness, numbness and loss of movement of the affected foot and limb. If a large embolus lodges at the bifurcation of the aorta (*saddle embolus*), both legs become acutely ischaemic. Occasionally, small emboli break up and dislodge themselves, resulting in a return of the circulation, but in most instances urgent surgical intervention is needed. If it is delayed, thrombosis distal to the embolus occurs, gangrene results and amputation becomes necessary.

Where embolisation has resulted from thrombi in the heart, recurrence is a real danger and can be prevented by treating these patients indefinitely with anticoagulant drugs. This therapy is of little benefit where there is pre-existing peripheral vascular disease, and the patient with intermittent claudication who suddenly develops acute limb ischaemia does not usually benefit from long term anticoagulant treatment. The importance of collateral circulation in the outcome of limb ischaemia may occasionally be seen in patients with a history of claudication in one limb, who suddenly develop acute ischaemia in both limbs. It is not uncommon to find that the previous good leg requires amputation whilst the claudicating leg survives.

Inflammatory arterial disease

The main types of this disease, producing lower limb ischaemia, are thromboangiitis obliterans and polyarteritis nodosa. Syphilitic aortitis produces angina, giant cell arteritis produces blindness and strokes and Takayasu's disease produces upper limb ischaemia and strokes.

Thromboangiitis obliterans (Buerger's disease)

This disease, sometimes called endarteritis obliterans, affects chiefly the peripheral arteries and veins. Segmental lesions are found along vessels, separated by normal areas. In affected areas there is intimal proliferation accompanied by thrombus formation and infiltration of all coats of the vessel and thrombus by inflammatory cells. Additional areas of vessels are affected at varying times, so that the process is characterised by exacerbations and remissions which may last from weeks to years. Old lesions become converted to fibrotic scar tissue and since veins, arteries and nerves run in close proximity in neurovascular bundles in the limbs, the peripheral nerves tend to be involved in this perivascular fibrous reaction. The late stages of the disease are not always distinguishable from atherosclerosis.

All races are prone to this disease but it is commoner in Jews and oriental races than in Caucasians. Men are affected far more frequently than women, in the ratio 75 to 1. Whilst it can present at all ages, it is perhaps commonest in young men in the 20 to 45 age group. The aetiology is unknown but there is a very strong association with cigarette smoking, which exacerbates and may even precipitate the disease in susceptible patients, probably because of an increased sensitivity to the vasoconstrictive effect of nicotine.

Clinical features. Patients are typically young cigarette smoking males and commonly present with rest pain, coldness of the feet, paraesthesia and trophic changes. Intermittent claudication does occur but less commonly than with atheromatous disease, and pain in Buerger's disease is often excruciating compared with other vascular disorders.

Migratory thrombophlebitis may precede or accompany arterial changes and occurs in almost half the cases at some stage in the disease. Red tender elevated skin lesions appear near the valves of superficial veins and disappear after about ten days to be followed by further crops during active periods of thrombophlebitis.

Arterial involvement tends to be distal, with loss of foot pulses, the disease sparing the aortoiliac and femoro-popliteal vessels with preservation of these pulses.

The outcome during paroxysms of thromboangiitis depends upon the frequency of the episodes and the speed of development of a collateral blood supply. Sooner or later surgery is required because of rest pain or gangrene. Lumbar sympathectomy may delay the time for amputation but ultimately this is required. It is often possible to be less radical with the amputation in this situation compared with atheromatous disease, and amputation of part of a foot is often followed by healing and relief of symptoms, until a further episode of inflammation produces more ischaemia.

In addition to the general measures for the care of the ischaemic foot and leg, it is important to withdraw tobacco from the patient. This is never easy to achieve and whilst the story of the bilateral amputee sitting in a wheelchair holding a cigarette in the two remaining fingers of his one hand may be apocryphal, it epitomises the problems doctors have in persuading these patients to give up smoking.

Polyarteritis nodosa

This is a rare collagen vascular disorder of unknown aetiology characterised by segmental involvement of the media of medium-sized and small arteries. There is oedema, fibrinoid necrosis of the vessel wall and infiltration of the adventitia and intima of the vessels with inflammatory cells. Secondary thrombosis on the vessel wall is common. Chronic lesions become fibrosed. The clinical manifestations are protean, since any system in the body can be affected. Constitutional symptoms such as fever, anorexia and malaise are common and patients often develop arthralgia and myalgia. In 25% of cases cutaneous involvement occurs. Subcutaneous haemorrhage and gangrene result from the necrotising arteritis and ulcerations develop on the feet and hands. Occlusion of digital vessels may produce localised areas of gangrene on the fingers and toes.

This disease is often fatal due to renal and cardiac involvement. Occasionally, patients respond to treatment when large doses of steroids are given.

Peripheral arteritis and gangrene in systemic infections

Symptoms and signs of peripheral vascular disease occasionally appear during bacterial and viral infection. Bacterial arteritis may occur when the heart valves become infected (bacterial endocarditis), the patient developing painful tender swellings on the tips of fingers and toes (Osler's nodes). These findings are uncommon since the advent of powerful antibiotics.

Conservative management of lower limb ischaemia

Irrespective of the cause of ischaemia, great care is needed in the management of patients with ischaemic feet. Measures for improving the circulation, or at least preventing further deterioration, have already been discussed. It is also important to educate the patient so that they do not further compromise the circulation to the feet by their own actions.

Patients should be advised that the feet should be washed daily in warm water with a bland soap, followed by careful drying with a soft towel, particular attention being paid to the interdigital spaces. Dry skin can be helped by the application of bland emulsifying ointment, and moist skin by a little surgical spirit. Exposure to cold should be avoided and suitable woollen clothing worn, especially on the limbs. Normal toenails should be cut straight across, keeping the scissors well away from the nail grooves. This should preferably be done after a warm bath when the nails have softened, and in a good light. Cutting the nails too short may result in paronychial infection which readily precipitates gangrene. Hypertrophied and deformed nails should be treated only by a podiatrist, as should any hyperkeratotic lesions producing symptoms. Patients should be firmly discouraged from applying any keratolytic preparations.

It is imperative that patients wear well-fitting shoes and stockings which do not cramp the feet or chafe the skin. Footwear must always be examined for any nails which may have penetrated the sole as these may stick into the foot and introduce infection.

Once ulceration has occurred, healing can be achieved by careful nursing. Further trauma has to be avoided and the ulcer cleared of debris and infected matter, dressed with non-adhesive material soaked in topical antiseptics and covered with protective padding. When the ulcer is clear of infection, the application of a mild astringent with dry dressings can be used. If there is any evidence of spreading infection with cellulitis and lymphangitis, antibiotics may be given, although penetration to the ischaemic area will not be easy because of the diminished blood supply.

Vasospastic disorders

This section includes a group of disorders characterised by abnormal vasoconstriction and vasodilatation.

Raynaud's phenomenon

This is paroxysmal bilateral ischaemia of the digits precipitated by cold or emotional stimuli and relieved by warmth. It is *primary* where there is no underlying pathology and this is commonest in young women. It is *secondary* when the phenomenon occurs as a result of (a) obliterative arterial disease, (b) pressure from cervical ribs, (c) certain occupations, especially pneumatic drill operators, or (d) in certain connective tissue disturbances.

Primary Raynaud's phenomenon occurs most often in the 15 to 40 age group and is five times commoner in women.

The ischaemia results from spasm of the digital, palmar and plantar arteries, which produces the initial pallor in the fingers and toes. Later there is dilatation of the digital capillaries and venules resulting in a sluggish return of blood to the skin, producing cold cyanotic digits. During this stage the affected areas are cold, numb and somewhat painful, but when the vasocontriction is relieved the extremities become very red (due to reactive hyperaemia) and warm. The patient develops a throbbing pain and tingling of the digits, occasionally with swelling of the fingers and toes.

Typically the paroxysms are precipitated by

cold and so tend to occur in winter or if the hands are immersed in cold water. More severe cases may occur at other times and paroxysms may become frequent and prolonged. The hands are always affected and in half the cases the feet are involved. The problem is sometimes progressive so that the hands have a permanent cold cyanotic hue. Trophic changes occur with loss of soft tissue, smooth shiny stretched skin and ridging and discolouration of nails with reduced growth. Recurrent infections and small areas of gangrene appear at times. These areas are extremely painful and eventually separate to leave small depressed scars. It is exceedingly uncommon for extensive gangrene to develop.

Diagnosis is made on the history and physical findings and the absence of any disease or anatomical abnormality responsible for digital ischaemia. The episodes must be bilateral and symmetrical and there should be no history of drug ingestion, e.g ergot compounds for migraine.

In mild cases, the avoidance of exposure to cold is all that is required. The provision of warm boots and gloves during the winter months is advisable. Tobacco should be withdrawn. In more severe cases, vasodilator drugs can be tried and are sometimes effective. Where paroxysms are frequent, protracted and resistant to medical treatment, sympathectomy (cervical for the arm, lumbar for the leg and foot) is usually beneficial, at least in the short term. Local treatment for any skin or nail infection should be given as the need arises.

Acrocyanosis

This is a symmetrical cyanosis of the hands and feet occurring in otherwise healthy individuals. There is increased arteriolar tone and secondary capillary and subpapillary venous plexus dilatation resulting in a sluggish flow of blood through the skin and thereby producing blue, cold extremities which sweat profusely and are worse in cold weather. Puffiness and hyperaesthesiae may occur but trophic changes and gangrene do not result. Unlike Raynaud's phenomenon, the digits are always discoloured except when warmed.

The patient should be reassured as to the nature of the problem and treatment should be aimed at avoiding exposure to cold and keeping the hands and feet warm by the wearing of warm gloves and footwear, especially in winter. Vasodilator drugs may be used if patients wish to abolish the discolouration for cosmetic reasons.

Erythrocyanosis

Chilblains and erythrocyanosis commonly occur in young adults, especially females with a history of cool limbs. The symptoms are only seen in cold damp climates and the incidence has fallen with the advent of central heating.

Chilblains occur on the dorsum of the fingers and toes and elsewhere on the feet. Erythrocyanosis involves the lower parts of the legs, particularly in women, perhaps because of their mode of dress. Localised warm red pruritic lesions with an area of swelling appear, especially when cold extremities are warmed. These lesions disappear within a few days but occasionally blood stained blisters which ulcerate may develop. In the warmer months symptoms improve. Treatment is nonspecific; steroid creams and vasodilator drugs may help, together with warm protective clothing and avoidance of extremes of temperature.

Glomus tumour

This consists of an hypertrophy of the glomus body, which contains an arteriovenous anastomosis with associated muscle and nerve fibres and it represents an abnormal communication between arteries and veins.

It presents as a slowly growing painful subcutaneous nodule most frequently beneath the nail, especially in the finger. The nodule is flat with reddish blue discolouration. Both local and referred burning, shooting pains occur either spontaneously or by direct pressure. In certain situations symptoms mimic peripheral ischaemic pain. Subungual glomus tumours in the feet may give a superficial clinical picture of rest pain and intermittent claudication. Rarely, because of changes in vasomotor tone, tissue atrophy may occur. If the diagnosis is to be made, the possibility of a glomus tumour must be considered and a search made for the lesion, which may be only a few millimetres in diameter. Surgical removal results in immediate relief of symptoms.

DISEASES OF VEINS

Disturbances in the function of veins occur because of thrombosis within the vein or because the veins develop incompetent valves (varicose veins).

Phlebothrombosis and thrombophlebitis

These terms are often interchangeable but etymologically, thrombophlebitis should be used for those situations where thrombosis and intimal damage result in an inflammatory response in the vein wall and phlebothrombosis when simple clotting within the vessel occurs. It is often very difficult to distinguish between the two clinically. The occurrence of thrombosis within veins poses two problems. There is the local one produced by the difficulty in removing blood from the tissues and also the danger that part of the thrombus may become dislodged from the vein and travel to the lungs—*pulmonary embolism*. At worst, this may be fatal—approximately 2500 people per annum in the United Kingdom die from this cause.

Aetiology and pathology. Venous thrombosis occurs most commonly in the legs and may occur in either the superficial or deep venous systems, or both. Whilst the thrombus may arise spontaneously there are often local or systemic reasons for its occurrence. Circulatory stasis is probably the most important single factor, and when varicose veins are present then there is a greater tendency to develop thrombosis. Debilitated patients who are confined to bed have reduced blood flow through the veins mainly because of the loss of the muscular pump, and it is in this group of patients that venous thrombosis is likely to occur. Injury to the vessel wall also enhances thrombus formation and this may result from infection, trauma, accidents, operations or intravenous injections. Finally, those situations characterised by increased coagulability of the blood may encourage venous thrombosis. These include tissue damage from operations or accidents, myocardial infarction and the oral contraceptive pill.

Deep leg vein thrombosis usually commences in the soleal arcade of the calf muscles. Further spread may not occur and the thrombus may resolve, producing no clinical symptoms. With extension to the major deep vessels, however, circulatory obstruction, damage to the valves and the risk of emboli result. The thrombus may extend into the popliteal, femoral and iliac veins, occasionally reaching the inferior vena cava. Healing occurs by recanalisation of the thrombus but this may be incomplete and give rise to a post-phlebitic limb.

The incidence of venous thrombosis in the general population is low but a high incidence occurs in those clinical situations already mentioned. It has been shown that about 75% of patients with femoral neck fractures develop some form of leg vein thrombosis, the majority of which do not produce symptoms.

Clinical features. In thrombophlebitis the vein is painful and tender, with local swelling or more generalised limb swelling if the deep veins are affected. Constitutional symptoms such as fever, malaise and anorexia occur but there is less risk of emboli because the clot is more adherent to the vessel wall as a result of the inflammatory response. The vein is tender and superficial veins are inflamed with redness and swelling of the overlying skin.

The phlebothrombotic process is relatively painless and unless obstruction to the venous drainage occurs it produces no signs until embolisation occurs. This complication is more likely because the clot is less firmly adherent to the vessel wall. Phlebothrombosis usually affects the deep veins in the legs. The symptoms are a sense of tightness in the leg, swelling and perhaps calf discomfort on walking. Whenever major deep veins are occluded, the leg becomes swollen and oedematous, and dorsiflexion of the foot produces calf tenderness (Homan's sign). Since blood tends to be diverted to the superficial veins these become distended and the skin is warm. If there is much swelling the leg becomes very tense and painful and sometimes arterial spasm occurs, producing a pale cold limb—the so called 'white leg'.

Following extensive or repeated venous thromboses, the venous valves become damaged and produce venous stasis and insufficiency which, of course, enhances the risk of further thrombotic episodes. The limb becomes chronically oedematous with induration of the subcutaneous tissues; pigmentation and trophic ulcers may develop.

Diagnosis. This is made on clinical grounds but the extent of thrombosis can be determined by venography and by injecting radio-opaque dyes into peripheral veins and taking radiographs. Other techniques include thermography (the use of infra-red photography), ultrasound and the use of radio-labelled fibrinogen, which becomes incorporated into the thrombus. These techniques are beyond the scope of this book but can be useful in the preclinical diagnosis of thrombosis in hospitals, where deep vein occlusion and pulmonary embolism remain a significant cause of both morbidity and mortality.

Treatment. Superficial thrombophlebitis and thrombosis in varicose veins is rarely life threatening, but because of the dangers of pulmonary emboli in deep vein thrombosis the aims of treatment are prevention of this potentially fatal complication. The prevention of further venous thromboses and emboli is achieved with anticoagulant drugs. Conventional treatment also includes bed rest and elevation of the limb to ease drainage, lessen oedema and discourage damage to the venous valves, which is of importance in the postphlebitic limb. The period of rest in bed varies depending on the severity of the condition but after about a week it is usually possible to begin mobilisation.

At this time, it is advisable to support the leg with bandages or elastic support stockings to prevent swelling in the dependent position until recanalisation and organisation of the thrombus has occurred. This may take several weeks and certain patients may be left with residual swelling and require continued support for the leg. Anticoagulants are currently continued for six to twelve weeks. Other forms of therapy for deep vein thrombosis have included agents to dissolve the clot (thrombolysins) but these are not without dangers to the patient. Occasionally it is necessary to ligate the vein proximal to the thrombus if there is evidence of ascending thrombosis despite anticoagulants.

Unless patients are bed-fast and liable to develop deep vein thrombosis, the occurrence of superficial thrombophlebitis does not usually demand anticoagulants. Analgesics, anti-inflammatory drugs and antibiotics if there is clear evidence of infection, together with local measures such as the application of lead and opium dressings should suffice. The patient should be mobilised quickly and symptoms are usually greatly improved within a week.

Patients who have recurrent problems may require long term anticoagulant drugs, and recurrent thrombophlebitis in superficial veins may require surgery if the deep venous system is sound. Occasionally patients with carcinoma, especially of the pancreas and bronchus, develop recurrent thrombophlebitis in the superficial veins in the limbs.

The post-phlebitic limb

Following extensive deep venous thrombosis, whilst the vein may recanalise, the valves in these deep and perforating veins become incompetent. As a result, when pressure rises in the veins, as it does on walking, blood is forced from the deep veins into the subcutaneous veins so that prolonged venous hypertension over many years gradually results in capillary dilatation, swelling, discomfort, discolouration and ulceration of the skin. The skin on the inner aspect of the ankle is very prone to necrosis.

Treatment. The aim should be to slow down or prevent the above changes by controlling the venous hypertension.

The simplest way is to elevate the limb so that the foot and ankle are above heart level. This means sleeping with the foot of the bed elevated and resting in the reclining position with the feet elevated. Since most mortals have to be ambulant other measures are also needed. Elastic pressure, usually as a one-way stretch elastic bandage or heavy duty stocking, applied evenly and firmly from toes to knee or thigh, including the heel and malleoli, is of great benefit when the patient is ambulant. This form of treatment is unsatisfactory for elderly patients because the pressure may damage the skin and lead to ulceration. Even younger patients with arterial insufficiency should not use this treatment.

In the early stages, surgery can be of benefit in preventing deterioration by ligating the perforating veins and thereby preventing blood flowing backwards from the deep to the superficial system. Unfortunately this procedure is of little use if the ilio-femoral veins have been involved.

The above principles also apply to the treatment of venous ulcers to which must be added specific treatment aimed at healing the ulcer. Any infection should be treated with systemic antibiotics and the wound dressed with non-adherent dry dressings followed by protective gauze and then the application of an elasticated bandage as described previously. The patient should rest with the foot elevated as much as possible. Failure to achieve healing usually means poor technique or failure of patient compliance. It is important to avoid the use of irritating antiseptic creams, topical antibiotics and steroids, as these delay healing.

Varicose veins

These are dilated, lengthened, tortuous veins and occur commonly in the legs due to our erect posture (animals do not suffer from this condition). The condition is precipitated by failure of one or more of the valves which guard the communications between the superficial and deep venous systems in the leg. Incompetence of the veins may be due to previous thrombotic episodes (q.v.) or congenital absence of valves. Pelvic tumours, including pregnancy (a self limiting but sometimes recurrent pelvic tumour) put increased pressure on the pelvic veins and may produce varicosities which improve with removal of the tumour. The effect of pregnancy may partly explain the greater incidence of varicose veins in women.

Clinical features. Patients usually present in the third to fifth decade. Earlier presentation usually implies a congenital defect of the venous valves and a positive family history is likely. Symptoms of varicose veins are mainly those of tiredness and aching of the legs after prolonged standing or walking. Sharp pains may be noted over the veins, and ankle swelling towards evening sometimes occurs. Calf cramp

on retiring to bed may be a symptom. The skin may become discoloured and itchy. Some patients, especially females, merely complain of the disfigurement.

Treatment. Support stockings and resting of the legs as detailed above may be all that is required. For the more severe cases, injection with sclerosant or ligation and stripping of the veins may be needed. Acute thrombophlebitis and previous deep vein thrombosis are contraindications to this treatment. Oral contraceptives are also contraindicated.

The complications, including thrombophlebitis, eczema and ulceration have already been discussed. Haemorrhage may follow rupture or injury. Both ends of the vein bleed and blood loss may be profuse. Fatalities have occurred. First aid measures are simple. Elevate the leg above the level of the heart to stop the profuse bleeding and then apply a firm pressure bandage.

Malignant change. Occasionally chronic venous ulcers undergo malignant change with the development of squamous cell carcinoma. This is usually after prolonged ulceration for many years. The ulcer develops raised edges and local invasion results. Progression is slow and the diagnosis may not be made for long periods. Biopsy of the ulcer including an area of normal skin confirms the diagnosis in suspected cases. Surgical treatment consists of local excision or amputation and radiotherapy.

Oedema

Foot and ankle oedema may occasionally be the first presenting symptom of systemic disease although it is due more often to local conditions in the limbs, e.g. varicose veins.

Lymph is formed by the transudation of plasma through the capillary wall at the arterial end of the capillary network. As the pressure of blood falls across this capillary network, fluid is reabsorbed into the venular end of the capillaries as a result of the osmotic pressure of the albumin within the intravascular compartment. Any fluid which is not reabsorbed in this way is collected by the lymphatic vessels, which drain to regional lymph nodes, and eventually the fluid is returned to the left internal jugular vein via the thoracic duct.

Oedema may result from disordered lymphatics (lymphoedema), from an increase in the hydrostatic pressure on the venous side of the capillary network (varicose veins, heart failure), or from a reduction in the oncotic pressure of the plasma proteins.

Lymphoedema

This is a form of chronic oedema of the extremities due to accumulation of lymph, secondary to blockage or abnormalities of the lymph vessels and nodes. Secondary lymphoedema most commonly occurs in inflammation and may follow recurrent episodes of lymphangitis. Malignant tumours invading or compressing lymph vessels and nodes, or fibrosis of lymphatics following irradiation for malignant disease, are other important factors.

Occasionally lymphoedema is a primary phenomenon, often inherited, and may appear at birth or in later life. Various anatomical abnormalities have been shown.

Clinical features. Primary lymphoedema is slow in onset and produces few symptoms other than swelling of one or both ankles and legs. The swelling tends to disappear overnight and is initially soft and pitting. Superimposed infection is common, when the limb will become painful, red and hot. As time passes the oedema becomes a constant feature with induration as a result of fibrosis, so that the limb is permanently swollen with little pitting and thick coarse skin in hard folds (elephantiasis).

Secondary lymphoedema is rarely bilateral and when due to malignant disease it produces painless swelling of a limb. Pelvic malignancy (prostate, rectum in men; cervix, uterus and rectum in women) not uncommonly presents in this manner.

Lymphoedema is to be distinguished from venous insufficiency by the lack of history of varicose veins, stasis dermatitis or ulceration.

Treatment. The underlying abnormality needs to be remedied if possible. Therapy is otherwise aimed at preventing infection and elephantiasis. Infection is best avoided by keeping the limb oedema free, i.e. keeping the leg elevated wherever possible.

Oedema due to raised hydrostatic pressure

Varicose veins have been dealt with previously. Congestive cardiac failure may produce bilateral pitting oedema of the feet and ankles. Its differentiation from other forms can be made from a history of previous heart disease (rheumatic, hypertensive or ischaemic), together with symptoms of breathlessness, especially on exercise or in the recumbent position, palpitations, tiredness and lethargy. Treatment is with digoxin and diuretics.

Oedema due to lowered plasma albumin

Starvation produces famine oedema, but it should be unknown in this country now. The cachectic nature of the patient should be obvious to most observers.

Certain renal disorders, by allowing protein to leak into the urine, produce oedema. In addition to ankle swelling, patients have puffiness of the face and pass frothy urine which contains large amounts of protein. Management is not easy but includes diuretic drugs, providing a high protein diet and restricting salt.

Liver disease produces oedema when the liver is so diseased that it cannot produce enough albumin. A history of alcoholism, or previous or present jaundice may be obtained. Management includes diuretics.

Miscellaneous causes

Certain situations characterised by salt and water retention by the body occasionally produce oedema.

During the latter half of the menstrual cycle, many women retain fluid and may develop ankle oedema. Nothing needs to be done other than to reassure the patient.

Pregnancy is commonly associated with some oedema of the lower limbs because of the tendency to develop varicose veins. A common complication of pregnancy called toxaemia is also associated with ankle swelling. Other features are hypertension and proteinuria. This is more sinister and requires prompt and expect medical care.

Certain drugs, including steroids and non-steroidal anti-inflammatory drugs, can produce mild to moderate fluid retention and oedema.

A rare and as yet undetermined but well documented syndrome — idiopathic cyclical oedema of women — deserves mention. The woman, who is usually rather highly strung and neurotic, has periods lasting several days when her weight may increase by several pounds due to fluid retention. Oedema may be so marked that she requires different sizes of shoes, bras and clothes to cope with these fluctuations. During the period of oedema formation patients are often tired, lethargic and dizzy. This is thought to be due to a diminished circulating blood volume resulting from the capillary leak of fluid. The hypovolaemia may be compounded by the diuretics prescribed to clear the oedema fluid. After a period, which varies from one to several days, the oedema resolves, weight falls and the patient feels better. Treatment is unsatisfactory but diuretics occasionally help the oedema.

FURTHER READING

MacLeod J (ed) 1985 Davidson's principles and practice of medicine, 15th edn. Churchill Livingstone, Edinburgh

Weatherall D J, Ledingham J G G, Warrell D A (eds) 1983 Oxford textbook of medicine. Oxford University Press, Oxford

21. Metabolic disorders

Michael Davies

All diseases have a metabolic basis. Custom dictates that certain unrelated disorders are grouped together as metabolic, despite the fact that often no metabolic abnormality has been identified. In this chapter some of these disorders are described because of their effects on the lower limb and, in particular, the foot.

OBESITY

Obesity is an excess of adipose tissue in the body and may be said to be present when the fatness of a person is beyond what is socially acceptable or when good health is likely to be affected by the degree of obesity. Using the latter definition, a large proportion of our society is mildly obese with between 25 and 35% of the population 9 kg (20 lb) or more overweight. In children, both sexes are affected equally but after puberty it is commoner in women than men, and is liable to arise after pregnancy and the menopause.

The body mass index (BMI) is a good method for deciding upon the presence or absence of obesity in adults and is derived by dividing body weight (in kilograms) by body height in metres squared. Thus a 70 kg person measuring 1.7 metres in height has a BMI of 24.2. The normal BMI is 20–25; people with BMI greater than 30 have significant obesity warranting individual attention and detailed management.

Aetiology

This is multifactorial but basically results from energy input (the calorific value of food) being greater than energy expenditure. As the young adult moves into middle life, there is a tendency to be less active but to retain the eating and drinking habits acquired in more active years. If this occurs, the excess calories are stored as fat which produces the well recognised middle-age spread.

Overweight parents tend to produce overweight children and whilst genetic factors have been invoked the obesity probably results from environmental factors, with the child developing similar eating habits to his/her parents, no doubt with their encouragement.

Psychological factors also have an effect on obesity in so far as certain individuals gain psychological comfort from eating. This appears particularly true of women who may eat excessively when depressed or anxious.

There is no evidence to support the common assertion, 'It's my glands, doctor'. Whilst obese patients may become diabetic, no biochemical abnormality has ever been found in obese patients which is responsible for the obese state.

There is some evidence to support the claims, of many obese people that they do not overeat, although in the author's experience many obese patients underestimate their calorie consumption. It has been suggested that some obese patients produce less heat and thus conserve energy upon glucose ingestion compared to thin subjects. Many overfed animals can avoid excess weight gain by increasing metabolic rate. These data suggest that some obese patients may gain weight because of reduced calorie expenditure as a result of an inability to increase heat production via the sympathetic activation of brown adipose tissue. However, calorie expenditure from physical activity is commonly greater than their normal-sized counterparts because the obese person carries more weight.

Although some of these factors may apply to some obese patients, there are no treatments available and obese subjects, if they are to lose weight, must reduce calorie intake (eat less) and increase expenditure (exercise more). Because of the difficulty in performing physical tasks, however, obese patients tend to be inactive apart from the physical act of eating.

Clinical features

That a person is obese will be obvious to anyone. The clinical features of obesity are really those of the complications brought about by the obese state.

Obese patients are more prone to psychological illness, musculoskeletal disease, hypertension, heart disease, chest disease, gout, diabetes, skin infections, accidents and, not surprisingly, have a reduced life expectancy.

They are more liable to develop varicose veins and their complications, and often complain of pains in the knees and feet, ultimately developing premature osteoarthritis and foot strain purely because of the increased mechanical load.

Treatment

This is aimed at calorie restriction of 800 to 1000 calories per day to achieve a 0.5–1.4 kg (1–3 lb) weight loss per week. Increased physical activity should also be encouraged to increase calorie expenditure. Success as assessed by a continued long term reduction in weight is extremely difficult to achieve. Most patients relax their diets; because of this, jaw wiring and intestinal by-pass operations have been devised, but these are not always successful. More recent interventions include intragastric balloons, which can remain in situ for months, and gastric stapling. Both methods reduce the capacity of the stomach for food, producing a feeling of satiety after small meals.

Complications must be treated when they arise but since the basic problem is rarely solved the prognosis from the complications is very poor.

GOUT

This is characterised by recurrent episodes of acute arthritis due to an abnormality of purine metabolism, resulting in the accumulation of uric acid in the tissues. Gout may be primary or secondary to diseases of the blood-forming tissues, occurring in leukaemia and other states of excessive tissue turnover. It may also occur in renal failure and following administration of certain drugs, in particular diuretics.

Primary gout has a genetic basis in just over half the cases and probably affects 1–3 individuals per 1000 population, men much more often than women. It is uncommon before the age of 40. Known precipitating factors include dietetic indiscretion, injury, surgical operations, excessive exercise and infection. Because of increased skin turnover, patients with psoriasis have a tendency to develop a high blood uric acid and gout.

Pathology

Uric acid, in the form of sodium urate crystals, becomes deposited in articular tissues, extra articular cartilage and kidneys. In acid urine, uric acid stones may occur. As a result of deposits of urate, especially in joints, an inflammatory reaction occurs and with time there is erosion of bone and cartilage in the joints resulting in a chronic arthritis in which osteoarthritis may develop. Tophi appear in the ears and around joints and bursae and produce a low grade chronic inflammatory response with disruption of tissues and fibrosis.

Clinical features

In over 90% of cases of acute gout, the first metatarsophalangeal joint is affected. Attacks commonly begin in the sleeping hours with sudden severe excruciating pain. The joint becomes hot, red and swollen. The patient will resist anyone or anything touching it because of the pain and tenderness. A fever is common. Pain subsides over a few days with flaking of the skin. Paroxysms occur more frequently with time and the joint becomes progressively damaged so that some degree of discomfort is always felt. Other joints becomes affected and tophi develop. This is the stage of *chronic tophaceous gout*.

Diganosis is obvious to the patient who has had previous attacks. First episodes are alarming, especially if not in the classical site, because of the similarities to an acute infective arthritis. When larger joints, such as the knee, are affected large effusions may develop and should be aspirated if doubt exists as to the diagnosis. The finding of urate crystals confirms the diagnosis. Occasionally pyrophosphate is found, leading to the diagnosis of pseudo-gout which is usually associated with chondrocalcinosis and may occur in certain metabolic and endocrine disorders. It is often associated with primary hyperparathyroidism.

Treatment

Acute episodes should be treated with anti-inflammatory drugs, such as indomethacin or steroids, until the pain subsides; this should then be followed by life long treatment with drugs aimed at preventing further episodes of arthritis. Two types of drug exist: so-called uricosuric drugs, which increase the excretion of uric acid by the kidneys, and a xanthine oxidase inhibitor. Xanthine oxidase is an enzyme which converts hypoxanthine and xanthine to uric acid. The two former compounds are more soluble than uric acid and so if one uses a xanthine oxidase inhibitor it is possible to lower the uric acid level in the tissues and cure tophi, which will dissolve away. The increased levels of xanthine and hypoxanthine are harmless because they remain in solution.

Aspirin should not be given to gouty patients because in low doses it blocks uric acid excretion and may therefore precipitate acute gout.

OSTEOPOROSIS

This disorder results in the fracture of bones either spontaneously or following minor trauma and arises from a situation where the skeleton contains too little bone but the bone which is present is entirely normal. Osteoporosis is most commonly acquired and usually idiopathic, although certain diseases are associated with osteoporosis and these need to be considered once osteoporosis is diagnosed.

After maturity, bone loss is a feature of all humans but in some individuals the rate of loss is excessive and results in easy fracture of bone. The skeletal loss is accelerated in women after the menopause and this probably accounts for the increased incidence of osteoporosis in women. Disease such as thyrotoxicosis, Cushing's disease, hypogonadism and malnutrition are associated with osteoporosis and patients receiving prolonged treatment with steroid drugs develop similar problems. More recently other risk factors have been identified and include excessive alcohol intake, cigarette smoking and lack of physical activity. Immobilisation of the whole or part of the body is also characterised by an increase in the loss of mineral from the skeleton. Patients with malignant disease occasionally develop spontaneous fractures.

Clinical features

The main problems relate to easy fracture of the bones, particularly of vertebrae, which results in back pain, curvature of the spine and loss of height after repeated spinal fractures. These episodes occur usually after minor trauma, e.g. lifting household objects. Fractures of the hip and wrist are also common following minor falls. Occasionally patients complain of painful feet and may develop metatarsal fractures. Between episodes, patients are well and the fractures heal normally.

If the osteoporosis is secondary to other disease then additional symptoms will be present. Malignant disease associated with bone fracture never remits; the patients are ill and in continual pain, often showing considerable weight loss.

Radiographs show decreased bone mass with cortical thinning and loss of trabeculae. This is most marked in the spine where compression fractures may be seen. Examination of other parts of the skeleton, particularly the hands and feet, will also show changes of osteoporosis. The blood biochemistry is normal in simple osteoporosis.

Treatment

This is aimed at any underlying disorder. If none

is found, no specific therapy is possible but it is important to avoid prolonged periods of bed rest and immobilisation. Adequate pain relief is important together with physiotherapy to encourage the development of muscle tone. Trauma needs to be avoided. Stooping and lifting anything but the lightest of objects must be discouraged.

Osteoporosis may be delayed or prevented in post-menopausal women by hormone replacement therapy. However women in whom the uterus is present must continue to have periods and this aspect of hormone replacement is sometimes unacceptable.

In patients with established osteoporosis, there is preliminary evidence that the diphosphonate drug, etidronate, can reduce the incidence of fracture. Research with this drug and other diphosphonates may offer some hope for reducing fractures in patients with established osteoporosis.

Because physical activity is actively encouraged in patients with osteoporosis, the author is seeing an increasing number of patients with pain in the feet as a result of stress fractures from walking. These hairline fractures in the metatarsals may not be visible on X-rays but are usually apparent on bone scans. Such patients should take less exercise until the pain subsides.

Sudeck's atrophy

This is a form of local osteoporosis which occurs after fracture in an extremity, especially the foot and ankle. It can also occur without fracture when it follows minor injury and immobilisation. The onset is acute with the development of pain and swelling in the foot and ankle. The foot is tender and the overlying skin is moist. X-rays show a patchy osteoporosis of the tarsal bones.

The precise aetiology is unknown but blockage of the sympathetic nerves to the limb may produce relief of symptoms, and therefore abnormal sympathetic vasomotor tone has been implicated as a factor in the pathogenesis of the condition.

The disease is self-limiting and usually resolves after a few weeks although a few cases run a more protracted course. Injections of calcitonin sometimes produce relief of symptoms. Diphospho-

nates are also being used with some success in difficult cases.

OSTEOMALACIA

The term literally means softening of bone and histological examination shows an excessive amount of unmineralised bone matrix or osteoid. Increased amounts of osteoid are also seen in Paget's disease and other bone diseases with a high turnover of bone, but in these latter situations there is no defect of mineralisation. It is important to emphasise that osteomalacia has many causes. Some of these are related to problems with the supply and metabolism of vitamin D. There are other causes where vitamin D is not implicated in the aetiology but where large amounts of the vitamin may bring about relief of symptoms. These are termed vitamin D resistant osteomalacias. They are often hereditary, rather rare and will not be mentioned again.

Rickets refers to the childhood counterpart of osteomalacia. Here the changes are seen at the growing ends of long bones so that children can suffer from rickets *and* osteomalacia, adults from osteomalacia only.

Rickets and osteomalacia due to vitamin D deficiency

Vitamin D_3 (cholecalciferol) is produced in the skin from sunlight (ultraviolet irradiation) acting on a substance called 7-dehydrocholesterol. Vitamin D_2 (ergocalciferol) is produced by plants and often used to supplement foods such as margarine and tinned milk. Both are metabolised in a similar way by the body: proportions are converted first by the liver to 25-hydroxyvitamin D and then by the kidney to 1,25-dihydroxyvitamin D. This latter compound is important for normal calcium absorption from the gut, skeletal mineralisation and muscle metabolism.

Vitamin D deficiency can arise therefore from:

(a) poor diet and insufficient exposure to sunlight—nutritional deficiency
(b) malabsorption of dietary vitamin D
(c) adequate percursors but poor kidney

function, resulting in diminished 1,25 dihydroxyvitamin D production.

Theoretically, liver disease may produce a similar block in synthesis but as yet no such syndrome has been described. Whatever the underlying factors, the final result is a lack of 1,25-dihydroxyvitamin D and the clinical manifestations in the skeleton are similar.

Clinical features

There will be features of nutritional deficiency, malabsorption or renal failure depending upon the basic aetiology which, in the early stages, may mask symptoms of bone disease. Almost imperceptibly the patients develop aching bone pains, especially of the ribs, arms and legs. These pains are worse on weight-bearing and may progress until the patient cannot even tolerate the pressure of bedclothes. The patient is weak due to myopathy affecting the shoulder and hip girdle muscles. This results in difficulty in getting out of a chair, bed or bath, climbing stairs, carrying shopping and combing hair. This proximal muscle weakness is best seen in the waddling gait of the patient.

In children, rickets will present with pains especially around joints, typically ankle, knees and hips, together with deformity of the legs, knock knee, bow legs and bowing of femora and tibiae. Compensatory varus and valgus changes occur at the ankle.

Occasionally, the blood calcium level becomes very low and symptoms of tetany may be experienced. These are tingling in the hands and feet and carpopedal spasm; the hands, fingers and wrists become flexed, the toes and ankles plantarflexed. These symptoms are more prominent after exercise. An adult with long-standing vitamin D deficiency, apart from having tender bones, may also have stigmata of previous rickets including deformities of the lower limb. Patients with malabsorption, life-long renal disease or nutritional deprivation tend to be of short stature.

The blood biochemistry shows low or low normal levels of calcium and phosphate and raised levels of alkaline phosphatase. Radiological examination may be normal. The pathognomonic sign of osteomalacia is the pseudofracture or Looser's zone through which complete fractures sometimes occur. These are commonly found in the scapulae, pelvis, femora and ribs. In the growing child there is widening, fraying and cupping of the growth plates.

Treatment

This is aimed at the primary disorder wherever possible and the provision of vitamin D by mouth. Very large doses are required for renal osteomalacia. In children osteotomies may be required to correct deformity. Because of changes in the weight-bearing forces through the deformed lower limb, secondary varus or valgus deformities of the foot and ankle may occur and these may be helped by providing medial or lateral bars in the shoes of children. In adults who did not receive corrective orthopaedic treatment as children, callosities may develop on the feet and toes and require attention. It is of course important to recognise these abnormalities as secondary events and refer the patients for expert medical advice. This is especially relevant to children.

OSTEITIS DEFORMANS (PAGET'S DISEASE OF BONE)

The aetiology of this condition remains unknown, the most recent theory being one of viral infection. It is rare before the age of 30 and increases in incidence from about 1% of the population at 40 years of age to 10% at 80 years. If affects men more often than women. Occasionally there is a familial tendency but the mode of inheritance, if present, is unknown.

The disease is characterised by an increase in the osteoclastic activity of bone which in turn gives rise to increased osteoblastic activity. Bone turnover is therefore accelerated but new bone collagen is laid down in a mosaic rather than the normal lamellar fashion.

Radiologically there is patchy increase in the density and size of affected bones and, where bone destruction exceeds formation, rarefaction results. The net effect of the increased bone turnover is reduction in the mechanical strength of bone so that fracture and deformity result. Any bone may be involved but pelvis, skull, spine, femora, tibiae and humeri are the commonest sites to be affected.

Clinical features

In the majority of patients the disease is symptomless and is usually a chance finding, perhaps on a routine chest X-ray. When symptoms occur, they may be due to the increased size or altered shape of the bone, resulting in bowing of a leg or a patient requiring a larger sized hat.

Occasionally pain occurs, bones may be tender to touch and the pain unremitting. If a joint is affected secondary osteoarthritis may produce pain, especially in the hips and knees. Pagetic bone is more liable to fracture. Compression of the auditory nerve may produce deafness and occasionally spinal cord compression results from spinal Paget's disease, producing spastic lower limbs.

Affected bones have an increased blood supply and Paget's disease in the lower leg results in an increase in skin temperature. Rarely, congestive cardiac failure occurs because of the increased cardiac work load in extensive Paget's disease.

The blood biochemistry reveals raised alkaline phosphatase activity. Rarely, a high blood calcium level results if patients with extensive disease are immobilised.

Osteogenic sarcoma is a rare complication.

Treatment

Analgesics may be all that is required. The bone pain and nerve entrapments may be improved by injections of calcitonin which are also of value for the hypercalcaemia of immobilisation. This treatment is expensive and its indications have to be carefully assessed for each patient. Diphosphonates are a group of drugs developed from detergents and when given systemically they inhibit bone resorption. These newer drugs may be useful in Paget's disease.

HYPERLIPIDAEMIAS

This is a group of disease resulting from abnormalities of lipid metabolism. They may be primary or result from other disorders including diabetes mellitus, thyroid and liver disease. Early diagnosis of primary lipid disorders may prevent premature vascular disease and since there is sometimes a familial incidence, treatment in childhood may prevent complications in adult life.

Mention is made of these disorders because manifestations include the development of xanthomas. These are cutaneous deposits of lipid-laden macrophages. Xanthelasma are xanthomas around the eyelids. These are yellowish flat plaques, usually in the inner corners of the eyelids. More extensive lesions appear in tendons and on bony prominences, in particular in the tendo Achilles and tibial tubercles. These plaques may be yellow or brown, become nodular and at times hard and indurated. In themselves they are of little consequence but denote underlying abnormalities which can include vascular disease resulting in premature death. Recognition of the lesions and their implications and appropriate referral for full delineation of the type of hyperlipidaemia and its possible treatment is of extreme importance.

DIABETES MELLITUS

This metabolic disorder is characterised by a relative or absolute deficiency of insulin affecting the metabolism of protein, fat, carbohydrate, water and electrolytes. These disturbances lead to progressive and sometimes irreversible functional and structural changes in all organs of the body despite improvements in the treatment available for diabetics.

Aetiology

There are two broad classifications of diabetes mellitus, namely idiopathic (or primary) diabetes and secondary diabetes.

Idiopathic diabetes mellitus

This is conveniently subdivided into *juvenile-onset (insulin-dependent) diabetes*, which is characterised by rapid weight loss, undernutrition and ketoacidosis, and *maturity-onset (insulin-indepen-*

dent) *diabetes*. Patients in the second group are often obese and do not normally develop ketoacidosis.

Idiopathic diabetes is the commonest form in Britain today. The precise aetiology remains uncertain but there are many known associations. It is principally a disease of the middle-aged and elderly, 80% of cases presenting after the age of 50. In this age group women are affected more often than men but there are more male juvenile diabetics than female.

Heredity plays a role in both types but is more important in maturity-onset diabetics. Infections, particularly viral infections, are now believed to precipitate juvenile-onset diabetes in susceptible individuals.

Obesity is associated with the development of maturity-onset diabetes, the incidence of which falls during periods of severe food rationing as occurred in both World Wars.

Secondary diabetes

A small proportion of cases of diabetes result from other diseases, especially endocrine disturbances characterised by an over-production of certain hormones:

1. Acromegaly, resulting from increased pituitary growth hormone
2. Cushings's syndrome, due to increased adrenal steroids
3. Phaeochromocytoma, due to increased adrenal adrenaline
4. Thyrotoxicosis, due to increased thyroid hormone
5. Pregnancy.

Liver and pancreatic diseases may produce diabetes. Drugs such as steroids can also produce diabetes mellitus.

Whatever the precipitating factors in diabetes mellitus, the failure of insulin action results in an increase in the level of glucose in the blood stream. The glucose spills over into the urine producing glycosuria and, because of the osmotic effect, the volume of urine is increased and the patient develops thirst. Finally, there is weight loss because of the loss of sugar and fluid from the body.

Clinical features

The disease may present in the classical manner with thirst, polyuria, tiredness, loss of weight, visual disturbances, or as ketoacidosis with nausea, vomiting and coma. More commonly, however, it is discovered on the chance finding of glycosuria on routine urine testing. Less commonly, patients present with symptoms due to the complications of diabetes.

Complications

These can be divided into ocular, renal, vascular and neurological complications and hyperglycaemic and hypoglycaemic coma. In addition diabetics are more prone to pulmonary tuberculosis, candida skin infections and other opportunistic infections. Diabetic involvement of the eye is now the commonest cause of blindness in middle-aged people. Renal infection is commoner in diabetics and occasionally leads to death from renal failure because of sclerotic renal disorders peculiar to diabetes.

Premature vascular disease is also a feature of diabetes so that myocardial infarction, hypertension and peripheral vascular disease are much commoner than in the general population. There are several neurological disturbances which may affect diabetics. They include: cranial nerve palsies, particularly affecting the eye muscles; autonomic neuropathy, which may produce impotence and postural hypotension because of denervation of blood vessels; peripheral neuropathy and isolated peripheral nerve lesions.

The diabetic foot and leg

The combination of vascular disease, impaired peripheral nerve function and increased risk of infection makes the diabetic prone to the development of gangrene, especially in the lower limb.

Clinical features. Vascular insufficiency results in intermittent claudication, rest pain and gangrene. Its features in diabetics are little different from those already described in Chapter 20, except that there is usually a neuropathic element in diabetic gangrene.

Peripheral neuropathy is a frequent complication and may be unnoticed by the patient. The acute form occurs in poorly controlled diabetics and improves with proper management of the condition. Pain and paraesthesia in the feet and legs are common symptoms. Chronic peripheral neuropathy does not appear to improve with treatment and is very common in elderly diabetics. It may be symptomless but, if the patient is aware of the problem, sensory rather than motor symptoms predominate, with pain and paraesthesia in the limbs often worse at night. Changes in the upper limbs are very rare. In the legs, and especially the feet, there is loss of all modalities of sensations in a stocking fashion and tendon reflexes are absent. Occasionally neuropathic joints occur due to loss of the sense of pain and proprioception.

The patient who is unaware of peripheral neuropathy may easily traumatise the feet and toes and in the presence of diminished tissue circulation, this produces superficial ulceration. Small bullae appear, rupture and leave a black area of superficial gangrene which sloughs leaving a granulating ulcer surrounded by healthy tissue. If the circulation is not too severely impaired these lesions can heal, but great care is always required.

As a result of the neuropathy, the toes become retracted and weight is thrown on to the metatarsal heads. Callosities are common and all too often ulceration follows attempts to remove them. Perforating ulcers of the sole of the foot are usually beneath the first metatarsophalangeal joint but others may be affected. This type of lesion may penetrate the joint and produce a chronic suppurative arthritis and osteitis. Ulcers develop on the heel as a result of pressure sores from prolonged bed rest or footwear. These lesions are often painless and patients may continue to traumatise the tissues, exacerbating ulcers and infection. Infection may be extensive before the patient experiences any discomfort. Indeed, it may be the smell of the putrefaction which compels the patient to seek help.

Management. The management of the diabetic foot is similar to that of the ischaemic foot (Ch. 20) but additional considerations are necessary. Vision may have deteriorated so badly that supervision of the feet and footwear by informed relatives becomes necessary. Patients need to be made aware of their diminished appreciation of pain, heat and cold so that they avoid walking barefoot and spending long periods in house slippers. New footwear should be worn for brief periods initially. All footwear should be inspected for nails and other foreign material which may injure the foot. Bath water temperatures need to be checked before bathing and hot water bottles should be discouraged.

Superficial ulcers should be cleaned with debridements and then covered with sterile non-adherent dressings and, if necessary, a pad applied to prevent further damage. Often normal footwear cannot be worn but a Plastazote shoe can be made to accommodate even bulky padding. More extensive penetrating ulcers require surgical debridement and systemic antibiotics. Regular irrigation and packing is necessary until the cavity granulates in; the lesion is then managed along the same lines as superficial ulceration. More extensive infection with osteitis requires more heroic surgery with wide excision of necrotic tissue, drainage, irrigation with antiseptics, packing and systemic antibiotics. If this fails, then amputation becomes necessary, the level depending upon the quality of the peripheral circulation and the extent of infection.

Special footwear can be used to help the misshapen foot produced by diabetic neuropathy. Patients with Charcot joints and retracted useless toes can easily further damage the foot with conventional standard footwear which will not protect and cushion these vulnerable parts of the feet. Rocker bars, Plastazote insoles and light-weight surgical shoes can be used with benefit in the appropriate situation. Bed boots in bed-fast patients can be moulded to protect heels from pressure to prevent decubitus ulceration (see also Ch. 8).

General management of diabetes

In addition to the management of complications, the glucose intolerance of diabetics is controlled in one of several ways. All diabetics must follow a carbohydrate and calorie-controlled diet to achieve an ideal body weight and limit the amount of carbodydrate taken. Obese diabetics require no more than this regimen. Young diabetics require insulin which has to be given by injection either once or twice a day.

Ideally, a twice a day regime is likely to achieve better control of the blood glucose levels. An increasing number of patients are using a regime where they can give themselves varying amounts of soluble insulin with meals using an insulin syringe which looks like a fountain pen. This gives the patient a more flexible lifestyle. At night, the patient administers a single injection of long-acting insulin to keep blood sugar under control whilst sleeping. This regime reflects more accurately the normal state, where the pancreas produces small quantities of insulin whilst fasting and larger quantities when food is taken. Patients using this method have to be fastidious in

monitoring their blood sugar levels until they are familiar with the techniques.

The non-ketotic maturity-onset diabetic who is not obese may require tablets which act by encouraging the pancreas to produce more insulin to control the hyperglycaemia. During intercurrent infections, operations and in pregnancy the insulin requirements are increased and patients who do not normally require insulin may need it during that time. It is therefore very important to control the diabetic state when treating ischaemic, infected or gangrenous limbs. Many patients will require insulin or extra insulin at this time and failure to appreciate this aspect can lead to more suffering by the patient, and occasionally death.

FURTHER READING

Bondy P K, Rosenberg L E 1982 Metabolic control and disease, 8th edn. Saunders, London
Connor H, Boulton A J M, Ward J Q 1987 The foot in diabetes. J Wiley, Chichester
Keen H, Jarrett J 1982 Complications of diabetes, 2nd edn. Edward Arnold, London
Levin M E, O'Neal L W 1982 The diabetic foot. Mosby, St Louis
MacLeod J (ed) 1987 Davidson's principles and practice
of medicine, 15th edn. Churchill Livingstone, Edinburgh
Oakley W G, Pyke D A, Taylor K W 1975 Diabetes and its management. Blackwell, Oxford
Weatherall D J, Ledingham J G G, Warrell D A (eds) 1983 Oxford textbook of medicine. Oxford University Press, Oxford
William R H 1981 Textbook of endocrinology, 6th edn. Saunders, London

22. Rheumatic disorders

M. I. D. Cawley   L. A. Smidt

Rheumatic diseases are those which present with symptoms predominantly in the musculoskcletal system, comprising the bones, joints, muscles, tendons, ligaments, bursae and undifferentiated connective tissue. Rheumatic diseases are very common in the population, especially in the older age groups. They are a major cause of ill health and disability. The feet are commonly involved in a number of important rheumatic diseases and may indeed often be the site of presenting symptoms. The mechanical strains of weight-bearing frequently appear to affect adversely the underlying rheumatic lesions in the feet. A basic understanding of the pathology, clinical features and management of these diseases, and of the prevention of local complications, is therefore of importance to everyone professionally concerned with foot problems. It will be logical to consider these disorders under the sub-headings of the individual diseases, and a system of classification of rheumatic diseases affecting the feet is therefore necessary:

1. *Mechanical or degenerative conditions.* These include primary and secondary osteoarthrosis (osteoarthritis).
2. *Inflammatory disorders.* Lesions in the feet are usually local manifestations of diffuse systemic inflammatory disease of the joints or other connective tissue structures. Important subgroups are:

   a. Rheumatoid disease
   b. Spondyloarthritis, i.e. ankylosing spondylitis and diseases related to it
   c. Other inflammatory connective tissue diseases with autoimmune features
   d. Crystal deposition disease, e.g. gout

   e. Miscellaneous arthritic disorders not classified above.

OSTEOARTHROSIS (OA)

This is a disease of the joints in which the hyaline cartilage appears to bc primarily involved. Secondary changes occur in subarticular bone and in the synovial membrane, ligaments and other soft tissue. It will be considered first because in one form or another it is the most common clinical rheumatic disorder. It is not, however, usually a serious problem in the foot, except in the special local instances of hallux abductovalgus, hallux rigidus, post traumatic arthropathy and sometimes osteoarthrosis following previous inflammatory joint disease. It may also be associated with congenital or acquired foot deformity.

Primary generalised osteoarthrosis

This is a disorder which most commonly presents in middle-aged women and in which genetic factors appear to play a part. The disease has a particular predilection for the distal interphalangeal joints of the fingers (Heberden's nodes), the first carpometacarpal joints, and to a lesser extent the proximal interphalangeal joints (Bouchard's nodes). The corresponding joints in the feet may also be affected but rarely cause serious problems, with the exception of the first metatarsophalangeal joint which is perhaps more commonly affected by osteoarthrosis than any other joint in the body. This joint may be affected individually or as part of the generalised disorder and the result may be either hallux abductovalgus or hallux rigidus. Other joints commonly affected by the generalised form of osteoarthrosis include the hip and the knee as well as the interfacetal joints of the spine. The generalised form of osteoarthrosis tends to go through a painful phase lasting a few months or even years whilst the characteristic bony lesions are evolving. It then becomes pain free although the bony nodules and deformities remain.

Secondary and localised forms of osteoartherosis

These can affect any joint and commonly follow previous joint damage due to trauma or inflammation, or in some cases minor developmental abnormalities. In this form of the disease, pre-existing mechanical derangement or cartilage damage appear to be the important factors. The hip is a very common site of this form of osteoarthrosis, as is the knee. In the case of the foot, as already mentioned, the first metatarsophalangeal joint is very commonly affected.

Hallux abductovalgus

This common abnormality comprises an arthritic disorder at the first metatarsophalangeal joint (MPJ) combined with an adductus deformity of the first metatarsal and an abductus deformity of the hallux. The first metatarsophalangeal joint is commonly the site of trauma, due either to specific major incidents, probably more common in males, or to repeated minor trauma and distortion such as is thought to occur particularly in females wearing footwear with tapering pointed toes, or secondary to pes plano-valgus. There is loss of articular cartilage, the bony margins of the joint enlarge, and the prominent medial side of the metatarsal head forms the so-called 'bunion'. A bursa often forms over this prominence which may become inflamed and trophic damage to the skin may also occur. The joint is commonly painful on weight-bearing.

Hallux rigidus

Hallux rigidus also occurs after trauma and progressive osteoarthrosis of the first MP joint results in marked painful restriction, the pain being provoked by the extension of the toe when the patient walks.

Localised osteoarthrosis in the hindfoot

Secondary osteoarthrosis also occurs in the tarsal joints, probably most commonly in the subtaloid or midtarsal joints, especially the talonavicular, following previous inflammation, traumatic damage or deformity. Subtaloid osteoarthrosis is often accompanied by a pes plano-valgus deformity. Midtarsal osteoarthrosis appears to occur more frequently in the highly-arched rigid foot. The ankle joint itself may also become affected by osteoarthrosis following fractures or other trauma involving this articulation.

Pathology

There is first fibrillation and then progressive loss and eburnation of the hyaline articular cartilage. This is followed by sclerosis and increased density of the subarticular bone, and the laying down of new bone at the joint margins, thus producing osteophytes, which appear to be a form of natural attempt at repair. These result in restriction of movement and sometimes distortion of the joint architecture. The hyaline cartilage itself is not pain sensitive and pain appears to arise from nerve endings in the joint capsule which is presumably subjected to strain, stretching or trauma. Such trauma to the soft tissues, which appears to be a secondary phenomenon in most cases, may be the cause of minor signs of inflammation including effusion and a few inflammatory cells in the joint fluid. Mild synovitis undoubtedly occurs in some OA joints and is also thought to be provoked by cartilage debris in the joint cavity. There has been interest in recent years in the possible role of calcium crystals (either calcium pyrophosphate dihydrate, or hydroxyapatite) in the pathogenesis of osteoarthrosis, and it is not yet clear whether such crystals are a primary or secondary phenomenon.

Treatment

Osteoarthrosis is not a multisystem disease and does not affect general health except through discomfort and there is no good evidence that drug therapy modifies the course of the disease in any beneficial way. Symptoms often remit spontaneously. Treatment is essentially symptomatic during painful phases and in the milder cases involves (a) the use of simple analgesic drugs and occasionally sedatives to control the pain; if significant secondary inflammation is present it may be logical to use mild non-steroidal anti-inflammatory agents (see below); and (b) various physical measures.

The physical measures include, in the case of the foot, the control of body weight to reduce weight-bearing activity, the provision of suitable footwear and appliances to redistribute body weight more evenly and to relieve any painful area such as the first metatarsophalangeal joint. Surgical treatment can be useful in some cases of osteoarthrosis of the foot, particularly such measures as the correction of hallux abducto-valgus deformities and the arthrodesis of the slightly mobile hallux rigidus. Occasionally arthrodesis of one or more of the hindfoot joints is necessary. The same general principles of management are applicable to osteoarthrosis elsewhere in the body. Replacement arthroplasty in the foot is still at an experimental stage and only in the ankle joint has there been any success with joint prostheses.

In association with well-fitting footwear, or footwear which has been modified to accommodate the deformed foot, durable appliances of a palliative nature should be provided. Hallux abductovalgus shields may be fabricated to protect the prominent joint and are very effective in relieving pain and preventing infection. Latex shields incorporating protective foam padding are built up on a positive plaster cast. Those made from silicone compounds are moulded directly on to the foot.

In hallux rigidus, the joint is painful while it retains some degree of mobility. The pain can be alleviated by reducing the range of movement either with a relatively inflexible insole or by the patient wearing shoes with rigid or rocker soles. Redistribution of weight from the painful joint is also necessary. This can be achieved by fitting a valgus insole (Fig. 22.1) with a winged metatarsal pad to reduce thrust on the joint.

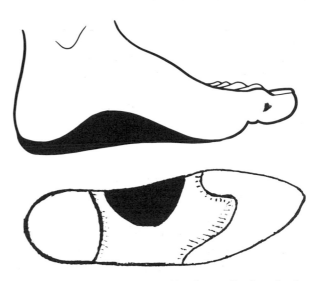

Fig. 22.1   Valgus and metatarsal insole to redistribute load on foot: (A) showing valgus support; (B) showing design of plantar padding.

In tarsal arthrosis, restriction of movement in the affected joints is also indicated. In the case of the subtaloid joint, a palliative valgus insole will help to maintain the foot in the most comfortable position. In midtarsal arthrosis this is best achieved by a combination of valgus padding with a tarsal platform which provides a 'tarsal cradle', thereby supporting both the medial and lateral borders of the foot and minimising the range of inversion and eversion of the forefoot.

RHEUMATOID ARTHRITIS (RA)

This is by far the most severe of the common rheumatic disorders affecting the feet. It frequently causes troublesome foot lesions. Rheumatoid arthritis or *rheumatoid disease*, as it is more correctly called, is a chronic inflammatory multisystem disease of unknown aetiology. Characteristic features include clinically obvious inflammation of synovial joints with effusion and thickening of the synovial membrane, radiological evidence of joint damage (loss of cartilage and bony erosions) by the inflammatory granulation tissue (pannus) and the presence in the serum of globulin antibody material reacting against the individual's own gammaglobulin. This abnormal antibody protein is called *rheumatoid factor* and is present in raised titres at some time or other in the

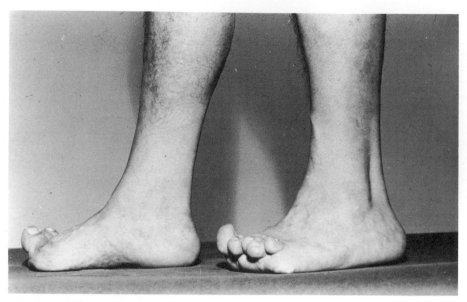

Fig. 22.2   Rheumatoid arthritis. Dorsal subluxation of toes.

great majority of patients with this disease. Subcutaneous fleshy nodules often occur over bony and other pressure points in the more severe cases and cutaneous ulcers are common.

RA is a common disease affecting perhaps 1% or more of the population. It can commence at any age but most commonly does so during the middle years of life and it is two to three times as common in women as it is in men. Although the clinical pattern of the disease varies considerably, it is typically symmetrical between the two sides of the body and the small joints of the hands and feet are nearly always involved. The pattern of involvement of the small joints, however, differs considerably from the generalised form of osteoarthrosis.

In rheumatoid arthritis the more serious lesions in the upper extremity usually involve the wrists and the metacarpophalangeal and proximal interphalangeal joints. In the feet, all the metatarsophalangeal joints are usually involved and the joints of the toes and the hindfoot are also often affected clinically. The characteristic clinical changes are again quite different from those of osteoarthrosis and are, in fact, those of inflammation associated with the secondary damage that occurs. Thus there is swelling of the soft tissues around the joints due to synovitis and

indeed the synovial lining membrane of the joint can become greatly thickened to hundreds of times its original dimensions. Effusions are often present in the affected joints and later there is destruction of articular cartilage with disorganisation of the joint architecture and secondary subluxation or even dislocation. Pain, stiffness and swelling are commonly noticed by the patient, and in the untreated case the pattern of stiffness is characteristic in that, along with the other symptoms, it is worse after periods of inactivity, producing 'early morning stiffness'.

In the foot, characteristic changes take place at the metatarsophalangeal joints (Figs. 22.2–22.4) which become painful, stiff and markedly tender. On weight bearing, this tenderness produces a sensation often akin to that of walking barefoot on pebbles. It seems likely that mechanical forces acting on the inflamed joints of the foot during standing or walking contribute to the characteristic deformity that occurs. This deformity consists of a dorsal subluxation of the toes at the metatarsophalangeal joints and a migration forwards of the fibro-fatty pad, which normally bears weight under the metatarsal heads (Fig. 22.2). This exposes the already inflamed metatarsophalangeal joints to a less protected position adjacent to the ground. There may also

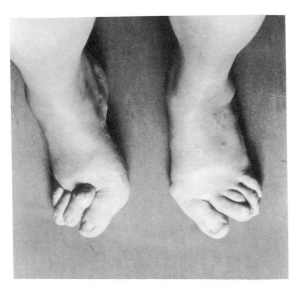

Fig. 22.3 Rheumatoid arthritis. Hallux abducto valgus and overriding of toes.

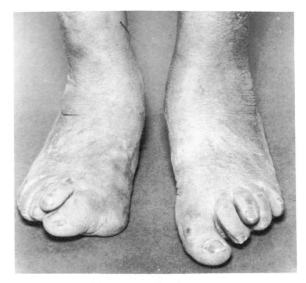

Fig. 22.4 Rhematoid arthritis Heloma durum and trophic changes secondary to toe deformities.

be hallux abductovalgus and overriding of one or more toes (Fig. 22.3). The toes themselves are displaced upwards, sometimes to the extent of being dislocated, and therefore tend to be traumatised by the shoe; secondary trophic lesions develop (Fig. 22.4). The toes may also develop flexion deformities at the interphalangeal joints. Once troublesome forefoot deformity of this type has occurred, ordinary retail shoes are unsatisfactory and special footwear is required.

Different problems may arise in the hindfoot. Many of the tarsal joints may be involved but the problems commonly arise from the subtaloid joint. The mechanical stresses of weight-bearing on this joint while it is inflamed often produce a valgus deformity. Even without this, arthritis of this particular joint is often very painful on weight-bearing. Varus deformities occur but are much less common. Valgus deformity in its early stages may be compensated for by the additon of wedging to the medial side of the shoes and by suitable insoles. The ankle joint itself may also be severely affected by rheumatoid arthritis, with marked restriction of movement, and bursitis may develop deep or superficial to the attachment of the Achilles tendon.

Rheumatoid nodules are inflammatory granulomatous lesions occurring subcutaneously at sites of repeated pressure or minor trauma. Thus they occur very characteristically on the ulnar border of the forearms. These nodules commonly develop under the pressure-bearing areas of the heels and also under the metatarsal heads, on the dorsum of the toes, and around the Achilles tendon. Occasionally, nodules ulcerate, either spontaneously or due to trauma, and then they provide a portal of entry for infection. Callosities tend to occur under the metatarsal heads and may be extremely tender.

Ulcers are a serious problem on the lower legs and feet in rheumatoid arthritis, and they occur at least twice as commonly as in degenerative rheumatic disorders. They appear to be multifactorial in aetiology and may be due to vasculitis, trauma, venous insufficiency, arteriosclerosis and local joint dysfunction, especially of the ankle joint.

Other complications of rheumatoid arthritis which can occur in the foot include bursitis or nodules over the first metatarsophalangeal joint, and peripheral neuropathy. The neuropathy is most commonly of an insidious symmetrical sensory-motor type. Less commonly a more severe mononeuritis multiplex may occur with predominant motor features due to vasculitis of the vasa vasora, with ischaemic infarction of the peripheral nerve trunks. Small periungual infarcts due to vasculitic obstruction of small blood vessels may also occur in the feet just as they do often and more obviously in the hands.

Treatment

As already indicated, rheumatoid arthritis is a systemic disorder often causing such manifestations as weight loss, malaise, anorexia and depression. In addition, specific lesions of various non-articular tissues may occur, including involvement of the lungs, heart, blood vessels, eye and peripheral nerves. Nevertheless, the predominant clinical changes usually occur in the joints and associated structures. The rational objective of therapy in rheumatoid arthritis — since the ultimate cause is unknown and cannot therefore be deliberately eliminated — is at least to suppress directly the destructive inflammation affecting the joints and other tissues or, better still, to induce a biological remission so that the abnormalities producing the inflammation are reversed. The wide range of anti-rheumatic drugs available are the principal means used in the attempt to achieve this aim. These drugs fall into two main groups and one or more members of each group are often given in conjuction.

1. Anti-inflammatory drugs (See Ch. 12)

These include a large group of non-steroid anti-inflammatory drugs (NSAIDs). They are compounds which behave pharmacologically like aspirin, i.e. their properties are mainly analgesic, anti-inflammatory and anti-pyretic. There are many different types of chemical compound which act in this way. In addition to aspirin and other salicylate compounds, there are propionic acid derivatives, indomethacin, pyrazole compounds and phenylacetic acid derivatives, to name those that are most widely used. The substances in this group have an analgesic effect in low doses but are usually given in higher doses to produce anti-inflammatory activity. Moreover, this latter effect requires continuous adequate blood and tissue levels. Regular medication in adequate dosage is therefore required to suppress inflammation continuously and, unfortunately, gastrointestinal side-effects are common with this form of continuous medication. NSAIDs act by suppressing the local release of humoral mediators of inflammation, especially certain prostaglandins derived from arachidonic acid, which is released from phospholipid in the cell membranes.

Corticosteroids (synthetic glucocorticoid analogues of cortisone and hydro-cortisone, such as prednisone and prednisolone) are more powerful agents in the direct suppression of inflammation and almost always achieve this effect in rheumatoid arthritis. However, the long term therapy, which is nearly always necessary in this disease, poses serious problems so far as the side effects of corticosteroid therapy are concerned. An important side-effect relevant to foot care is that the suppression of inflammatory changes by corticosteroids may mask or reduce the natural response to infection in local superficial lesions on the feet. If this form of therapy is necessary, the maintenance dose is kept as low as possible.

2. 'Disease-modifying' drugs

A number of slow-acting 'disease-modifying' drugs have been shown to be capable of facilitating a biological remission over a period of time. These drugs do not appear to have any direct suppressive effect on the joint inflammation at its local site, but act indirectly in more subtle biological ways which are at present not well understood. Drugs in this group include gold compounds such as gold sodium thiomalate (Myocrisin) and auranofin, D-penicillamine, chloroquine compounds, some of the cytotoxic and immunosupressive drugs used otherwise in the treatment of malignant disease, and two sulphonamides: dapsone and sulphasalazine. Full or partial remission may occur when drugs in this group are given in appropriate dosage, but the effect often takes several months to become fully apparent. These drugs all have potential severe toxic effects and careful monitoring of the patient is necessary.

Physical aspects of treatment

While the inflammatory process in rheumatoid arthritis is active, periods of general rest or local immobilisation of joints by special splints are often necessary since rest—local or general—facilitates the resolution of the inflammatory process. After inflammation subsides, expert physiotherapy becomes important to re-establish adequate muscle and joint function. In the special case of the feet, during active inflammation it seems reasonable to maintain normal anatomy as far as possible and to protect the feet from trauma by the provision of made-to-measure lightweight footwear with such special features as arch supports and plentiful toe room. During severe exacerbations, periods of enforced hospitalisation and b rest are often indicated to avoid weight-bearir altogether.

Podiatric treatment

As a result of the vasculitis, the local tissue ischaemia, the immunosuppressive effects of the disease, as well as possible side-effects from systemic drug therapy, the patient with rheumatoid arthritis is at risk from infection. Therefore utmost pre- and postoperative antisepsis is of paramount importance, as is skilful and cautious operating. All padding and appliances should be aimed at relieving pressure and reducing friction. Because of its thermoplastic properties, expanded polyethylene (Plastazote) is used extensively for the fabrication of cushion insoles and lightweight footwear. (The techniques are described in Ch. 13). Toe deformities require permanent protection by durable non-adhesive appliances. Adhesive padding and strapping cannot be used for long because of problems of maceration and sensitivity and the difficulty of normal hygiene. It is therefore essential for the patient suffering from rheumatoid arthritis to have digital appliances of a detachable type. Hallux abductovalgus shields and digital splints made from silicone rubber or Plastazote are extremely useful and add considerably to the patient's comfort.

Surgical treatment

This may be indicated when deformity and pain in the foot do not respond to the measures described above. Careful assessment is required before surgery is recommended and this is best done in a combined clinic where the patient can be seen by both rheumatologist and surgeon. Subcutaneous nodules may be excised or injected with hydrocortisone acetate if their position makes shoe fitting difficult. The painful subtalar joint which goes into valgus may be stabilised by triple arthrodesis. Isolated toe deformities such as hallux abductovalgus, hallux rigidus, hammer toe and claw toe can be helped by proximal hemiphalangectomy.

However, in rheumatoid arthritis there are usually multiple toe deformities, a common problem being hallux abductovalgus accompanied by clawing of the lesser toes and severe metatarsalgia secondary to dorsal dislocations of the metatarsophalangeal joints. Relief from metatarsalgia and secondary correction of the toe deformities can be obtained by resecting the heads of the metatarsals. Plantar, dorsal or combined incisions may be used depending on the preference of the surgeon. Most surgeons would agree that it is important to draw the thick pad of plantar tissue that lies distal to the exposed metatarsal heads into a more proximal weight-bearing position. Despite removal of the weight-bearing metatarsal heads, the relief of metatarsalgia and the realignment of the deformed toes improves the overall function of the foot. Full weight-bearing in sandals is allowed when the incisions are healed.

Finally, when there are gross, rigid deformities of all toes, amputation may be carried out through the metatarsophalangeal joints or the necks of the metatarsals. Normal footwear may then be worn if a suitable insole with toe block is fitted.

In properly selected patients, operation on a foot affected by rheumatoid arthritis can produce a substantial improvement in overall function.

ANKLOSING SPONDYLITIS AND OTHER FORMS OF SPONDYLOARTHRITIS

Seronegative spondyloarthritis is a term now widely used to include ankylosing spondylitis and a number of other inflammatory disorders which show negative tests for rheumatoid factor in the serum, and which, in varying degrees, resemble spondylitis clinically and are related to it genetically and pathologically. It includes arthritis occurring in association with other well defined non-rheumatic diseases such as psoriasis and chronic inflammatory bowel diseases. Thus, apart from ankylosing spondylitis, this group includes *Reiter's syndrome, psoriatic arthritis,* the arthropathies associated with *ulcerative colitis* and *Crohn's disease,* as well as certain rarer disorders. Most of these diseases are more common in males than females and tend to arise in early adult life, although they can also present at other ages. The genetic influence is stronger than with most other rheumatic diseases and there is often a positive family history of one or more of these related disorders.

In *ankylosing spondylitis* itself, the dominant clinical features are usually seen in the spine with inflammation and ossification of the ligaments resulting in marked limitation of movement. The sacroiliac joints are always involved in this disease and commonly in other members of the disease group as well. Peripheral joint lesions are also common in ankylosing spondylitis and other members of the group. These joint lesions differ somewhat from the arthritis of rheumatoid arthritis in that the synovitis is less proliferative and erosive; the feet are likewise commonly involved in these diseases in a way not characteristic of rheumatoid arthritis.

A characteristic lesion in these seronegative disorders is the formation of *calcaneal spurs.* These arise at the origin of the small muscles of the sole of the foot and the plantar fascia from the inferior surface of the calcaneus. This lesion is often painful on weight-bearing and also on waking in the morning due to inflammation at the ligament-bone junction. This junction area is known as an *enthesis* and the lesion therefore as *enthesopathy.* Such lesions, often called *plantar fasciitis,* heal by new bone formation and a spur is thus formed (Fig. 22.5). They may be unilateral or bilateral. Methods of treatment include sorbo pads in the heel of the shoe, combined with a tarsal platform, anti-inflammatory drugs, local injection of steroids, or occasionally a single dose of radiotherapy. The various synovial joints of the feet may also be inflamed in these diseases, especially the metatarsophalangeal joints.

In *Reiter's disease* and *psoriatic arthritis,* 'sausage like' inflammation of one or more toes may occur and these often assume a dusky red colour. In association with this, the toe-nails may show the changes of psoriasis (pitting and onycholysis) and there may be *pustular psoriasis,* or, in Reiter's disease, *keratoderma blenorrhagica* on the soles of the feet. The joints of the hindfoot may be inflamed with pain, swelling and subsequent

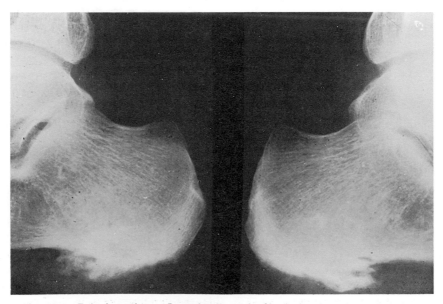

Fig. 22.5   Reiter's syndrome. Lateral radiograph of heels showing calcaneal spurs on inferior aspect.

erosions. In the arthritis accompanying ulcerative colitis or Crohn's disease there is often predominant involvement of a few lower limb joints.

The cause of this group of disorders is unknown but patients with ankylosing spondylitis and Reiter's disease and other conditions in which sacroileitis is present often have the HLA-B27 histocompatibility antigen, indicating an inherited predisposition to this type of musculoskeletal inflammation. It is likely that infection with microorganisms is a trigger factor in at least some of these diseases, especially Reiter's syndrome.

Reiter's syndrome in its fully developed form is a triad comprising arthritis, urethritis and ocular inflammation which may follow either non-specific genital infection or dysentery. The acute features usually resolve after a few weeks or months but some articular lesions may persist for years. The arthropathies associated with chronic inflammatory bowel disease often fluctuate in severity in parallel with the degree of inflammation in the intestine. Ulcerative colitis is a chronic inflammatory disease of the colon and rectum of unknown aetiology. Crohn's disease, or regional ileitis, is a granulomatous inflammatory disorder, also of unknown aetiology, predominantly affecting the small intestine but which may also involve the large intestine. Apart from local treatment of the feet, the spondyloarthritides are often considerably improved by non-steroid anti-inflammatory drugs, indomethacin and various propionic acid derivatives being widely used.

GOUT

Classically, acute gout most commonly affects the first metatarsophalangeal joint of either foot and this is the first clinical manifestation of the disease. However any other joint may be the site of this type of inflammation which is due to the deposition of sodium urate crystals in or around the joint. This occurs in patients with hyperuricaemia, which is usually a constitutional anomaly, more common in men but also occurring in women after the menopause. It is seen rarely in younger women or children. It can also occur secondarily due to increased cell division and nucleic acid turnover, e.g. in leukaemia, and, more commonly, due to the effect of diuretics on clearance of urate by the renal tubules. In acute attacks, the intense inflammation at the site can prevent the patient from putting their foot to the ground and there are marked local changes with swelling, warmth and exquisite tenderness. The attacks are usually intermittent initially, with full resolution in between, and most acute attacks subside rapidly after large doses of non-steroid anti-inflammatory drugs. Aspirin should not be given as it may elevate the uric acid level.

Chronic gout can also affect the foot with signs of chronic arthritis and deformity of a number of joints, and occasionally gouty tophi which are due to urate crystal deposits under the skin. However the long-term control of hyperuricaemia with the drug allopurinol, which inhibits the enzyme xanthine oxidase and thereby reduces the synthesis of urate, means that chronic gouty-arthritis nowadays is a largely curable and increasingly rare disorder. Dietary restriction is very rarely necessary.

THE INFLAMMATORY CONNECTIVE TISSUE DISEASES

In this relatively uncommon group of inflammatory diseases, sometimes alternatively called *collagen-vascular diseases*, a variety of foot lesions may occur.

This group of disorders includes *systemic lupus erythematosus*, *systemic sclerosis* or *scleroderma*, *polyarteritis nodosa*, and *dermatomyositis*. In these diseases, various features indicate an autoimmune process, i.e. the body appears to be reacting immunologically against its own constituents, a situation which is also true to some extent in rheumatoid arthritis. The clinical picture varies according to the tissue or tissues mainly affected. The inflammatory lesions are often based on small or medium sized blood vessels. Although in some of these diseases foot problems are not numerically important, a number of lesions can occur in the feet and these will be mentioned briefly.

Raynaud's phenomenon is blanching and numbness of the fingers due to excessive vasospasm and, less commonly, cold sensitivity of this type can also occur in the foot with any of the diseases in this group, but especially scleroderma and systemic lupus erythematosus. Inflammation in small blood vessels with *vasculitic infarcts* can also occur in any of the group, especially systemic lupus erythematosus and polyarteritis nodosa, and this may lead to healing with small depressed scars in the pulp of the toes after the painful acute phase has subsided. In scleroderma *tethering* and *fibrosis* of the skin may occur particularly at the extremities, with a tendency to secondary restriction of joint movement. Subcutaneous *calcinotic nodules* can also occur in this disease. The systemic management of this group of diseases is beyond the scope of this book, but it is worth pointing out that potentially powerful and toxic drugs such as corticosteroids and immunosuppressive agents are commonly used, either separately or in combination. Local treatment may be important, especially for lesions of the foot, in order to protect them from trauma and infection. In these diseases and in rheumatoid arthritis, peripheral neuropathy can also occur and this may involve the feet. Individual peripheral nerves can also be involved, e.g. the anterior tibial nerve, with resulting foot drop which may need a toe spring or caliper for control.

SEPTIC ARTHRITIS

Septic arthritis nowadays is often a complication of some other disease, particularly rheumatoid arthritis, but can also occur as a feature of septicaemia from any cause and sometimes as a complication of certain specific infections, e.g. in the case of gonococcal arthritis. Patients who are debilitated or immunosupressed for any reason are at special risk. Feet are as susceptible as other joints to blood-borne infection of this type. In addition, there is the risk of direct access of organisms if the feet have become deformed or traumatised, with trophic ulcers occurring as has already been mentioned in relation to rheumatoid arthritis. In cases of septic arthritis or potential septic arthritis, it is important to ascertain whether the infection has spread to the bone and this may require serial radiographs and radioisotope scintigraphy. *Staphylococcus aureus* is the most common causative organism but many other bacteria are sometimes responsible. Treatment is by the systemic administration of antibiotics and may also on occasions require surgical drainage. Apart from this, the local care of the feet is largely the application of protective measures and during the infected phase weight-bearing should be prohibited.

ARTHRITIS IN CHILDREN

The arthritic disorders occurring in children are mainly the same as those occurring in adults, but they may present in different ways and are less common. The joints of the feet are liable to be involved in many of the disorders. A number of different patterns of joint involvement are recognised in what is now called juvenile chronic arthritis and was formerly referred to as *Still's disease*. A small proportion of children have what appears to be adult rheumatoid arthritis presenting in early life. This group has the worst prognosis and is probably the most likely to have chronic damage to the foot joints. Of those with other forms, many improve but a few go on to develop typical adult diseases such as ankylosing spondylitis and psoriatic arthritis. The management of local foot problems in children is essentially the same as for adults except that allowance should be made for growth.

FURTHER READING

Dixon A St J 1971 The rheumatoid foot. In: Hill A G S (ed) Modern trends in rheumatology 2. Butterworth, London, ch 11

Jayson M V, Smidt L A (eds) 1987 The foot in arthritis. Ballierès Clinical Rheumatology 1 (2) August

Mason M, Currey H L F (eds) 1986 Mason and Currey's clinical rheumatology, 4th edn. Churchill Livingstone, Edinburgh

Scott J T (ed) 1986 Copeman's textbook of the rheumatic diseases, 6th edn. Churchill Livingstone, Edinburgh

23. Neurological disorders

Peter Sandercock

For ease of discussion, those diseases of the nervous system which affect the innervation of the lower limbs and, either directly or indirectly, the control of the feet, are best divided into disorders of the upper motor neurones (or *pyramidal system*) and disorders of the lower motor and sensory neurones (or *peripheral nervous system*). The clinical features of these two groups of diseases are very different and they also have contrasting effects upon the function of the feet.

THE PYRAMIDAL SYSTEM: UPPER MOTOR NEURONES

Disorders affecting upper motor neurones in the cerebral cortex and their axons which pass to the anterior horn cells of the lumbosacral expansion of the spinal cord produce characteristic changes in the function of the lower limb(s). There is an increase in the passive resistance to movement which is normally present in muscles (*hypertonia*), particularly in the extensor muscles of the hip and knee and the plantar flexors of the ankle. In contrast, weakness is more marked in the flexors of the hip and knee and the dorsiflexors and evertors of the ankle. This distribution of weakness and hypertonia reduces spontaneous flexion of the knee when walking and also causes dragging of the toe along the ground in an arc-like movement producing characteristic wearing of the anterior and lateral aspect of the shoe. The sound of the gait is unmistakable with a regular prolonged scraping sound as the leg is slowly dragged forward, the patient tending to trip over minor obstacles due to an inability to lift the foot clear of the ground. Patients may complain that the foot seems 'stuck to the ground'.

The foot is held in a position of plantarflexion and also partial inversion. This causes most of the body weight to be transmitted to the anterior and lateral aspect of the foot in the region of the metatarsal heads and the metatarsophalangeal joints rather than being evenly distributed over the sole of the foot. The anterior part of the foot first comes into contact with the ground during weight transfer and the heel becomes a secondary weight-bearing area. Partial inversion of the foot causes increased lateral stress on the ankle joint and this deformity is increased during maximum weight-bearing. In addition to these usual bony and ligamentous stresses, greater pressure is also applied to parts of the skin which are not usually the main areas of contact with the ground or the side walls of the shoe.

An upper motor neurone lesion affecting one leg is often accompanied by an upper motor neurone weakness affecting the arm and face on the same side (*hemiplegia*). When both legs are affected, the patient's walking difficulty is greatly increased and the term *paraplegia* is used. Complete paralysis is usually referred to as '—plegia' (hemiplegia or paraplegia), whereas patients who are still able to move a limb are said to have—paresis' (*hemiparesis or paraparesis*). It is convenient to consider neurological disorders using this form of classification.

Hemiplegia/hemiparesis

Cerebrovascular disease

In those parts of the world which enjoy a higher standard of living, the stroke syndrome is by far the commonest cause of a hemiplegia. Despite an ever increasing range of medical terminology, the term 'stroke' is still the most apt description of the sudden onset of a focal neurological deficit due to vascular disease affecting the cerebral hemispheres or brainstem. The deficit typically resolves over several weeks or months but in one third to a half of cases, recovery is never complete. A stroke may be preceded by warning episodes or 'little strokes' which have identical symptoms to the more persistent lesion but resolve completely within minutes or hours. Less commonly, cerebrovascular disease may present insidiously in a series of minor events which go unnoticed until their gradual accumulation gives the impression of a steadily progressive disorder.

About 80% of patients with strokes have hemiparesis. If it is accompanied by other signs and symptoms, accurate localisation of the site of the lesion is possible. Damage to one cerebral hemisphere may result in *hemianaesthesia* (loss of sensation over half of the body) or *hemianopia* (inability to see to one side of the mid-line), and with involvement of the dominant side of the brain, the addition of speech and language disturbance (*dysphasia*, *dyslexia*) and memory impairment. The brain stem is a highly concentrated region of neural activity containing most of the cranial nerve nuclei and also linking the cerebral hemispheres, spinal cord and cerebellum. Common accompaniments of a hemiplegia or, not uncommonly in this site, a quadriplegia (weakness of all four limbs) are paralysis or eye movements causing *diplopia*, *ataxia* (loss of balance), weakness of the muscles permitting speech and swallowing (*dysarthria* and *dysphagia*) and vertigo.

About 85% of strokes are due to blockage of an artery; the lack of blood supply to that part of the brain supplied by the artery causes irreversible brain damage. The damaged area is called a *cerebral infarction*. The remaining 15% of strokes are due to bursting of an artery. The blood can enter the brain substance, causing local damage (intracerebral haemorrhage), or it can enter into the fluid spaces around the brain (subarachnoid haemorrhage). Strokes due to cerebral infarction and intracerebral haemorrhage cannot be reliably distinguished by bedside examination, but computerised tomographic scanning (CT) can do so quickly and easily.

In the majority of cases, haemorrhage is secondary to arterial hypertension and the most vital aspect of management is the control of the elevated blood pressure. Infarction is often due to the formation of emboli. These are accumulations of platelets and fibrin which form on the surface of irregular atheromatous blood vessels (e.g. at the origin of the internal carotid artery) or on the wall of the heart damaged by rheumatic fever or a myocardial infarct. They may subsequently break loose and pass downstream to occlude an intracranial artery. In patients with stroke due to cerebral infarction, the mainstay of treatment is to control high blood pressure, which is the single most important cause of atheromatous arterial disease. Reduction in blood fats and getting patients to stop smoking are also important. Regular aspirin therapy can reduce the risk of subsequent stroke or heart attack by about 30%. Anticoagulant treatment may be needed in the few patients whose strokes were due to embolism from the heart to the brain. Surgical removal of atheromatous narrowing in the carotid artery (carotid endarterectomy) may prevent stroke in carefully selected patients.

Cerebral tumour

Headache is a common symptom which often makes patients and their doctors worry about the possibility of a brain tumour. Tension headache and migraine are extremely common, affecting perhaps 20% of the population, whereas brain tumours are rare; so the vast majority of headache patients do not turn out to have tumours.

In a similar manner to a stroke, a tumour may present with a hemiplegia together with other features which depend upon the siting of the lesion. In contrast to the sudden onset of a stroke, the symptoms and signs gradually evolve over weeks, months or even years. Unlike most other organs, the brain is enclosed in a rigid cover for protection, and so, when the contents increase in volume, a rise in intracranial pressure soon follows to produce increasing headache, vomiting and a deteriorating conscious level. Ophthalmoscopy may enable the clinician to conform the presence of raised intracranial pressure by looking for swelling of the optic nerves (*papilloedema*) as they enter the retinae.

Computer-assisted tomography is now the most reliable and least hazardous method of confirming the presence of a cerebral tumour. The majority of tumours are due to spread of cancer from other organs (e.g. bronchus, breast, stomach, bowel) or to neoplastic proliferation of nerve cells (gliomas); as such, they usually infiltrate into the brain, making complete surgical removal impossible in most cases. Radiotherapy and chemotherapy may extend the patient's survival time by a few months, but rarely is the quality of life improved. When investigating for a possible tumour, the physician hopes to find a benign lesion, such as a meningioma, which grows from the meninges over the surface of the brain. This is more amenable to surgery.

Paraplegia/paresis

Symptoms and signs

Patients with a severe hemiplegia may still remain ambulant with the use of a walking aid. The normal functioning half of the body permits adjustment of the gait to protect the foot by leaning away from the side of the lesion and raising the heel as the palsied leg is brought forward. In contrast, the presence of a bilateral pyramidal lesion considerably decreases the chances of remaining mobile. The effort of dragging each leg forward is greater due to the impairment or absence of any compensatory action by the opposite leg. Bony and ligamentous stresses in the feet and trauma to the skin are increased compared with those in the hemiplegic foot.

The term paraplegia does not specify any particular type of pathological process. Broadly, there are two types of diseases which can cause paraplegia: those which damage the spinal cord by compressing it, and those which affect the nerve cells and connections of the cord itself. It is very important to distinguish the two since the treatment of the two different types is quite different. Operations to relieve cord compression can be curative. Accurate diagnosis of the cause of paraplegia is absolutely essential. Furthermore, even if investigation does not show evidence of cord compression, there are several treatable conditions which must be looked for.

Compression of the spinal cord

Cervical spondylosis

In late middle and old age, degenerative changes in the cervical intervertebral discs and the adjacent vertebrae (*cervical spondylosis*) gradually compress the spinal cord, causing paraparesis or paraplegia. In this older age group, cervical spondylosis is the commonest cause of paraparesis. Some degree of cervical spondylosis occurs in 90% of the population over the age of 65 years but only a small proportion develop compression of the spinal cord. While sensory loss is not uncommon, the major deficit in the lower limbs is a combination of spasticity and weakness, producing a stiff-legged gait. Lateral compression of the cervical motor and sensory nerve roots as they emerge through the intervertebral foramina is frequently associated and causes pain in the arms, paraesthesia (tingling) in the fingers and wasting of the small muscles of the hands.

Plain X-rays of the cervical spine and contrast radiology with radio-opaque dye, to outline the spinal cord and internal contours of the spinal canal (*myelography*), are required to establish the diagnosis. Commonly, the first line of treatment is a plastic cervical collar to restrain neck movement but, in those patients with a moderate to severe progressive paraplegia, surgery is often necessary to relieve the compression.

Tumours

Compression of the spinal cord by a tumour is usually due to secondary spread of a cancer from another site in the body to either the meninges or vertebral bodies via the bloodstream. Primary tumours of the lung, breast and prostate gland (in men) are the commonest to spread in this way. The resulting paraplegia is often rapidly progressive and accompanied by considerable pain. Primary tumours of the spinal cord, spinal nerve roots or meninges (glioma, neurofibroma or meningioma) are much less common. Myelography is necessary to outline the site of spinal cord compression prior to surgery but the prognosis is usually poor except after removal of a benign tumour, such as a neurofibroma or meningioma.

Tuberculosis

In underdeveloped parts of the world, tuberculosis of the bony spine is the commonest cause of spinal cord compression. Bony weakness may result in severe spinal deformity (*kyphosis*). Treatment involves bed rest, immobilisation of the spine in a plaster jacket and antituberculous drugs. Surgery is best avoided if at all possible.

Non-compressive cord diseases

Multiple sclerosis

Excluding trauma, multiple—or disseminated—sclerosis (the terms are synonymous) is the commonest cause of paraplegia presenting in the third, fourth and fifth decades of life. It is more common in women. By definition, the term multiple or disseminated indicates the patients have evidence of neurological symptoms and signs which result from disease affecting several parts of the central nervous system. The part that may be affected and their related manifestations are as follows: optic nerves (causing temporary or permanent loss of vision in one eye); brain stem (causing double vision, loss of facial sensation, facial weakness, slurred speech and difficult swallowing); cerebellum (resulting in unsteady gait and uncoordinated limb movements) and spinal cord (causing paraplegia, poor control of micturition and sensory loss in the limbs). Usually the symptoms are acute in onset, occur at different times and are followed by a partial or complete remission. Some patients, typically middle-aged, present only with a progressive paraplegia and here the diagnosis has to be made by a process of exclusion of other disorders such as spinal cord compression. The term sclerosis is an unfortunate label for the condition since it fails to emphasise that the prime disturbance is one of demyelination of axons, which is followed by inflammation and finally scar tissue or sclerosis.

The cause of multiple sclerosis remains unclear and currently three theories hold strong support. One suggests an abnormal response of the nervous system to a viral infection. To support this view, high antibody titres to measles virus are found in some patients with multiple sclerosis, and epidemiological studies show areas of high incidence of the disease in temperate zones and a possible parallel between multiple sclerosis and other central nervous system disorders which are well established as being due to a virus infection. The second is that an autoimmune response results in the abnormal production of antibodies which selectively destroy the myelin sheath of nerve fibres. The third theory suggests that some people inherit a susceptibility to develop the condition. Certain genetic markers (HLA types) are found more commonly in patients with MS than in the general population. Studies of twins are also compatible with the theory that genetic factors may increase the risk of developing the disease, though genetic factors probably interact with other, perhaps environmental, factors.

There is no specific test available which reliably confirms the clinical diagnosis so the diagnosis must be made on the basis of a history of a relapsing and remitting disorder with evidence of lesions in different parts of the central nervous system at different times. New investigative techniques, such as magnetic resonance imaging, may provide dramatic evidence of disseminated lesions, but are unfortunately not necessarily diagnostic of MS.

Treatment is empirical and mainly supportive with courses of steroids being used for the acute relapse. Steroids speed recovery by reducing the inflammatory response but unfortunately they do not reduce long-term disability. Immunosuppressive drugs (such as azathioprine) may reduce the risk of relapse, but treatment does carry a significant risk of side effects. Where power is well preserved in the legs, stiffness (spasticity) can be relieved by drugs which act on spinal cord reflexes. Despite these gloomy inferences, however, it is important to maintain a balanced perspective of multiple sclerosis since over half the patients manage to lead a full life with either no persisting symptoms or only a moderate disability. Life expectancy is not significantly reduced.

Vitamin B₁₂ deficiency

This is usually associated with pernicious anaemia and caused by deficient absorption from the small bowel. Vitamin B_{12} is important for neurone metabolism and, almost invariably, deficiency results in both spinal cord and peripheral nerve degeneration, hence the term *subacute combined degeneration of the spinal cord.* There is a characteristic combination of proximal weakness at the hip and knee due to the pyramidal deficit, with a distal lower motor neurone weakness and absent ankle jerks caused by the neuropathy. Prompt recognition of the condition is important to enable treatment with intramuscular vitamin B_{12} to proceed as soon as possible. With early diagnosis, the prognosis is good but increasing delay leads to permanent spinal cord and peripheral nerve damage. The basic failure to absorb vitamin B_{12} cannot usually be rectified and monthly intramuscular replacement therapy is needed for the reminder of the patient's life.

Infections

Certain infections agents, both bacterial and viral, can damage the spinal cord. The bacterial infections must be recognised since they require specific treatment with antibiotics, so, when clinically indicated, a series of tests for syphilis, *Borrelia Burgdorferi* and other rarer infections must be performed. Several viruses, including the human immunodeficiency virus (HIV), which is responsible for the acquired immunodeficiency syndrome (AIDS), can attack the spinal cord. In tropical countries, a closely related virus (HTLV–1) causes a clinical syndrome known as tropical spastic paraparesis. The herpes zoster virus, which causes shingles, sometimes affects the spinal cord. Specific treatments for these different virus infections are now becoming available. In many parts of the world, polio virus, rare in the UK, is still a common cause of spinal cord damage (see below).

Poliomyelitis

As a result of the introduction of vaccination, the last major epidemic of poliomyelitis in this country was over 20 years ago and only very isolated cases are now seen. The disorder is caused by an enterovirus which spreads from the bowel to invade the nervous system, particularly the anterior horn cells of the spinal cord. It is acute in onset and associated with fever, headache, meningism (neck stiffness) and photophobia. Within several days of the onset of these prodromal symptoms, asymmetrical weakness, hypotonia and loss of reflexes occur in groups of muscles in either the upper or lower limbs or the thoracic cage. Assisted ventilation may be required. In the lower limbs involvement of the muscles of the leg and foot causes weakness of eversion, inversion and plantarflexion of the ankle and also foot drop. Recovery is often incomplete and associated with contracture (shortening and fibrosis) of muscles causing an equino-varus deformity, pes cavus or permanent foot drop. This may require surgical correction but it will certainly demand considerable attention by the podiatrist due to the abnormal load bearing of the foot and the need for special appliances and shoes.

Other non-compressive causes

Motor neurone disease is a rapidly progressive disorder involving degeneration of both upper and lower motor neurones. Patients can present with any possible combination of weakness, wasting and spasticity affecting the bulbar muscles (larynx, pharynx, tongue and face) and the limbs; but typically the weakness in the arms and hands is mainly of a lower motor neurone type, whereas in the legs pyramidal features predominate. The disease usually leads to death within a few years due to difficulty in swallowing and respiratory failure. The cause is unknown and no treatment is available, though much supportive care can and should be devoted to these patients.

Syringomyelia is a rare cause of paraplegia which typically occurs in the third and fourth decades of life. The cervical spinal cord becomes cavitated due to enlargement of the central canal and this causes damage to the crossing spinothalamic pathways, the anterior horn cells and lateral pyramidal pathways. The resulting clinical features are a loss of pain and temperature awareness in the upper limbs, wasting of the hands and a spastic paraplegia. In 80 to 90% of patients, syringomyelia is associated with a congenital abnormality at the junction of the cervical spinal cord and brainstem which prevents the normal flow of cerebrospinal fluid from the brain and central canal of the spinal cord (Chiari malformation). Surgical correction of this often prevents the disorder progressing and allows some recovery of function.

Spina bifida

Failure of complete development of the spinal canal is most commonly asymptomatic and associated with lack of fusion of the posterior arches of the lower lumbar vertebrae which can only be detected radiologically (spina bifida occulta). It may, however, be associated with a spinal cord abnormality such as a dermoid cyst or lipoma, causing compression of the lumbosacral nerve roots with weakness of the leg and intrinsic foot muscles, absent ankle reflexes and pes cavus. Myelography is required to visualise such an abnormality prior to surgery.

THE PERIPHERAL NERVES

Damage to or degeneration of peripheral nerves supplying the lower limbs most commonly presents as a mixed sensory and motor peripheral neuropathy, but in some disorders the motor or sensory neurones can be affected in isolation (e.g. peroneal muscular atrophy, tabes dorsalis). The diseases which affect peripheral nerves fall into two broad categories: those which diffusely affect all the peripheral nerves, which are called *peripheral neuropathies*, and those affecting a single nerve, which are called *mononeuropathies*.

Peripheral neuropathies

Symptoms and signs

The presenting features are a combination of muscular weakness and sensory loss. Since in the majority of cases the longest nerves are the earliest to be affected and eventually the most severely damaged, weakness is mainly confined to the intrinsic hand and foot muscles, the anterior tibial, peroneal and calf muscles and the forearm flexors and extensors of the fingers and wrist joints. In contrast to a pyramidal lesion, muscle wasting is prominent and associated with fasciculation (spontaneous contraction of groups of muscle fibres) and hypotonia. The ankle reflexes are lost, the knee reflexes may be reduced and the plantar responses are normal or non-reacting. All or some of the modalities of sensation (light touch, pain, temperature and proprioception) are lost over the hands, feet and distal part of the legs and forearms in a glove and stocking distribution. As a result of denervation, the skin becomes atrophic, the articular ligaments weakened and there is often interstitial oedema of the feet.

Weakness and hypotonia in the leg and intrinsic foot muscles cause distortion of the normal architecture of the foot with reduction of the longitudinal and transverse arches and undue stress on the interosseous ligaments. The ankle joints are unstable and there is a tendency to develop excessive inversion and eversion when walking over uneven ground. Weakness of the main extensor muscle of the ankle joint (tibialis anterior and extensor digitorum longus) causes foot drop with a characteristic high stepping, slapping gait. Inevitably, the anterior border of each foot catches against minor obstacles causing repeated trauma directly to the feet and indirectly to the inadequately supported ankle joints.

These motor deficiencies are compounded by the sensory disturbance. The loss of proprioception causes an unsteady (ataxic) gait. Repeated and excessive trauma to the feet go unheeded because of the lack of pain awareness and burning and scalding may also occur due to the absence of temperature sensation. The skin over the feet becomes ulcerated, joint spaces are damaged and, particularly at the ankle, tarsometatarsal and metatarsophalangeal joints, overgrowth of bone around the joint produces gross deformity and crepitus (Charcot joint).

There are many possible causes of a mixed sensory and motor neuropathy. These include endocrine and metabolic disorders (e.g. diabetes mellitus, renal failure and myxoedema), toxic factors (e.g. industrial solvents, glue sniffing), drugs (e.g. anti-tuberculosis therapy), deficiency states (e.g. pernicious anaemia, thiamine deficiency) and the non-invasive effects of cancer. In practice none of these factors can be demonstrated in approximately half of patients investigated, and by a process of exclusion the neuropathy is labelled as a primary degenerative condition of unknown cause (idiopathic), for which there is no direct form of treatment. In the remaining patients the most commonly demonstrated causes are diabetes mellitus, alcoholism, drugs, cancer and pernicious anaemia.

Metabolic causes

The neuropathic manifestations of *diabetes mellitus* can occur as an early complication of the disorder or present many years after diagnosis. The disorder of glucose metabolism is probably the main factor producing nerve degeneration, with ischaemia due to associated arterial degeneration as a contributory factor. Rigorous control of the blood sugar with diet, oral hypoglycaemic drugs and insulin may offer some protection. Many years of careful management may still be followed by the appearance of neuropathy. Apart from the motor and sensory manifestations previously described, pain is also a common feature. It is typically severe at night and presents as a burning sensation over the feet, aching discomfort in the calves or sometimes a transient shooting pain throughout the legs. Before sensation is completely lost, the skin becomes very sensitive to light touch which produces an intensely unpleasant feeling (*dysaesthesia*) to the extent that patients are terrified of any form of contact with their feet and legs and go to great lengths to protect them. The neuropathic complications of the feet, such as skin atrophy and ulceration and joint degeneration, are aggravated in diabetic patients by the associated arterial disease. The part played by the podiatrist is vital if amputation is to be postponed or avoided.

Toxic causes

Excess *alcohol* probably has a direct toxic effect upon peripheral nerves but the main cause of the associated neuropathy is a dietary deficiency of thiamine (vitamin B_1). This results from appetite suppression due to the high liquid intake and the limited financial resources for nutritious types of food due to overspending on alcohol. Alcohol and diabetes mellitus are the two commonest causes of a painful neuropathy and the patient often complains that his feet seem to be on fire or that he is walking over broken glass. These symptoms compel the alcoholic to seek medical help. Prompt treatment with large doses of vitamin supplements, and adequate diet and abstinence from alcohol bring relief and a good prognosis but unfortunately memory impairment is not uncommonly associated with the neuropathy and as the agony of the condition fades, the tendency for the alcoholic to relapse increases.

Many *drugs* may cause a peripheral neuropathy but the major offenders are isoniazid, which is used for the treatment of tuberculosis, the antimetabolites vincristine and vinblastine, required for the chemotherapy of leukaemia, and the urinary antibiotic nitrofurantoin. Diagnosis demands a continual awareness of the complications with these and other drugs and, where possible, other forms of therapy should be substituted as soon as neuropathic features appear. Usually these are reversible if recognised early and if the drug is stopped.

Cancer of the bronchus, breast and gastrointestinal tract may be complicated by a peripheral neuropathy presenting at the same time or after the diagnosis of malignancy has been made, or even several years before its clinical recognition. The mechanism is unclear but it is probably due to toxic metabolites or antibodies to peripheral nerve tissue produced by the tumour. Unfortunately, the condition often persists or progresses despite removal of the primary lesion.

Pernicious anaemia is due to deficient absorption of vitamin B_{12} from the small intestine. It is usually caused by an acquired loss of secretion by the stomach of 'intrinsic factor', which links to vitamin B_{12} and facilitates its absorption in the terminal part of the small intestine. Less commonly the loss of absorption is due to primary disease of the small intestine (e.g. Crohn's disease). Vitamin B$_{12}$ deficiency causes anaemia and degeneration of the peripheral nervous system and spinal cord (q.v.). The first symptom of the neuropathy is paraesthesia in the feet and hands followed by distal muscle weakness and wasting in the upper and lower limbs. The disability is compounded by the degeneration of the corticospinal tracts and posterior columns in the spinal cord, producing a spastic paraparesis and ataxia.

Infections

Leprosy

Leprosy is a chronic infectious granulomatous disease affecting superficial tissues, especially the skin, the nasal mucosa and the peripheral nerves. It is caused by *Mycobacterium leprae*.

Epidemiology

The number of people with leprosy in the world is unknown, but was estimated by the World Health Organisation in 1977 to exceed 12 million, almost all of whom live in the tropics or subtropics.

The condition was endemic in Britain and Western Europe in the Middle Ages, but with improved standards of living and freely available medical facilities, the disease is now only seen in immigrants or those who have lived in the tropics for long periods.

Transmission occurs primarily from lepromatous leprosy patients, who excrete millions of bacilli per day from the upper respiratory tract. The portal of entry is unknown, but is likely to be the nasal mucosa or skin. Prolonged exposure is required and the incubation period is 3 to 5 years. Other methods of transmission have been postulated, including insect carriers, sexual intercourse and via breast milk.

Classification

The classification of leprosy is based on clinical findings, histopathological features and the Lepromin test.

The classification consists of a spectrum, with lepromatous leprosy at one end and tuberculoid leprosy at the other. Borderline leprosy is a combination of the two polar types and may shift to either end of the scale.

In tuberculoid leprosy there is a single hypo-pigmented anaesthetic skin lesion and extensive nerve involvement. As one moves towards the lepromatous end of the scale, the skin lesions become more numerous and fleshy and the skin becomes diffusely thickened. Nerve damage is less prominent. Other tissues are often involved in lepromatous leprosy, particularly the nasal mucosa, the testes, the eye and the lymph nodes. The Lepromin test is strongly positive in tuberculoid leprosy and negative in lepromatous leprosy.

Lepromatous leprosy occurs when the cellular immune response is poor, and tuberculous leprosy when the response is stronger.

The three major problems associated with the feet are: 1. anaesthesia, 2. deformities and 3. ulceration.

Anaesthesia

Loss of sensation, particularly loss of the appreciation of pain and/or temperature, is potentially hazardous to the tissues of the foot. Minor injuries or cuts to the skin may go unnoticed and repeated damage to ligaments may weaken joints without causing symptoms. The damage to joints may become so severe as to disrupt completely the joint and its surrounding structures; this is known as a Charcot's joint.

Deformities

These results from various causes:

1. *Nerve damage* results in foot drop with inability to evert the foot at the subtalar joint or to dorsiflex the foot at the ankle.

2. *Trauma* is common and traumatic lesions heal slowly because of poor blood supply due to endarteritis.

3. *Bone changes* commonly occur and affect primarily the distal phalanges and the metatarsals. The phalanges become rarified, living a thin needle of bone and in advanced cases the bone

totally disappears with subsequent shortening of the digits. The metatarsals become pointed at the distal end, a condition affecting mainly the fifth metatarsals.

The causes of *bone loss* include repeated trauma, disuse, osteoporosis, endarteritis, leprous osteitis with cystic formation and pathological fractures, secondary osteomyelitis and androgen deficiency in male patients with lepromatous leprosy.

Ulceration

Three types of ulcer occur on the foot and lower leg in leprosy, namely 1. *stasis ulcers*, 2. *lepromatous ulcers* and 3. *plantar ulcers*.

Stasis ulcers. These occur on the ankle and the dorsum of the foot and are due to chronic lymph stasis, fibrosis, ischaemia and secondary infection.

The differential diagnosis includes varicose ulcers, ulcers due to peripheral vascular disease and other causes of vascular insufficiency, such as sickle cell anaemia, Raynaud's phenomenon and macroglobulinaemia.

Treatment is often difficult and prolonged, requiring immobilisation in a posterior plaster cast, daily dressings and parenteral antimicrobial therapy with an appropriate antibiotic. Occasionally excision and skin grafting may be required.

Lepromatous ulcers. Patients with advanced lepromatous leprosy, where much of the skin surface is infiltrated with papular lesions, are prone to the development of lepromatous ulcers. The lesions have a predilection for the extremities, but tend to avoid palms and soles. Numerous papules occur on the end of the foot and these break down because of repeated trauma, to form ulcers.

Treating the leprosy with systemic therapy resolves the lesions within a few weeks. Local treatment consists of keeping the feet clean and preventing further trauma.

Plantar ulcers. These occur on the weight-bearing area of the anaesthetic sole and are the commonest and most serious foot ulcers occurring in leprosy.

Pathogenesis. Muscle paralysis and foot deformities, e.g. foot drop and claw toes, lead to a loss of the subcutaneous tissue which normally acts as a protective cushion. Walking leads to repeated trauma to the metatarsal heads and toe ends. The skin eventually blisters and breaks down into ulcers. External trauma occurs particularly in areas where people walk barefoot and are thus prone to penetrating injuries from stones, thorns or glass. Anaesthesia of the foot means that damage may go unnoticed by the patient. Poor blood supply leads to delayed healing which may in turn predispose to secondary infection or absence of sweating and the skin becomes dry, brittle and cracked, resulting in further damage. Callus formation is common in leprous feet and the callosities frequently blister and ulcerate. They may also become secondarily infected, thus perpetuating a vicious cycle of trauma, callus formation, ulceration and infection.

Sites of occurrence. Plantar ulcers may arise under the first metatarsal head, under the head of the proximal phalanx of the big toe, under the second and lateral metatarsal heads, and, less commonly, ulcers may occur on the heel, the tips of the toes and on the plantar surface of the midfoot.

Differential diagnosis. Trophic, perforating plantar ulcers are seen in various nonlepromatous conditions, such as diabetic neuropathy, spina bifida, and hereditary sensory neuropathy. However, in the majority of cases leprosy is readily diagnosed and differentiated from these conditions.

Types of plantar ulcer. There are simple and complicated ulcers, which can be either acute or chronic. An *acute* ulcer is newly formed with little or no fibrous tissue. It may become *chronic* when neglected as when infected with an organism of low virulence. These ulcers are lined with fibrous tissue and have heaped up edges. *Simple* ulcers are either acute or chronic and are confined to the subcutaneous tissue. A *complicated* ulcer has penetrated the underlying bone or tendon sheath with subsequent osteomyelitis or tenosynovitis.

Treatment of plantar ulcers. When treating a patient with an *uncomplicated ulcer*—*acute* or *chronic*—the general principles for treating a neuropathic ulcer apply:

a. Clean the area.

b. Remove any slough, obvious dead tissue and any foreign bodies, and ensure drainage of pus. This will require careful surgery.

c. Infection should be vigorously treated with an appropriate antibiotic. Topical application is contraindicated.

d. Immobilisation. Once infection, dermatitis and discharge have been controlled, the leg should be immobilised with a below-knee plaster with a walking wood with rocker. This prevents contamination, keeps the patient mobile, and distributes the weight over the entire foot. It has the disadvantage of hiding any infection or other problems. Meticulous care must be taken during application of a plaster cast. It should be remembered that the patient will not complain of any discomfort in the anaesthetic foot.

For *complicated ulcers*, the general principles applied to uncomplicated ulcers must be adhered to. Additional measures may be necessary including more radical surgery. Metatarsectomy, metatarsophalangeal joint excision and sequestrectomy are indicated where there is bone or joint infection, or a separated sequestrum. It is important to preserve as much of the weight-bearing area as possible. Total destruction of the ankle joint or the subtalar region is the only absolute indication for amputation. The amputation should leave a stump for which a prosthesis is available and should aim to preserve as much of the foot as possible.

Prevention of plantar ulcers. Most complicated ulcers heal adequately with the appropriate therapy, but keeping the foot ulcer free is far more difficult. Shoes should be worn constantly, preferably with socks. The outer layer must be impervious to stones and thorns and the insole should be made of microcellular rubber. The patients must be taught to examine their own feet daily looking for blisters, haematomas, fissures and hyperkeratotic lesions. These should be treated in the normal way. Blisters, fissures and subcuticular haematomas require the foot to be rested. Patients should avoid walking long distances.

Leprosy chemotherapy

The drug of choice for treating leprosy is a sulphone drug called dapsone (DDS 4, 4-diaminodiphenyl sulphone). It is given in a dose of 50 to 100 mg per day. In tuberculoid leprosy, treatment is for 3 to 5 years and in lepromatous leprosy, it is for life. Other useful drugs are rifampicin, clofazamine, ethionamide and thiacetazone.

Summary

Leprosy, now uncommon in the developed world, is still one of the major causes of morbidity in the tropics and subtropics. Foot deformities, anaesthesia and ulceration are all common forms of disability and may be seen in immigrants. Plantar ulceration, in particular, is one of the most serious complications of leprosy. It results not only in severe crippling, but is one of the major causes of ostracism from the community.

With improved living conditions and modern chemotherapy, leprosy is a preventable and curable condition.

Tabes dorsalis (neurosyphilis)

Tabes dorsalis is an example of the chronic effect of syphilis upon the nervous system (tertiary syphilis) occurring 15 years or more after an untreated or inadequately treated acute venereal infection. Degeneration of posterior root sensory ganglia causes spontaneous shooting pains in the lower limbs. Pain sensation over the feet is lost, resulting in unnoticed trauma, burning and scalding and eventually skin ulceration and Charcot joints. Absence of proprioception causes an ataxic gait. Usually there is no associated motor weakness but the degeneration of sensory neurones interrupts the spinal reflex arc causing hypotonia and loss of ankle reflexes. Often other manifestations of tertiary syphilis, such as general paresis of the insane, may combine with tabes causing intellectual impairment and extensor plantar responses.

With the introduction of penicillin for the treatment of venereal disease the tertiary manifestations of syphilis are less commonly seen. When tabes is diagnosed it usually means that irreversible sensory nerve damage has occurred although treatment at this late stage with penicillin may reduce or abolish the shooting pains.

Post-infectious polyneuritis (Guillain-Barre syndrome)

This is a rapidly progressive but self-limiting disease of the peripheral nervous system which can occur at any age. The pathological changes occur predominantly in the proximal parts of the nerves adjacent to the spinal cord and consist of acute inflammation and demyelination, which is usually associated with a marked rise in the cerebrospinal fluid protein concentration. The disorder seems to be due to an autoimmune phenomenon with the body producing antibodies to peripheral nerve tissue, and is usually triggered by a viral or bacterial infection.

The symptoms are mainly motor and typically occur in an ascending fashion, starting with weakness of the legs followed by involvement of the muscles of the thighs, spine, arms and forearms and even of the facial and bulbar muscles. Symptoms develop over several days to several weeks and examination usually confirms fairly severe weakness of a lower motor neurone type with generalised areflexia. There may be sensory loss ranging from a peripheral glove and stocking deficit to more severe involvement extending proximally on to the body.

The main objective of management is one of supportive physiotherapy until spontaneous recovery occurs, usually within 3–6 months. Severe motor weakness may cause respiratory embarrassment and require a period of assisted ventilation. Severe cases should be treated with plasmapheresis, a technique which extracts the plasma (the cell-free part of the blood containing proteins, including the antibodies thought to be responsible for the illness) and replaces it with antibody-free albumin.

Inherited diseases

One of the commonest inherited neuropathies is peroneal muscular atrophy (Charcot-Marie Tooth disease, Fig. 23.1). The term *muscular atrophy* is an unfortunate one since it suggests a primary muscle disorder for what is in fact an inherited degenerative neuropathy. Inheritance is often dominant but it can be recessive.

The symptoms and signs are predominantly motor and typically just affect the lower limbs and present in the second and third decades of life. Patients may complain of either unsteadiness of walking due to marked instability of the ankle joints or of foot drop, a tendency to trip easily and a slapping gait. Because of the family history, they are often reluctant to seek medical advice.

Neuropathic wasting is usually marked and affects the intrinsic foot muscles, anterior tibial, peroneal and calf musculature. Typically, the muscle wasting starts in the distal third of the leg muscles producing an inverted 'Indian club' appearance. Sometimes it extends more proximally above the knees, and there may be associated wasting of the intrinsic muscles of the hands. The longitudinal arches of the feet are commonly exaggerated (pes cavus) and the ankle reflexes are absent. Sensory loss is rarely marked and when present is localised to a short stocking distribution. Occasionally the disorder is severe, more generalised and associated with thickening and hypertrophy of peripheral nerves (Déjerin-Sottas type).

Typically, peroneal muscular atrophy produces

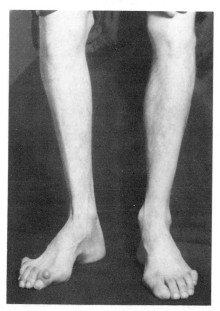

Fig. 23.1   Charcot-Marie-Tooth disease: typical cavus deformity of feet.

only a slight or moderate disability in early or middle age but its slow progression may result in a more severe disability in later life. There is no treatment for the condition but polypropylene foot splints can greatly improve walking by reducing the degree of foot drop. The patient should also receive genetic counselling.

Mononeuropathies

Lateral popliteal nerve palsy

Unlike a symmetrical and generalised peripheral neuropathy, damage to the lateral popliteal nerve, either in the popliteal fossa or as it winds around the head of the fibula, is usually acute in onset and associated with spontaneous partial or complete recovery. It can occur without any precipitating factor and as such is probably due to impairment of the blood supply to the nerve but it may also result from compression (from fractures, badly fashioned plaster casts, excessive kneeling and a variety of other mechanisms). Muscle weakness is limited to the anterior tibial and peroneal muscles with preservation of the ankle reflex. Any sensory disturbances is often slight and localised to the dorsum of the foot opposite the first and second toes.

The effect of such a lesion upon the foot is naturally less than with a more generalised neuropathy. The main problem relates to the fairly severe foot drop and a polypropylene splint is often needed until recovery occurs.

THE EXTRAPYRAMIDAL SYSTEM

In evolutionary terms, the extrapyramidal system is a much older collection of nuclei, known as the *basal ganglia*, which provides the foundation for movement and permits the expression of pyramidal activity. Diseases of this older system fall into two categories, the first characterised by poverty of movement and known as parkinsonism and the second by an excess of involuntary activity termed chorea.

Parkinsonism

Parkinsonism was first described in 1817 by James Parkinson but one hundred years passed before it was recognised as being due to degeneration of one part of the basal ganglia, the *substantia nigra*, and another forty years before it was realised that depletion of the neurotransmitter dopamine was the main consequence of this degeneration. This has led to the most important advancement in the treatment of this condition, namely the administration of L-dopa, the precursor of dopamine. Degeneration of the substantia nigra may be primary or secondary to arteriosclerosis or encephalitis, particularly the type known as sleeping sickness which was prevalent in Europe after the first World War.

The clinical features of parkinsonism can be divided into three types. The most disabling is the lack of spontaneous movement known as *hypokinesia*, reflected in the still, expressionless face, loss of fine movements of the hands causing difficulty in writing, dressing and eating and the monotonous quiet voice. The posture becomes stooped and the patient leans forward and walks with small shuffling steps, the feet hardly lifting from the ground. The anterior displacement of the centre of gravity causes most of the body weight to be transferred to the anterior part of the foot in the region of the metatarsophalangeal joints. The impoverishment of movement is accompanied by increased muscle tone and a coarse tremor affecting one or both hands and sometimes the legs. Muscular pain and cramps are not uncommon. Painful dystonic flexion movements of the foot are an unusual feature, but are distressing to the patient and difficult to treat.

The diagnosis is based solely upon the clinical findings. Treatment with L-dopa commonly results in improvement which can sometimes be striking and result in virtual complete disappearance of all restriction of movement. Surgical treatment of tremor is now rarely required.

Chorea

Chorea is the complete opposite of parkinsonism and is associated with involuntary uncontrolled jerking movements of the face, head, shoulders, arms and legs. The patient has the appearance of extreme fidgetiness and an inability to keep still which, to the observer, can be both disturbing and infective. The term chorea relates to the gait which is like a dance, the interjected involuntary movements of the legs causing a combination of halting and lurching steps. In childhood, chorea is usually associated with rheumatic fever (*Sydenham's chorea*) and is typically self-limiting.

In adult life, chorea can be part of a dominantly inherited progressive degenerative disorder of the brain known as *Huntington's chorea*, which is associated with the development of severe dementia. Genetic counselling and antenatal diagnosis can be offered, with abortion of affected foetuses where appropriate.

FURTHER READING

Jopling W H 1984 Handbook of leprosy, 3rd edn. Heinemann, London

Matthews W B, Miller H 1982 Diseases of the nervous system, 4th edn. Blackwell, Oxford

Ross Russell R W, Wiles C M 1985 Neurology. Heinemann, London

Walton J N 1984 Brain's diseases of the nervous system, 9th edn. Oxford University Press, Oxford

Orientation and terminology

1. The cardinal body planes

The anatomical relationships of parts of the body to each other, and also their movements and positions, are denoted in terms which relate them to the three cardinal body planes which correspond to the three dimensions of space. These arc the *sagittal*, *frontal*, and *transverse* planes, which intersect at the centre of gravity of the body, located at the level of the pelvis. Planes parallel to these cardinal planes are then imagined at any desired point in order to aid descriptions of movements or positions (Fig. A1-1).

A *sagittal plane* is an anteroposterior vertical

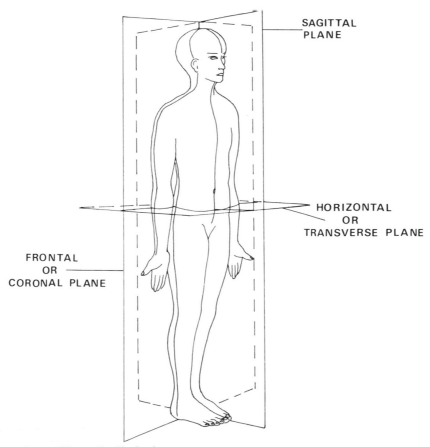

Fig. A1-1   The cardinal body planes.

plane which divides the body into right and left sections and divides the foot into medial and lateral sections. Movement of the foot (or toes) in this plane hinges on a horizontal axis either upwards or downwards from the horizontal (or transverse) plane, i.e. dorsiflexion or plantarflexion of the foot at the ankle joint, and extension or flexion of the toes at the metatarsophalangeal joints.

A *transverse (or horizontal) plane* is a plane parallel to the horizon (or floor) which divides the body into upper (superior) or lower (inferior) sections, and divides the foot into upper (dorsal) and lower (plantar) sections. Movement of the foot (or part) in this plane turns on a vertical axis either towards (adduction) or away from (abduction) the midline of the body, the cardinal sagittal plane.

An exception to this general rule applies to the muscles and movements of the toes, which are related to the sagittal plane bisecting the second metatarsal segment. This makes no difference to the terminology applicable to the muscles and movements of the three lateral toes. In the case of the hallux, however, 'abduction' denotes movement away from the second metatarsal line and towards the midline of the body, and 'adduction' denotes the opposite movement. The corresponding muscles are denominated as 'abductor hallucis' and 'adductor hallucis' respectively.

A *frontal (or coronal) plane* is a side-to-side vertical plane which divides the body into front (anterior) and back (posterior) sections, and divides the foot into hindfoot (proximal) and forefoot (distal) sections. Movement of the foot (or part) in this plane turns on a longitudinal axis and is either towards (inversion) or away from (eversion) the midline of the body.

2. Joint movements

Movements in a joint are determined by its intrinsic structure, which may permit motion in one, two or three planes. Such motion is depicted as occurring around axes perpendicular to the plane of motion. The knee and the ankle are hinge-like joints, allowing movement only in the sagittal plane and around a single axis for each joint (Fig. Al-2). The first metatarsophalangeal

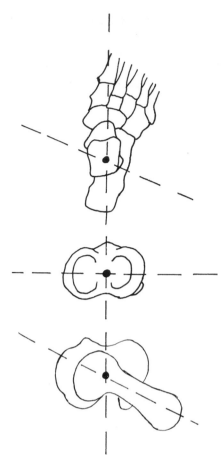

Fig. A1-2 Frontal plane axes of hip, knee and ankle joints. With the knee axis aligned on the frontal plane as shown, the head and neck of the femur are externally rotated on the shaft to a variable extent (the angle of anteversion). The ankle axis is also externally rotated because of the normal torsion in the lower end of the tibial shaft. This also varies in extent individually, and at different ages in the same subject.

joint moves in both the sagittal and transverse planes around two axes, while the hip, being a ball-and-socket joint, allows movement in all three planes around three axes. The peritalar joints (ankle, subtalar and midtarsal) also provide collectively for movements in all three planes.

Joint movements may thus be *simple* (motion in one plane) or *complex* (motion in two or three planes simultaneously).

Simple movements in each of the three planes result in *positions*, which are denoted in the following summary in both traditional and biomechanical terminology (Table Al-1). *Fixation* of any such position which prevents the foot (or part) from assuming a normal attitude indicates a structural abnormality.

Complex movements of the foot or its parts occur on all three planes simultaneously and are denoted by the terms *supination* and *pronation*.

Supination denotes a compound movement of

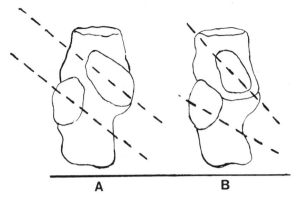

Fig. A1-4   The articular facets of the talonavicular and calcaneocuboid components of the midtarsal joint. In eversion (A), they are more congruent with each other, thereby facilitating flexibility for shock-absorption. In inversion (B), they are less congruent, thus 'locking' the joint and imparting rigidity to the foot for leverage purposes.

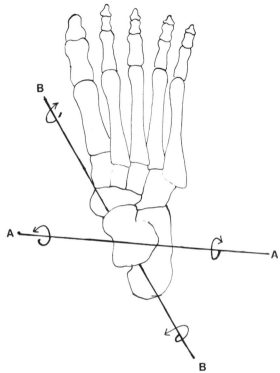

Fig. A1-3(i)   The axes of the ankle (AA) and the subtalar joint (BB) (dorsal view).

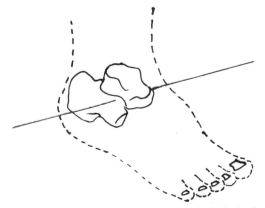

Fig. A1-3(ii)   The subtalar joint axis round which the foot pronates and supinates. Normally angled at 42° from the transverse plane and 16° from the sagittal plane, but individually variable.

inversion, adduction and plantarflexion of the foot or parts of the foot taking place at the peritalar joints (the ankle, subtalar and midtarsal joints). Pronation denotes a compound movement of eversion, abduction and dorsiflexion of the foot or parts of the foot taking place at the peritalar joints. Both of these movements turn on an oblique axis which passes through the foot from the posterior, lateral and plantar aspect to the anterior, medial and dorsal aspect of the tarsus (Figs A1-3(i) & (ii)).

The midtarsal joint, being compounded of the talonavicular and the calcaneocuboid joints, is regarded as having two resultant axes, providing for reciprocal longitudinal torsion of the forefoot on the hindfoot in order to maintain the metatarsus in a correct relationship to the ground as the hindfoot supinates/pronates in locomotion. The position of the subtalar joint dictates the range of movement in the midtarsal joint. In eversion, the axes of the separate components become parallel, thereby facilitating movement and hence flexibility in the foot for shock absorption. In inversion, the separate axes diverge, thus restricting movement and inducing greater rigidity in the foot for purposes of leverage (Fig. Al-4)

The five metatarsal segments (or rays) distal to the midtarsal joint provide dorsoplantar movement for the metatarsal heads, enabling them to adjust to the surface as required by motions

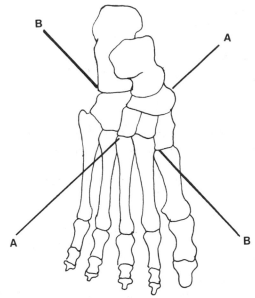

Fig. A1-5   The axes of the first (AA) and fifth (BB) metatarsal segments (dorsal view).

within the foot or by varying and irregular terrain. The three medial segments are comprised of both cuneiforms and metatarsals, the lateral two of metatarsals only. While each is capable of some independent movement, their function of adapting to the ground surface is essentially a collective one. The first and fifth have the greatest range of movement about their respective oblique axes (Fig. A1-5), including some capacity for inversion and eversion.

3. Terminology

Traditionally, the terms *valgus* and *varus* have been applied to fixed positions of the lower limb and its parts in relation to *both* the vertical and horizontal dimensions of the cardinal sagittal plane, i.e. to deviations in *both* the frontal and transverse planes. Hence the terms coxa valga and vara, genu valgum and varum, talipes equinovarus and calcaneovalgus, pes valgus, hallux valgus, metatarsus varus and digiti quinti varus have all denoted variations from the normal towards (varus) or away from (valgus) the cardinal sagittal plane.

Current biomechanical usage departs from the traditional in confining *varus* and *valgus* to positional deviations of the foot or its parts in the frontal plane only. Thus hindfoot valgus and hindfoot varus denote positions of eversion and inversion of the hindfoot respectively, and similarly for the forefoot. Hence also metatarsus adductus and hallux abductus in preference to metatarsus varus and hallux valgus. When applied to the toes, these terms denote axial rotations, varus in an inverted direction and valgus in an everted direction, corresponding to similar frontal plane movements of the foot. This usage leads logically to hallux abductovalgus (lateral deviation of the hallux with an everted axial rotation) instead of hallux valgus, and to digiti quinti adductovarus (medial deviation of the fifth toe with an inverted axial rotation) instead of digiti quinti varus.

Though entirely logical, this usage may be initially confusing, particularly in the case of the hallux, where it conflicts with the traditional anatomical nomenclature which relates movements of the hallux and actions of its abductor and adductor muscles to the sagittal plane bisecting the second metatarsal segment. If the term *hallux abductovalgus* is used, it must be remembered that the abduction element is in

Table A1-1:   Summary of orientation terminology.

	Sections of body	Sections of foot	Simple movement of foot or part	Fixed position of foot or part	
				Traditional terminology	*Biomechanical terminology*
Sagittal plane	Right	Medial	Dorsiflexion (extension of toes)	Calcaneus	Calcaneus
	Left	Lateral	Plantarflexion (flexion of toes)	Equinus	Equinus
Transverse (horizontal) plane	Superior	Dorsal	Adduction	Varus	Adductus
	Inferior	Plantar	Abduction	Valgus	Abductus
Frontal (coronal) plane	Anterior	Distal	Inversion	Inverted (varus)	Varus
	Posterior	Proximal	Eversion	Everted (valgus)	Valgus

relation to the *midline of the body* and not to the line through the second metatarsal segment from which the muscles are denominated. Similarly, the *valgus* element refers to the everted axial rotation of the hallux, and not to its abduction from the midline of the body.

It should also be borne in mind that terms are often descriptive rather than specifically diagnostic. For example, *pes cavus* describes the main clinical feature of a deformity which has various different causes, and similarly with *pes plano-valgus*. Both traditional and biomechanical forms of terminology have their uses and will co-exist. Both forms are given where necessary, the biomechanical terminology being given preference in the general text.

For ease of reference, a list of the main terms which are related, though not necessarily interchangeable, is given below:

Traditional terms	*Related biomechanical terms*
Pes planus; flatfoot congenital flatfoot	Calcaneovalgus; hindfoot valgus
Talipes equinus; short tendo Achilles	Ankle equinus
Pes valgus; valgus foot acquired flatfoot; supinated forefoot	Pronated foot
Pes cavus	Forefoot valgus; plantarflexed 1st metatarsal

Metatarsus varus	Metatarsus adductus
Metatarsus primus varus	Metatarsus primus adductus
Hallux valgus	Hallux abductovalgus
Digitus quintus varus	Digitus quintus adductovarus

Compensations

The degree of compensation depends in each case on the degree of the primary skeletal deformity.

Calcaneovalgus is usually compensated by supination of the forefoot, resulting in a low-arched foot.

Ankle equinus is usually compensated by pronation of the hindfoot to permit additional dorsiflexion at the midtarsal joint.

Calcaneovarus is usually compensated by sufficient pronation of the foot to enable the heel and forefoot to reach the horizontal plane.

Forefoot varus is usually compensated by pronation of the hindfoot to enable the forefoot to reach the horizontal plane.

Forefoot valgus, when it is an intrinsic deformity, is usually compensated by supination of the hindfoot, resulting in a high-arched foot. It may, however, be caused for other reasons, particularly neuropathies.

Ossification timetable

| Bone | Appearance of centres of ossification | | Fusion | Remarks |
	Primary centres	Secondary centres		
Tibia—diaphysis	7th week			
Tibia—upper epiphysis	—	At birth	20th yr	
Tibia—lower epiphysis	—	2nd yr	18th yr	Sometimes a separate centre for the medial malleolus appears at the same time
Fibula—diaphysis	8th week	—	—	
Fibula—upper epiphysis	—	4th yr	25th yr	
Fibula—lower epiphysis	—	2nd yr	20th yr	
Calcaneum body	6th month	—	—	
Calcaneum epiphysis	—	6–10th yr	13–15th yr	
Talus	7th month	—	—	
Cuboid	At birth			
Lat. cuneiform	1st yr	—	—	
Med. cuneiform	3rd yr	—	—	
Int. cuneiform	4th yr	—	—	
Navicular	4th yr	—	—	
1st metatars. shaft	8–9th week	—	—	
1st metatars. base	—	3rd yr	17–20th yr	Sometimes a separate centre for the head appears at the same time
Other metatars. shafts	8–9th week	—	—	Sometimes a separate centre for the base of the 5th metatars. appears at the same time
Other metatars. heads				
Prox. phals. shafts	12–16th week	—	—	
Prox. phals. bases	—	3–6th yr	17–18th yr	
Int. phals. shafts	4–9th month	—	—	That for the 5th toe does not appear until shortly after birth
Int. phals bases	—	3–6th yr	17–18th yr	Distal phal. of hallux
Dist. phals. shafts	8th week	—	—	
Dist. phals bases	—	6th yr	17–18th yr	

Clinical emergencies

Emergencies are relatively rare in podiatric practice but the more widespread use of local anaesthetics has slightly increased the risk which exists in any situation involving patient treatment. Most emergency situations can be prevented by good practice and careful preparation coupled with close monitoring of the patient's state and reactions. The good practitioner should be prepared to deal effectively with any such problems and this section is designed to outline the best procedures to be followed.

The most common emergency is fainting, which is often attributable to apprehension in the patient; therefore it is important to put patients at ease, consider their problems with interest and explain the treatment carefully. The patient is more relaxed in a semirecumbent position during treatment, and patients' chairs which allow this are of considerable value. A well ventilated surgery maintained at a comfortable temperature is also a good precaution. An essential preparation which should be made when local anaesthetics will be used is the provision of oxygen apparatus for resuscitation.

This account of emergency resuscitation will be confined to the management of unconsciousness in patients. For a more comprehensive review of first aid procedures, the reader is recommended to refer to one of the standard texts on first aid.

ASSESSMENT OF CONSCIOUSNESS

There are four main levels of consciousness to be considered:

• Full consciousness — the patient is fully orientated, usually able to speak and to answer questions sensibly
• Drowsiness this is the first level of unconsciousness. The patient can be roused easily, is usually orientated but can lapse back into the unconscious state
• Stupor — in the second level of unconsciousness, the patient can only be roused with difficulty and with painful stimuli; the patient is usually disorientated and not able to answer questions sensibly
• Coma—the patient is deeply unconscious and cannot be roused by any means.

The Glasgow Coma Scale

The Glasgow Coma Scale is internationally recognised as a highly valuable method of recording the conscious state of a patient and can be used for both initial and continuous assessment. It is based upon eye opening, verbal and motor responses.

For first aid in clinical emergencies, an adaption of the Glasgow Coma Scale may prove useful—see Table A3-1. This initial assessment will accompany the patient to hospital.

RESUSCITATION

Resuscitation is the restoration of breathing and circulation. Asphyxia is due to a decrease in the amount of oxygen and an increase in carbon dioxide in the body as a result of some interference in the respiratory process.

A clear airway

Any foreign object in the mouth must be

Table A3-1   Glasgow Coma Scale (adapted).

Name of patient:		Date:
Time:		
Eyes open:	Spontaneously To speech To pain No response	
Movement:	Obeys command To painful stimulus No response	
Verbal responses:	Normal Confused Nonsensical words No response	
Pulse:		
Respiration:		
Pupil size:		R L R L R L R L

removed, e.g. dentures, broken teeth, blood, saliva or debris. Neck wear must be loosened and the neck placed in the fully extended position (Fig. A3-1). The lower jaw of the patient is held in a forward position by pressure of the thumb behind the angle of the jaw. This forces the tongue into a forward position and so maintains a clear airway. Should the tongue fall to the back of the throat, it would obstruct the airway.

Very often, clearing of the airway will lead to the return of spontaneous breathing. Cyanosis and asphyxia will improve and consciousness will frequently return. Thereafter, the patient is kept comfortable and their condition carefully observed. Should spontaneous respiration not occur, artificial respiration is administered.

Artificial respiration

This is the maintenance of respiratory movements and oxygenation of the lungs by artificial means. The most effective procedure is mouth to mouth breathing (Fig. A3-2).

Mouth to mouth method

a. The airway is cleared and the patient put on their back.
b. The soft lower part of the nose is pinched in order to prevent escape of air.
c. The operator gives five sharp pants with their mouth over the mouth of the patient. This in itself may initiate spontaneous breathing.
d. If not, air is breathed directly into the mouth of the patient at a rate of 20 breaths per minute. After each exhalation, the operator observes the patient's chest to see whether it expands, indicating that air has entered the lungs.
e. In a young child, the nostrils need not be pinched since the area of the adult mouth easily covers mouth and nostrils.

Artificial respiration may be required for a considerable period of time, and should certainly be continued until a doctor or ambulance arrives or until the patient is certified dead by a doctor. Since the procedure may be long and tiring, it is important for the operator to be comfortable,

Fig. A3-1   Resuscitation. Fully extended position of neck.

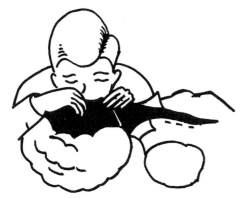

Fig. A3-2   Resuscitation. Mouth to mouth lung ventilation.

removing their jacket or coat and loosening their own neck wear.

External cardiac massage

When the heart has stopped beating, the pupils of the eyes remain dilated, the carotid and femoral pulses cannot be palpated and cyanosis persists despite artificial respiration.

In such cases, external cardiac massage should be started immediately to maintain circulation of oxygenated blood.

a. The patient should be placed on a firm base. The legs are raised to 90° for 10 seconds in order to help venous return to the heart.
b. A sharp blow should be given to the left lower third of the sternum. This sometimes stimulates the heart to beat spontaneously.
c. If this does not occur, the heels of the hands should be placed one over the other on the lower third of the sternum and the sternum depressed 4 cm ($1\frac{1}{2}$") at the rate of 60 times per minute (Fig. A3-3).

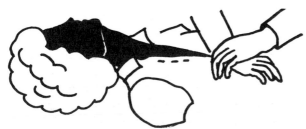

Fig. A3-3   Resuscitation. External cardiac massage.

External cardiac massage must be continued until:

a. the carotid pulse returns
b. resuscitation is taken over by the medical team
c. the operator is asked to discontinue by a doctor.

Mouth to mouth lung ventilation and cardiac massage combined

In this instance, it is preferable that there be two operators maintaining one lung inflation to five sternal depressions. If one operator only is present, two lung inflations to ten sternal depressions should be performed.

Cardiac arrest

When the heart stops beating suddenly, with immediate loss of consciousness, cyanosis, absence of pulses and dilatation of pupils, a cardiac arrest has occurred. The most common causes are heart attack, severe shock or anaphylactoid reaction. The patient is rested supine on a firm support and the airway cleared. In external cardiac massage, the heart is compressed between the operator's hands from above and below the vertebral column in order to pump blood forwards to maintain the circulation. Artificial ventilation (mouth to mouth) must also be administered.

UNCONSCIOUSNESS

In podiatric practice, loss of consciousness is relatively rare and is mainly due to reasons other than direct trauma. The likely possibilities are faints, cerebrovascular accidents, epilepsy, hyper- or hypoglycaemic coma, anaphylaxis, heart conditions, etc. The major consideration is to ensure the patient's ability to breathe and tight clothing should be loosened. If the patient continues to breath without trouble, they should be placed in the recovery position or three-quarters prone (Fig. A3-4).

If there is difficulty in breathing, oxygen should

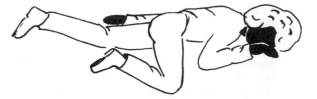

Fig. A3-4 Unconsciousness. Three-quarter prone recovery position.

be administered. It may be necessary to use resuscitative measures as described previously.

Vascular emergencies

Cerebral haemorrhage, clot, embolus or subarachnoid haemorrhage can lead to unconsciousness with shock. Resuscitation may be required. If breathing is stable, place the patient in the three-quarter prone recovery position. Partial paralysis is usually present and medical attention is essential.

Faints

A faint occurs when there is a temporary inadequate supply of blood to the brain. Commonly, people faint in hot airless rooms, but in podiatric practice they may do so from anxiety. The patient may have forewarning, feeling hot and clammy with yawning or nausea. This is followed by giddiness and fainting. The patient may, however, turn ashen grey and drop down without any warning.

Treatment

Lay the patient flat, loosen neckwear and ensure a clear airway. They will usually recover in one or two minutes. An older person may take longer to recover due to poorer cerebral circulation. On recovery, rest the patient and administer sips of water or tea. A check-up by the family doctor is a wise precaution.

Epilepsy

Fits indicate a disturbance of brain function and are of two types: in a *minor* fit, the patient stares into space and appears to be in a day dream. One part of the body may quiver, e.g. a hand or arm.

Such a fit usually lasts about a minute and on recovery the patient has no recollection of the event. In a *major* fit, the patient loses consciousness and falls to the ground. They foam at the mouth and the face becomes congested. Muscle convulsions and incontinence may occur. On recovery, they are exhausted and fall into a deep sleep.

Treatment

During a fit, the patient has to be protected form inadvertent injury. Remove any sources of danger from the patient's vicinity. Do not attempt to force the mouth open. Loosen all neckwear and check the breathing. Always advise such patients to see their doctor, particularly if they have never had a fit before. Ensure they are escorted home.

Diabetic emergencies leading to unconsciousness

Insulin excess resulting in hypoglycaemia

This can occur when the patient has missed as meal or inadvertently had too much insulin. The signs and symptoms are profuse sweating and a feeling of hunger, followed by nausea and confusion which may lead to unconsciousness.

Treatment. If the patient is conscious, administer a sugary drink, but beware of a tendency to vomit and only give sips at a time. Never give an unconscious patient anything to eat or drink. Obtain medical help or arrange transport to hospital; the patient requires emergency drug treatment. While waiting for the ambulance, maintain a clear airway, loosen neckwear and maintain the patient in the three-quarter prone recovery position (Fig. A3-4).

Insulin lack resulting in hyperglycaemia

This can occur when the patient has had insufficient insulin or has failed to comply with the prescribed diet. It also occurs in diabetics with an infection, e.g. a carbuncle or pneumonia. The skin is dry and the patient smells of acetone (similar to nail polish or apples).

Treatment. Such patients must go to hospital

immediately. If there is doubt as to whether the patient is hypoglycaemic or hyperglycaemic, a sugary drink may be given, provided they are not unconscious. They will only improve if they are hypoglycaemic, but no harm will be done if the condition is due to hyperglycaemia.

Medi–Alert bracelets or chains

Patients who are on special treatment may have a bracelet or chain giving this information. They may also carry cards giving details of their condition, treatment and the name of their family doctor.

Index